Principles of
Radiological Physics

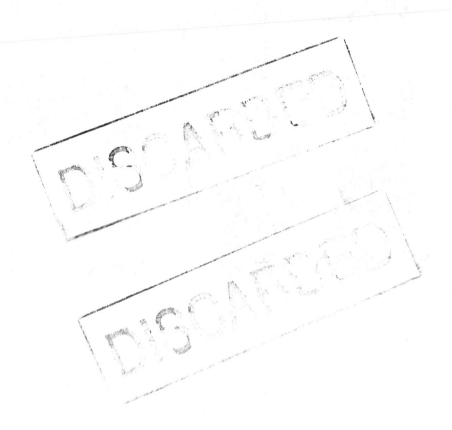

For Elsevier

Commissioning Editor: Dinah Thom
Project Manager: Nancy Arnott
Design: Erik Bigland
Illustration Manager: Bruce Hogarth

Principles of
Radiological Physics

Donald T. Graham MED TDCR

Former Director, Radiography, School of Health Sciences, The Robert Gordon University,
Aberdeen, UK

Paul Cloke MSc TDCR

Former Lecturer in Diagnostic Imaging, Centre for Radiographic and Medical Studies,
Department of Materials and Medical Science, Cranfield University, Shrivenham Campus, Swindon,
Wiltshire, UK

Martin Vosper MSc HDCR

Senior Lecturer, Department of Radiography, University of Hertfordshire, Hatfield, UK

FIFTH EDITION

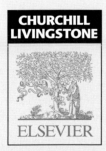

EDINBURGH LONDON NEW YORK OXFORD PHILADELPHIA ST LOUIS SYDNEY
TORONTO 2007

First edition 1981
Second Edition 1987
Third Edition 1996
Fourth Edition 2003
Fifth Edition 2007
 Reprinted 2008, 2009

ISBN: 978 0 443 10104 5

British Library Cataloguing in Publication Data
A catalogue record for this book is available from the British Library

Library of Congress Cataloging in Publication Data
A catalog record for this book is available from the Library of Congress

Note
Knowledge and best practice in this field are constantly changing. As new research and experience broaden our knowledge, changes in practice, treatment and drug therapy may become necessary or appropriate. Readers are advised to check the most current information provided (i) on procedures featured or (ii) by the manufacturer of each product to be administered, to verify the recommended dose or formula, the method and duration of administration, and contraindications. It is the responsibility of the practitioner, relying on their own experience and knowledge of the patient, to make diagnoses, to determine dosages and the best treatment for each individual patient, and to take all appropriate safety precautions. To the fullest extent of the law, neither the publisher nor the authors assume any liability for any injury and/or damage to persons or property arising out of or related to any use of the material contained in this book.   *The Publisher*

The Publisher's policy is to use **paper manufactured from sustainable forests**

Printed in China

Contents

Preface   vii

Part 1 Radiography and mathematics   1
1   Principles of radiography   3
2   Geometric radiography   9
3   The inverse square law   19
4   The exponential law   25

Part 2 General physics   37
5   Laws of physics (classical)   39
6   Units of measurement   44
7   Experimental error and statistics   52
8   Heat   62
9   Electrostatics   72
10   Electricity (DC)   80
11   Magnetism   93
12   Electromagnetism   106
13   Electromagnetic induction   112
14   Alternating current flow   120
15   The motor principle   134
16   Capacitors   141
17   The AC transformer   150
18   Semiconductor materials   163
19   Rectification   177
20   Exposure and timing circuits   185

Part 3 Construction and operation of X-ray tubes   193
21   Diagnostic X-ray tubes   195
22   Monitoring and protection of X-ray tubes   207
23   Orthovoltage Generators and Linear Accelerators   214

Part 4 Atomic physics   221
24   Laws of modern physics   223
25   Electromagnetic radiation   228
26   Elementary structure of the atom   237
27   Radioactivity   246

Part 5 X-rays and matter   267
28   The production of X-rays   269
29   Factors affecting X-ray beam quality and quantity   277
30   Interactions of X-rays with matter   284
31   Luminescence and photostimulation   298
32   The radiographic image   306

Part 6 Dosimetry and radiation protection   317
33   Radiation dosimetry   319
34   Radiation protection   333

Appendices, tables and answers to self-tests   355

Appendix A   Mathematics for radiography   357
Appendix B   Scintillation counters   371
Appendix C   CT scanning   376
Appendix D   Magnetic resonance imaging   382
Appendix E   Digital imaging   386
Appendix F   Ultrasound imaging   390
Appendix G   Positron emission tomography (PET) scanning   394
Appendix H   Modulation transfer function (MTF)   397
Appendix I   SI base units   401

Tables   403
Table A   Powers of 10   403
Table B   Physical constants   403
Table C   Important conversion factors   403
Table D   Greek symbols and their common usage   404
Table E   Periodic table of the elements   405
Table F   Electron configuration of the elements   406

Answers to self-tests   409

Index   437

Preface

The fourth edition of Principles of Radiological Physics was produced in 2003 mainly in response to changes in legislation for radiation protection and the increasing use of new technologies in the production of the radiographic image. Change continues in the profession and more recent changes have seen role expansion with the effective formation of a four-tier professional structure from assistant to consultant practitioner. This change in career structure has allowed radiographers increased responsibility both in clinical and technical decision making. In parallel with this change in the professional career ladder there have been significant technical changes and we have tried to reflect these in this edition. Such changes include the development of digital techniques with the potential to make greater use of teleradiology. This gives radiographers at satellite locations improved access to technical and clinical support when required.

The layout and content of the fourth edition were well received by students and academics, and the layout of the fifth edition remains basically the same. As in previous editions, redundant material has been removed and replaced by more up-to-date material but some material, which is not current practice, has been left in the text if it shows the historical development of legislation or technology. The addition of Martin Vosper to the team of authors has also facilitated the expansion of some previous chapters and the addition of new material. A new chapter with an overview of orthovoltage generators and linear accelerators has been added, as has an appendix outlining the principles of positron emission tomography. In addition the appendices on ultrasound, computed tomography and magnetic resonance imaging have been expanded.

The production of a new edition would be an impossible task without the help and constructive criticism received from present and past colleagues and the publishing team at Elsevier, and we acknowledge this with gratitude.

Regardless of changes in technology and clinical grading, the most important role of the radiographer remains unchanged, namely ensuring the production of high quality images and optimal treatments. These should be performed with the minimum of radiation hazard to the patient, the radiographers themselves and others whose presence is a necessary part of the examination or treatment. An understanding of physics and the basics of radiographic technology is essential to enable us to do this effectively.

Donald T Graham
Paul Cloke
Martin Vosper
Aberdeen, Bicester and Hatfield, 2007

Part 1

Radiography and Mathematics

PART CONTENTS

1. Principles of Radiography   3

2. Geometric Radiography   9

3. The Inverse-Square Law   19

4. The Exponential Law   25

1

Chapter 1

Principles of Radiography

CHAPTER CONTENTS

1.1 Aim 3

1.2 Diagnostic and Therapeutic Radiography 3
  1.2.1 Diagnostic Radiography 3
  1.2.2 Therapeutic Radiography 5

1.3 Radiation Protection 7

Further Reading 7

1.1 AIM

The aim of this chapter is to consider the basic principles of diagnostic radiography, therapeutic radiography and radiation protection. This should allow the reader to appreciate how the individual chapters within the text form part of a whole study.

1.2 DIAGNOSTIC AND THERAPEUTIC RADIOGRAPHY

X-rays (and other forms of radiation) can have two main uses in medicine. They can be used to investigate the patient's illness or physical state – this forms *diagnostic radiography*; or they can be used to produce cell changes in certain body tissues – this is the basis of *therapeutic radiography*.

1.2.1 Diagnostic Radiography

In diagnostic radiography an image of a structure within the patient's body is produced on a film or a television monitor. Normally, of course, we cannot see inside each other's bodies because light photons, to which our eyes are sensitive, are absorbed and reflected very close to the surface of body tissues.

INSIGHT

To examine internal body structures using light, an instrument called an endoscope must be inserted

3

into the body. This consists of fibreoptic bundles that transmit the light to and from the region of interest and so allow the operator to view the organ. Such techniques are used in keyhole surgery. This type of imaging does carry some risk, or it may be uncomfortable for the patient, and so radiography will often be considered as an alternative.

Light is a form of *electromagnetic radiation* (see Ch. 25) and it seems logical to suggest that, if we can take photons of electromagnetic radiation which have higher energies than light photons, then these may have sufficient energy to penetrate body tissues and allow us to visualise internal organs. *X-rays* are in this part of the electromagnetic spectrum and so will penetrate body tissues and allow us to image internal organs. Unfortunately, the retina of the eye cannot detect X-rays and so we cannot see an image of an organ just by shining an X-ray beam on it. This means that the X-rays that have passed through the body must be made to strike an image receptor which will produce a visible image, e.g. a piece of film.

Figure 1.1 shows the basic requirements for the formation of a radiographic image. The X-rays are produced in the X-ray tube by accelerating electrons and causing these to collide with an anode. To understand how this works we need to know about *energy* (see Ch. 6) and *electricity* (see Chs 10 and 14) as well as the construction of the *X-ray generator* (see Chs 17 and 19) and the *X-ray tube* (see Ch. 21). The X-rays so produced are over a wide band of energies. Most of the photons that have insufficient energy to be of diagnostic value are removed from the beam *using filtration* (see Ch. 29) and the area of the patient irradiated is restricted using a *diaphragm* (see Ch. 21).

The beam now interacts with the patient and a number of things may happen to the X-ray photons. These may be:

- *transmitted* (T in Figure 1.1): these photons pass through the patient without interacting with the patient's tissues. They are thus unaffected by their passage through the patient

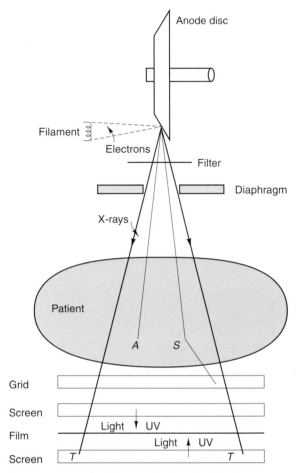

Figure 1.1 Principal interactions involved in the production of a radiographic image. *A* represents absorbed photons, *S* represents scattered photons and *T* represents transmitted photons. UV, ultraviolet.

- *absorbed* (*A* in Figure 1.1): these photons interact with the patient's tissues and as a result lose all of their energy. As the photon consists only of energy, then these photons disappear from the spectrum of radiation transmitted through the patient
- *scattered* (*S* in Figure 1.1): these photons interact with the patient's tissues and are then deflected from their original path. Such a deflection may or may not result in a loss of some of the photons' energy.

Different tissues will absorb different amounts of radiation (see Ch. 30) and so a differentiated radiation pattern leaves the patient. The scattered radiation is not helpful to the image, so when the scatter production is significant, as much as possible of this is removed using a *secondary radiation grid* (see Ch. 32). Finally the radiation interacts with the image receptor. In this case a screen made of a material that will fluoresce (see Ch. 31) the light produced from this interaction strikes the film to create a radiographic image (see Ch. 32). Other image receptors form the latent image directly from the interaction of the radiation with the image receptor.

1.2.2 Therapeutic Radiography

In therapy radiography, we are not trying to produce images but are using the *biological effects* of radiation to kill tumour cells. At the same time, we try to cause as little damage as possible to the healthy cells in the body.

INSIGHT

There are four main methods of cancer treatment:surgery, chemotherapy, alteration of the hormone balance and radiotherapy. They may be used in isolation or together to give the optimum treatment regimen for a given cancer in a given patient. The treatment may be *radical* or *palliative*. The former is an all-out effort to achieve a cure and the latter is used to relieve pain and other distressing symptoms when no cure for the disease is possible. This is normally in the terminal stages of the disease.

The relative success of radiotherapy in the management of cancer lies in the fact that malignant cells are more sensitive to radiation than healthy cells in the same organ. The reasons for this will be discussed in Chapter 34. In spite of this, a number of healthy cells are affected by radiation and so must be given time to recover. Thus the radiation dose is delivered as a number of treatments rather than as a single dose. This technique is known as fractionation and may mean that a patient has 15–30 treatments over a period of 3–6 weeks.

1.2.2.1 Methods of Radiation Treatment

A detailed description of the different methods of radiation treatment is beyond the scope of this introductory chapter and the reader is directed to some of the more specialised texts on the subject. In considering the overview of radiation treatment methods we can, however, identify some distinct types which we will discuss further. These are:

- teletherapy
- brachytherapy
- nuclear medicine.

Teletherapy. Here an external source of radiation (normally X-rays or gamma-rays) is directed at the tumour. The aim is to give the maximum dose to the tumour and the minimum dose to the healthy tissue. This is often achieved by treating the tumour from a number of fields (Figure 1.2). The areas in the patient that receive doses of equal value are joined by lines called *isodose lines*. The shape and the position of these lines may be altered by the use of absorbing wedges and compensators and also by altering the energy of the beam (where this is possible). When the treatment plan has been produced, the positions of the treatment fields on the patient are checked in a *simulator* where the treatment angles can be set up and the fields marked. In areas of the patient around the head and the neck, accurate positioning and immobilisation are achieved by placing this part in a specially prepared clear plastic shell.

Brachytherapy. When we use external radiation beams, the radiation must travel through healthy tissue to reach the tumour. There are some situations where tumours are relatively accessible from the body surface or are in body cavities where sealed *radioactive sources* (see Ch. 27) may be inserted. This technique is known as brachytherapy. The technique can often mean that a large dose can be delivered to the tumour while a much smaller dose strikes the surrounding tissues because of the effects of the inverse-square law (see Ch. 3). If the sources are implanted directly by the radiotherapist, the dose to the hands of the operator could be quite large. This is overcome by inserting a number of

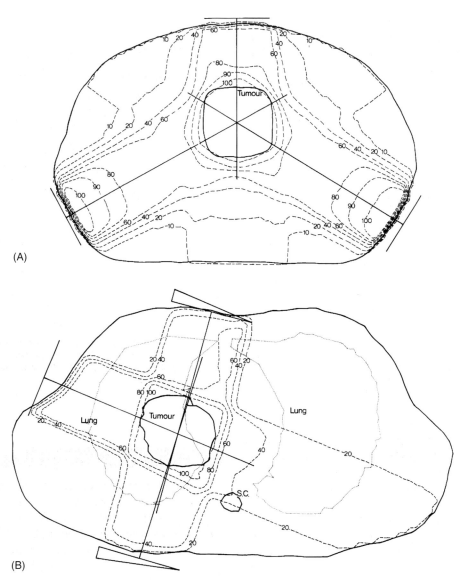

Figure 1.2 Examples of radiotherapy treatment plans. A, Three-field plan for a pelvic tumour; B, three-field plan for a mediastinal tumour (note how the fields minimise dose to the spinal cord (SC) on plan).

guides into the correct position and mechanically inserting the sources over the guides for the required treatment. This technique is called *afterloading* and is often used in the treatment of pelvic cancers.

Nuclear medicine. A third possibility is that the radiation can be delivered to the tissue by allowing the tissue to absorb a certain radionuclide (see Ch. 27). This is probably best illustrated by considering the treatment of an overactive thyroid gland. The activity of the gland can be reduced by surgical removal of part of the gland, or some of its tissue may be destroyed using radiation. To allow the thyroid to produce the required hormones it must absorb iodine. The patient may be given sodium iodide (where the iodine is in the form of ^{131}I) as a capsule or in an oral solution. Some of this isotope (see Ch. 27) is taken up by the gland and the rest is secreted in the urine. ^{131}I is a beta-particle emitter (see

Ch. 27) and this results in a radiation dose to the thyroid tissue which reduces its metabolic rate to normal. Because of the limited range of the beta-particles produced, there is less radiation dose to structures around the thyroid than there would be if we used an external radiation beam. ^{131}I also has a relatively short half-life (8 days; see Ch. 27) and so the radiation hazard posed by the patient to others can be minimised.

1.3 RADIATION PROTECTION

All radiation to the cells which make up our bodies carries a risk of damage to those cells. It is also true that some tissues are more sensitive to radiation than others (see Ch. 34). The use of radiation in medicine is of great value to humans, but it is the single largest factor which contributes to the *artificial radiation dose* received by the human race. The contribution of the various radiation sources is shown in Figure 1.3.

Because of this we have a duty to minimise the dose to our patients and colleagues and so minimise the risk of radiation damage. The radiation dose is composed of *primary radiation* and *secondary radiation*, and so we need to look at the ways in which these are produced and absorbed. This will be considered in Chapters 28 and 30. Because of the known hazards of radiation, there are certain statutory requirements for *radiation protection* and *monitoring* in diagnostic and therapy departments (see Ch. 34). In terms of assessing the risk it is important to know the dose received by both patients and radiation workers and this will be discussed in Chapter 33, which deals with the topic of *radiation dosimetry*.

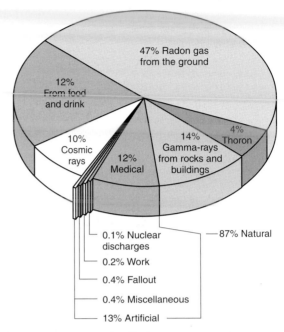

Figure 1.3 Sources of radiation exposure to humans. (Based on data from the Radiation Section of the Health Protection Agency (formerly the National Radiological Protection Board.)

SUMMARY

This brief overview should enable the reader to understand certain physical principles that underpin diagnostic radiography and therapy radiography. Patients and staff should be exposed to the minimum risk from the radiation and the principles governing this have been outlined.

FURTHER READING

This overview covers a very large subject area and so only the principal texts are identified. Further reading in specialised topics will be covered in the chapter bibliographies.
Diagnostic radiography
Carlton R, McKenna Adler A 2000 Principles of radiographic imaging: an art and a science, 3rd edn. Delmar, Thomson Learning, Albany, New York

Lisle D A 2001 Imaging for students, 2nd edn. Arnold, London
Therapeutic radiography
Bomford C K, Kunkler I H 2003 Walter and Miller's textbook of radiotherapy, 2nd edn. Churchill Livingstone, Edinburgh
Souhami R, Tobias J 2005 Cancer and its management, 5th edn. Blackwell Publishing, Oxford

Wang C C 2000 Clinical radiation oncology: indications, techniques and results, 2nd edn. Wiley, New York

Radiation protection

Dowd S B, Tilson E R 1999 Practical radiation protection and applied radiobiology, 2nd edn. W B Saunders, Philadelphia, PA

Statutory Instrument 2000/1059 The ionising radiation (medical exposure) regulations 2000. HMSO, London

UK National Radiological Protection Board website: http://www.hpa.org.uk/radiation/

Chapter 2

Geometric Radiography

CHAPTER CONTENTS

2.1 Aim 9

2.2 Introduction 9

2.3 Effective (apparent) and Real Focal Spot Sizes 10

2.4 Field Size and FFD 11

2.5 Image Magnification 12

2.6 Geometric Unsharpness (penumbra) 13

2.7 Penumbra from Diaphragms 15

2.8 Tomography 15
    2.8.1 Principles of Linear Tomography 15
    2.8.2 Fulcrum Height Adjustment 15
    2.8.3 Tomographic Angle Adjustment 16

Self-test 18

Further Reading 18

2.1 AIM

The aim of this chapter is to explore the geometry involved in the production of certain radiographic images.

2.2 INTRODUCTION

The very nature of this chapter involves a basic knowledge of mathematics and especially geometry. If this fills you with foreboding, please read Appendix A before proceeding with the rest of the chapter.

Many of the concepts and calculations encountered in radiography are based on the application of geometry and trigonometry to the production of the image. These will be discussed in this chapter. To allow us to apply these to radiography there are some commonly used terms, defined here.

DEFINITIONS

Field size	This defines the size and the shape of the X-ray beam. As we will see later in this chapter (Sect. 2.4), the field size varies with the distance from the source of the radiation or *focus* of the X-ray tube
FFD	focus to film distance
FSD	focus to skin distance
FOD	focus to object distance
OFD	object to film distance
FDD	focus to diaphragm distance

The influence of these quantities on the image production will be described in the rest of this chapter.

2.3 EFFECTIVE (APPARENT) AND REAL FOCAL SPOT SIZES

As described in Chapter 21, X-rays are produced when a beam of electrons is accelerated from the cathode to the anode of the X-ray tube. At the anode the electrons are decelerated and their kinetic energy is converted to approximately 99.5% heat and 0.5% X-rays. The small area of the anode bombarded by the electrons is known as the *focus*. Because of the large amount of heat produced, the focus should occupy as large an area as possible, thus limiting the temperature rise. The size of the focus also affects the image sharpness (see Sect. 2.6) and so, from an imaging point of view, the focus should be as small as possible. These seemingly contradictory requirements are accommodated using the *line focus principle*. This is shown in Figure 2.1.

The electron beam from the cathode is represented by *AB* and this strikes the anode at *XZ*. The distance *XZ* is one dimension of the *real focal spot*. The central ray of the X-ray beam is represented by *CD*. By viewing the focus along this line the *effective focal area* is seen. One dimension of this is represented by the line *YZ*. The angle between the central ray and the anode, θ (theta), is referred to as the anode angle or target angle.

Consider the triangle *XYZ* in Figure 2.1.

Since the lines *XY* and *CD* are parallel, the angle *YXZ* is also θ. Also:

$$\sin \theta = \frac{YZ}{XZ}$$

By cross-multiplying (see Appendix A Sect. A3.7) this can be arranged as:

$$XZ = \frac{YZ}{\sin \theta}$$

$$\text{real focus} = \frac{apparent\ focus}{\sin \theta}$$

Equation 2.1

This means that if the apparent focal spot and the target angle are known for an X-ray tube, the real focal spot can be calculated using the above formula.

It is important to remember that the focal spot has two dimensions (it has breadth as well as length), as can be seen from Figure 2.2.

But, because the breadth of the focal spot is at right angles to the electron beam and the central ray, it is not affected by the target angle.

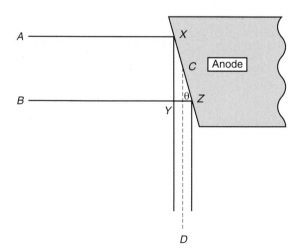

Figure 2.1   Relationships between the real and the effective focal spot sizes. The length *AB* represents the electron beam, the length *XZ* the real focal spot and the length *YZ* the effective focal spot. *CD* shows the midpoint of apparent focus.

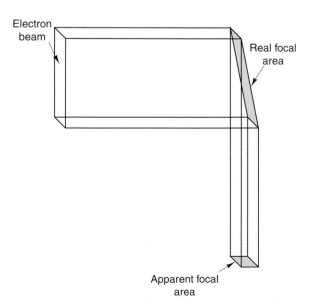

Figure 2.2   Three-dimensional nature of real and apparent (effective) focal spots.

EXAMPLE

An X-ray tube has an apparent focal spot of 0.6×0.6 mm and the target angle of this tube is $17°$. Calculate the size of the real focal spot.

Using Equation 2.1 we can say that:

$$\text{real focus} = \frac{\text{apparent focus}}{\sin \theta}$$

$$= \frac{0.6}{0.292}$$

$$= 2.05 \text{ mm}$$

As the breadth of the focus is unaffected by the target angle, the dimensions of the real focal spot will be 2.05×0.6 mm.

As the sine of an angle increases with the angle, it can be seen that the dimensions of the real focal spot (and hence the loading which can be applied to the X-ray tube) increase with smaller target angles. (Try the above calculation using a target angle of $10°$.) The significance of this will be discussed in Chapters 21 and 22.

2.4 FIELD SIZE AND FFD

Figure 2.3 shows the divergence (in two dimensions) of the X-ray beam with increasing distance from the focus of the X-ray tube. Using the principles of similar triangles a number of deductions can be made.

Consider the triangles FCD and FAB. It can be seen that:

$$\frac{CD}{FG} = \frac{AB}{FJ}$$

or

$$\frac{S_1}{FFD_1} = \frac{d}{FDD}$$

Thus, by cross-multiplication (Appendix A Sect. A3.7):

$$S_1 = (d \times FFD_1) \, FDD \qquad \textit{Equation 2.2}$$

From this it can be seen that the size of the field for a given X-ray tube with a given FDD is related to the size of the diaphragm aperture and the FFD.

Now consider the triangles FCD and FEP. It can be seen that (see Appendix A Sect. A9.2 similar triangles):

$$\frac{CD}{FG} = \frac{EP}{FH}$$

or

$$\frac{S_1}{FFD_1} = \frac{S_2}{FFD_2} \qquad \textit{Equation 2.3}$$

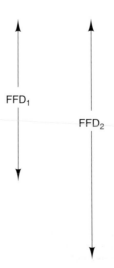

Figure 2.3   Variations of field size with focus to film distance (FFD). FDD, focus to diaphragm distance.

From the above it can be seen that, if the diaphragm aperture is left unaltered, the field size is proportional to the FFD.

Many *light-beam diaphragms* used in radiography have a scale indicating the size of the field which will be covered at various FFDs. Similar techniques are applied in radiotherapy where the treatment field is altered by altering the *applicator size* or the position of the *jaws* on the unit.

EXAMPLE

An X-ray beam has a field size of 20 × 20 cm at an FFD of 100 cm. At what FFD will the field size be 30 × 30 cm?

It may be helpful to draw the triangles so that you can visualize the situation (Figure 2.4).

Using Equation 2.3:

By cross-multiplication:

$$\text{FFD}_2 = \frac{S_2 \times \text{FFD}_1}{S_1}$$

$$\text{FFD}_2 = \frac{30 \times 100 \text{ cm}}{20}$$

$$= 150 \text{ cm}$$

(*Useful check:* The field size has increased by 50% (i.e. from 20 to 30 cm) so the FFD, which is directly proportional, must also have increased by 50% (i.e. from 100 to 150 cm)).

2.5 IMAGE MAGNIFICATION

Figure 2.5 represents the geometry of an imaging situation either in diagnostic radiography or on a radiotherapy simulator. *AB* is an object within the patient (e.g. a piece of bone or a tumour) and *CD* is the radiographic image of that object. *BD* is the OFD and FD is the FFD.

Obviously *CD* is greater than *AB* and so we can say that the image of the object will be magnified. There are occasions where it is necessary to measure the size of a structure and so the degree of magnification must be calculated.

Consider the triangles *FAB* and *FCD*:

$$\text{magnification} = \frac{\text{size of the image}}{\text{size of the object}}$$

$$= \frac{CD}{AB}$$

$$= \frac{FD}{FB}$$

$$= \frac{\text{FFD}}{(\text{FFD} - \text{OFD})}$$

$$\text{magnification} = \frac{\text{FFD}}{(\text{FFD} - \text{OFD})}$$

Equation 2.4

Note that the magnification factor does not depend on the position of the object related to the central ray but only on the FFD and OFD. To limit

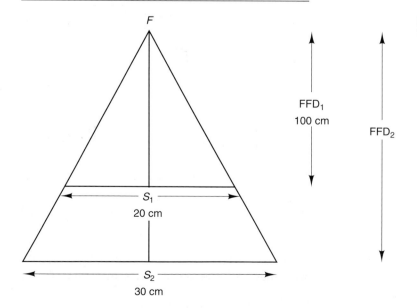

Figure 2.4   Field sizes at given focus to film distances (FFDs).

F

FFD₁
100 cm

FFD₂

S₁
20 cm

S₂
30 cm

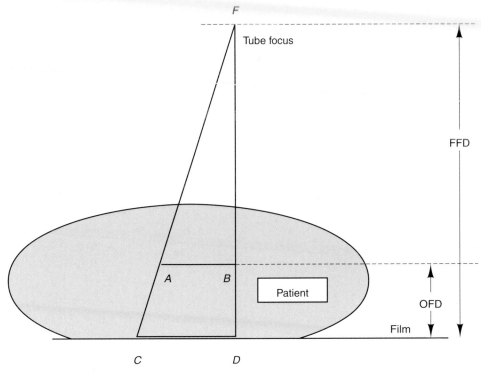

Figure 2.5   Magnification of the radiographic image. *AB* is an object within the patient and *CD* is the image of this object. FFD, focus to film distance; OFD, object to film distance.

the degree of magnification there are two possibilities:

1. The patient should be positioned so that the object of interest is as close to the film as possible
2. If it is impossible to position the object close to the film (e.g. in the lateral view of the cervical spine), then the magnification can be limited by increasing the FFD.

EXAMPLE

Radiography of a child's femur is undertaken using the following exposure factors. The FFD is 100 cm and the OFD is 6 cm. The length of the radiographic image of the femur is 25 cm. Calculate the true length of the femur.

Using Equation 2.4 the magnification can be stated as:

$$\text{Magnification} = \frac{\text{FFD}}{(\text{FFD} - \text{OFD})}$$

$$= \frac{100}{(100 - 6)}$$

$$= 1.064 \text{ (Note that magnification has no units)}$$

$$\text{size of the object} = \frac{\text{size of the image}}{\text{magnification}}$$

$$= \frac{25 \text{ cm}}{1.064}$$

$$= 23.49 \text{ cm}$$

2.6 GEOMETRIC UNSHARPNESS (PENUMBRA)

The focal spot in the X-ray tube is a finite size. Figure 2.6 represents the situation that exists because of this. (*Note* that the focal spot used for the calculation of image distortion is the apparent focal spot.)

AB represents the focus, *CD* the object and *FG* the image of the object. At either end of this

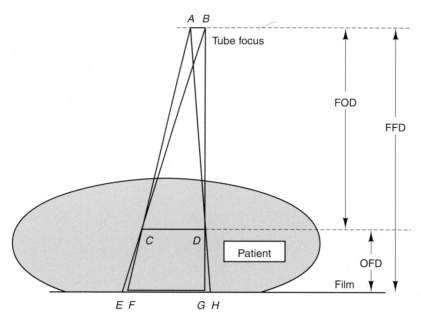

Figure 2.6 Geometry of penumbra or geometric unsharpness. *AB* is the effective focal spot, *CD* is the object, *FG* is the image and *EF* and *GH* represent the penumbra. FOD, focus to object distance; FFD, focus to film distance; OFD, object to film distance.

image there is *penumbra* or *geometric unsharpness* represented by *EF* and *GH*. (For simplicity it is assumed that the X-ray beam is centred to end *D* of the object.)

Using similar triangles the following can be seen:

$$\frac{GH}{AB} = \frac{GD}{BD}$$

$$= \frac{OFD}{FOD}$$

$$GH = \frac{AB \times OFD}{(FFD - OFD)}$$

or

$$penumbra = \frac{focus \times OFD}{(FFD - OFD)}$$

Equation 2.5

A similar situation exists for the value of the penumbra at *EF*.

In most radiographic imaging situations it is desirable to keep the penumbra as low as possible (or at least below 0.3 mm, where it is below the resolution of the eye at normal viewing distances) and so we can deduce from Equation 2.5

that the following methods might accomplish this:

- The apparent focal spot should be as small as possible
- The OFD should be as small as possible
- The FFD may be increased if the previously identified techniques are impossible.

Note: The unsharpness on a radiograph *(Ut)* is a combination of three types of unsharpness:

1. geometric unsharpness *(Ug)*
2. movement unsharpness *(Um)* – this is unsharpness of the image caused by movement of the patient or the imaging equipment
3. photographic unsharpness *(Up)* – this type of unsharpness is caused by the film and intensifying screens used to produce the image.

These are linked by the equation:

$$Ut^2 = Ug^2 + Um^2 + Up^2 \qquad \textit{Equation 2.6}$$

Care must be taken in considering ways of reducing geometric unsharpness if these have an effect on the other types of unsharpness that contribute to the total unsharpness.

EXAMPLE

The following conditions exist for a lateral projection of the cervical spine.

FFD = 200 cm; OFD = 20 cm; focal spot size = 1.2 mm. Calculate the size of the penumbra.

Using Equation 2.5:

$$\text{penumbra} = \frac{\text{focus} \times \text{OFD}}{(\text{FFD} - \text{OFD})}$$

$$= \frac{1.2 \times 200}{(2000 - 200)} \text{ mm}$$

$$= 0.13 \text{ mm}$$

2.7 PENUMBRA FROM DIAPHRAGMS

Figure 2.3 showed us how a movable diaphragm could be used to delineate the field size of an X-ray beam. This diagram, however, assumes that the radiation was produced at a point source. The situation for a focus of finite size is shown in Figure 2.7.

Here D_1 and D_2 represent one pair of leaves of a diaphragm. As an alternative to a diaphragm,

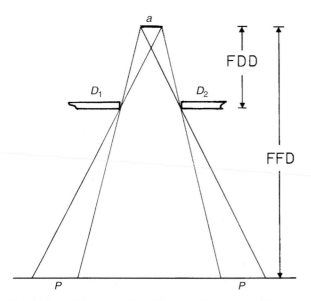

Figure 2.7 Penumbra, P, due to the diaphragms (D_1 and D_2). FDD, focus to diaphragm distance; FFD, focus to film distance.

detachable cones may be used but the principle is still the same.

The penumbra, P, is the 'shadow' of the edge of the diaphragm or cone formed because of the finite size of the focal spot. The calculation shows exactly the same progression as the calculation in the previous section. By substituting the appropriate values in Equation 2.5 then:

$$P = \frac{F \times (\text{FFD} - \text{FDD})}{\text{FFD}}$$

Equation 2.7

This particular penumbra has very little significance in diagnostic radiography except that it explains why the edges of a long cone (e.g. the type used for imaging of the paranasal sinuses) are more clearly defined than the image of the leaves of a light-beam diaphragm. *The calculation of the diaphragm penumbra is important in teletherapy radiation treatment* (see Ch. 1), where it is necessary to know the radiation dose to the whole treatment volume within the patient.

2.8 TOMOGRAPHY

Tomography is a technique used to produce sharp images of a plane or section within the patient. This allows the clinician to identify the anatomy of this section of tissue without the distraction of superimposed shadows; for example, if the clinician is only interested in the renal areas, the shadows cast by the bowel in the abdominal radiograph may make these more difficult to visualise.

Tomography may be performed using a variety of techniques, many of which are outside the scope of this text. For the purpose of this discussion about the geometry of image production, only linear tomography will be considered.

2.8.1 Principles of Linear Tomography

In linear tomography the X-ray tube and the film holder are linked by a rod mechanism. During the exposure the tube moves in one direction and the film holder moves in the opposite direction. This movement is around a fulcrum. The height of the fulcrum and the angle through which the tube moves during the exposure can be adjusted by the radiographer. We will now consider the effect of each of these adjustments.

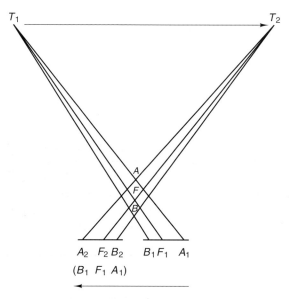

Figure 2.8 Images produced in linear tomography for a tube movement from position T_1 to position T_2. See text for further explanation.

2.8.2 Fulcrum Height Adjustment

Figure 2.8 shows the imaging situation in linear tomography. Points A, F and B are within the patient, with the point F being on the plane of the fulcrum. During the exposure the tube moves from position T_1 to T_2 and the film holder moves in the opposite direction from position 1 to position 2. The projection of the points A, F and B on the film produces images A_1, F_1 and B_1 when the tube is in position T_1 and A_2, F_2 and B_2 when the tube is in position T_2. From Figure 2.8 it can be seen that the projection of point F moves with the same velocity as the film and so F_1 and F_2 are superimposed and will appear sharp on the radiograph. The projection of point A moves at a higher velocity than the film and so A_1 and A_2 are not superimposed and will appear unsharp. Similarly, the projection of point B moves at a lower velocity than the film and so will also appear unsharp. Thus we can conclude that:

The images of points on the plane of the fulcrum will be sharp on the radiograph, whereas the images of points above and below this plane will be unsharp.

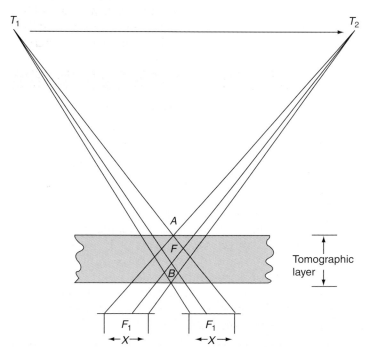

Figure 2.9 Tomographic layer thickness for a large tomographic angle. X represents the unsharpness tolerance of the eye when the image is viewed.

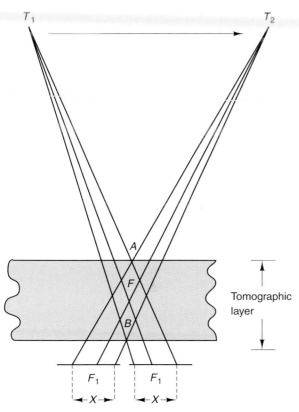

Figure 2.10 Tomographic layer thickness for a small tomographic angle. X represents the unsharpness tolerance of the eye when the image is viewed.

By raising or lowering the fulcrum height, the radiographer can control the level of the layer within the patient which produces sharp images on each radiograph.

2.8.3 Tomographic Angle Adjustment

The eye is not a perfect optical instrument and so will tolerate a certain amount of movement unsharpness around a point. Consider the situation in Figure 2.9. If the eye will tolerate a movement unsharpness of X around the point F_1, then the projection of any point within the layer A and B will be accepted as sharp. Thus the tomographic layer has a finite depth, with the fulcrum being at the centre of this layer.

Now consider the situation where the tube moves through a smaller tomographic angle during the exposure. This situation is shown in Figure 2.10. If we accept that the tolerance of the eye is still a distance X around the point F_1, then we can see that the thickness of the tomographic layer is increased. Thus we can establish the relationship between layer thickness and tomographic angle, namely:

> **The thickness of the tomographic layer can be increased by reducing the tomographic angle and can be reduced by increasing the tomographic angle.**

Calculation of the exact thickness of the tomographic layer is a somewhat complex exercise as this also varies with the height of the fulcrum (the higher the fulcrum, the thinner the layer) and the focal spot selected (the broader the focus, the thinner the layer). This is beyond the scope of this introductory chapter. Students should refer to the manufacturers' literature for various tomographic units to note the layer thickness produced at different tomographic angles.

EXAMPLE

Draw an imaging situation similar to the one shown in Figure 2.10.

Now, allowing the same tolerance for movement unsharpness and the same tomographic angle, repeat the drawing with the fulcrum set at twice the height in the original drawing. Verify that the tomographic layer within the patient is thinner.

SUMMARY

In this chapter you should have learnt:

- The relationship between the apparent and real focal spot sizes (see Sect. 2.3)
- The relationship between the field size and the FFD (see Sect. 2.4)
- The factors that affect image magnification (see Sect. 2.5)
- The factors that affect geometric unsharpness and how to minimise this form of unsharpness in the radiographic image (see Sect. 2.6)
- The factors that affect the height and thickness of the tomographic layer (see Sect. 2.8).

SELF-TEST

a. An X-ray tube used in a skull unit has a target angle of 10°. The apparent focal spots available on this tube are 0.6 × 0.6 mm (fine focus) and 1.2 × 1.2 mm (broad focus). Calculate the size of the real focal spots.

b. What are the dimensions of a diaphragm placed at a distance of 10 cm from the focal spot which will allow a field of 25 × 30 cm to be covered at an FFD of 1 m?

c. A lateral radiograph of a patient's spine was taken at an FFD of 1 m. The distance between the spine and the film was 15 cm. On the resultant radiograph the height of a particular intervertebral disc was measured as 1.2 cm. Calculate the true height of the disc.

d. If the effective focal spot size is 0.5 mm and an object is 8 cm from the film, what would be the size of the penumbra if the FFD was:

(i) 1 m

(ii) 2 m?

e. With respect to linear tomography:

(i) Why are the images of points on the plane of the fulcrum sharp on the radiograph, whereas images of points above and below this plane are unsharp?

(ii) What is the relationship, at a given fulcrum height, between the tomographic angle and the tomographic layer thickness?

FURTHER READING

Effective and real focal spots
Further information on this topic is available in Chapter 21 of this text. The following may also prove useful:
Carter P H 1994 Chesney's equipment for student radiographers, 4th edn. Blackwell Scientific, Oxford, ch 1
Dendy P P, Heaton B 1999 Physics for diagnostic radiology, 2nd edn. Institute of Physics Publishing, Bristol, ch 2
Webb S (ed) 2000 The physics of medical imaging, 2nd edn. Institute of Physics Publishing, Bristol, ch 2, sect. 2.5
Image magnification
Bushong S C 2004 Radiologic science for technologists: physics, biology and protection. Mosby, New York, ch 20

Dendy P P, Heaton B 1999 Physics for diagnostic radiology, 2nd edn. Institute of Physics Publishing, ch 5
Fauber T 2005 Radiographic imaging and exposure, 2nd edn. Mosby, New York, ch 5
Tomography
Carter P H 1994 Chesney's equipment for student radiographers, 4th edn. Blackwell Scientific, ch 12

Chapter 3

The Inverse-Square Law

CHAPTER CONTENTS

3.1 Aim   19

3.2 Intensity of Radiation   19

3.3 Statement of the Inverse-Square Law   20

3.4 Mathematical Proofs of the Inverse-Square Law   20
   3.4.1 Similar-Triangles Proof   20

3.5 The Inverse-Square Law and the X-ray Beam   21

3.6 mAs and the Inverse-Square Law   21

Self-Test   24

Further Reading   24

3.1 AIM

The aim of this chapter is to introduce the reader to the inverse-square law and to explore its applications in radiography and radiation protection.

3.2 INTENSITY OF RADIATION

To understand the inverse-square law we must first understand what is meant by the term *intensity*.

As we will see in Chapter 25, electromagnetic radiation is composed of quanta, each of which has an energy. If we draw a square of unit area at right angles to the path of a uniform beam of electromagnetic radiation (such as X-rays), then the total energy per second from all the quanta passing through the square is defined as the *intensity* of the beam, so that:

DEFINITION

The intensity of a beam of electromagnetic radiation at a point is the total energy per second flowing past that point when normalised to a unit area.

It is not necessary at this stage to understand the units of energy or exposure to allow us to apply the inverse-square law; these will be dealt with in later chapters.

3.3 STATEMENT OF THE INVERSE-SQUARE LAW

The intensity of the radiation emitted from a small isotropic source is inversely proportional to the square of the distance from the source, provided there is negligible absorption or scattering of the radiation by the medium through which it passes.

Note that this statement of the inverse-square law also gives the conditions under which the law may be directly applied:

- *Small source* – in practice this means small compared to the distance from the source to the point of measurement
- *Isotropic source* – this means that it emits radiation in all directions. This is necessary in order that the intensity of the radiation is independent of the *direction* from the source
- *No absorption or scattering of radiation* – this ensures that the radiation passing through an area is not affected by the medium through which the radiation passes. It is important to remember that back-scattering of the beam from objects beyond the point of measurement must also be eliminated as this would produce an increase in the intensity.

As we will see, it is not possible to meet all of these conditions in many situations in radiography. In such cases the law must be applied with caution or even with appropriate correction factors (e.g. absorption due to air may be important when we consider low-energy beams of X-rays).

INSIGHT

A situation where the inverse-square law does not apply is in the case of a laser beam. This is because the light is essentially parallel, so the intensity is constant and does not depend on distance from the source.

3.4 MATHEMATICAL PROOFS OF THE INVERSE-SQUARE LAW

3.4.1 Similar-Triangles Proof

It is sometimes easier for radiographers to use the similar-triangles proof of the inverse-square law as this relates more closely to the geometry considered for image production.

Consider the situation shown in Figure 3.1. The radiation is produced at a point *P* and is allowed to fall on the square of side *CD* and the square of side *EF*.

PB is twice the length of *PA*.

From our consideration of similar triangles in Chapter 2, we can say that *EF* must therefore be twice the length of *CD*.

Thus the area of the square of side *EF* is four times the area of the square of side *CD*.

Remembering that the intensity is the total energy per unit time divided by the area, we can calculate that I_1 must be four times the value of I_2.

Thus, by doubling the distance between the point and the source of radiation, we can see that the intensity of the radiation is reduced to one-quarter.

Stated mathematically, this is:

$$\frac{I_1}{I_2} = \frac{d_2^{\,2}}{d_1^{\,2}}$$

Equation 3.1

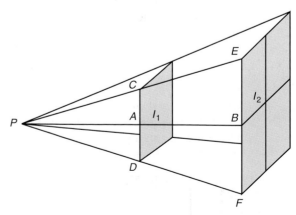

Figure 3.1   Similar-triangles proof of the inverse-square law. Note that the radiation at I_2 is spread over four times the area of I_1, and so the intensity at I_2 is one-quarter of the intensity at I_1.

Using the relationship established in equation 3.1 we can produce a table of intensities at given distances (see Table 3.1).

Table 3.1 Relationships between *distance* and *intensity*

Distance	Area	Intensity	1/(distance)^2
X	1	I_x	$1/X^2$
$2X$	4	$I_x/4$	$1/4X^2$
$3X$	9	$I_x/9$	$1/9X^2$
$4X$	16	$I_x/16$	$1/16X^2$
$5X$	25	$I_x/25$	$1/25X^2$
$10X$	100	$I_x/100$	$1/100X^2$

3.5 THE INVERSE-SQUARE LAW AND THE X-RAY BEAM

If we consider the three conditions listed earlier for the inverse-square law to be applied we can see that, strictly speaking, the X-ray beam does not satisfy these conditions because:

- X-rays are not emitted from a true point source (see Sect. 2.3) as the focal spot has a finite size
- They are not emitted equally in all directions as the anode heel effect (see Ch. 21) causes the intensity to vary across the beam
- Absorption and scattering of the X-ray beam (see Ch. 30) occur as it passes through air.

These effects are, however, small for X-ray beams generated above 50 kVp so the inverse-square law may be applied to such beams.

EXAMPLES

a. The absorbed dose rate in air at a distance of 60 cm from the focal spot of an X-ray tube is 0.5 mGy·s^{-1} (do not worry about the unit, as this does not affect the calculation!). What is the absorbed dose rate at 75 cm from the focus?

Using Equation 3.1 we can say that:

$$\frac{I_1}{I_2} = \frac{d_2^2}{d_1^2}$$

where I_1 = 0.5 mGy·s^{-1}, d_1 = 60 cm and d_2 = 75cm. I_2 is what we need to calculate.

The equation can be rearranged thus:

$$I_2 = \frac{I_1 \times d_1^2}{d_2^2}$$

(If you are unable to follow this, look at Section A3.7 on cross-multiplication in Appendix A.)

$$= \frac{0.5 \times (60)^2}{(75)^2} \text{ mGy·s}^{-1}$$

$$= 0.32 \text{ mGy·s}^{-1}$$

Thus, the absorbed dose rate at 75 cm will be 0.32 mGy·s^{-1}.

b. In the above example, at what distance would the exposure rate be 2.0 mGy·s^{-1}?

Again we start with Equation 3.1:

$$\frac{I_1}{I_2} = \frac{d_2^2}{d_1^2}$$

where I_1 = 0.5 mGy·s^{-1}, d_1 = 60 cm and I_2 = 2.0 mGy·s^{-1}. This time d_2 is unknown.

We can arrange the equation in terms of d_2 thus:

$$d_2^2 = \frac{I_1 \times d_1^2}{I_2}$$

$$= \frac{0.5 \times (60)^2}{2.0}$$

$$= \frac{(60)^2}{4}$$

$$d_2 = \sqrt{\frac{(60)^2}{4}} \text{ cm}$$

$$= 30 \text{ cm}$$

Thus the absorbed dose rate will be 2.0 mGy·s^{-1} at a distance of 30 cm from the tube focus. (*Note:* By the inverse-square law, if we halve the distance the intensity will increase by a factor of 4, so the calculation is correct.)

3.6 MAS AND THE INVERSE-SQUARE LAW

In radiography, if the kVp is unaltered, the radiation output from the tube is altered by altering the mAs (defined in Table 6.3) – if the mAs is doubled, then the output will be doubled. We can see how this is affected by the inverse-square law from the discussion following.

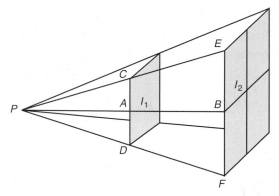

Figure 3.2 Radiographs taken at different focus to film distances. If we wish to get the same intensity of radiation on both radiographs then the mAs for *PB* must be four times the mAs required for *PA*.

Suppose a given setting of mAs produces a satisfactory radiograph at a given focus to film distance (FFD). How will this setting of mAs have to be altered for a different value of FFD?

Consider the situation shown in Figure 3.2. If a radiograph was taken using an FFD of *PA* and the image produced was satisfactory, then this means that the film received the correct amount of radiation. If the film was repositioned for an FFD of *PB* and the exposure factors remained unaltered, then the amount of radiation received by the film would be one-quarter of the correct exposure (the distance has been doubled and so the intensity is quartered). This second radiograph would be too light or *underexposed*. In order that the film at *B* receives the same exposure as the original film at *A*, the amount of radiation leaving the tube must be increased by a factor of 4. This means that both these radiographs would have the same *optical density* or blackening.

From the above we can see that:

The mAs required to produce radiographs of the same density at different FFDs is proportional to the FFD squared.

This can be expressed mathematically as:

$$\frac{mAs_1}{mAs_2} = \frac{FFD_1^{\,2}}{FFD_2^{\,2}} \qquad \textit{Equation 3.2}$$

It is important to form a mental picture of the difference between the straightforward measure-

ment of the intensity of the radiation at a point where the amount of radiation leaving the source is constant (this involves applying the inverse-square law) and this second case where the amount of radiation at a point is kept constant by altering the output from the X-ray tube (this involves using Equation 3.2).

EXAMPLE

A chest radiograph was produced at an FFD of 2 m and required the following exposure factors: 65 kVp and 16 mAs. If this radiograph is to be repeated at an FFD of 1 m at the same kVp, what mAs will be required?

Using Equation 3.2 we can say that:

$$\frac{mAs_1}{mAs_2} = \frac{FFD_1^{\,2}}{FFD_2^{\,2}}$$

where mAs_1 = 16 mAs, FFD_1 = 2 m and FFD_2 = 1 m. mAs_2 is unknown.

The equation can be arranged in terms of mAs_2 thus:

$$mAs_2 = \frac{mAs_1 FFD_2^{\,2}}{FFD_1^{\,2}}$$

$$= \frac{16 \times (1)^2}{(2)^2} \; mAs$$

$$= 4 \; mAs$$

Note: By the inverse-square law, if we halve the distance then we will have four times the intensity. If we want to have the same intensity to the film, then we need one-quarter of the original mAs. So the answer is correct.

The influence of the FFD on the mAs required can be seen by comparing the radiographs of a wrist phantom in Figure 3.3. Radiograph A was exposed at an FFD of 100 cm and was given an exposure of 16 mAs. Radiograph B was exposed at an FFD of 200 cm and was given an exposure of 16 mAs. Radiograph C was exposed at an FFD of 200 cm and was given an exposure of 32 mAs. Radiograph D was exposed at 200 cm and was given an exposure of 64 mAs. Note that radiographs A and D have the same optical densities.

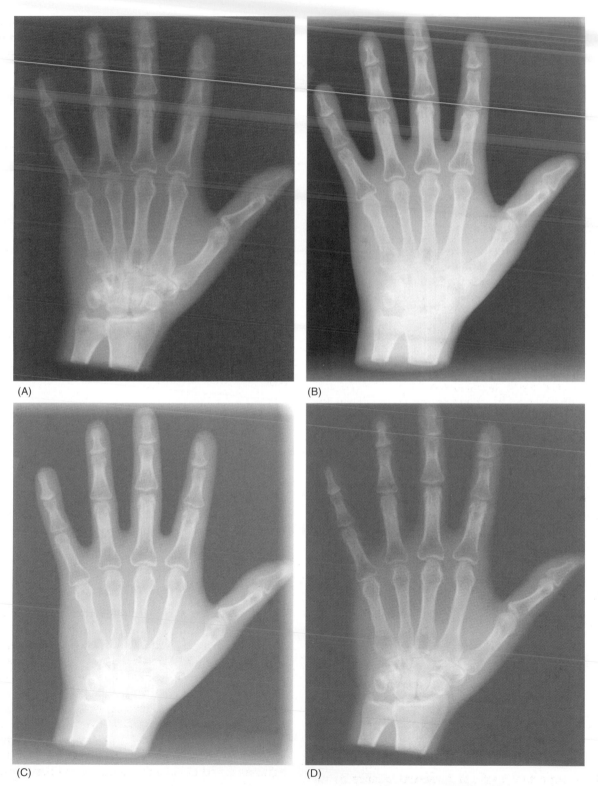

(A)   (B)

(C)   (D)

Figure 3.3 The effect of mAs and inverse-square law on the radiographic image. (A) 100 cm focus to film distance (FFD), 16 mAs; (B) 200 cm FFD, 16 mAs; (C) 200 cm FFD, 32 mAs; (D) 200 cm FFD, 64 mAs.

SUMMARY

In this chapter you should have learnt:

- The definition of radiation intensity (see Sect. 3.2)
- The inverse-square law and its use in calculating the intensity of radiation at a given distance from a source (see Sects 3.3–3.5)
- How the mAs given for a radiograph is influenced by the FFD used because of the inverse-square law (see Sect. 3.6).

SELF-TEST

a. What is meant by the intensity of electromagnetic radiation?

b. State the inverse-square law as applied to a beam of electromagnetic radiation.

c. The absorbed dose rate in air at a distance of 100 cm from the target of an X-ray tube is 1.8 mGy.s^{-1}.

   (i)   What will be the absorbed dose rate in air at a distance of 150 cm?

   (ii) At what distance from the focus will the absorbed dose rate in air be 0.2 mGy.s^{-1}?

d. A radiograph of a lateral cervical spine required an exposure of 65 kVp and 24 mAs at an FFD of 200 cm. A repeat radiograph was later required but this time the distance was restricted to 100 cm. If all other factors remained unchanged, calculate the new mAs required to produce the same density on the radiograph.

FURTHER READING

Intensity of radiation
Ball J L, Moore A D 1997 Essential physics for radiographers, 3rd edn. Blackwell Scientific Publications, London, ch 15
Inverse-square law
Ball J L, Moore A D 1997 Essential physics for radiographers, 3rd edn. Blackwell Scientific Publications, London, ch 14

mAs and the inverse-square law
Ball J, Price T 1995 Chesney's radiographic imaging, 6th edn. Blackwell Scientific Publications, London, ch 17
Fauber T 2005 Radiographic imaging and exposure, 2nd edn. Mosby, New York, ch 10

Chapter 4

The Exponential Law

CHAPTER CONTENTS

4.1   Aim   25

4.2   Description of the Exponential Law   25

4.3   Radioactive Decay and the Exponential Law   27

4.4   Measures of Radioactivity   28

4.5   Half-life and Decay Constant   28

4.6   Physical Half-Life, Biological Half-Life and Effective Half-Life   30

4.7   Attenuation of Electromagnetic Radiation by Matter   31

4.8   Half-Value Thickness   32

4.9   Tenth-Value Thickness   33

4.10 The Use of the Logarithmic Form of the Exponential Law   33

Self-Test   34

Further Reading   35

4.1 AIM

The aim of this chapter is to introduce the exponential law and consider its applications to radiographic science. The law is fundamental to an understanding of radioactive decay and the attenuation of certain electromagnetic radiations (e.g. X-rays and gamma-rays).

4.2 DESCRIPTION OF THE EXPONENTIAL LAW

Perhaps the best everyday example of the exponential law concerns money. If £100 is invested with a financial institution which gives a fixed interest rate of 5% per annum then the growth of that money over a 25-year period is shown in Table 4.1.

Notice that the net increase per year is initially quite small (£5.00 in the first year) but the rise increases with time (£16.13 in the 25th year). This is an example of exponential growth in that as the time increases by *equal amounts* (1 year) the money increases by *equal fractions* (5%). If we draw a graph of the total money with the financial institution we get a smooth curve, as shown in Figure 4.1. This is the typical shape of an increasing exponential.

For a second example, consider a situation where we possess an initial sum of £100. If we consider a tax system where 5% of this money is removed each year as a tax, then the fate of the original £100 is shown in Table 4.2.

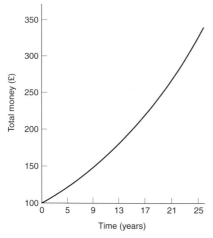

Figure 4.1 Growth of £100 at 5% per annum. Note that the rate of growth becomes greater with time. This is an example of *exponential growth*.

Again we can note that the net decrease is greatest during the first year (£5.00) and is least during the 25th year (£1.46). The rate of decrease is, however, the same, at 5% per annum. This is an example of exponential decay in that as the time increases by *equal amounts* (1 year) the money left will decrease by 5% of that remaining, but will never reach zero (i.e. there will always be some money left). If we draw a graph of the total money left, we get a smooth curve, as shown in Figure 4.2. This is the typical shape of a decaying exponential.

The common factor in these two examples is that the change each year is 5%. This is characteristic of all exponential change and may be expressed as follows:

Table 4.1	Growth of £100 at 5% per annum		
Year	Interest rate	Money at end of year	Net increase for year
1	5%	£105	£5.00
2	5%	£110.25	£5.25
3	5%	£115.76	£5.51
4	5%	£121.55	£5.79
5	5%	£127.63	£6.08
6	5%	£134.01	£6.38
7	5%	£140.71	£6.70
8	5%	£147.74	£7.03
9	5%	£155.13	£7.39
10	5%	£162.90	£7.77
11	5%	£171.03	£8.13
12	5%	£179.59	£8.56
13	5%	£188.56	£8.97
14	5%	£197.99	£9.43
15	5%	£207.89	£9.90
16	5%	£218.29	£10.40
17	5%	£229.90	£10.91
18	5%	£240.66	£11.46
19	5%	£252.70	£12.04
20	5%	£265.33	£12.63
21	5%	£278.60	£13.27
22	5%	£292.53	£13.93
23	5%	£307.15	£14.62
24	5%	£322.51	£15.36
25	5%	£338.64	£16.13

Table 4.2	Decrease of £100 at 5% per annum		
Year	Tax rate	Money at end of year	Net decrease for year
1	5%	£95.00	£5.00
2	5%	£90.25	£4.75
3	5%	£85.74	£4.51
4	5%	£81.45	£4.29
5	5%	£77.38	£4.07
6	5%	£73.51	£3.87
7	5%	£69.83	£3.68
8	5%	£66.34	£3.49
9	5%	£63.02	£3.32
10	5%	£59.87	£3.15
11	5%	£56.88	£2.99
12	5%	£54.04	£2.84
13	5%	£51.33	£2.70
14	5%	£48.77	£2.57
15	5%	£46.33	£2.44
16	5%	£44.01	£2.32
17	5%	£41.81	£2.20
18	5%	£39.72	£2.09
19	5%	£37.74	£1.99
20	5%	£35.85	£1.89
21	5%	£34.06	£1.79
22	5%	£32.35	£1.70
23	5%	£30.74	£1.62
24	5%	£29.20	£1.54
25	5%	£27.74	£1.46

DEFINITION

A quantity *y* is said to vary *exponentially* with *x* if equal changes in *x* produce equal *fractional* (or *percentage*) changes in *y*.

INSIGHT

For students familiar with calculus the mathematical equivalent of the above statement is:

$$\frac{dy}{y} = k \times dx$$

or

$$\frac{dy}{dx} = ky$$

If we integrate this equation then we get:

$$y = y_0 \times e^{kx}$$

Here the independent variable *x* forms part of the exponent of the number e and hence the term *exponential law*.

Note also that the equation $y = y_0 \times e^{kx}$ represents exponential growth. The equivalent for exponential decay would be expressed as $y = y_0 \times e^{-kx}$.

The two major examples of the exponential law in radiographic science are radioactive decay and the attenuation of electromagnetic radiation by matter. Both of these are described in the following sections.

4.3 RADIOACTIVE DECAY AND THE EXPONENTIAL LAW

Radionuclides are said to *decay* when they change from one nuclear configuration to another. This decay takes several forms, including the ejection of alpha-particles, beta-particles (both positive and negative) and gamma-rays from the nucleus. These and other modes of decay are discussed more fully in Chapter 27. The particular mode of decay is, however, not important to our discussion in this section as the application of the exponential law is valid for all the modes. It can be stated as:

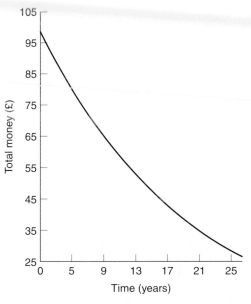

Figure 4.2   Decay of £100 at 5% tax per annum. Note that the rate of decay decreases with time and the amount of money left never reaches zero. This is an example of *exponential decay*.

DEFINITION

The *law of radioactive decay* states that the rate of decay of a particular nuclide (i.e. the number of nuclei decaying per second) is proportional to the number of such nuclei left in the sample (i.e. it is a fixed fraction of the number of nuclei left in the sample).

It can be seen that this is exactly analogous to the changes which occurred in the decaying exponential sum of money, in that a fixed fraction (or percentage) will decay each unit time (similar to the loss of money from the lump sum). Figure 4.3 shows a graph depicting the above situation. You will note that the initial fall in number of atoms is steep but slows down as fewer and fewer of the original nuclei are left. Also note that the number of original nuclei never reaches zero. This is exactly the same as happened in the case of the lump sum of money and you should note the similarities between Figure 4.3 and Figure 4.2.

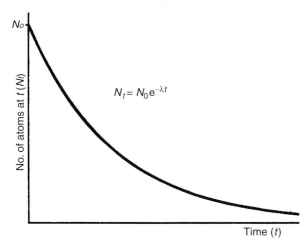

Figure 4.3 Exponential decay of the *number of atoms* of a particular radionuclide. Note the similarity to Figure 4.2.

4.4 MEASURES OF RADIOACTIVITY

In practice it would be extremely difficult to measure the number of nuclei remaining and draw a graph like Figure 4.3. What we can measure more easily is the *effects* of the nuclear disintegrations by counting the number of gamma-rays (for example) emitted, using a suitable counter. In this way we may make an estimate of the total number of disintegrations per second occurring within the radioactive sample at any given time. This quantity is known as the *activity* of the sample and is measured in becquerels, where 1 Bq is 1 nuclear disintegration per second. We may now plot *activity* against *time* (Figure 4.4) and we obtain exactly the same curve as in Figure 4.3.

The equation for this curve is expressed as:

$$A_t = A_0 e^{-\lambda t} \qquad \text{Equation 4.1}$$

where A_t is the activity after a time t, A_0 is the initial activity, e is the exponential constant, λ is the decay constant and t is the time after the initial measurement.

INSIGHT

In practice it is often easier to use Equation 4.1 in its logarithmic form. Consider the equation:

$$A_t = A_0 e^{-\lambda t}$$

If we take logarithms to the base e of both sides of the equation then we get:

$$\log_e A_t = \log_e A_0 - \lambda t \qquad \text{Equation 4.2}$$

This equation and its use with logarithmic graph paper will be considered further at the end of this chapter.

Figure 4.4 shows the decay curves for radionuclides which have different rates of decay. As we cannot consider the time it will take a nuclide to reach zero as a measure of its rate of decay, a quantity called the *half-life* is used to describe the rate of decay. This is further considered in the next section.

4.5 HALF-LIFE AND DECAY CONSTANT

DEFINITION

The *half-life of* a radionuclide is the time required for the activity of the radioactive sample to decay to one-half of its original value.

An illustration of the half-life of a particular radionuclide is shown in Figure 4.5. The activity

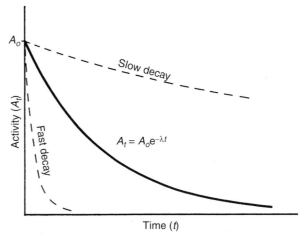

Figure 4.4 Exponential decay of the *radioactivity* of a particular radionuclide.

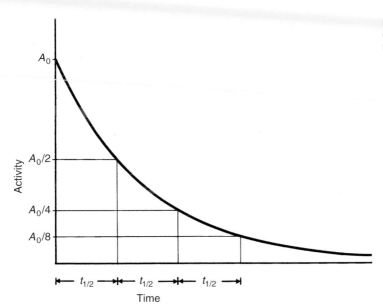

Figure 4.5 Half-life ($t_{1/2}$) and the radioactive decay. Note that each $t_{1/2}$ reduces the level of radioactivity by one-half.

of the sample when $t = 0$ is A_0. When the activity is reduced to $A_0/2$ then the radionuclide has undergone one half-life. This is indicated by the time $t^{1/2}$. If another half-life passes, then the activity is reduced by a further factor of 2 and is now $A_0/4$, and so on for further half-lives. Notice that, as in our monetary example (Figure 4.2), the curve never reaches zero activity, so no radioactive source is ever completely *dead*.

If we now consider Equation 4.1 we can use this to establish a relationship between the decay constant and the half-life:

$$A_t = A_0 e^{-\lambda t\frac{1}{2}}$$

Now, by definition, at the half-life, $A_0/2 = A_0 e^{-\lambda t1/2}$. Thus the equation can be rewritten in the form:

$$\frac{A_0}{2} = A_0 e^{-\lambda t\frac{1}{2}}$$

$$\frac{1}{2} = e^{-\lambda t\frac{1}{2}}$$

$$2 = e^{\lambda t\frac{1}{2}}$$

$$\log_e 2 = \lambda t\frac{1}{2}$$

$$0.693 = \lambda t\frac{1}{2}$$

$$\lambda = \frac{0.693}{t\frac{1}{2}} \qquad \text{Equation 4.3}$$

The decay constant is thus measured in time^{-1} since it is inversely related to the half-life.

EXAMPLE

The half-life of $^{99}Tc^m$ is 6 h. What is its decay constant?

From Equation 4.3:

$$\lambda = \frac{0.693}{t\frac{1}{2}}$$

$$\lambda = \frac{0.693}{6} \text{ h}^{-1}$$

$$= 0.1155 \text{ h}^{-1}$$

Because of this relationship between the half-life and the decay constant, we may also write Equation 4.1 as follows:

$$A_t = A_0 e^{-(0.693t/t\frac{1}{2})} \qquad \text{Equation 4.4}$$

Another important point is that it does not matter from which time measurement of the half-life is begun. Figure 4.6 shows the decay of a radionuclide over a time of one half-life starting from an arbitrary time, T. Note that the value of $t_{1/2}$ shown in Figure 4.6 is exactly the same as the value shown in Figure 4.5. Thus, over an interval of $t_{1/2}$ the activity is reduced by a factor of 2, independent of the starting time, T.

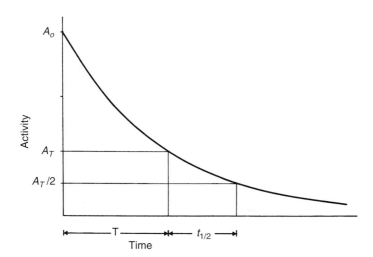

Figure 4.6 The half-life ($t_{1/2}$) is measured from an arbitrary time, *T*. It is found that the value of $t_{1/2}$ so obtained does not depend on the value of *T*, so the half-life may be measured from any starting time.

EXAMPLE

A radioisotope of iodine, ^{131}I, has a half-life of 8 days. Its activity was measured as 14.4 MBq at 09:00 on 3 February. What will be its activity at 09:00 on 27 February?

The time interval over which we are considering the decay of the nuclide is 24 days. With a half-life of 8 days, this represents decay through three half-lives.

After one half-life the activity will be reduced by a factor of 2.

After two half-lives the activity will be reduced by a factor of $(2 \times 2) = 4$.

After three half-lives the activity will be reduced by a factor of $(4 \times 2) = 8$

i.e. each successive half-life reduces the activity by a factor of 2.

Thus the activity after three half-lives = 14.4/8 = 1.8 MBq.

The activity at 09:00 on 27 February will therefore be 1.8 MBq.

This example gives some clue as to the general method of solving such problems. Assuming *n* half-lives of decay, the decayed activity A_n can be calculated from the formula:

$$A_n = \frac{A_0}{2^n} \qquad \text{Equation 4.5}$$

where A_0 is the original activity.

Similarly, we can use this equation to *look back* to consider how much original activity would be required on a certain date to give us the required activity at the time of use of the isotope. Here the unknown is A_0 and the equation can be rearranged as follows:

$$A_0 = 2^n \times A_n \qquad \text{Equation 4.6}$$

EXAMPLE

An activity of 36.5 MBq of ^{99}Tc^m is required at 17:00 on 22 March. The radionuclide has a half-life of 6 h. What activity of the isotope must be dispensed at 05:00 on 22 March to give the required activity?

Using Equation 4.6:

$$A_0 = 2^n \times A_n$$
$$= 2^2 \times 36.5 \text{ MBq}$$
$$= 146 \text{ MBq}$$

4.6 PHYSICAL HALF-LIFE, BIOLOGICAL HALF-LIFE AND EFFECTIVE HALF-LIFE

In all the considerations of radioactive decay so far we have considered the *physical half-life* of an isotope – the half-life as it would be measured using a quantity of isotope in the laboratory. In *nuclear medicine* there are two other types of half-life we need to consider:

1. The *biological half-life* is the time taken for the concentration of a certain chemical in an organ to be reduced to half its original concentration. In this case, the concentration of the chemical is the important part and its activity is not important. This value is affected by the body's ability to excrete the chemical
2. The *effective half-life* is the time taken for the activity of a certain radionuclide in a certain organ to be reduced to half of its original activity. This will be affected by the physical half-life and the biological half-life.

The three types of half-life are connected by the equation:

$$\frac{1}{t_{\frac{1}{2}(\text{eff})}} + \frac{1}{t_{\frac{1}{2}(\text{phys})}} + \frac{1}{t_{\frac{1}{2}(\text{bio})}}$$

Equation 4.7

4.7 ATTENUATION OF ELECTROMAGNETIC RADIATION BY MATTER

The attenuation of electromagnetic radiation by matter constitutes the other major application of the exponential law in radiography.

The types of interactions which electromagnetic radiation undergoes when it passes through matter are explained in Chapter 30. A detailed knowledge of these mechanisms is not required at this stage. If we consider a slab of material which has 100 units of radiation incident on it and the transmitted radiation measures 90 units, then we can say that the material *attenuates* 10 units of radiation (the differences between absorption and attenuation will be explained in Ch. 30).

For the exponential law to be applied, certain conditions must be satisfied:

- The radiation beam must be parallel. This means that it is not affected by the inverse-square law
- The radiation beam must be homogeneous (i.e. the photons must all have the same energy). This means that the beam is not 'hardened' by the removal of low-energy photons by the attenuating material

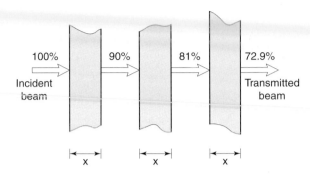

Figure 4.7   Exponential attenuation of a parallel beam of electromagnetic radiation by matter. Equal thickness (*x*) of the attenuator will transmit equal fractions (in this case 9/10) of the incident radiation.

- The attenuator must be homogeneous. This means that the attenuating properties must be the same in different parts of the attenuator.

Consider the situation in Figure 4.7. Here, a parallel beam of radiation (e.g. gamma-rays) is incident on a slab of uniform attenuating material of thickness *x*. Suppose there is 10% attenuation in the first slab, then 90% of the original beam is transmitted. If we put a further identical attenuator in the path of the beam, then it is found that it also attenuates 10% of the radiation incident upon it and 81% ($0.9 \times 90\%$) will be transmitted. A third identical attenuator transmits 90% of this amount (72.9%), and so on for further attenuators. Thus we can say that *equal changes in x produce equal fractional (or percentage) changes in the transmitted radiation intensity*. This is again an exponential relationship so we can say that:

> **The attenuation of a monoenergetic parallel beam of electromagnetic radiation by a uniform attenuator will vary exponentially with the attenuator thickness.**

A graph of the transmitted intensity I_x through the attenuator of thickness *x* is shown in Figure 4.8. The incident radiation I_0 is the value of I_x when there is no attenuator ($x = 0$). Note the similarities between this curve and the other exponential curves shown in this chapter. The mathematical relationships between the quantities can be given using the equation:

$$I_x = I_0 e^{-\mu x}$$

Equation 4.8

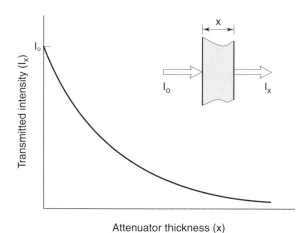

Figure 4.8 Graph showing changes in transmitted intensity due to exponential attenuation of radiation by a uniform attenuator. Note the similarity to Figure 4.3.

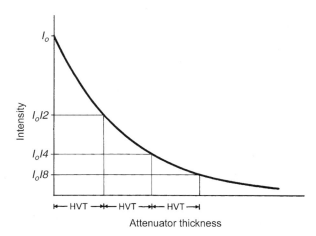

Figure 4.9 Half-value thickness (HVT) of a beam of electromagnetic radiation. Each HVT of the attenuator reduces the intensity by one-half. Note the similarity to Figure 4.5.

where μ (mu) is the *total linear attenuation coefficient* and so takes into account all the processes of attenuation. The equation therefore refers to variations of transmittance within *linear distance, x*.

DEFINITION

The *total linear attenuation coefficient* is the fractional change in the intensity of a parallel beam of monoenergetic radiation per unit thickness of homogeneous attenuator.

Note the similarities between the exponential relationships for radioactive decay (Equation 4.1) and exponential attenuation (Equation 4.8). This would suggest that there is a term similar to *half-life* which can be used to describe the penetrating properties of a beam of radiation. This term is the *half-value thickness* (often abbreviated to HVT).

4.8 HALF-VALUE THICKNESS

If we consider Figure 4.9, we can see that successive HVTs reduce the intensity by factors of 2. We are therefore in a position to define HVT more precisely.

DEFINITION

The *half-value thickness* is that thickness of a substance which will transmit one-half of the intensity of radiation incident upon it.

The HVT therefore depends on the attenuating properties of the substance itself and the penetrating power of the beam of electromagnetic radiation incident upon it. Thus in diagnostic radiography we might compare the penetrating properties of two beams using aluminium to calculate the HVTs, whereas in therapy radiography we would do this using copper as our attenuator.

To complete the analogy with radioactive decay, Equation 4.3 is paralleled by:

$$\mu = \frac{0.693}{HVT} \qquad \textit{Equation 4.9}$$

EXAMPLE

a. The HVT for a beam of radiation is found to be 2.8 mm of aluminium. What is the total linear attenuation coefficient of this beam in aluminium?

From Equation 4.9:

$$\mu = \frac{0.693}{HVT}$$

$$= \frac{0.693}{2.8}\text{mm}^{-1}$$

$$= 0.2475 \text{ mm}^{-1}$$

b. The HVT for a particular beam of gamma-rays is 3 mm of lead. What thickness of lead must be placed in the beam such that only 0.1% of it is transmitted?

There are several ways of tackling this and similar problems. Below is one method.

100% of the beam is incident on the lead and 0.1% is transmitted. This gives a reduction factor of 100/0.1 = 1000.

Now each HVT gives a reduction factor of 2 between the incident and the transmitted radiation, as shown in the table below:

Number of HVTs	Intensity reduction factor
1	2
2	4 (i.e. 2 × 2)
3	8
4	16
5	32
6	64
7	128
8	256
9	512
10	1024

This sort of table is very easy to check so there should be little chance of arithmetic errors.

After 10 HVTs the intensity reduction factor is 1024, which is very close to the required factor of 1000.

Thus 30 mm of lead (10 HVTs) must be used to reduce the transmitted intensity to 0.1% of the incident intensity.

As was the case with radioactive decay (see Equation 4.5), we can use a formula to calculate the intensity (I_n) after n HVTs:

$$I_n = \frac{I_0}{2^n}$$

Equation 4.10

4.9 TENTH-VALUE THICKNESS

It should be clear at this stage that values of absorber thickness other than the HVT will produce equal fractional changes in transmission and so it is possible to define a 'fifth-value thickness' or a 'tenth-value thickness' (TVT), etc. Although the HVT is a very common method of measuring the attenuation of electromagnetic radiation through matter, the TVT is also used when considering large amounts of attenuation. An example of this would be when designing the walls of a radiotherapy treatment room when a very high intensity of radiation from the treatment machine must not be allowed to penetrate through the wall in significant quantities. One TVT would reduce the intensity by a factor of 10; two would reduce the intensity by a factor of 100, and so on.

4.10 THE USE OF THE LOGARITHMIC FORM OF THE EXPONENTIAL LAW

Consider Equation 4.2, which is the logarithmic form of the exponential law:

$$\log_e A_t = \log_e A_0 - \lambda t$$

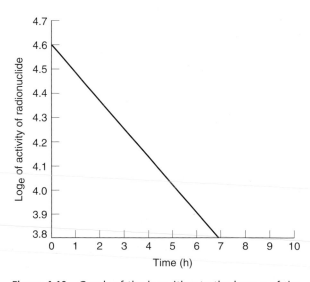

Figure 4.10 Graph of the logarithm to the base e of the activity of a radionuclide plotted against time. Note that the previous *exponential* curve (see Figure 4.4) is now a *straight line*.

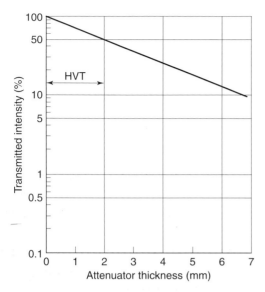

Figure 4.11 An example of the use of logarithmic graph paper to plot an exponential relationship. Note that the previous *exponential curve* (see Figure 4.8) has become a *straight line*. The half-value thickness (HVT) for the beam of radiation is 2 mm, as read from the graph. Half-lives may also be determined in this manner.

If we look at this equation, we see that it is in the form of $y = c - mx$ and so we would expect its graph to be in the form of a straight line. If we plot $\log_e$ of the activity on the y-axis and time on the x-axis, we get the graph shown in Figure 4.10.

The requirement to calculate the logarithm for each result and the antilogarithm for each reading from the graph is overcome by the use of logarithmic graph paper (for a fuller description, see Appendix A). Suitable graph paper in this case is log/linear graph paper, i.e. the y-axis is logarithmic and the x-axis is linear.

An example of such a graph for the attenuation of a beam of electromagnetic radiation is shown in Figure 4.11. Note that equal spaces on the log scale represent changes by factors of 10, and so the logarithmic scale never reaches zero. This type of paper allows us to plot the points directly on the paper and then draw the best straight line through them. Such a linear graph makes it easier to interpolate and to extrapolate (see Appendix A) information from the graph.

SUMMARY

In this chapter we have considered the following factors pertinent to the exponential law:

- The description of the exponential law (see Sect. 4.2)
- Radioactive decay and the exponential law (see Sect. 4.3)
- Measures which can be made of the activity of a radionuclide (see Sect. 4.4)
- The relationship between the half-life and the decay constant for a radionuclide (see Sect. 4.5)
- The relationships between the physical half-life, the biological half-life and the effective half-life (see Sect. 4.6)
- How the attenuation of electromagnetic radiation by matter obeys the exponential law (see Sect. 4.7)
- The HVT for a beam of radiation and a given attenuator (see Sect. 4.8)
- The use of the TVT (see Sect. 4.9)
- The use of the logarithmic form of the exponential law (see Sect. 4.10).

SELF-TEST

a. Some swabs have been contaminated with $^{99}Tc^m$ at 09:00 on 16 February. The half-life of the isotope is 6 h. The level of activity from the swabs was measured at 64 MBq. If the activity of the swabs must be 1 MBq or less before they can be disposed of, what is the earliest time the swabs can be sent for disposal?

b. The decay constant for ^{75}Se is 0.0057 day^{-1}. What is its half-life?

c. An isotope of iodine, ^{131}I, has a half-life of 8 days. 16.8 MBq is required for a study starting at 10:00 on 19 March. If this isotope is to be dispensed of at 10:00 on 3 March, what activity should be dispensed?

d. What is the equation which links the *biological half-life*, the *effective half-life* and the *physical half-life*?

e. The HVT for a particular beam of gamma radiation is 1.8 mm of lead. The absorbed dose in air at the front of a barrier is 15 mGy.h^{-1}. We wish the dose at the far side of the barrier to be 7.5 µGy.h^{-1} or less. What is the minimum thickness of lead required in the barrier?

f. (For this final item it is desirable to have access to 3 cycle log/linear graph paper. If this is not available, it is possible (but less convenient) to plot the line using log$_e$ of the activity against time on linear graph paper.)

Below is a set of readings of the activity of a certain isotope at the stated time intervals:

Time (h)	Activity (MBq)
0	78.2
5	43.9
10	24.6
15	13.8
20	7.8
25	4.4
30	2.4
35	1.4
40	0.8

(i) Draw a graph of the activity against time (preferably on logarithmic graph paper).

(ii) Using the graph, estimate the half-life of the isotope.

(iii) What is the decay constant for this isotope?

(iv) Using the graph, estimate the activity of this isotope after 50 h.

FURTHER READING

Radioactivity and the exponential law
Chapter 27 of the current text contains more information on this topic.
Ball J L, Moore A D 1997 Essential physics for radiographers, 3rd edn. Blackwell Scientific Publications, London, ch 20
Bushong 2004 Radiologic science for technologists: physics, biology and protection. Mosby, New York, ch 4
Dendy P P, Heaton B 1999 Physics for diagnostic radiology, 2nd edn. Institute of Physics Publishing, ch 1

Webb S (ed) 2000 The physics of medical imaging, 2nd edn. Institute of Physics Publishing, Bristol, ch 6
Exponential attenuation of radiation
Ball J L, Moore A D 1997 Essential physics for radiographers, 3rd edn. Blackwell Scientific Publications, London, ch 17
Bushong S C 2004 Radiologic science for technologists: physics, biology and protection. Mosby, New York, ch 13
Dendy P P, Heaton B 1999 Physics for diagnostic radiology, 2nd edn. Institute of Physics Publishing, ch 3

Part 2

General Physics

PART CONTENTS

5. Laws of Physics (Classical)   39

6. Units of Measurement   44

7. Experimental Error and Statistics   52

8. Heat   62

9. Electrostatics   72

10. Electricity (DC)   80

11. Magnetism   93

12. Electromagnetism   106

13. Electromagnetic Induction   112

14. Alternating Current Flow   120

15. The Motor Principle   134

16. Capacitors   141

17. The AC Transformer   150

18. Semiconductor Materials   163

19. Rectification   177

20. Exposure and Timing Circuits   185

Chapter 5

Laws of Physics (Classical)

CHAPTER CONTENTS

5.1 Aim   39

5.2 Law of Conservation of Matter (mass)   39

5.3 Law of Conservation of Energy   40

5.4 Law of Conservation of Momentum   40

5.5 Newton's Laws of Motion   40

5.6 Avogadro's Hypothesis, the Mole and Avogadro's number   42

Self-Test   42

Further Reading   43

5.1 AIM

The aim of this chapter is to introduce the reader to some of the laws of classical physics. An understanding of these laws will aid an understanding of some of the physics discussed in later chapters of the book. (Some of the physics in the later chapters of this book (e.g. pair production as an absorption mechanism) cannot be explained in terms of the laws of classical physics. Before these concepts are considered (Ch. 25 onwards) the laws of modern physics will be considered in Ch. 24.)

5.2 LAW OF CONSERVATION OF MATTER (MASS)

Statement of the law

Matter is neither created nor destroyed, but it may change its chemical form as the result of a chemical reaction.

This law tells us that the total mass of the ingredients after a chemical reaction is equal to their mass before the reaction.

INSIGHT

Let us consider the reaction:

$$AgNO_3 + KBr = AgBr + KNO_3$$

Here silver nitrate is mixed with potassium bromide to form silver bromide (used as the light-sensitive salt in the photographic emulsion) and potassium nitrate. The total mass of silver nitrate plus potassium bromide is equal to the total mass of silver bromide plus potassium nitrate. Matter has neither been created nor destroyed by the reaction.

5.3 LAW OF CONSERVATION OF ENERGY

Statement of the Law

Energy can neither be created nor destroyed but can be changed from one form to another. The amount of energy in a system is thus constant.

This law tells us that energy is never used up but changes from one form to another.

INSIGHT

When an electron is released from the filament of an X-ray tube it has potential energy. As it is accelerated across the tube, this potential energy is converted to kinetic energy. When it makes contact with the target of the tube, this kinetic energy is converted to heat and X-ray energy. At any time the sum of all the energies remains constant.

Some of the common forms of energy are listed below:

Chemical	Kinetic
Gravitational	Sound
Electrical	Radiation
Potential	Heat.

These two laws of conservation of mass and energy are combined into one law by modern physics (see Ch. 24).

5.4 LAW OF CONSERVATION OF MOMENTUM

Statement of the Law

The total linear or rotational momentum in a given system is constant.

This law is important when we consider collisions between two bodies.

INSIGHT

There are two types of collision which occur, elastic and inelastic. An *elastic* collision is one where all kinetic energy is conserved, as in the case of a 'perfect' billiard ball colliding with a similar but stationary billiard ball; the moving ball stops, while the ball which was previously stationary moves with the same velocity as the first ball had before collision. In an *inelastic* collision the total kinetic energy is not conserved, as in the case of two billiard balls colliding with a glancing blow, so that both continue to move after the collision. In both cases the *momentum* is conserved, although the velocities of the bodies in each case will be different.

In radiographic science, conservation of momentum is mainly concerned with the interactions of X-rays with matter and these will be dealt with in Chapter 30.

5.5 NEWTON'S LAWS OF MOTION

Newton's laws of motion can be derived from the above laws, but they are so useful that they merit a separate section. They are defined as follows:

Law 1

A body will remain at rest or will travel with a constant velocity unless acted upon by a net external force.

Law 2

The rate of change of momentum of a body is proportional to the applied force.

Law 3

The action of one body on a second body is always accompanied by an equal and

opposite action of the second body on the first.

Note: The terms *velocity* and *momentum* in the first two laws imply direction, as both are vector quantities (see Ch. 6).

A body of mass m and velocity u has a force F applied to it. After a time t its velocity has changed to v. Then the second law of motion can be stated thus:

$$\frac{(mv - mu)}{t} \propto F$$

$$\frac{m(v - u)}{t} \propto F$$

Now $(v - u)/t$ is the rate of change of velocity or the acceleration, a, of the body (see Sect. 6. 3).

Hence we can say that:

$ma \propto F$ or F = kma, where k is the constant of proportionality (see Appendix A).

If we choose suitable units it can be arranged that k is equal to 1 and we finally have:

F = ma Equation 5.1

In International System of Units (SI) units (see Sect. 6.3.4) F is measured in newtons, m is measured in kilograms and a is measured in ms^{-2}. This makes Equation 5.1 the familiar mathematical statement of Newton's second law and can also be used as the basis for the definition of the newton (1 N = 1 kg $\times$ 1 m.s^{-2}).

INSIGHT

As an illustration of the use of this law, we are now in a position to calculate the kinetic energy of a body of mass m travelling with a velocity v. If we apply a steady force F in the opposite direction to that of v, the body will slow down and eventually come to rest. The work done in bringing the body to rest must be equal to its kinetic energy. This we can state mathematically as:

$E = -F \times s$ Equation 5.2

where s is the distance taken for the body to come to rest. (The force, F, and its associated acceleration, a, are regarded as negative as they are applied in the opposite direction to v.)

From Equation 5.1 we can now change Equation 5.2 as follows:

$E = -m \times a \times s$ Equation 5.3

The acceleration, a, is the change in velocity per unit time. Stated mathematically, this is:

$$-a = \frac{(v - 0)}{t}$$

$$a = \frac{-v}{t}$$

As the action of the force is consistent throughout the deceleration, the time taken for the body to stop can be calculated by dividing the distance travelled by the average velocity (v/2). So:

$$t = \frac{s}{\frac{1}{2}v}$$

$$= \frac{2s}{v}$$

Thus we get:

$$a = \frac{-v}{t}$$

$$= \frac{-v}{(2s/v)}$$

$$= \frac{-v^2}{2s}$$

$$as = -\tfrac{1}{2}v^2$$

If we now consider Equation 5.3, this can be rewritten:

$$E = \frac{-m(as)}{\frac{1}{2}}$$

$$= -m(-\tfrac{1}{2}v^2)$$

$E = \tfrac{1}{2}mv^2$ Equation 5.4

Newton's third law is usually paraphrased as: 'To every action there is an equal and opposite reaction'. There are many examples of this in everyday life, such as a hammer hitting a nail, but it is important to realise that there need not necessarily be physical contact between the two bodies for one to act on the other. If we take two charged bodies and bring these close together (but not actually touching), the forces between the two bodies will be equal and opposite. The significance of this in the design of the cathode of the X-ray tube will be considered in Chapter 21.

5.6 AVOGADRO'S HYPOTHESIS, THE MOLE AND AVOGADRO'S NUMBER

As we will see in Chapter 26, all substances consist of atoms or molecules. These may react chemically with the atoms or molecules of other substances. These reactions occur with fixed proportions in order to produce a given chemical compound and it is possible to predict the number of molecules of the compound from a knowledge of the number of molecules of the original elements or compounds, for example:

$$2H_2 + O_2 = 2H_2O$$

In the case of gases, Avogadro's hypothesis postulated that *equal volumes of gases at the same temperature and pressure contain equal numbers of molecules*. This hypothesis was first postulated in the early nineteenth century and has been verified by a number of experiments since then.

This is taken one stage further within the SI system in the more general statement that *the number of molecules per mole is the same for any substance*. The mole is the SI unit of the amount of substance and is defined as:

DEFINITION

The *mole* is the amount of substance which contains as many elementary particles as there are atoms in 0.012 kg of carbon-12.

Here, carbon-12 is used as the standard for technical experimental reasons. From this we can predict the number of atoms or molecules in a substance by knowing its atomic mass number and comparing this with carbon-12. For example, if we consider cobalt-60, then there will be the same number of atoms in 0.060 kg of cobalt-60 as there will be in 0.012 kg of carbon-12, as each consists of one mole of substance.

The number of molecules in a mole is given by *Avogadro's number* (or constant) and is 6×10^{23} molecules.

INSIGHT

If we consider X-ray photons being attenuated by matter, this is a reaction between the photons and the electrons of atoms of the material through which they pass. If we know the number of atoms per mole of the material we can calculate the number of atoms per unit mass. By knowing the atomic number of the material it is then possible to establish the electron density and so predict the likelihood of an X-ray photon interacting with an electron. This will be further discussed in Chapter 30.

SUMMARY

In this chapter you should have learnt:

- The law of conservation of matter (see Sect. 5.2)
- The law of conservation of energy (see Sect. 5.3)
- The law of conservation of momentum (see Sect. 5.4)
- Newton's laws of motion (see Sect. 5.5)
- Avogadro's hypothesis, the mole and Avogadro's number (see Sect. 5.6).

SELF-TEST

a. State the law of conservation of matter.

b. State the law of conservation of energy.

c. State the law of conservation of momentum.

d. State Newton's laws of motion.

e. The rest mass of an electron is 9.11×10^{-31} kg. Such an electron is accelerated across the X-ray tube and at the point of contact with the target its kinetic energy is 1.6×10^{-14} J. Calculate its velocity at the point of contact.

f. Iodine-131 is a common isotope of iodine which is used in thyroid studies (its mass number is 131). Calculate the mass of the substance required to give 12×10^{23} atoms.

FURTHER READING

Further reading on the laws of classical physics can be found in most textbooks which are used in schools for the study of AS level or A2 level physics. In addition the following may prove useful:

Allan E, Harris J 1999 New higher chemistry. Hodder Gibson, London, ch 3

Ball J L, Moore A D 1997 Essential physics for radiographers, 3rd edn. Blackwell Scientific Publications, London, ch 1

Chapter 6

Units of Measurement

CHAPTER CONTENTS

6.1 Aim   44

6.2 Units of Measurement   44

6.3 SI Base Units   45
    6.3.1 Derived SI Units   45
    6.3.2 Speed and Velocity   46
    6.3.3 Acceleration   46
    6.3.4 Force   46
    6.3.5 Pressure   46
    6.3.6 Weight and Mass   47
    6.3.7 Work and Energy   47
    6.3.8 Power   48
    6.3.9 Momentum   48

6.4 Units Used in Radiography   48
    6.4.1 kVp   49
    6.4.2 mA and mAs   49
    6.4.3 keV   50
    6.4.4 Heat Units   50

Self-Test   51

Further Reading   51

6.1 AIM

The aim of this chapter is to introduce the reader to the main units that are used in measurement in radiographic science.

6.2 UNITS OF MEASUREMENT

Science has three fundamental tools that are used in its attempts to understand the external world:

1. experimental measurements
2. logic
3. theory.

These will be discussed in this chapter and in Chapter 7.

Problems arise when making experimental measurements as to what quantities to measure and how to measure them. In particular, the *units* in which these quantities are expressed must be defined so that, when two people make the same measurement, they get the same results. Also there are obvious advantages if one set of units is universally adopted as the basis for all measurements.

Each of the *base* units discussed in the next section relies on the appropriate *standard* to which each measurement is compared. Thus there are units of standard length, standard mass, standard time interval and so on. Without such standards no really accurate measurements can be made. This in turn retards the development of adequate theories, or models, of the world.

6.3 SI BASE UNITS

There are a plethora of units of measurement used throughout the world. The International System of Units (SI) attempts to replace this with seven standard units. These standards are termed *base units* (Table 6.1) and represent the fundamental measurements which we might wish to make of a body:

- What is its size? (unit of *length – metre*)
- How massive is it? (unit of *mass – kilogram*)

Table 6.1 SI base units

Quantity	Unit of measurement	Symbol
Length	metre	m
Mass	kilogram	kg
Luminous intensity	candela	cd
Electric current	ampere	A
Amount of substance	mole	mol
Temperature	kelvin	K
Time	second	s

- How bright is it? (unit of *luminous intensity – candela*)
- How much electrical current flows through it? (unit of *electrical current – ampere*)
- How many elementary particles does it contain? (unit of *amount of substance – mole*)
- How hot is it? (unit of *temperature – kelvin*)
- How do all the quantities vary with time? (unit of *time – second*).

The very precise definitions of the units are not required for the rest of this text but if you wish to see them they are given in Appendix I.

The base units of mass, length and time are termed *fundamental units* since one or more of them is always involved in the measurement of any other quantity.

These seven SI base units may be combined to give *derived units*, as described in the next section.

6.3.1 Derived SI Units

A number of derived SI units can be formed by the combination of the seven base units. Some of these are sufficiently important to be given their own names and they are listed in Table 6.2

Table 6.2 Derived SI units and their definitions

Quantity	Definition	SI unit	Scalar/vector
Speed	Distance travelled in unit time	metre per second ($m.s^{-1}$)	Scalar
Velocity	Distance travelled in unit time in a given direction	metre per second ($m.s^{-1}$)	Vector Vector
Acceleration	Change of velocity in unit time	(metre per second)/per second ($m.s^{-2}$)	Vector
Force	The application of unit force to unit mass produces unit acceleration	newton (N) ($kg.m.s^{-2}$)	Vector
Pressure	Force applied per unit area	pascal (P) ($N.m^{-2}$)	Vector
Weight	Force acting on a body due to gravity	newton (N) ($kg.m.s^{-2}$)	Vector
Work	Product of the force acting on a body times the distance the body moves	joule (J) (N.m)	Scalar
Energy	Kinetic energy: work which can be done by a system because of its velocity	joule (J)	Scalar
	Potential energy: work which can be performed because of the position or state of a system	joule (J)	Scalar
Power	Rate of doing work	watt (W) ($J.s^{-1}$)	Scalar
Momentum	Product of the mass and the velocity of the body	($kg.m.s^{-1}$)	Vector

and discussed in the rest of this chapter. Further derived units are of a more specialised nature (e.g. absorbed radiation dose) and will be discussed in the specific chapters which require such measurement.

INSIGHT

For some quantities we can consider a body moving between two points. For certain measurements it is important to know how far the body has travelled between the two points. In other cases we wish to know how far it has travelled and also the direction it has travelled. Measurements where the direction is important are termed *vector* quantities whereas those where the direction is not important are known as *scalar* quantities.

6.3.2 Speed and Velocity

The speedometer in a car is calibrated in terms of kilometres per hour (kph) or miles per hour (mph). Either of these shows that *speed* means distance travelled in unit time.

In SI units, speed (S), distance (d) and time (t) are related by the equation:

$$S = \frac{d}{t}$$ *Equation 6.1*

where d is in metres, t is in seconds and S, therefore, is in metres per second ($m.s^{-1}$). The speedometer in a car gives no indication of the *direction* in which the car is moving so we can see that speed is a scalar quantity. *Velocity* is measured in the same units as speed ($m.s^{-1}$) but this time the *direction* of movement is also measured. Thus a car travelling at a constant speed around a roundabout is continuously changing its velocity.

6.3.3 Acceleration

Acceleration implies a change in velocity and is defined as the *change in velocity per unit time*. For example, the acceleration due to gravity is approximately 9.8 metres per second per second ($9.8\ m.s^{-2}$). This means that for a free-falling body the velocity increases by $9.8\ m.s^{-1}$ after each second. Thus, if a body is dropped, its downward velocity is $9.8\ m.s^{-1}$ after the first second, $19.6\ m.s^{-1}$ after the next second and so on.

The acceleration due to gravity causes a free-falling body to increase its velocity, but if the accelerating force is in the opposite direction to the direction of movement of the body, then it will cause it to lose velocity. This force causes a negative acceleration or a *deceleration*.

Also notice that acceleration is a vector quantity as the acceleration has direction.

6.3.4 Force

Newton's second law of motion (see Sect. 5.5) shows that the net force acting on a body is proportional to the mass of the body multiplied by the acceleration produced on the body. The units of force are therefore $kg.m.s^{-2}$ in SI units. However, this quantity is sufficiently important to be given its own special name and is known as the *newton*. This can be defined as follows:

DEFINITION

A net force of 1 *newton* acting on a body of mass 1 kg causes it to have an acceleration of $1\ m.s^{-2}$.

Force is a vector quantity as it has direction. The acceleration produced by the action of the force (also a vector quantity) is in the same direction as the force.

6.3.5 Pressure

Pressure is defined as the *force exerted per unit area*. The units of pressure would therefore be $N.m^{-2}$. Again it is sufficiently important to merit its own unit, known as the *pascal*, and is defined as follows:

DEFINITION

The pressure acting on a body is 1 *pascal* if 1 newton of force is applied per square metre of body surface.

The difference between force and pressure can be readily appreciated if one considers crossing some snow wearing either shoes or skis. In both cases the force is the same but this force is applied to a smaller area in the case of shoes (the pressure on the snow is greater) so they tend to sink into the snow.

6.3.6 Weight and Mass

As we have already seen, mass is a base SI unit and is defined as *the amount of matter in a body* and is defined against the standard kilogram. This is sometimes confused with the mole (the amount of substance in a body) and so it is possibly easier to understand the concept of mass if we consider it in terms of inertia. We know that a force acting on a body will produce an acceleration and that the force, the mass and the acceleration are linked by the equation $F = m \times a$ (see Equation 5.1) so that inertia can be defined as the body's resistance to acceleration. From the equation it can be seen that, as the mass of the body increases, so the force required to produce a given acceleration also increases, i.e. *the inertia of the body increases with mass*.

The *weight* of a body is the downward force on the body due to the gravitational attraction of earth. Hence, the weight of a body is expressed in newtons, not in kilograms. An equation similar to Equation 5.1 links weight, mass and gravity:

$$w = m \times g \qquad\qquad Equation\ 6.2$$

From the above discussion and equation we can see that a body always has mass but it only has weight in the presence of a gravitational field. Hence, a body in deep space has no weight (because of the zero gravitational field) but it has mass as it still requires a force to cause it to change its velocity (i.e. it has inertia).

6.3.7 Work and Energy

Both *work* and *energy* are measured using the same units. A force is said to do work if it moves its point of application in the same direction as the applied force. This can be expressed as:

$$W = F \times d \qquad\qquad Equation\ 6.3$$

Thus, the units of work are newtons and metres (N.m). Again, the concept of work is sufficiently important to merit its own unit, which is the *joule*.

DEFINITION

1 *joule* of work is performed when a force of 1 newton moves its point of application through a distance of 1 metre.

Energy can be considered as the capacity of a body to do work. There are two types of energy that we need to consider separately:

1. kinetic energy
2. potential energy.

6.3.7.1 Kinetic Energy

Kinetic energy is energy that a body possesses by virtue of its motion. This motion may be translational (movement along a path) or rotational or a combination of both types. The kinetic energy is simply the work that must be done in the process of bringing the body to rest. We have already looked at this when we considered Newton's laws of motion and established an equation (Equation 5.4) for the kinetic energy of a body of mass m having a velocity of v.

$$E = \tfrac{1}{2}mv^2$$

INSIGHT

Consider an electron which has been accelerated across the X-ray tube and is travelling with a velocity *v* at the point when it starts to collide with the atoms of the target. It has a kinetic energy (= $\frac{1}{2}mv^2$) and then starts to liberate some of that energy in the form of X-ray photons.

6.3.7.2 Potential Energy

Potential energy is energy possessed by a body (or a system) by virtue of its condition or state. Thus a stationary body has potential energy if it is in a condition which allows it to release its stored energy. The potential energy of the system can be thought of as the work which the system will perform in bringing its potential energy to zero. If we consider a body of mass m which is at a height h above the ground, then we can apply Equation 6.3 to this situation:

$$W = F \times d$$

The force at work here is the weight of the body (mg) and the distance it can move its height above the ground, so we now have the equation for the potential energy (PE):

$$PE = mgh \qquad \text{Equation 6.4}$$

INSIGHT

Consider the case of a hospital lift sitting at the ground floor. Attached to this lift, over a pulley system, is a counterweight. This counterweight has potential energy because of its position. If the brakes on the lift are released, it will assist in moving the lift up to the top floor (i.e. the counterweight performs work).

Work and energy are both scalar quantities as they do not have direction.

6.3.8 Power

A particular car may reach a speed of 60 mph in 6 s while another car of the same mass does the same speed in 20 s. The first car is said to be more *powerful* than the second. If we assume that the cars are both travelling in the same direction, then their velocity is the same and so their kinetic energy (= $\frac{1}{2}mv^2$) is the same, but the first car reached that energy more quickly. Hence *power* can be expressed as the *rate at which energy is expended* and, since energy and work are basically the same thing, we can say that:

DEFINITION

Power is the rate at which work is done.

Thus, power is measured in joules per second ($J.s^{-1}$) but is again an important enough concept to merit its own unit, the *watt*. Thus:

$$\text{watts} = \frac{\text{joules}}{\text{seconds}}$$

or 1 *watt* is 1 joule of work per second.

6.3.9 Momentum

In everyday speech, *momentum* expresses the ability of a moving body to 'keep going'. This depends on the mass of the body and its velocity and so momentum is defined:

DEFINITION

The *momentum* of a body is the product of its mass and its velocity.

We have already, briefly, come across the concept of momentum in the law of conservation of momentum (Sect. 5.4).

INSIGHT

Consider the situation where a projectile (e.g. a bullet) strikes a barrier. The depth to which it penetrates the barrier is dependent on the *mass* of the projectile and its *velocity* at the point of impact. This fits in with our concept of *momentum* as the ability of a body to keep going.

6.4 UNITS USED IN RADIOGRAPHY

Many derived SI units (such as the joule, coulomb, etc.) are used in radiographic science. However, other units that do not strictly adhere to the SI system are especially useful to radiography

Table 6.3	Units used in radiography
Unit	Definition
kVp	The maximum kilovoltage applied across an X-ray tube in a forward direction during an exposure
mA	The average electrical current passing through an X-ray tube during an exposure (measured in milliamperes)
mAs	The average current passing through the tube during an exposure multiplied by the exposure time in seconds (1 mAs = 1 millicoulomb)
keV	The energy imparted to an electron when passing through a potential difference of 1 kV in a vacuum
HU	Heat unit: a measure of the heat energy deposited in the anode by an exposure: the product of the kVp and the mAs

and are unlikely to be discontinued, because of their practical convenience. These are shown and defined in Table 6.3.

6.4.1 kVp

The potential difference (see Ch. 9) existing between the cathode and anode of an X-ray tube is measured in kilovolts, where $1 \text{ kV} = 10^3 \text{ V}$. In many X-ray generators, however, this potential difference is not constant but varies, with a given frequency, during the exposure time. Hence, it is conventional practice to quote the *peak* (i.e. maximum) value of the potential difference across the X-ray tube. Thus, when a radiographer selects 50 kVp, he/she is selecting a maximum voltage of 50 kV to be applied to the tube during the exposure. The effects of this voltage on the beam will be discussed in later chapters (Chs 28 and 29) and also later in this chapter when we consider keV.

6.4.2 mA and mAs

X-rays are produced in an X-ray tube when electrons from the cathode, with high kinetic energy, strike the anode (see Chs 28 and 29). If we assume that each electron has a chance of producing X-rays, then the intensity of X-ray production is proportional to the number of electrons striking the anode per second. The number of electrons flowing per second is related to the *current* flowing through the tube (see Ch. 10). The SI unit of current is the ampere (A), as we saw earlier in this chapter, and it is equivalent to a current of 6×10^{18} electrons per second. This unit of current is too large a unit for radiography so current is measured in milliamperes ($1 \text{ mA} = 10^{-3} \text{ A}$).

We only wish the tube to produce X-rays in sufficient quantity to produce the image on the recording medium (e.g. film) and so an exposure time is set by the radiographer. It can be seen that, all other factors remaining constant, the amount of blackening (or optical density) of the film will be determined by the number of X-rays leaving the tube. From the above arguments this is determined by the total number of electrons striking the anode of the tube.

The total number of electrons striking the target (and hence the X-ray output) is determined by the number of electrons flowing in unit time (related to the mA) and the length of time for which the current flows (the exposure time in seconds, *s*). Thus the X-ray output from a tube (if all other factors remain unaltered) is determined by the mAs.

Any combination of mA and time which produces a given mAs will result in the same quantity of X-rays being emitted by the tube. If 60 mAs was required to produce an acceptable image, this could be delivered in the ways listed in Table 6.4.

The reasons why we might wish to use the different combinations of mA and time will be discussed in Chapters 29 and 32.

As we shall see in Chapter 10, the mAs is equivalent to the *millicoulomb* (10^{-3} C), which is the unit of electrical charge. The mAs is, however,

Table 6.4 Different combinations of mA and time to produce a given mAs		
Current (mA)	Exposure time (s)	mAs
10	6.0	60
20	3.0	60
100	0.6	60
200	0.3	60
300	0.2	60
600	0.1	60

used in preference to the millicoulomb as it makes it more obvious that this can be altered by altering the tube current (mA) or the exposure time (s).

6.4.3 keV

As we have already seen in this chapter, energy is measured in joules. When we come to consider the energies involved in the atom or the energies of the photons of the X-ray beam, the coulomb is an extremely large unit. The electron-volt (eV) and the kiloelectron-volt (keV = 10^3 eV) are much more convenient units of measurement for such energies.

DEFINITIONS

If an electron is accelerated from rest across a potential difference of 1 volt in a vacuum, it gains a kinetic energy of 1 *electron-volt*.

Similarly, an electron accelerated from rest across a potential difference of 1 kilovolt in a vacuum gains a kinetic energy of 1 *kiloelectron-volt*.

The energy (E) in joules can be calculated from the equation:

$$E = e \times V \qquad \textit{Equation 6.5}$$

In this equation e is the charge on the electron (1.6×10^{-19} C) and V is the potential difference measured in volts. Thus:

1 eV = 1.6×10^{-19} J
1 keV = 1.6×10^{-16} J

INSIGHT

If 75 kVp is selected by a radiographer for a specific exposure then some of the electrons travelling across the X-ray tube will have a kinetic energy of 75 keV when they strike the anode. If we assume that some of these electrons give up all their energy as a single X-ray photon, then the energy of this photon will be 75 keV and it will represent the maximum photon energy in

this beam. Thus, by altering the kVp, the radiographer can alter the maximum photon energy of the X-ray beam.

6.4.4 Heat Units

When electrons strike the anode of the X-ray tube, their kinetic energy is given up in a small area of the anode known as the focus (see Chs 2 and 28). Some of this energy is converted into X-ray photons but most of it (about 99%) is converted into heat. It is important to know how much heat an exposure or series of exposures produces, as too much heat could produce sufficient temperature rise to melt the focal spot. In the case of most modern X-ray tubes, this is quoted by the manufacturer in kilojoules and will be considered in Chapter 22. For some of the older X-ray tubes, rating is quoted in heat units (HU) which give a useful measure of the heat energy imparted to the anode. In Chapter 10 we will show that the total energy (joules) dissipated by a current I (amperes) driven by a potential difference V (volts) for a time t (seconds) is given by the equation:

$$E = V \times I \times t$$

This equation is only correct if V and I remain constant for the time t, which is not necessarily the case for the X-ray tube. Thus, to find an absolute value of the heat produced (in joules) we would need to know the effective values for the tube voltage (kV) and tube current (mA). As we have already seen, the kV selector allows us to select the kVp and we will see that the value of the mA which we select is the *average* value. Thus we can adapt the above equation to give:

$$\text{Heat units} = \text{kVp} \times \text{mA} \times t \qquad \textit{Equation 6.6}$$

But we already know that the product of the *mA* and the *exposure time* is the *mAs* and so we can say that:

$$\text{Heat units} = \text{kVp} \times \text{mAs} \qquad \textit{Equation 6.7}$$

Provided the manufacturer quotes the maximum permissible heat loading in heat units, this allows us to check if an exposure or a series of exposures is within the permissible rating for a particular focal spot. The importance of the rating of a particular focal spot will be considered in more detail in Chapter 22.

SUMMARY

In this chapter we considered the following factors related to units of measurement:

- The SI base units for length, mass, luminous intensity, electric current, amount of substance, temperature and time (see Sect. 6.3)

- The SI derived units for speed, velocity, acceleration, force, pressure, weight, work, energy, power and momentum (see Sect. 6.3.1)
- Units of measurement used in radiography in the form of kVp, mA, mAs, keV and heat units (see Sect. 6.4).

SELF-TEST

a. Give the derived SI unit in which each of the following are measured: velocity; acceleration; force; pressure; weight; work; energy; power.

b. Calculate the heat generated (in heat units) by the following exposure: 75 kVp, 200 mA, 0.5 s.

If the maximum heat storage capacity of the anode disc is 10 000 HU, state why this exposure cannot be repeated immediately.

FURTHER READING

Ball J L, Moore A D 1997 Essential physics for radiographers, 3rd edn. Blackwell Scientific Publications, London, ch 1

Thompson M A, Hattaway R T, Hall J D, Dowd S B 1994 Principles of imaging science and protection. W B Saunders, London, chs 2 and 6

Chapter 7

Experimental Error and Statistics

CHAPTER CONTENTS

7.1 Aim 52

7.2 Introduction 52

7.3 Experimental Errors 52
    7.3.1 How Exact is Accurate? 52
    7.3.2 Random and Systematic Errors 53
    7.3.3 Fractional and Percentage Errors 54
    7.3.4 Combining Errors 54
    7.3.5 Examples of Errors in Practical
          Radiography and Radiotherapy 55

7.4 Statistics 56
    7.4.1 Measures of Location and
          Deviation 57

7.5 Assessment of a Procedure/Examination 59

Self-Test 60

Further Reading 61

7.1 AIM

The aim of this chapter is to introduce the reader to techniques that allow the accuracy and precision of various experimental measurements to be calculated and also to consider basic statistical methods that allow us to manipulate experimental data. The chapter will conclude by mentioning the importance of the methods used to assess the treatment or examination, giving an example of a method that could be used.

7.2 INTRODUCTION

Much of the knowledge in radiographic science is based on experimentation. It is important in dealing with such experiments that we know the limitations of our measurements and that we have sufficient statistical skill to allow us to draw correct conclusions from the measurements we take.

7.3 EXPERIMENTAL ERRORS

7.3.1 How Exact *is* Accurate?

As we saw in Chapter 6, physics attempts to be an exact science based on accurate measurements of defined quantities such as mass, length, temperature and time. However no instrument is able to give a truly exact value of the quantity being measured since errors of measurement or observation will always be present. Used in this sense, an error in measurement is not the same as a mistake but just an uncertainty as to the correct value of the measured quantity. It is also possible that the act of undertaking a measurement may alter the quantity we are trying to measure. For example, suppose that we are using a non-digital meter to measure an electric current. Among many possible sources of error, the following may be present:

- an observational error due to the thickness of the pointer on the scale
- an observational error due to incorrect interpolation between scale markings
- an observational error due to poor technique (e.g. not looking at right angles to the scale)
- a measurement error due to an incorrect 'zero', i.e. the pointer is not on the scale zero mark when no current flows
- a measurement error due to the scale being incorrectly calibrated
- a measurement error due to the act of measuring the current changing the current being measured.

Finding and reducing the effects of possible sources of error in a measurement are essential if an accurate – even if not exact – reading is to be taken. How accurate do we need to be? Well, this depends upon why a particular measurement is being performed. If we make an error of 2 mm in a focus to skin distance (FSD: see Ch. 2) setting of 50 cm, then the effect will be negligible on a conventional radiograph. However a fault in an X-ray tube which produced the same error of 2 mm in an effective focal spot size of 1 mm (Sect. 2.3) will have the observable effect of increasing the unsharpness (Sect. 2.6) quite markedly. The fractional (or percentage) error is important, therefore, and is discussed in more detail in this chapter (Sect. 7.3.3).

Basically, the errors of measurement are sufficiently small if they do not affect the conclusions drawn from a result of a measurement or affect a procedure being undertaken (e.g. radiograph or radiotherapy treatment). In radiography or radiotherapy practice, errors of 1 mm when setting a distance or 1° when setting an angle are usually considered to be sufficiently accurate.

7.3.2 Random and Systematic Errors

Random errors are those errors which, on repeated measurements of the same quantity, are variable in size and have no discernible pattern or sequence. This may be due to the quantity itself varying in a random manner (e.g. number of radioactive disintegrations per second; see Ch. 27) or due to slight differences in the measurement technique of the observer on each occasion. Alternatively, the ambient conditions of temperature, pressure or humidity may affect the instrument being used in an apparently random manner.

Systematic errors may arise either from the observer or from the instrument itself, and may be constant or vary in some regular (i.e. non-random) manner. For example, the measurement of length using a ruler with the zero incorrectly positioned will give rise to results that are systematically in error by a constant amount, e.g. 10.3 cm and 4.6 cm when the correct values are 10.0 cm and 4.3 cm respectively, when the zero is displaced by 3 mm.

Many sources of error are either wholly random or wholly systemic, but most errors encountered in practical situations are the result of both types. You may like to inspect the list of meter errors in the previous section and decide where the random and systematic errors might lie. The existence of random and systematic errors leads to the concept of accuracy versus precision. *Precision* is a measure of the repeatability of a series of measurements, while *accuracy* is a measure of the correspondence between the result obtained and its exact value. The precision of a series of readings may be quite high in that they all might lie close to each other, but the accuracy may be poor if there is a significant systematic error involved. A faulty scale on a meter or a ruler, for example, will give the 'wrong' answers even though the readings taken from the scale may be highly repeatable. Precision leads to accuracy, therefore, if the systematic errors have been eliminated or corrected. It is the usual practice in physics to record a result with the estimated error in the form:

True value = measured value ± estimated error

If we have the statement that FSD = 50.0 ± 0.2 cm, then it is implied that the true value of FSD lies somewhere between 49.8 cm and 50.2 cm.

Mathematically, if the error is e, the measured value is m and the true value is t, then $e = m - t$, since the error is just the difference between the measured and true values. Rearranging this we have:

$$m = t + e \qquad \text{Equation 7.1}$$

where the error e may be positive or negative. The magnitude of e may be reduced by careful measurement technique and, where possible, the recording of a large number of readings so that a mean value (see Sect. 7.4.1) may be taken.

7.3.3 Fractional and Percentage Errors

In practice, it is often useful to express an error in relation to the magnitude of the quantity being measured. If it is possible to measure to within 1 mm when using a particular ruler, then this error will become progressively less important as lengths of 1 cm, 10 cm, 1 m, 1 km are taken. Expressing the error of 1 mm as a fraction of the measured value, we obtain 0.1, 0.01, 0.001 and 0.000001 or 10%, 1.0%, 0.1% and 0.0001% respectively. This concept of a fractional or percentage error is important because it helps us to predict the accuracy we need for our individual measurements in order to achieve a given percentage error in the final result. If we wish to measure the area of a rectangle to within 1%, for example, then it may be shown (Sect. 7.3.4) that it is necessary to measure the sides to an accuracy of 0.5%. Hence, a 10% error would be much too high while a 0.001% error would be unnecessarily restrictive for our purpose. A knowledge of the accuracy required also has an effect on the experimental apparatus used: for a 0.5% error in a 1 mm length is 0.005 mm – well beyond the capabilities of a ruler, so that a travelling microscope would be more suitable, while a 0.5% error in a length of 10 cm is 0.5 mm, enabling an accurate ruler to be used.

If we give the fractional error in a quantity the symbol f then f is just the size of the error

(i.e. measured value, m, minus true value, t) divided by the true value t, of the quantity, so that $f = (m - t)/t$. Rearranging this equation, we have:

$$m = t(1 + f) \qquad \text{Equation 7.2}$$

7.3.4 Combining Errors

This section illustrates how to combine errors in some simple examples to obtain an error in the final result.

7.3.4.1 Error in a Product

Taking the previous example of measuring the sides of a rectangle, then the measured area A is just the product of the measured lengths of the sides. Now, if the exact lengths are a and b, and the fractional errors are taken as f_a and f_b, then from Equation 7.2 the measured lengths are just $a(1 + f_a)$ and $b(1 + f_b)$ respectively.

Hence:

$$A = a(1 + f_a) \times b(1 + f_b)$$
$$= ab(1 + f_a) \times (1 + f_b)$$
$$= ab(1 + f_a + f_b + f_a \times f_b)$$

Now, the product $f_a \times f_b$ is very small compared with f_a and f_b (e.g. if f_a and $f_b = 0.01$, then $f_a \times f_b = 0.0001$) and may be neglected, so that we obtain:

$$A = ab(1 + f_a + f_b)$$

We now relate this to f_A, which is the fractional error in the exact area, ab, due to the errors involved in measuring the sides a and b. Equation 7.2 gives us: $A = ab(1 + f_A)$. Thus, by comparison with the above formula, we can say that $ab(1 + f_A) = ab(1 + f_a + f_b)$. This simplifies to $f_A = f_a + f_b$: hence, the fractional error in area f_A is just the sum of the fractional errors f_a and f_b produced when measuring the two sides. Generally, if we have a product involving several terms then, in words:

The fractional (or percentage) error in product is the sum of the individual fractional (or percentage) errors of each term in the product.

As another example, if the mA is in error by +5% and the exposure time is in error by –2%, then the percentage error in the mA (Sect. 6.4.2) is +3%. Frequently, however, the signs of the errors are unknown, so they are both taken as either positive or negative to obtain an error band about the measured value. This constitutes the 'worst-case' size of the error.

7.3.4.2 Error in a Quotient

If we divide one measured value of an exact quantity, a, by another measured value of an exact quantity, b, then the result obtained, R, is given by:

$$R = \frac{(a(1+f_a))}{(b(1+f_b))}$$

where f_a and f_b are the fractional errors in a and b.

$$R = \frac{a}{b} \times (1+f_a)\,(1-f_b) \qquad \text{(approximately)}$$

Expanding the two brackets and ignoring $f_a \times f_b$, as described above, we have:

$$R = \frac{a}{b}\,(1 + f_a - f_b)$$

so that the fractional error in R is $f_a - f_b$.
Hence:

The fractional error in a quotient is obtained by subtracting the fractional error of the denominator from that of the numerator.

If the signs of the errors are unknown, however, then the worst case is obtained by *adding* the fractional errors.

7.3.4.3 Error in a Sum

If S is obtained by summing the various measured quantities a and b (whose exact values are $a0$ and $b0$, and whose errors are e_a and e_b) then:

$$\begin{aligned} S &= (a0 + e_a) + (b0 + e_b) \\ &= a0 + b0 + e_a + e_b \end{aligned}$$

Hence, as may be expected:

The error in a sum is the sum of the individual errors.

As in the two previous cases, if the signs of the errors are unknown, then the worst-case error is still obtained by adding the errors, i.e. assuming both are either positive or both negative. The fractional error in S, f_s, is given by the formula:

$$F_s = \frac{a0 \times f_a + b0 \times f_b}{a0 + b0}$$

so that the fractional error in the sum depends on the relative magnitude of the individual terms and their fractional errors.

7.3.5 Examples of Errors in Practical Radiography and Radiotherapy

Whenever a measurement is made or a procedure undertaken, inexact quantities will be involved. These are present in even the best and most careful of techniques and do not necessarily invalidate the results of the measurements or procedures performed. It is important to be aware of the magnitude of the errors, however, in order to be confident of the validity of the procedure. This is particularly important in radiotherapy where the dose delivered to the patient over a course of treatment must be as accurate and as reproducible as can realistically be achieved. For example, an inherent 'chain of errors' exists in the calibration procedure of a radiotherapy machine, involving errors in the following:

- errors of measurement from an ionisation chamber (see Ch. 33) placed in the beam
- errors in correcting the above reading for temperature and pressure
- errors in correcting for various calibration factors
- errors in the positioning of the chamber
- errors in the reproducibility of the therapy machine's output dose rate 'switch-on' and 'switch-off' errors, i.e. the output dose rate does not immediately assume its steady value at switch-on nor immediately drop to zero at switch-off
- errors relating the measured dose rate to the 100% value of an isodose distribution (see Ch. 1), since in many cases it is not practicable to measure the 100% value, but some known percentage depth dose at, say, 5 cm in water.

Table 7.1   Areas of significant potential error

Measurement/procedure	Method	Potential source of error	Comment
FSD/SSD setting (see Ch. 2)	Applicator	Incorrect length	Systematic
	Pointer	Reading error	Random and systematic
	Optical indicator	Incorrect alignment	Systematic
Radiation field size adjustment	Adjustable collimator	Calibration or mechanical error	Random and/or systematic
Image magnification	Measurement of image of an object of known size placed in the appropriate position	Incorrect positioning of the object	Affects magnification
		Incorrect angulation of object to the central ray	May cause elongation or foreshortening of the image
		Inaccurate measurement of image size	Results in an incorrect magnification formula

FSD, focus to skin distance; SSD, source to skin distance.

If all of these errors act in the same direction, for example, all tending to make the dose rate seem larger than it really is, then an overall error of 5% or greater is possible. Hence great attention to detail is required in order to reduce the percentage error to 1% or less.

Further examples of areas where significant errors may occur are shown in Table 7.1.

7.4 STATISTICS

In the preceding sections it was described how repeated measurements of the same quantity will reduce, but not eliminate, the errors of measurement associated with that quantity. This is the situation where a quantity (e.g. a length) has an exact value but where the measured values are clustered around the exact value.

There is another class of measurements which involves a cluster (or population) of values and that is when measurements are made of different objects belonging to the same category. In this case the errors of measurement on an individual object may be completely negligible when compared to the magnitude of the natural variation among the objects themselves. For example the heights of all the radiographers within a given department will probably exhibit quite a large variation and certainly more than the errors involved in measuring the height of one radiographer.

The body of knowledge which concerns itself with the analysis of information (data) obtained from observations is known as *statistics*. There are two types of statistics: *descriptive* and *inferential*. Descriptive statistics is concerned solely with such things as the organisation of the data, its graphical display and numerical calculations of means, while inferential statistics may be described as the science of making decisions in the face of uncertainty (i.e. on the basis of incomplete information). The latter is the situation frequently encountered in the field of medical statistics where complete information is rarely available.

A group of items belonging to the same category is known as a *population*. A population may be very large (e.g. the number of atoms in a radioactive sample) or small. Note that 'population' as used here does not necessarily imply that people are involved.

Where it is difficult or impossible to collect data on every member of a population, it is necessary only to select a representative sample of that population such that the smaller and more manageable sample has all the important characteristics of the population from which it was drawn, except that of size. This technique is known as *random sampling,* and is much used in public opinion polls, for example. If the sample were not random then there would be a *bias* in the data collected which would not be present in the larger population, and false conclusions may be drawn.

For example, we would not get a reasonable indication of the average weight of patients attending the X-ray department if we happened to select our 'random sample' from patients who were attending a clinic for unexplained weight loss – our sample is not representative of the typical patient population of the X-ray department.

7.4.1 Measures of Location and Deviation

The graphical representation of the data associated with a population is usually drawn with the measured values on the x-axis and the number of each measured value on the y-axis. The position of the graph so obtained is known as the *location* of the population and the width of the graph as its *deviation.* The statistical quantities (usually just called 'statistics') that are used to measure location are the *mean, mode* and *median,* while the statistic used to measure deviation is the *standard deviation.* These are described below, together with some other statistical measures.

7.4.1.1 The Mean, Mode and Median of a Population

The mean value of a population is the same as the average value. It is obtained by dividing the sum of all the data by the number of items in the population. This is shown by the formula:

$$\bar{x} = \frac{\sum_{i=1}^{n} x_i}{n}$$

Equation 7.3

The value which occurs most frequently in a population is not necessarily the mean value however. Figure 7.1A–D shows there are two other measures or statistics of curve location: the *mode* and the *median.* The mode is defined as the value that occurs most frequently and the median is the middle value of all the measurements in a series (e.g. in the series 1, 2, 4, 4, 5, 6, 6, 6, 7 the median is 5 and the mode is 6). The figures show how these statistics vary with asymmetrical distributions of values: Figure 7.1(B) demonstrates positive skewness while Figure 7.1(C) demonstrates negative skewness.

The *standard deviation,* a function found in most spreadsheets and calculators, is a measure of the variation of the values of a distribution, i.e. by how much the distribution varies from the mean value. Two symmetrical distributions with the same mean but different standard deviations are shown in Figure 7.2.

The *coefficient of variation* expresses the standard deviation as a percentage of the mean of a distribution and is equal to $100\sigma/\bar{x}\%$.

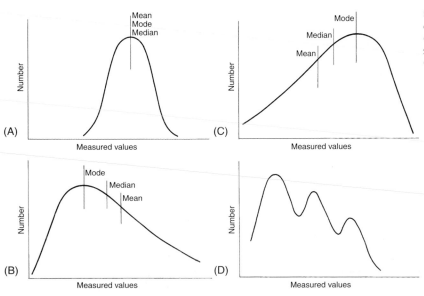

Figure 7.1   Measures of location of a population. (A) Symmetrical ('normal') distribution; (B) positive skewness; (C) negative skewness; (D) multimodal distribution.

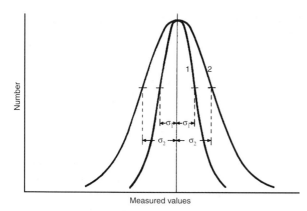

Figure 7.2 A graphical representation showing the standard deviation of two populations 1 and 2 where both distributions have the same mean.

7.4.1.1 Standard Error of the Mean

There will inevitably be an uncertainty, even if small, in the practical measurement of a mean value, due to the errors inherent in the original observations (Sect. 7.3.2). This uncertainty may be expressed as the standard error of the mean (SEM), and is given as:

$$\text{SEM} = \frac{\sigma}{\sqrt{n}} \qquad \text{Equation 7.4}$$

It may be shown that there is a 68% probability that the value of the mean (ignoring systematic errors) lies within 1 SEM above or below the measured mean. Notice that both the standard deviation and SEM become smaller as the number of measurements (*n*) increases.

7.4.1.3 Statistics in Diagnostic and Therapeutic Radiography

Statistical methods are widely used in all aspects of diagnostic imaging and radiotherapy. This section touches on a few examples.

Quality control. **The analysis of the reject images produced, and the reasons for rejection, is a useful method of reducing patient dose. The reasons for repeated investigations may be itemised and numbered in a reject analysis, leading to a clearer understanding of the commonest causes of faulty radiographs. From this** analysis, steps may be taken to reduce the number of repeated investigations, leading to reduced film wastage, better financial management and a lower radiation dose to the patient.

This example does not impose a complex mathematical or statistical burden on the department, but there are real advantages to be gained in using it.

Quantum noise. A rather more fundamental (and visible) example of statistics in X-ray imaging is the so-called 'quantum mottle' seen on a television monitor during a fluoroscopic examination of a patient using an image intensifier system. This mottle, or quantum noise, is potentially noticeable at low mA or when short-persistence phosphors are used in the intensification system. It is due to the statistical variation of the video signal, which in turn is caused by the random variation in the production of electrons from the faceplate of the image intensifier. At the desired low-dose rates for fluoroscopic examination there is random variation in the mean value of the X-ray intensity transmitted through the patient, and in the production of electrons from the faceplate of the image intensifier and thus the light emitted from the intensifier output phosphor and reaching the television camera tube. This in turn causes variations in the generation of an electrical video signal from the target of the television camera tube. The standard deviation of an average of N electrons per second is just $\sqrt{N}$, so that increasing the mA by a factor of 4 increases the mottle by an absolute factor of 2 (i.e. $\sqrt{4}$). However, the *relative* quantum mottle has been reduced from $\sqrt{N}/N = 1/\sqrt{N}$ to $\sqrt{4N} = \frac{1}{2}\sqrt{N}$, so that there has been a halving of the perceived 'noise' on the television monitor. Hence, the effect of quantum mottle on the image is reduced as the mA (or quantity of radiation) is increased. Obviously a balance must be struck between using such a low dose rate that the picture obtained is not adequate for diagnostic purposes and using such a high dose rate that the patient receives an unnecessarily high radiation dose. A high-output X-ray tube is required on a computed tomographic (CT) scanner, for example, in order to reduce the quantum noise in the reconstructed sectional image which would otherwise hide structural detail.

Assessment of fetal maturity. A measurement of the fetal biparietal diameter or the crown–rump distance may be used to estimate the age of the fetus. However, not all fetuses grow at the same rate, so a range of normal values for different fetal ages in ethnic groups is first determined by ultrasonic methods, and an unknown age may then be read from an appropriate graph. This is a simple technique, but how may we assess the accuracy of the age read from such a graph – is it within 1 day, 1 week or 1 month? Figure 7.3 shows a plot of the mean biparietal diameter against age together with a pair of lines separated from the mean by 2 standard deviations. This means that, at any given age, the biparietal diameter will be about 95% certain to lie somewhere between the -2σ line and the $+2\sigma$ line. A measured biparietal diameter may be used to estimate an age by drawing a horizontal line on the graph and reading the intersections of the three lines on the age axis. We may then say that a normal fetus's age is 95% likely to lie between these three lines, with the most likely age given by the mean value. Note that the lines separate more as the age increases, so that there is more uncertainty closer to 40 weeks than at 16 weeks. A typical age estimated by the graph will be accurate to within 1–2 weeks, and it is quite unrealistic to expect to be more accurate than this, not because the measurement technique needs improvement, but because of the natural variation of biparietal diameter in the population.

Calculation of radiotherapy dose. In radiotherapy, the absorbed radiation dose to a tumour volume is specified by the radiotherapist. However, in a practical situation, it may be known that the absorbed dose is not constant over the whole of the volume to be treated. The radiotherapist may therefore specify a particular dose to a given point, a mean dose or a modal dose depending upon the clinical situation. The mean or modal dose to a volume may be calculated from a computer printout of the dose distribution.

Evaluation of procedures. Statistical methods may be used to select between two different diagnostic or treatment regimes in order to discover which gives better diagnostic information or treatment results. It is important to select appropriate parameters to measure the relative performance of the two techniques. These may include the number of false positives or false negatives for a diagnostic procedure or the 5-year survival rate or suitably defined quality of life for a therapeutic regime. Such evaluations should assess the *sensitivity*, i.e. the ability of the examination to detect the condition's presence, and *specificity*, i.e. the accuracy with which the condition is detected.

A method that may be used for such a purpose is shown in Table 7.2.

Epidemiology. Finally, statistical methods are employed to find correlations between disease and the environment. This branch of study is known as epidemiology and it is valuable in suggesting causal links between our way of life, or the pollution in our environment, and the diseases we suffer. This may be performed on a local, national or international level. Obvious examples include smoking and lung cancer or diet and heart disease.

7.5 ASSESSMENT OF A PROCEDURE/EXAMINATION

A requirement of the Ionising Radiations (Medical Exposure) Regulations 2000 (see Ch. 34) is that existing procedures must be reviewed periodically to ensure that the minimum radiation dose is

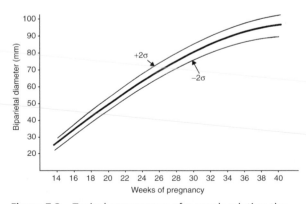

Figure 7.3 Typical appearance of a graph relating the age of a fetus to its biparietal diameter. Also shown are the 2 standard deviation limits, within which 95% of the normal values lie.

Table 7.2 A simple table to assess sensitivity and specificity of an examination/procedure

Name of examination/procedure

		Present	Absent
Result	Positive	A	B
	Negative	C	D
Sensitivity = A/(A + C)	%		
Specificity = D/(B + D)	%		

delivered to the patient. This involves comparing the doses delivered by the procedures with the mean doses achieved for similar examination in other hospitals of the UK.

SUMMARY

In this chapter we have considered the following factors which relate to experimentation and statistics:

- Experimental measurements are always subject to errors, both random and systematic (see Sect. 7.3.2)
- The precision of a set of measurements is a measure of their repeatability, while their accuracy is how close they are to the exact result (see Sect. 7.3.2)
- Accuracy is improved by taking a large number of measurements and correcting for the sources of systematic errors (see Sect. 7.3.2)
- The fractional error is the error divided by the mean value (see Sect. 7.3.3)

- The fractional error in a product is obtained by adding the individual fractional errors of each term in the product, and the fractional error in a quotient by subtracting them. If the signs of the errors are unknown, they are added to obtain the 'worst-case' error (see Sect. 7.3.4)
- The location of a distribution of measurements (a population) may be defined by the mean, the mode or the median (see Sect. 7.4)
- A measure of the spread of a population is given by the standard deviation, where 68 % of all values lie between −1 and +1 standard deviation from the mean, and 95% of values lie within −2 and +2 standard deviations (see Sect. 7.4.1).

SELF-TEST

a. What are the fractional and percentage errors in an mA value which is set to 20 but which is really 22?

b. If a kVp setting is in error by +5%, the mA by −1% and the timer overestimates by 2%, what is the percentage error in the heat units delivered during an exposure? (For the calculation of heat units, use Equation 6.7.)

c. A particular exposure-timer is always in error by 0.01 s. What is the percentage error in the actual exposure time for the following set times:

(i)   0.01 s

(ii) 0.02 s

(iii) 0.1 s

(iv) 0.5 s

(v)   1.0 s?

d. Which condition results in a greater effect on the intensity of an X-ray beam:

(i)   an error of 10% in the mA

(ii) an error of 10% in the kV?

(*Note*: Intensity is proportional to mA $\times$ kVp^2; see Ch. 29.)

e. Find the mean and the median of the following samples:

   (i)   37, 34, 40, 35, 33, 36, 37

   (ii) 10, 4, 6, 11, 13, 8, 11

   (iii) 52, 70, 37, 55, 42, 31, 47

f. The following readings are taken with a dose-measuring system for a series of 1-min exposures on a therapy machine: 69.92, 70.20, 69.95, 70.14, 70.14, 69.97, 70.02, 70.24, 70.10, 70.00. Calculate the mean, standard deviation and SEM of this population. State the range within which 95% of all such readings would lie.

FURTHER READING

There are many specialised textbooks which deal with the topics of experimentation and statistics. Below is a list of titles which may be found in a radiography education library:

Altman D G 1990 Practical statistics for medical research. Chapman & Hall, London

Anderson A J B 1991 Interpreting data – a first course in statistics. Chapman & Hall, London

Northedge A, Thomas J, Lane A, Peasgood A 1997 The sciences good study guide. Open University, Milton Keynes

Rowntree D 2003 Statistics without tears – a primer for non-mathematicians. Allyn & Bacon, London

White B 1991 Studying for science – a guide to information, communication and study techniques. E & F M Spon, London

Chapter 8

Heat

CHAPTER CONTENTS

8.1 Aim   62

8.2 Introduction   62

8.3 Heat Energy and Temperature   63
   8.3.1 Temperature Scales   63
   8.3.2 Units of Heat Energy, Specific Heat
         Capacity and Thermal Capacity   63

8.4 Transfer of Heat   64
   8.4.1 Conduction   65
   8.4.2 Convection   65
   8.4.3 Radiation   66
   8.4.4 Black-Body Radiation   66

8.5 Thermal Expansion   67

8.6 Evaporation and Vaporisation   68

8.7 Heat Loss From an X-ray Tube   68
   8.7.1 The Stationary Anode Tube   68
   8.7.2 The Rotating Anode Tube   69

Self-Test   71

Further Reading   71

8.1 AIM

The aim of this chapter is to consider heat as a transfer of energy. Links between heat and temperature are also established. The mechanisms of transferring heat are explored and their applications to the cooling of the stationary anode and rotating anode X-ray tube are considered.

8.2 INTRODUCTION

We are familiar with the feelings of hot and cold; indeed, we are crucially dependent on our bodily temperature staying within a very limited range in order to survive. Compared to the vast ranges of temperature which exist across the universe, our experience of 'hot' and 'cold' is very limited indeed.

INSIGHT

We are, in fact, better at noticing 'hotter' or 'colder' than we are at determining an absolute value of 'hot' or 'cold'. This can readily be shown from a simple experiment for which you require a bowl of hot water, a bowl of cold water and two bowls of tepid water. Place your right hand in the bowl of hot water and your left hand in the bowl of cold water and leave them in position for about 1 min. Now transfer both hands to the bowls of tepid water. You will note that this water feels cold to the right hand and warm to the left hand. This shows that we are better at detecting changes in temperature than we are at detecting absolute values of temperature.

In order to investigate heat further, we must use objective measures of heat and cold, as described in the following sections.

8.3 HEAT ENERGY AND TEMPERATURE

When heat is given to a body its atoms or molecules are given increased kinetic energy in the form of increased lattice vibration (this is the reason why substances expand when heated). Thus, a body whose atoms have a higher kinetic energy than those of another body is said to be hotter or at a higher temperature. If two bodies are placed in contact, then heat will be transferred from the hotter body to the cooler body by collisions between the molecules at the point of contact. Thus the molecules of the cooler body receive a net increase in kinetic energy and so its temperature rises. The molecules of the hotter body have lost kinetic energy and so its temperature falls. This process continues until the two bodies are at the same temperature when no further exchange of energy takes place. The bodies are now in a state of *thermal equilibrium*. Notice that the thermal energy is always transferred from the body at the higher temperature to the body at the lower temperature, irrespective of the size of the bodies. Also note that the temperature existing at thermal equilibrium will always lie somewhere between the initial temperatures of the two bodies.

INSIGHT

If a body is made to give away thermal energy, then the lattice vibrations of its atoms or molecules will decrease. It is logical to assume that there must therefore be a temperature at which no lattice vibration exists. As all movement of molecules ceases to exist at this temperature, this is the lowest temperature that we can attain. This temperature is known as *absolute zero* and will be further discussed in the next section.

8.3.1 Temperature Scales

There are two temperature scales used in modern physics: Celsius (also called centigrade) and kelvin. The Celsius scale is defined as 0°C at the temperature of melting ice, and 100°C at the temperature of boiling water at an atmospheric pressure of 1.01×10^5 newtons per square metre (76 mm of mercury). On this scale the temperature of absolute zero (see previous Insight) is approximately −273.15°C. This temperature is zero on the kelvin scale (0 K) while the temperature of melting ice is 273.15 K. From this we can see that the units of temperature are the same on both scales but the scales have different starting points, i.e. one unit on the Celsius scale is equivalent to one unit on the kelvin scale. Note that temperature on the kelvin scale does not have the degree symbol in front of the K. It is a convenient approximation to assume that 0°C = 273 K, so that the simple conversion formula may be used:

$$T°C = (T + 273) \text{ K} \qquad \textit{Equation 8.1}$$

8.3.2 Units of Heat Energy, Specific Heat Capacity and Thermal Capacity

As we have already discussed, if heat is given to a body, then its molecules will have a higher kinetic energy and its temperature will rise. Hence it is convenient to express a quantity of heat in terms of the temperature change it produces in a given body. Consider the situation where we wish to apply an amount of energy (Q) which will raise the temperature of a body by 1 kelvin unit (for simplicity, assume that this does not change the state of the body, i.e. it does not change from a solid to a liquid). This will be affected by the mass and the type of material of the body. It also seems logical to assume that we would need twice the amount of heat to raise the temperature of the body by 2 kelvin units. If we take all these factors together we can write the equation:

$$Q = mc(T_2 - T_1) \qquad \textit{Equation 8.2}$$

where Q is the heat energy required to raise the temperature of a body of mass m from T_1 to a temperature T_2. The factor c is approximately constant for a particular material and is known as the specific heat capacity of the material. We can rearrange Equation 8.2 to get:

$$c = \frac{Q}{m(T_2 - T_1)} \qquad \textit{Equation 8.3}$$

so that c, the specific heat capacity, is in units of joules per kilogram per kelvin ($J.kg^{-1}K^{-1}$). Specific heat capacity can be defined thus:

DEFINITION

The specific heat capacity of a body is the energy in joules which is required to raise the temperature of 1 kilogram of the body by 1 kelvin unit.

The specific heat capacity is thus unique to a substance and it allows us to predict the behaviour of different masses of the same substance.

EXAMPLE

The specific heat capacity of water is about 4.2 ($J.kg^{-1}K^{-1}$). How much heat energy is required to raise a mass of 10 g of water from 280 K to 285 K? (Remember that the unit of energy is the joule and the unit of mass is the kilogram.)

Using Equation 8.2 we have:

$Q = mc(T_2 - T_1)$
  $= 10^{-2} \times 4.2 \times 10^3 \times (285 - 280)$
  $= 210$ J

In the situations considered so far we have considered the amount of heat required to raise the temperature of 1 kg of the material. Another unit of heat energy which is useful in practice is the thermal capacity.

DEFINITION

The thermal capacity of a body is the heat energy in joules which is required to raise the temperature of the body by 1 kelvin unit.

Note that this definition differs from the previous one for specific heat capacity in that no mention is made of unit mass. Thus the thermal capacity refers to the whole of the body and not just 1 kg of it. It should also be noted that the thermal capacity of a body is the specific heat capacity of the body multiplied by the mass of the body. The units of thermal capacity are joules per kelvin.

EXAMPLE

The anode discs of two X-ray tubes are made of the same material but one has twice the mass of the other. If the same amount of heat is applied to each anode, which will have the higher temperature rise at the end of the exposure?
  The thermal capacity is the product of the mass and the specific heat. Thus the larger anode will have twice the thermal capacity of the smaller one. If the same amount of heat is applied to each, the smaller one will experience twice the temperature rise of the larger one. The importance of this will be considered when we consider the rating of the X-ray tube (see Ch. 22).

8.4 TRANSFER OF HEAT

As we mentioned at the beginning of this chapter, heat can be given to a body from some other structure with greater thermal energy than the body. Similarly, if a body can be isolated from its environment or is in a state of thermal equilibrium with its surroundings, there is no net gain or loss of heat from the body.
  The mechanisms of heat transfer form an important part of the study of radiography because of the large amounts of heat energy produced at the target of the X-ray tube. The mechanical and thermal stresses associated with this make it possible to damage the X-ray tube unless adequate precautions are taken. The anodes of all X-ray tubes must therefore be designed to transfer the heat away from the focal spot area as quickly as possible in order to minimise the temperature rise in this region. To understand how this is achieved,

we must first understand the different mechanisms of heat transfer and then we will look at the practical application of this knowledge to the design of X-ray tubes. The three methods of heat transfer are *conduction*, *convection* and *radiation*.

8.4.1 Conduction

Conduction is the transfer of heat between bodies by physical contact of those bodies and therefore results in a transfer of kinetic energy by interatomic collision, thus forming the main process by which heat is transferred through a solid. If we apply heat to one end of a metal bar, the atoms at this end of the bar receive copious supplies of kinetic energy. These atoms, because of their increased vibrational energy, collide with neighbouring atoms and so kinetic energy is gradually transferred along the bar. This method of heat flow along the bar is known as *conduction* of heat.

We can find by experiment that the rate of flow of heat, q (joules per second or watts; see Sect. 6.3.7), by conduction is controlled by a number of things:

- $q \propto A$ (the cross-sectional area of the rod)
- $q \propto (T_1 - T_2)$ (the temperature difference between the ends of the rod; this is known as the temperature gradient)
- $q \propto (1/l)$ (where l is the length of the rod)
- q depends on the material of the rod.

Combining all these factors we have:

$$q \propto \frac{A(T_1 - T_2)}{l}$$

$$q = \frac{kA(T_1 - T_2)}{l} \qquad \text{\textit{Equation 8.4}}$$

Here k is the constant of proportionality and this is a constant for any given material. This is known as the thermal conductivity of the material. Materials are classed as 'good' or 'bad' conductors depending on the value of k. Typical values of k are shown in Table 8.1.

Also note that the rate of flow of heat along a bar can be altered by altering the length, the cross-sectional area and the temperature gradient as well as by altering the material.

8.4.2 Convection

Convection is the main process by which heat is transferred in fluids (i.e. liquids and gases). If we consider heat being applied to a liquid in a beaker (Figure 8.1), then the liquid near the source of heat has thermal energy transferred to it by conduction. This increase in thermal energy causes the liquid to expand and consequently become less dense than the surrounding liquid. This causes the heated liquid to rise (as a result of hydrostatic pressure) and, as it rises, it transfers heat to the surrounding molecules by conduction. Thus the temperature of the small section of heated liquid returns to the same temperature

Material	Thermal conductivity (W.m^{-1}.K^{-1})	Comments
Table 8.1 Thermal conductivity of materials		
Copper	386	Excellent conductor – used as the anode material in the stationary anode tube
Tungsten	202	Fairly good conductor – used as the target material in X–ray tubes
Molybdenum	147	Relatively poor conductor – used as the anode stem in the rotating anode tube
Glass	1.0	Poor conductor – involved in the transfer of heat to the oil in the tube housing
Rubber	0.05	Very poor conductor
Air	0.02	Very poor conductor – removes heat from the housing of the X-ray tube by convection

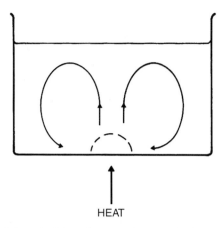

Figure 8.1 Principles of convection. Applied heat causes the broken-line region of fluid to expand, become less dense and rise, being replaced by cooler parts of the fluid. This sets up convection currents.

as the surrounding liquid and so sinks back into the beaker, to be heated a second time. Thus convection currents are established, as shown in Figure 8.1. The overall effect is that the whole volume of fluid is heated and not just the region where the heat is applied.

Some interesting points emerge from this:

- Convection can only occur where the molecules are free to move through the medium, i.e. in liquids and gases
- It is not possible to have convection currents without some conduction
- It is necessary to have a gravitational field in order for the convection currents to be initiated as the warm fluid moves in the opposite direction to the gravitational force, by hydrostatic pressure.

8.4.3 Radiation

In this process, heat is lost from a body with high thermal energy in the form of electromagnetic radiations. Radiation is the only heat transfer process which will take place through a *vacuum*. The most obvious and striking example is the heat we can feel from our sun where the radiation must pass through a near-perfect vacuum for 93 million miles (approximately 150 million km). Light and heat also reach us from other stars but we are only able to discern the light, as we are not sufficiently sensitive to small amounts of heat (although the latter can be detected with infrared sensors).

We are able to feel heat by radiation because it imparts kinetic energy to molecules of our tissues, which we discern as an increase in temperature. Heat radiations occur in a band of energies just below the red part of the visible spectrum (see Ch. 25 for further detail of the electromagnetic spectrum). This band of energies is known as infrared radiations. All bodies radiate electromagnetic energies if their temperature is above absolute zero. This does not necessarily mean that we can discern the radiations, as we perceive only a narrow band of energies extending from violet light to infrared. Bodies of different colours and different surface compositions radiate somewhat differently and so it is conventional to consider *black-body radiation*. This we will do next.

8.4.4 Black-Body Radiation

A body looks black because very little of the light incident upon it is reflected or transmitted. A black body is defined as one that will absorb 100% of all radiations at all frequencies incident upon it. If such a black body is in a state of thermal equilibrium with its surroundings, then equal amounts of radiation must be absorbed and emitted per second. Hence it can be deduced that the black body must radiate more energy than any other type of body since no other body absorbs 100% of the energy incident upon it. The foregoing statements can be summarised thus:

- All bodies are capable of emitting radiation
- A black body absorbs 100% of all radiations incident upon it
- A black body is the most efficient emitter of radiation of any body.

We now need to know in more detail the spectrum of radiations emitted by a black body. Figure 8.2 shows such a spectrum for a black body at different temperatures. The following should be noted from the graph:

- The wavelength corresponding to the peak radiation progressively decreases as the temperature of the body increases

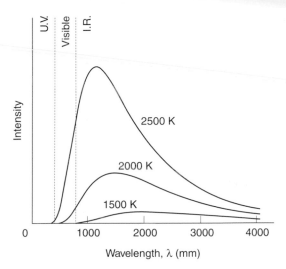

Figure 8.2 The spectrum of electromagnetic radiation emitted by a black body at different temperatures. The total intensity is a function of the kelvin temperature ($I \propto T^4$). UV, ultraviolet; IR, infrared.

- The height of the graph (intensity of radiation) is very sensitive to changes in temperature
- The spectrum of the radiation is a smooth curve, of which we perceive only a small part (violet to infrared)
- The total intensity of the radiation emitted by a body at a given temperature is the sum of the intensities at each wavelength. This is therefore related to the area under the curve in each case. *Stefan's law* states that the total intensity of the emitted radiation is proportional to the *fourth power* of the *kelvin temperature*. Thus:

$$I \propto T^4$$
$$\text{or } I = \sigma T^4 \qquad \qquad Equation\ 8.5$$

where σ is Stefan's constant.

Thus a doubling of the kelvin temperature results in the amount of heat radiation emitted being increased by a factor of $2^4 = 16$ times. As we can see from this, the intensity of the radiation emitted varies greatly with the body temperature. This has important consequences in the design of the rotating anode X-ray tube disc, as we shall see later in this chapter.

A curve of emitted radiation at about 1000 K is equivalent to a metal rod which has been heated until it is glowing cherry-red. As the temperature

increases, the colour changes through light-red to white since an increasing amount of the violet end of the spectrum is emitted along with the red (see 2000 K and 2500 K lines in Figure 8.2). At higher temperatures, objects emit white light: this is true of the filament of an electric light bulb or the anode disc of the rotating anode tube after a large exposure.

INSIGHT

The mechanism that causes the emission of radiation is the acceleration and deceleration of the charged particles which make up the atoms or molecules of the body involved. An example particularly relevant to radiography is the sudden deceleration of electrons when they strike the anode of the X-ray tube – the *Bremsstrahlung* or braking radiation. Here some (or all) of the kinetic energy of the electron is transformed into an X-ray photon (see Ch. 28). Another example is the production of radiowaves, where electrons are forced to oscillate at high frequencies in a radio-transmitting aerial.

Thus the interactions of energetic atoms produce a broad band of emitted quanta wavelengths because of the range of interactions that are possible. All of these radiations form part of the electromagnetic spectrum. A narrow range of frequencies (in the infrared part) is capable of being absorbed by the whole atom (as opposed to the electron shells or the nucleus) and so these atoms gain kinetic energy. This increase in the kinetic energy of the atoms is in the form of heat. Higher frequencies of radiation interact with the electrons in the orbitals and even higher frequencies will interact with the atomic nuclei.

8.5 THERMAL EXPANSION

Most substances expand when heated, owing to the increased kinetic energy of the atoms. The *linear expansivity* is a measure of this thermal expansion and is defined as the *fractional change in unit length per unit change in kelvin temperature*. The thermal expansion of different parts of the X-ray tube is an important design consideration as the tube is subject to large temperature variations during its working life. If materials of very different thermal expansivity are used, this can cause mechanical stress which could result in fracture of one of the components. A particularly weak point in this respect is the seal between the glass and the copper anode in a stationary anode tube. A special type of glass with a thermal expansivity very similar to copper is chosen. This reduces the mechanical stress and thus the chances of fracture of the glass envelope and loss of vacuum in the tube.

8.6 EVAPORATION AND VAPORISATION

We are all familiar with the evaporation of liquids which occurs when heat is applied to them, e.g. boiling kettles. Evaporation is caused by the loss of *whole atoms* from the surface of the liquid. Some of the atoms are given sufficient kinetic energy to escape from the forces of attraction of their neighbours near the surface of the liquid and produce a vapour in the free space above this surface.

Whole atoms may also be liberated from the surfaces of solid materials under the action of heat. There is a stronger force of attraction between the atoms in a solid compared to a liquid and so liberation of the atoms is more difficult to accomplish. This means that in a solid the atoms require higher kinetic energy for liberation, i.e. solids need to be subjected to a higher temperature. The tungsten at the target and in the filament of the X-ray tube is subjected to such high temperatures that a certain amount of *vaporisation* takes place. The tungsten vapour can condense to form a thin layer of tungsten on the inside of the glass of the envelope (Figure 8.3). The major effect of this is to reduce the electrical insulation provided by the glass, as tungsten is a reasonable conductor of electricity. This can produce an effect called a 'gassy tube', which renders the X-ray tube inoperable. Fortunately this does not occur readily as tungsten has a low *vapour pressure* so does not readily vaporise at its normal working temperatures.

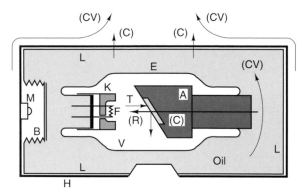

Figure 8.3 Stationary anode X-ray tube and housing. Heat is lost from the target mainly by conduction (C) but convection (CV) and radiation (R) also play a part in the dissipation of heat from the target to the atmosphere of the room. H, housing; L, lead lining; M, microswitch; B, expansion bellows; E, envelope; V, vacuum in envelope; K, cathode; F, filament; T, tungsten target; A, copper anode.

8.7 HEAT LOSS FROM AN X-RAY TUBE

The mechanisms of heat loss discussed earlier in this chapter will now be discussed in relation to the heat loss from the anode of both a stationary anode and a rotating anode X-ray tube. In the case of all X-ray tubes, a large amount of heat is generated during the X-ray exposure and so efficient heat loss is necessary to protect the tube against thermal damage and to allow short exposures of high intensity.

8.7.1 The Stationary Anode Tube

Figure 8.3 shows the construction of a typical stationary anode tube in its housing. Superimposed on the figure are arrows originating from the focal spot which represent the paths taken by the heat energy to remove the heat from this small area of high temperature. The arrows marked (R) represent heat loss by radiation, while those marked (C) represent heat loss by conduction and those marked (CV) represent convection. The sequence of events is as follows:

• An exposure is made, resulting in a considerable amount of heat energy being deposited at the focal spot of the tungsten target. This energy must be quickly dispersed, otherwise the temperature rise at the target will cause thermal damage

- Some of the heat is lost from the focal spot by radiation through the vacuum, to be absorbed by the glass envelope and the oil
- The main heat loss is by conduction through the tungsten target into the copper anode block and along the anode stem
- The end of the stem is in contact with the oil and so sets up convection currents that warm up the whole of the oil. The oil expands as its temperature increases and, at a certain temperature, it will cause the expansion bellows to trip the microswitch, preventing further exposures
- Heat from the oil passes through the metal casing by conduction
- The warm casing sets up convection currents in the air of the room.

Thus all three processes of conduction, convection and radiation are involved in the removal of heat from the focal spot. However, the stationary anode tube is designed to remove the majority of the heat from the target by *conduction*. From Equation 8.3 we can see that conduction depends on the type of material, the cross-sectional area, the temperature gradient and the length of the conductor. To maximise heat transfer by conduction:

- a material of high thermal conductivity (copper) is chosen
- a large cross-sectional area of anode block is used
- one end of the anode stem is surrounded by oil to achieve a temperature gradient
- the anode length is as short as possible.

The tungsten insert itself is not as good a thermal conductor as copper, so it is kept as thin as possible. The melting point of copper is 1083°C and this imposes a practical limit on the amount of heat which can be applied to the anode. The anode is, however, constructed with a fairly large mass, thus increasing its thermal capacity and limiting the temperature rise in the copper.

8.7.2 The Rotating Anode Tube

All three processes are again involved in the heat loss from the focal spot of the rotating anode

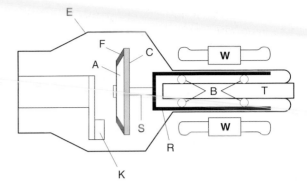

Figure 8.4   Rotating anode insert. Key: E, glass envelope; F, focal track; C, graphite disc; A, anode disc; S, anode stem; R, rotor; K, cathode assembly; W, stator coils; B, bearings; T, anode spindle.

tube, but in this case the main mechanism of heat loss is *radiation*, not conduction.

Figure 8.4 shows a simplified diagram of the construction of the insert of a rotating anode X-ray tube. The focal track is made of a mixture of tungsten and rhenium. Both have a high atomic number and melting point. However, tungsten has a low linear expansivity and is prone to crazing with repeated expansion and contraction; rhenium has a higher linear expansivity and slows the rate at which this crazing occurs. The anode disc itself is a tungsten molybdenum alloy, which is often backed (as shown) by a graphite disc. Molybdenum has approximately twice the specific heat capacity and half the density of tungsten; graphite has an even higher thermal capacity and is a quarter of the density of molybdenum (see Table 8.2). This permits the thermal capacity of the anode to be increased, without any increase in its mass. As we saw earlier (see *Stefan's law*), the heat loss from a body is proportional to T^4 and so heat loss from the anode by radiation can be encouraged by allowing it to reach a high temperature; during large exposures it gets white-hot. During longer exposures thermal equilibrium may be achieved when the rate of heat transfer balances the rate of heat production.

The radiated heat is absorbed by the insert envelope, which in turn heats the surrounding oil, setting up convection currents in it. Heat is then conducted through the casing and convected in the air of the room, as in the case of the stationary anode X-ray tube.

Table 8.2 Materials used in the construction of a rotating anode insert

	Symbol	Atomic no.	Density	Melting point (°C)	Specific heat capacity (cal.mol^{-1}.°C^{-1})	Thermal conductivity
Rhenium	Re	75	21.0	3180	0.033	0.17
Molybdenum	Mo	42	10.2	2610	0.061	0.35
Carbon (graphite)	C	6	2.5	3727	2.038	0.057
Tungsten	W	74	19.3	3410	0.032	4.00

While we wish the anode to dissipate its heat by radiation, we also wish to prevent heat travelling along the anode stem by conduction, as this would overheat the bearings and the rotor, preventing rotation of the anode. This is achieved in three ways:

1. the stem is made from molybdenum, which has a lower thermal conductivity than tungsten
2. the cross-sectional area is made as small as possible
3. the anode stem is made as long as mechanically practicable.

The anode rotor is also blackened to encourage the black-body radiation of any heat which reaches it.

Overheating of the anode may result in mechanical damage to it (e.g. pitting or cracking); softening of the anode stem may result in instability of the anode or expansion of the rotor or rotor bearings, which would in turn prevent the anode from rotating (thus increasing the risk of thermal damage to the target).

SUMMARY

In this chapter you should have learnt:

- That heat is a form of energy produced by the kinetic energy of atoms in a body (see Sect. 8.3)
- The greater the kinetic energy of the atoms, the higher the temperature and vice versa (see Sect. 8.3)
- That bodies which are in thermal equilibrium with their surroundings lose heat as fast as they gain heat and so experience no change in temperature (see Sect. 8.3)
- Absolute zero temperature corresponds to zero atomic kinetic energy and has a temperature of 0 K (see Sect. 8.3.1)
- On the kelvin scale, the temperature at which ice melts is approximately 273 K (see Sect. 8.3.1)
- The link between heat and temperature provided by specific heat capacity and thermal capacity (see Sect. 8.3.2)

- Heat may be transferred from one point to another by conduction (mainly in solids), convection (in fluids) and radiation (may travel through a vacuum) (see Sects 8.4.1–8.4.3)
- Heat must be transferred quickly from the focal spot of an X-ray tube if thermal damage is to be avoided (see Sect. 8.7)
- For a stationary anode tube *conduction* is the main mechanism of heat loss, therefore a copper anode with a large cross-sectional area is used (see Sect. 8.7.1)
- For a rotating anode tube *radiation* is the main mechanism of heat loss. Higher anode temperatures are required to give efficient heat loss (Stefan's law: intensity $\propto$ T^4) (see Sect. 8.7.2).

SELF-TEST

a. Why does a metal bar expand if it is heated?

b. The boiling point of water is 100°C. What is this in kelvin units?

c. The specific heat capacity of water is 4.2 kJ.kg^{-1}.K^{-1}. Calculate the power required to raise the temperature of 10 l of water from 20°C to 32°C in 10 min.

d. The specific heat capacity of molybdenum is approximately twice the specific heat capacity of tungsten. If the same amount of heat is applied to two discs, one made of tungsten and one made of molybdenum, each having the same mass, what will be the relationship between the temperature change produced in each disc?

e. Describe the mechanism by which heat is transferred by conduction.

f. Describe the mechanism by which heat is transferred by convection.

g. Describe the mechanism by which heat is transferred by radiation.

h. Compare the methods of heat loss from the target of the stationary anode and the rotating anode X-ray tubes.

FURTHER READING

Further information on X-ray tube design and rating is available in Chapters 21 and 22 of this text. The following may also prove useful:

Heat and heat transfer processes
Ball J L, Moore A D 1997 Essential physics for radiographers, 3rd edn. Blackwell Scientific Publications, London, ch 2

X-ray tube design and cooling pathways
Ball J L, Moore A D 1997 Essential physics for radiographers, 3rd edn. Blackwell Scientific Publications, London, ch 12

Bushong S C 2004 Radiologic science for technologists: physics, biology and protection. Mosby, New York, ch 10
Carter P H 1994 Chesney's equipment for student radiographers, 4th edn. Blackwell Scientific, ch 1
Dendy P P, Heaton B 1999 Physics for diagnostic radiology, 2nd edn. Institute of Physics Publishing, ch 2

Chapter 9

Electrostatics

CHAPTER CONTENTS

9.1 Aim 72

9.2 Introduction 72

9.3 Properties of Electrical Charges 72

9.4 Force Between two Electrical Charges in a Vacuum 73

9.5 Permittivity and Relative Permittivity (Dielectric Constant) 74

9.6 Electrical Field Strength 74

9.7 Electrostatic Induction of Charge 74
    9.7.1 Induction of a Conductor 75
    9.7.2 Induction of an Insulator (Dielectric) 75

9.8 Electrical Potential 76
    9.8.1 Zero Electrical Potential 76
    9.8.2 Absolute Potential and Potential Difference 76
    9.8.3 The Volt 76
    9.8.4 Electrical Potential Due to a Point Charge 77
    9.8.5 Electrical Potential Due to a Conducting Sphere 77

9.9 Distribution of Electrical Charge on an Irregularly Shaped Conductor 77

Self-Test 79

Further Reading 79

9.1 AIM

The aim of this chapter is to introduce the reader to the concepts involved in understanding the electrostatics which is relevant to radiographic science. This involves the consideration of electrical charge, charge distribution and electrical potential and potential difference.

9.2 INTRODUCTION

Electrostatics, as the name implies, is the study of static electrical charges. We are familiar with many examples of electrostatics from our ordinary lives, from sparks which may occur from our clothes when undressing, to the large discharges of electricity which occur during lightning strikes. Much of the early experimentation with electricity involved electrostatics. It was discovered at a fairly early stage that there were two types of electrical charge, one called negative, and the other positive. While it is mathematically convenient to regard charge in this way, it does not explain what electrical charge actually is and how it behaves. This will be the subject of this chapter.

9.3 PROPERTIES OF ELECTRICAL CHARGES

The general properties of electrical charges are as follows:

- Charges can be considered as being of two types: positive and negative
- The smallest unit of negative charge which can exist in isolation is that possessed by an electron, and the smallest unit of positive charge which can exist in isolation is that possessed by the proton
- Electrical charges exert forces on each other even when they are separated by a vacuum. The forces are mutual, equal and opposite, as expected by Newton's third law (see Sect. 5.5)
- Like charges (i.e. charges of the same sign) repel each other while unlike charges (of opposite signs) attract each other
- The magnitude of the mutual forces between the charges is influenced by:
  - the magnitude of the individual charges
  - the medium in which they are embedded, being greatest when the medium is a vacuum
  - the inverse square of the distance between the charged bodies – this is another application of the inverse-square law (see Sect. 3.3)
- Electrical charges may be induced in a body by the proximity of a charged body, leading to a force of attraction between the two bodies
- Electrical charges may flow easily in some materials (called *electrical conductors*) and with difficulty in other materials (called *electrical insulators*). Both types of material are capable of having charges induced in them
- When electrical charges move they produce a magnetic field.

9.4 FORCE BETWEEN TWO ELECTRICAL CHARGES IN A VACUUM

Consider two charges, q_1 and q_2, separated by a distance d in a vacuum, as shown in Figure 9.1.

If we assume that both charges are of the same sign, then q_1 will exert a force of repulsion (F) on q_2 and q_2 will exert the same force of repulsion on q_1. As we have already stated above, it can be shown that:

1. $F \propto q_1$
2. $F \propto q_2$
3. $F \propto 1/d_2$.

Thus, F is proportional to the magnitude of each charge and to the inverse square of the distance separating them.

If we combine the factors in 1, 2 and 3 above, we can produce the equation:

$$F \propto \frac{q_1 q_2}{d^2} \qquad \text{Equation 9.1}$$

If q_1 and q_2 both have the same sign, then F will be positive and will represent a force of repulsion. If the charges have opposite signs, then F will be negative and will represent a force of attraction.

If we wish to replace the proportionality sign in Equation 9.1 by an equals sign then we need to introduce a constant of proportionality (see Appendix A). This equation now reads:

$$F = \frac{q_1 q_2}{4\pi\varepsilon_0 d^2} \qquad \text{Equation 9.2}$$

This equation is often referred to as *Coulomb's law of force* between two charges and has particular relevance when we consider the charges between subatomic particles (see Chs 26 and 27).

The constant of proportionality is $^1/_4\pi\varepsilon_0$, where ε_0 is the *permittivity of a vacuum* and has a value of 8.85×10^{-12} F.m^{-1}. The charges q_1 and q_2 are expressed in coulombs, the separation d is in metres and the force F is in newtons.

The coulomb corresponds to the charge carried by 6×10^{18} electrons or protons. An alternative (and more practical) definition of the coulomb is:

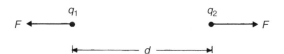

$$F \xleftarrow{\quad q_1 \quad} \bullet \qquad\qquad \bullet \xrightarrow{\quad q_2 \quad} F$$
$$\longmapsto\!\!-\!\!-\!\!-\!\! d \!\!-\!\!-\!\!-\!\!\longmapsto$$

Figure 9.1 The forces (F) between two electrical charges, q_1 and q_2, separated by a distance d are equal and opposite.

DEFINITION

A charge of 1 coulomb is possessed by a point if an equal charge placed 1 metre away from it in a vacuum experiences a force of repulsion of $^1/_4\pi\varepsilon_0$ newton.

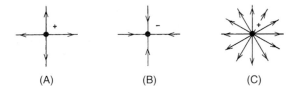

Figure 9.2 Electric 'lines of force' associated with (A) a weak positive charge, (B) a weak negative charge and (C) a strong positive charge.

INSIGHT

The influence of the inverse-square law on the force between charged bodies may be grasped if we assume that charged bodies emanate lines of force in all directions similar to the light emission from a point source of light obeying the inverse-square law. The number of such lines of force is proportional to the magnitude of the charge (analogous to the brightness of the light source). This is shown diagrammatically in Figure 9.2, where the arrows point in the direction of the force experienced by a positive charge if placed at that point. There will be further discussion of lines of force in the section of this chapter dealing with electrical field strength (see Sect. 9.6).

9.5 PERMITTIVITY AND RELATIVE PERMITTIVITY (DIELECTRIC CONSTANT)

Equation 9.2 only holds true when the charges are in a vacuum, as ε_0 is the permittivity of a vacuum. In any other medium the equation requires to be modified to:

$$F = \frac{q_1 q_2}{4\pi\varepsilon d^2} \qquad \text{Equation 9.3}$$

where ε is the permittivity of the medium

It is, however, often convenient to compare the permittivity of the medium relative to that of a vacuum, e.g. if the permittivity of the medium is twice that of a vacuum, then the *relative permittivity* (K) is 2. This can be obtained from the simple formula:

$$K = \frac{\varepsilon}{\varepsilon_0}$$

or by cross-multiplying:

$$\varepsilon = \varepsilon_0 K \qquad \text{Equation 9.4}$$

so Equation 9.3 may be rewritten as:

$$F = \frac{q_1 q_2}{4\pi\varepsilon_0 K d^2} \qquad \text{Equation 9.5}$$

K is known as the *dielectric constant* of the medium and so we can see that the relative permittivity and the dielectric constant are the same. *Note* that as the dielectric constant is a comparative number, it does not have any units. (The dielectric constant is further discussed in Ch. 16, where we consider its importance in capacitors.)

9.6 ELECTRICAL FIELD STRENGTH

We have already seen that an electric charge is capable of influencing other charges placed at a distance from it. This influence on other charges at a distance is known as a field and, for the purpose of comparing electrical charges, E is measured as the force on a unit positive charge. E is therefore measured in units of newton/coulomb. Consider the electric field around a point charge. If we wish to know the field strength at a point we simply place a unit positive charge at that point and measure the magnitude and direction of the force exerted upon it. If we consider Equation 9.5 and have $q_2 = 1$ (unit charge) then we can say that:

$$E = \frac{q_1 \times 1}{4\pi\varepsilon_0 K d^2}$$

$$E = \frac{q_1}{4\pi\varepsilon_0 K d^2} \qquad \text{Equation 9.6}$$

We have already considered a diagrammatic representation of the field around a point charge (Figure 9.2). The arrows represent the direction of the force acting on a unit positive charge (if placed at that point) and the line density represents the intensity of the electrical field.

9.7 ELECTROSTATIC INDUCTION OF CHARGE

As mentioned earlier, a charge may be induced on an electrical conductor or on an insulator. Each will now be considered.

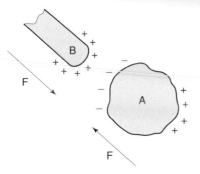

Figure 9.3   Induction of a charge on a conducting body, *A*, results in a force of attraction, *F*, with the inducing body (*B*).

9.7.1 Induction of a Conductor

The situation which exists if an electrically charged body (*B*) is placed close to a conductor (*A*) is shown in Figure 9.3. A conductor is a body which will allow a flow of electrons. The positive charge on *B* attracts electrons to it and leaves equal numbers of positive charges on the opposite surface of *A*. Notice that the opposite charge is induced on the surface of the conductor closest to the inducing charge. Also note that equal numbers of positive and negative charges are induced. There is eventually a state of equilibrium where the electrons on the surface of *A* experience an equal force of attraction from the two sets of positive charge. When this happens, no further electron flow takes place.

The charge distribution results in a net force of attraction as the unlike charges are closer to the charged body than the like charges.

Withdrawal of the charged body results in uniform distribution of the charges in *A*.

9.7.2 Induction of an Insulator (Dielectric)

If we bring a charged body close to an insulator, a similar force of attraction occurs – this can be demonstrated by running a comb through your hair and holding it close to a small piece of paper, which will be attracted to it. This result is somewhat surprising, as electrons cannot move as freely through an insulator as a conductor. Some insulators are more efficient at producing induced charges than others and it is found that this varies

with the dielectric constant (see Sect. 9.5) of the material. There are two explanations of the induced charge in an insulator, *molecular distortion* and *polar molecules*.

9.7.2.1 Molecular Distortion

A body is composed of atoms or molecules. These contain equal numbers of protons (+ve) and electrons (−ve), thus making the body electrically neutral. As can be seen in Figure 9.4A, the electrons normally form symmetrical orbits around the nucleus so that the average position of the electron is over the nucleus, and so the two sets of charges cancel each other out. If a charged body is placed close to the atom (Figure 9.4B), then the electron orbits are distorted relative to the atomic nucleus. The average position of the electrons is now displaced to one side of the atom, and so the atom has been *polarised* into an *electrical dipole*.

9.7.2.2 Polar Molecules

Some molecules exist in which the atoms are so arranged that the average position of the electrons is not coincident with that of the nuclei, even when the atoms are not subject to an electrical field.

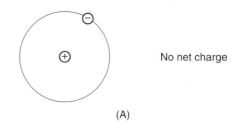

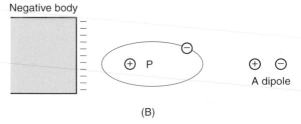

Figure 9.4   The effect of an external field on an atom. (A) The atom with no external field applied; (B) the polarisation of the atom to form a dipole caused by the proximity of a negatively charged body.

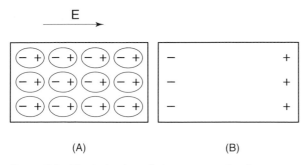

Figure 9.5 The induction of charge on an insulator containing polar molecules. (A) The alignment of the polar molecules; (B) the net charges at the ends of the body.

These molecules are polarised even when not subject to an electric field. The effect of an external electric field is to rotate these molecules such that they tend to become aligned with the field. This means that the structure now has a definite positive end and a definite negative end, as shown in Figure 9.5. Within the body, the dipoles are so close together that the positive and negative ends of adjacent dipoles cancel each other's effects. Practical dielectrics use such materials as they produce a much stronger effect than molecular distortion alone.

9.8 ELECTRICAL POTENTIAL

There are a number of similarities between electrical potential and potential energy. In the case of potential energy this represents the work done in raising the body through a height h with reference to zero level. Similar concepts will now be discussed for electrical potential.

9.8.1 Zero Electrical Potential

The most convenient point to choose as having zero electrical potential is the point at which the force exerted by the charged body on a unit positive charge would be zero. This point is *infinity* and all work performed on a unit charge is measured from there. Obviously infinity is chosen for its mathematical convenience rather than its practicality!

INSIGHT

It is often stated that 'the earth is at zero potential'. The earth is assumed to be electrically neutral in that it contains equal numbers of positive and negative charges. Thus there is no force between neutral earth and a unit positive charge and so no effort is needed to move the latter towards earth. Hence no work is done and the electrical potential of earth, or any other neutral body, is zero.

9.8.2 Absolute Potential and Potential Difference

From the discussion so far, we may define the *absolute electrical potential* at a point as follows:

DEFINITION

The *absolute electrical potential* at a point is the work done in moving a unit positive charge from infinity to that point.

In practice it is often more convenient to compare the potential at one point relative to another rather than know its absolute potential. If the potential at point A is V_A and the potential at point B is V_B, then the potential difference (PD) between A and B is $V_A - V_B$ and represents the difference in the work done in moving a unit positive charge from infinity to point A and from infinity to point B. It can be seen that this is the same as the work which would be required to move a unit positive charge from point A to point B. This leads to the definition of potential difference:

DEFINITION

The *potential difference* between two points is the work done on a unit positive charge in moving it from one point to the other.

9.8.3 The Volt

The volt is the International System of Units (SI) unit of potential and is defined as:

DEFINITION

1 volt of potential exists at a point if *1 joule of work* is performed in moving *1 coulomb of positive charge* from infinity to that point.

Similarly, for potential difference we have:

DEFINITION

1 volt of *potential difference* exists between two points if *1 joule* of work is done in moving *1 coulomb of positive charge* from one point to the other.

These definitions can be shown in the form of an equation:

$$\text{volts} = \frac{\text{joules}}{\text{coulombs}}$$
    Equation 9.7

9.8.4 Electrical Potential Due to a Point Charge

Consider a point charge Q, as shown in Figure 9.6, where a unit positive charge has been moved from infinity to a distance r from Q. The nearer the unit charge comes to Q, the greater the force of repulsion (if Q is positive) or attraction (if Q is negative). Thus the potential is positive if Q is positive and negative if Q is negative since the potential is the work done on the unit positive charge. If we consider that the work done on all unit positive charges which are equidistant from Q will be the same, then it is logical to assume

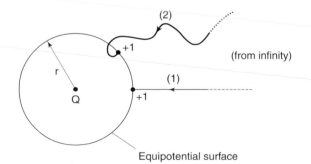

Figure 9.6   The electrical potential energy of a point charge Q.

that equipotential surfaces will be concentric spheres with Q as the centre. It is also worth noting that the particular path chosen to bring a unit positive charge from infinity to the point r is of no importance and so paths (1) and (2) give exactly the same electrical potential.

Electrical potential is usually given the symbol V and so we can produce the equation:

$$\text{work} = \text{force} \times \text{distance}$$

$$V = \frac{Q \times r}{4\pi\varepsilon_0 r^2}$$

$$V = \frac{Q}{4\pi\varepsilon_0 r}$$
    Equation 9.8

where V is in volts, Q is in coulombs and r is in metres.

The electrical potential due to a point charge is given the term *coulomb potential* and the force between two charges is the *Coulomb force* (see Sect. 9.4).

9.8.5 Electrical Potential Due to a Conducting Sphere

If we place a charge Q on a conducting sphere, then the charged particles will mutually repel each other and so the charges will be evenly distributed on the outer surface of the sphere – this is true whether the sphere is hollow or solid. Thus no potential difference exists between any points either on the surface or within the sphere (if a potential difference did exist, the charge would redistribute in such a way that the whole body was at a constant potential). When we consider the potential which exists outside the sphere, it may be shown mathematically that the sphere behaves as though all the charge Q is placed at its centre. This is shown in the graph in Figure 9.7. Thus Equation 9.8 can be used to calculate the potential of points outside the sphere where r is the distance from the centre of the sphere.

9.9 DISTRIBUTION OF ELECTRICAL CHARGE ON AN IRREGULARLY SHAPED CONDUCTOR

Having considered the charge distribution on a sphere, it is now useful to consider the

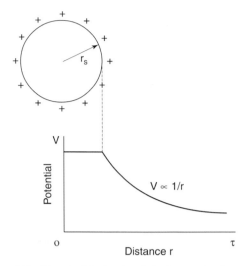

Figure 9.7 The electrical potential of a conducting sphere of radius r_s. The potential is constant within the sphere and reduces outside it ($V \propto 1/r$).

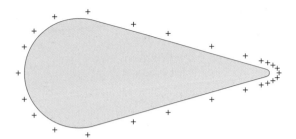

Figure 9.8 The distribution of positive charge on an irregularly shaped conductor. Note the high intensity of charge at the area of low radius of curvature.

distribution of charge on a conducting body of irregular shape. Such a body is shown in Figure 9.8. Again the charge is distributed so that no potential difference exists between any points

within the body. This gives the charge distribution shown in Figure 9.8. Note that there are large collections of charge at parts of the body which have a small radius of curvature. This is important in the design of the X-ray tube both in the prevention of coronal discharge (where electrons are forcibly removed from their orbits to create an electrical spark) from sharp corners and also in the use of a sharp-edged focusing cup for electron focusing (see Ch. 21).

SUMMARY

In this chapter you should have learnt:

- The properties of electrical charges (see Sect. 9.3)
- The force between two electrical charges in a vacuum (see Sect. 9.4)
- The meaning of permittivity and relative permittivity (dielectric constant) (see Sect. 9.5)
- The concept of electrical field strength (see Sect. 9.6)
- The meaning of electrostatic induction (see Sect. 9.7)
- Electrostatic induction of a conductor (see Sect. 9.7.1)

- Electrostatic induction of an insulator or dielectric (see Sect. 9.7.2)
- The concept of electrical potential (see Sect. 9.8)
- The meaning of zero electrical potential (see Sect. 9.8.1)
- The meaning of absolute potential and potential difference (see Sect. 9.8.2)
- The definition of the volt (see Sect. 9.8.3)
- Electric potential due to a point charge (see Sect. 9.8.4)
- Electric potential due to a conducting sphere (see Sect. 9.8.5)
- Electrical charge distribution on an irregularly shaped conductor (see Sect. 9.9).

SELF-TEST

a. List the properties of electrical charges.

b. List the factors that determine the force between two point charges in a vacuum.

c. Discuss the induction of charge on:

(i) a conductor

(ii) an insulator

when a positively charged body is brought into close proximity with it.

d. Discuss the statement 'earth is at zero potential'.

e. Describe the distribution of charge on a conducting:

(i) sphere

(ii) irregularly shaped body.

FURTHER READING

Ball J L, Moore A D 1997 Essential physics for radiographers, 3rd edn. Blackwell Scientific Publications, London, ch 3

Chapter 10

Electricity (DC)

CHAPTER CONTENTS

10.1   Aim   80

10.2   Introduction   80

10.3   Simple Electron Theory of Conduction   81
        10.3.1 Electron Arrangements in a
                Conductor   82
        10.3.2 Electron Arrangements in a
                Semiconductor   83
        10.3.3 Electron Arrangements in an
                Insulator   83

10.4   Electric Current   83

10.5   mA, mAs and Millicoulombs   84

10.6   Potential Difference and Electromotive
        Force   84

10.7   Resistance   85
        10.7.1 Factors Affecting Resistance   85

10.8   Ohm's Law   86
        10.8.1 Resistors in Series   87
        10.8.2 Resistors in Parallel   87
        10.8.3 Calculations Using Ohm's Law   88

10.9   Electrical Energy and Power   89
        10.9.1 The Joule   89
        10.9.2 The Watt   89
        10.9.3 Power in a Resistor   89

10.10   Power Loss in Cables   90
        10.10.1 Reducing the Current Flowing
                Within the Cable   90
        10.10.2 Reducing the Resistance of the
                Cables   90
        10.10.3 Mains Cable Resistance and X-ray
                Exposures   90

Self-Test   91

Further Reading   92

10.1 AIM

The aim of this chapter is to introduce the reader to the concept of electron flow as a means of conducting electricity. Factors affecting the resistance to this flow will be explored and Ohm's law will be discussed. The consequences of resistance in terms of electrical 'power loss' will be discussed and the practical implications of this in the design of X-ray-generating apparatus will be considered.

10.2 INTRODUCTION

In Chapter 9 we considered the behaviour of static electrical charges. This chapter considers the behaviour of electrical charges which are unidirectional in their movement – *direct current* or *DC electricity*. In a vacuum, gas or liquid (e.g. in an air ionisation chamber; see Ch. 33) both positive and negative charges move with relative freedom. These charges are called *ions*. In a solid, however, the atomic nuclei are relatively tightly bound to other atoms and so take no part in the flow of charge. The electrical properties of a given solid are thus determined by the way in which the orbiting electrons behave. This behaviour will form the initial discussion in this chapter.

10.3 SIMPLE ELECTRON THEORY OF CONDUCTION

To explain why some materials readily allow a flow of electrons (i.e. are good electrical conductors) and other materials will only allow electron flow in extreme conditions (i.e. are good insulators) we need to look more closely at the structure of the atom. This chapter will only look at atomic structure in terms of explaining the electrical properties of the material and there will be a fuller description of the atom in Chapter 26.

The nucleus of the atom contains protons (+ve charge) and around this in orbitals are electrons (–ve charge). If we consider a single atom (see Figure 10.1), we can appreciate that electrons near the nucleus experience a high level of attraction (unlike charges attract) and are thus said to be *tightly bound*. Electrons in the more remote orbitals experience less force of attraction from the nucleus (remember $f \propto 1/d^2$) and are also repelled by other electrons which lie between them and the nucleus and so are said to be more *loosely bound*. Because the electrons in a given single atom are influenced by only that atom, the electrons lie at discrete energy levels, as shown in Figure 10.2A.

When electrons are brought closer together, as in a solid, the orbitals of the electrons are strongly influenced by the proximity of neighbouring atoms. This means that electrons are no longer at discrete energy levels but that they are

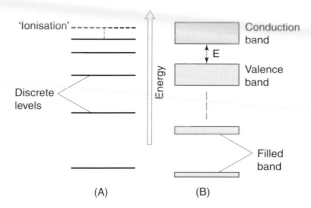

Figure 10.2   (A) Electron energy levels in a solitary atom. (B) Electron energy bands in an atom of a solid.

now within a band of energies. This situation is shown in Figure 10.2B.

For the purpose of this discussion, only the outer two energy bands are of interest to us: the *valence band* and the *conduction band*. The valence band is that band which contains the outermost electrons of the atom and may be partially or completely full of its permitted maximum number of electrons. The configuration of electrons in this band determines the *chemical properties* of the atom, i.e. its ability to form *chemical bonds* with other atoms. If electrons exist further away from the nucleus than the valence band, then their energies lie in the conduction band. This band is populated with electrons which have, for some reason, become free from their original atoms. Because of this, once an electron is in the conduction band of a solid, it is able to move relatively freely and hence may take part in electrical conduction through the material. Thus a material with a large number of electrons in the conduction band is a *good electrical conductor* whereas a material with no electrons in the conduction band is a *perfect electrical insulator*. Whether or not a material is a conductor, an insulator or a semiconductor is thus determined by the number of electrons in the conduction band. This number is in turn determined by the size of the *forbidden energy gap* (E) which exists between the top energy of the valence band and the bottom energy of the conduction band. The arrangement of the valence and conduction bands for conductors, semiconductors and insulators is shown in

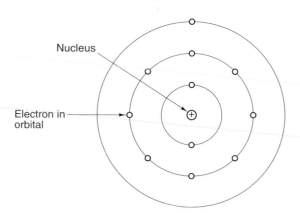

Figure 10.1   Diagrammatic representation of the sodium atom. Note the positive charge on the nucleus and that the electrons occupy specific orbitals.

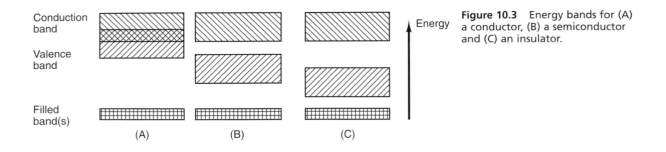

Figure 10.3   Energy bands for (A) a conductor, (B) a semiconductor and (C) an insulator.

Figure 10.3. Each of the above will now be considered individually.

10.3.1 Electron Arrangements in a Conductor

As can be seen from Figure 10.3A, the conduction band and the valence band of energies overlap in a conductor.

As a result, a large number of electrons always exist in the conduction band and because of this there is a ready exchange of electrons between the valence and conduction bands. This means that these electrons can be moved through the solid with *little resistance* to their flow. The main opposition to their flow arises from collisions with other electrons or atoms. If the temperature of the conductor is increased, there is an increase in the vibration of the atoms and a corresponding increase in the likelihood of collision with moving electrons. Thus we can see that *the opposition (or resistance) to the flow of electrons in a conductor will increase with an increase in its temperature.*

INSIGHT

As mentioned in Section 10.3.1, the main cause of resistance to the flow of electrons in a conductor is collisions with other atoms. It would therefore seem logical to suggest that, if the vibration of the atoms could be reduced, or even stopped, then the resistance of the conductor could be reduced. This is done by cooling the conductor to temperatures close to absolute zero. At these temperatures, atomic vibration ceases to exist and so flow of electrons through the conduction band is virtually unimpeded. Materials operating in this mode are known as *superconductors* and this technique is used to produce the large magnetic field required for magnetic resonance imaging (MRI).

10.3.1.1 Superconductivity

As can be seen from the insight (above), superconductivity is a phenomenon whereby electrical resistivity falls to zero at a critical temperature. Its main application is in the magnets used to produce the main (or static) magnetic field in magnetic resonance scanners. Materials such as niobium-tin or niobium-titanium alloy are used for the coils, which are maintained at a temperature of 4.2 K (roughly –269°C). Liquid helium is used as a cooling agent or cryogen. The advantage of this is that a current can be made to flow indefinitely in the closed loop of a superconducting coil without electrical resistivity losses, continually generating a magnetic field. This in turn means that, provided the temperature of the superconductor is maintained below the critical temperature of 4.2 K, the magnet will be 'persistent' once energised. Thus, due to the absence of resistance in the coil, heat losses ($H = I^2R$) are zero. Hence high magnetic field strengths can be obtained. In addition, the magnetic field is extremely stable. These characteristics are ideal for MRI.

Researchers have developed high-temperature superconductors such as ruthenium-oxyocuprate ($RuSr_2(Gd,Eu,Sm)Cu_2O_8$), which is a superconductor at temperatures in the region of 58 K (about –215°C!). However, at the time of writing these are not used in MRI magnets.

10.3.2 Electron Arrangements in a Semiconductor

In a semiconductor there is a gap between the maximum energy of the valence band and the minimum energy of the conduction band (Figure 10.3B) and so electrons need to be given energy to bridge this gap and flow through the material (this will be discussed in more detail in Ch. 18, which deals with semiconductors). Thus *semiconductors have a greater resistance to the flow of electrons than conductors*. If we increase the temperature of the semiconductor, we will increase the energy of the electrons in the valence band and so make it easier for them to transfer to the conduction band and move through the solid. Thus, *increasing the temperature of a semiconductor will reduce its resistance to the flow of electrons*.

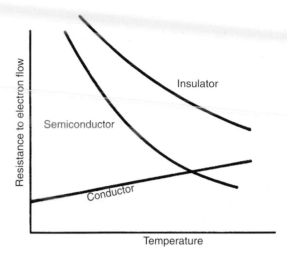

Figure 10.4   Effect of temperature on the electrical resistance of a conductor, a semiconductor and an insulator.

10.3.3 Electron Arrangements in an Insulator

In an insulator there is a significant gap between the maximum energy of the valence band and the minimum energy of the conduction band (Figure 10.3C). This means that electrons cannot readily bridge this energy gap, and so the conduction band contains no electrons, making conduction impossible. If the material is heated, then the electrons in the valence band gain energy, and so the gap between the valence and the conduction bands is narrowed, making it more likely that electrons can jump the gap. Thus *increasing the temperature of an insulator reduces its resistance*.

The effect on the resistance to the flow of electrons of increasing the temperature is shown in Figure 10.4.

10.4 ELECTRIC CURRENT

Electricity is the flow of electrons in a material. The rate of flow of electrons is a measure of the *electric current*. In order to produce a current the following conditions must be satisfied:

• There must be a source of electric *potential difference* (see Sect. 9.8.2)

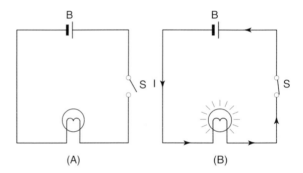

Figure 10.5   (A) The switch S is open and so no current flows through the circuit. (B) When the switch is closed, current will flow through the circuit and the bulb will light. This shows that a continuous circuit is necessary for electrical current to flow.

• There must be a *complete circuit* around which the electrons are able to travel.

These two points are illustrated in Figure 10.5. The battery (*B*) is a source of potential difference, but if the switch (*S*) is open (as in Figure 10.5A), no electric current flows and the bulb does not light up. When the switch is closed (Figure 10.5B), a complete circuit exists around which electrons are able to flow and so the bulb lights up. The *potential difference* may be thought of as the *driving force* which causes electrons to flow, while the *current* is the rate of flow of electrons, i.e. the number of electrons passing a given point in unit time.

DEFINITION

An *electric current of 1 ampere* (A) flows at a point if a charge of *1 coulomb* (C) flows past that point *per second*.

Thus we can say mathematically:

$$\text{amperes} = \frac{\text{coulombs}}{\text{seconds}} \qquad \textit{Equation 10.1}$$

From Section 9.4 we know that a charge of 1 coulomb is equivalent to approximately 6×10^{18} electrons so 1 ampere is simply this number of electrons passing a point in 1 second.

INSIGHT

We are accustomed to an instant response when we close an electrical switch and so it is surprising to discover that the average velocity of electrons in a circuit is only in the order of 0.5 mm.s^{-1}. When the switch is closed, electrons start to flow through the whole circuit and so the bulb in Figure 10.5 will light up even if the electrons from the battery have not yet reached it – this is similar to the situation where water enters a pipe from a reservoir when a tap is opened; water leaves the tap immediately, although it might be some time before the water from the reservoir reaches it.

10.5 mA, mAs AND MILLICOULOMBS

The electric current through an X-ray tube is a small one and so it is measured in *milliamperes* (mA) rather than in amps: 1 mA $= 10^{-3}$ A. This measures the rate of flow of electrons through the tube. If we wish to measure the number of electrons which have travelled across the tube during a given radiographic exposure, then we need to multiply the rate of flow by the time of the exposure. This unit is in *milliampere-seconds* (mAs) where:

$$\text{mAs} = \text{mA} \times \text{seconds} \qquad \textit{Equation 10.2}$$

Now the total number of electrons which have crossed the X-ray tube is just a measure of the charge, measured in *coulombs*. From Equation 10.1:

$$\text{amps} = \frac{\text{coulombs}}{\text{seconds}}$$

By cross-multiplying (see Appendix A):

$$\text{coulombs} = \text{amps} \times \text{seconds}$$

so:

$$\text{millicoulombs} = \text{milliamps} \times \text{seconds} \qquad \textit{Equation 10.3}$$

So we can say that:

$$1 \text{ mAs} = 1 \text{ millicoulomb} \qquad \textit{Equation 10.4}$$

10.6 POTENTIAL DIFFERENCE AND ELECTROMOTIVE FORCE

We have already considered potential difference in Section 9.8.2 and defined the potential difference in volts:

DEFINITION

The potential difference in volts is the work done in moving 1 coulomb of positive charge from one point to another.

Thus:

$$\text{volts} = \frac{\text{joules}}{\text{coulombs}} \qquad \textit{Equation 10.5}$$

In electricity we are concerned with moving charges and, as mentioned previously, we can regard the potential difference as the 'driving force' which moves the electron along a conductor.

Electromotive force (EMF) is also expressed in *volts* and is a measure of electrical potential energy developed across a *source* of electricity (e.g. a battery or a generator). Thus the EMF is the 'driving force' behind the electron flow in the circuit.

It is therefore possible to speak about the potential difference (PD) across any part of the circuit including the source of electricity, whereas the term EMF is reserved solely for the latter. It would not therefore be correct to use the term 'EMF across a resistor' as a resistor is not a *source* of electricity – the appropriate terminology would be 'PD across a resistor'.

INSIGHT

It is interesting to note that the PD across the terminals of a battery is less than the EMF when a current flows. This is due to the internal resistance of the battery. The effect is known as *regulation*. A similar effect is observed with transformers and will be discussed more fully in Chapter 17.

10.7 RESISTANCE

The elementary theory of conduction discussed earlier in this chapter refers to two mechanisms that impede electron flow:

1. lack of 'free' electrons in the conduction band – as in an insulator
2. collisions between flowing electrons with other vibrating electrons in the material.

This impedance to the flow of electrons is given the term *electrical resistance* or simply *resistance* and is measured in *ohms*. Obviously, from the earlier discussion, insulators have much higher resistance than conductors of the same shape and size. The resistance of a conductor can vary depending on a number of factors, which will be discussed below.

10.7.1 Factors Affecting Resistance

The resistance of a substance will be affected by:

- the *shape* of the substance
- the *type* of the substance
- the *temperature* of the substance.

Note that the resistance of the substance is not affected by either the potential difference across it or by the current flowing through it.

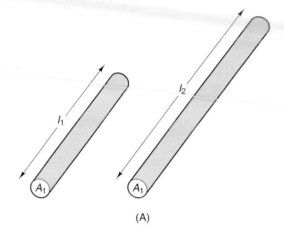

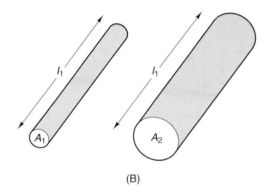

Figure 10.6   Factors affecting resistance of a conductor. In (A) the conductors are of different lengths and the resistance increases with the length. In (B) the conductors have differing cross-sectional areas and the resistance is inversely proportional to the cross-sectional area.

10.7.1.1 Shape

The shape of a body is capable of infinite variation, so for simplicity we shall consider circular conductors of constant cross-sectional area.

Figure 10.6 illustrates such a body and the effect on the resistance R of altering its length l and its cross-sectional area A.

The resistance is proportional to the length of the conductor ($R \propto l$). If we consider a situation where the length of the conductor is doubled, then electrons travelling along the conductor have twice as many vibrating atoms to get past, so the resistance to their flow will be doubled.

The resistance is inversely proportional to the cross-sectional area ($R \propto 1/A$). If the area is doubled, there are twice as many electrons capable of conducting charge. The number of atoms each electron must get past for the length of the conductor remains the same and so doubling the area will halve the resistance.

10.7.1.2 Type of Substance

By definition, good electrical conductors will have a lower resistance than insulators. Different metals also have different values of resistance. As we have just seen, the shape of the substance also affects its resistance, so that a standard shape and size must be used when comparing the resistance of different materials. The standard used is a cube of side 1 metre and the resistance is measured when a current is passed between opposing faces of the cube. The value of the resistance so obtained is called the *resistivity* or the *specific resistance* of the material and is measured in ohm-metres. Resistivity is given the symbol ρ (Greek rho) and it is clear that the resistance of the material will be directly proportional to its resistivity – $R \propto \rho$.

If we now consider all the factors discussed above we have:

$$R \propto \frac{\rho l}{A} \qquad \qquad \textit{Equation 10.6}$$

In the International System of Units (SI) system ρ is defined so that the constant of proportionality in the above equation is unity and we can say:

$$R = \frac{\rho l}{A} \qquad \qquad \textit{Equation 10.7}$$

The resistivities of insulators are about 1 million times greater than those of semiconductors, which in turn are about 1 million times greater than those of metallic conductors.

10.7.1.3 Temperature

As we have described at the beginning of this chapter, a change in temperature affects the resistance of a body. This effect is different for conductors, semiconductors and insulators, as shown in Figure 10.4. Because of these variations, resistance is usually quoted at a particular temperature (e.g. 20°C). The *temperature coefficient* of resistance, α, is defined as *the fractional change in resistance (or resistivity) per unit temperature change*.

$$\alpha = \frac{\text{change in resistivity}}{\text{original resistivity}}/\text{temperature change}$$

α is different for different conductors.

10.8 OHM'S LAW

Ohm's law applies to metallic conductors and combines, in a particularly simple and elegant way, the relationship between *current, potential difference* and *resistance*. It is found experimentally that the current flowing through a conductor is proportional to the potential difference applied across it – *as the driving force on the electrons is increased, so the number of electrons passing a point in unit time increases by a proportional amount.* Thus, if a potential difference of 2 volts causes a current of 1 amp to flow through a conductor, then a potential difference of 4 volts will cause a current of 2 amps to flow. Ohm's law may be formally stated as:

> The *current* flowing through a *metallic conductor* is *proportional* to the *potential difference* which exists across it provided that all *physical conditions* remain constant.

The main *physical condition* which must remain constant is the temperature of the conductor, as an alteration in the temperature will cause an alteration in the resistance (see Sect. 10.7.1).

Ohm's law may be stated mathematically thus:

$$I \propto V \qquad \qquad \textit{Equation 10.8}$$

where I and V are the magnitude of the current and the potential difference respectively.

Note that Ohm's law does not mention the word *resistance*. The resistance of the body (R) is introduced into Equation 10.8 as a constant of proportionality (see Appendix A) and so the equation may now be rewritten:

$$V \propto I$$
$$\therefore V = R \times I$$
$$\therefore V = I \times R \qquad \textit{Equation 10.9}$$

As we have already established, R is a *constant* for a given conductor at a given temperature and *does not depend on V or I.*

R is measured in ohm (Ω) and we can see from Equation 10.9 that when $V = 1$ volt and $I = 1$ amp, then R will be 1 ohm. The ohm may be defined as follows:

DEFINITION

A body is said to have an electrical resistance of *1 ohm* if a potential difference of *1 volt* across it produces an electrical current through it of *1 ampere.*

(*Note* that a potential difference always occurs *across* a body, never through it. Likewise, an electrical current always flows through a body and *does not exist across it.*)

Although Ohm's law is simple in its formulation, it has far-reaching implications which can be applied to radiological physics. The most important of these will now be discussed.

10.8.1 Resistors in Series

If we join resistors *in series* (end-to-end) and apply a potential difference of V volts across the unit, then a current of I amps flows through it. This is shown in Figure 10.7. Note that the same current flows through each resistor since the whole unit may be regarded as a continuous circuit and so electrons are neither lost nor gained throughout the circuit. Also note that the potential difference across the ends of the unit is equal to the sum of the potential differences across each resistor ($V = V_1 + V_2 + V_3$). We wish to calculate the effective resistance of the unit (R), i.e. *what would be the*

value of a single resistor which would behave in exactly the same way as the whole unit?

If we apply Ohm's law to each resistor in turn then we get:

$$V_1 = IR_1; \; V_2 = IR_2; \; V_3 = IR_3$$

We already know that:

$$V = V_1 + V_2 + V_3$$
$$V = IR_1 + IR_2 + IR_3$$
$$V = I(R_1 + R_2 + R_3) \qquad \text{Equation 10.10A}$$

If we apply Ohm's law to the total unit then:

$$V = I \times R$$

$$R = \frac{V}{1}$$

By substituting this value of V/I into Equation 10.10A, we get:

$$R = R_1 + R_2 + R_3 \qquad \text{Equation 10.10}$$

Thus, when resistors are connected in series the total resistance may be obtained simply by adding together the values of each separate resistor.

10.8.2 Resistors in Parallel

A potential difference of V exists across points A and B in Figure 10.8 and, since each resistor is connected to A and B, the potential difference across

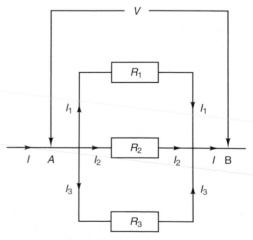

Figure 10.8 Combining resistors in parallel to produce a total resistance, R.

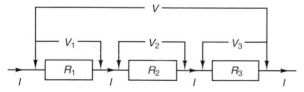

Figure 10.7 Combining resistors in series to produce a total resistance, R.

each resistor is also V volts. Electrons flow into the circuit at point A and then some will pass through each resistor to meet again at point B. Since electrons are neither gained nor lost in the circuit:

$$I = I_1 + I_2 + I_3 \qquad \text{Equation 10.11A}$$

If we apply Ohm's law to each of the resistors we get:

$$V = I_1 R_1; \; V = I_2 R_2; \; V = I_3 R_3$$

By substituting these values in Equation 10.11A:

$$I = \frac{V}{R_1} + \frac{V}{R_2} + \frac{V}{R_3}$$

$$\text{or } I = V\left(\frac{1}{R_1} + \frac{1}{R_2} + \frac{1}{R_3}\right)$$

so

$$\frac{I}{V} = \frac{1}{R_1} + \frac{1}{R_2} + \frac{1}{R_3} \qquad \text{Equation 10.11B}$$

If we apply Ohm's law to the whole unit (assuming it has a resistance R), then we get:

$$V = IR$$

$$\text{or } \frac{I}{V} = \frac{1}{R}$$

If we now substitute this value in Equation 10.11B, we get:

$$\frac{1}{R} = \frac{1}{R_1} + \frac{1}{R_2} + \frac{1}{R_3} \qquad \text{Equation 10.11}$$

10.8.3 Calculations Using Ohm's Law

a. A 30 Ω resistor is connected into a circuit and has a PD of 10 V across its ends. What is the current flowing through the resistor? By Ohm's law:

$$V = IR$$

$$I = \frac{V}{R}$$

$$= \frac{10}{30} \text{ A}$$

$$= 0.33 \text{ A}$$

b. A 6 V battery is connected across a 10 Ω and a 20 Ω resistor connected in series. What current flows in the circuit and what is the potential difference across each resistor? When resistors are connected in series:

$$R = R_1 + R_2$$
$$= 10 + 20 \; \Omega$$
$$= 30 \; \Omega$$

By Ohm's law:

$$V = IR$$

$$I = \frac{V}{R}$$

$$= \frac{6}{30} \text{ A}$$

$$= 0.2 \text{ A}$$

We know that the same current flows through each resistor and so we can apply Ohm's law to each.

$$V_1 = IR_1 \qquad \text{and} \qquad V_2 = IR_2$$
$$= 0.2 \times 10 \text{ V} \qquad\qquad\quad = 0.2 \times 20 \text{ V}$$
$$= 2 \text{ V} \qquad\qquad\qquad\quad = 4 \text{ V}$$

Note that the sum of the PDs across the resistors is equal to the PD across the battery terminals (6 V).

c. A 6 V battery is connected across a 10 Ω and a 20 Ω resistor connected in parallel. What is the total resistance of the circuit, the current flowing through the whole circuit and the current flowing through each resistor?

For resistors in parallel:

$$\frac{1}{R} = \frac{1}{R_1} + \frac{1}{R_2}$$

$$= \frac{1}{10} + \frac{1}{20}$$

$$= \frac{3}{20}$$

$$R = \frac{20}{3} \; \Omega$$

$$= 6.67 \; \Omega$$

From Ohm's law:

$$V = IR$$

$$I_1 = \frac{V}{R_1} \qquad \text{and} \qquad I_2 = \frac{V}{R_2}$$

$$= \frac{6}{10} \text{ A} \qquad\qquad\qquad = \frac{6}{20} \text{ A}$$

$$= 0.6 \text{ A} \qquad\qquad\qquad = 0.3 \text{ A}$$

The total current flowing in the circuit is the sum of the current values for each resistor:

$I = I_1 + I_2$
$= 0.6 + 0.3$ A
$= 0.9$ A

10.9 ELECTRICAL ENERGY AND POWER

To get an electric current to flow through a conductor the electrons must be driven by a potential difference. As the electrons move through the conductor they are involved in collisions with the atoms of the conductor and so *work* must be done to keep all the electrons moving in the same direction. The electrons dissipate energy to the atoms of the material which they pass through and so heat is produced in the material – this is the mechanism by which the filament of the X-ray tube is heated to produce electrons by thermionic emission (see Chs 21 and 28).

10.9.1 The Joule

As already discussed (Sect. 6.3), the joule is the SI unit of energy. The key to the method of calculating electrical energy lies in the definition of potential difference. As we discovered in Section 9.8.3, *the potential difference between two points is 1 volt when 1 joule of work is done in moving 1 coulomb of positive charge from one point to the other*. Thus we can say:

$$\text{volts} = \frac{\text{joules}}{\text{coulombs}} \qquad \textit{Equation 10.12}$$

or:

$$\text{joules} = \text{volts} \times \text{coulombs} \qquad \textit{Equation 10.13}$$

Since the ampere is a rate of flow of charge of 1 coulomb per second, then we can say:

$$\text{joules} = \text{volts} \times \text{amperes} \times \text{seconds}$$
$$\textit{Equation 10.14}$$

10.9.2 The Watt

We also saw in Section 6.3 that the SI unit of power is the watt, where 1 watt = 1 joule per second. Thus we can say that:

$$\frac{\text{joules}}{\text{seconds}} = \frac{\text{volts} \times \text{amperes} \times \text{seconds}}{\text{seconds}}$$

or:

$$\text{watts} = \text{volts} \times \text{amperes} \qquad \textit{Equation 10.15}$$

This is a general equation used in the calculation of electrical power which applies to any electrical system. It is, however, particularly useful to apply this formula to a metallic conductor which obeys Ohm's law.

10.9.3 Power in a Resistor

Consider a current I passing through a metallic resistor of resistance R when a potential difference V is applied across its ends. As previously discussed:

$$W = V \times I$$

However, we can apply Ohm's law to the resistor:

$$V = I \times R$$
$$\text{so } W = I \times I \times R$$
$$\text{or } W = I^2 R$$

By similar manipulations of Ohm's law we can get three possible equations for the electrical power in a resistor:

$$W = VI$$
$$W = I^2 R$$
$$W = \frac{V^2}{R} \qquad \textit{Equation 10.16}$$

The second of the three equations is probably the most useful one in radiography. Some calculations may clarify the use of these equations.

EXAMPLES

a. 10 A flows through a 2 Ω resistor. What power is generated in the resistor?

Using the equation:

$W = I^2 R$
$= (10)^2 \times 2$ W
$= 100 \times 2$ W
$= 200$ W

b. If a potential difference of 20 V is applied across a 2 Ω resistor, what power is generated in the resistor?

Using the equation:

$$W = \frac{V^2}{R}$$

$$= \frac{(20)^2}{2} \text{ W}$$

$$= \frac{400}{2} \text{ W}$$

$$= 200 \text{ W}$$

c. If a potential difference of 20 V is applied across a resistor and this causes a current of 10 A to flow through the resistor, what will be the power generated in the resistor?

Using the equation:

$$W = VI$$

$$= 20 \times 10 \text{ W}$$

$$= 200 \text{ W}$$

10.10 POWER LOSS IN CABLES

If we consider electricity in the form of a current I passing through a cable with a resistance R, it becomes apparent that some of the available electrical power will be 'lost' in the cable. The term lost does not imply that there is a breach of the law of conservation of energy but that the power is not available for the user at the far end of the cable – the 'lost' energy is in fact converted into heat.

It is obviously desirable that the power which is lost in the cables be kept to a minimum as this is not available to the user. If we consider that the power loss is given by the equation $P = I^2R$, then it can be seen that the power loss can be kept to a minimum in one of two ways:

1. reducing the current flowing within the cable
2. reducing the resistance of the cables.

10.10.1 Reducing the Current Flowing Within the Cable

Electrical power is a combination of the potential difference (V) across the cables and the current (I) flowing through them, i.e. $P = VI$. Thus, if we

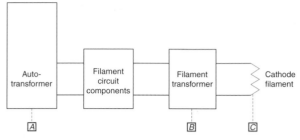

Figure 10.9 Transmission of electrical power from the autotransformer to the X-ray tube filament. Between points A and B, power is in the optimum form for transmission with minimum power loss – high voltage and low current. Thus 100 watts of power would be transmitted in the form of 100 volts and 1 ampere. Between points B and C, power is in the optimum form for heat generation at the filament. Thus 100 watts of power would be transmitted in the form of 10 volts and 10 amperes.

wish to transmit a given amount of electrical power with the minimum loss in the cables, this can be done by using a high voltage and a low current. This is shown in Figure 10.9, where a power of approximately 100 watts is required to heat the filament of the X-ray tube. This power is transmitted from the autotransformer to the filament transformer (see Ch. 17) in the form of a relatively high voltage and low current. At the filament we wish to use this power to generate heat, so it is converted to a relatively low voltage and high current at the filament transformer. Similar techniques are used in transmitting power from the generating stations to our homes.

10.10.2 Reducing the Resistance of the Cables

This is achieved in two ways: making the cables of a material with a low resistivity (usually copper) and making the cables as thick (large cross-sectional area) as possible. Because the cables are required to transmit power from one point to another there is little scope for the third possibility – reducing the length of the cables.

10.10.3 Mains Cable Resistance and X-ray Exposures

As we have previously discussed, there is a potential difference across any resistor which is related to the current through the resistor ($V = IR$). This volt drop is removed from the EMF available when a current flows to an X-ray unit. This can be seen in Equation 10.17:

$$V = EMF - IR_c \qquad \text{Equation 10.17}$$

where R_c is the resistance of the mains cables and V is the PD available at the mains supply when the unit is 'on load'. It is also worth noting that this volt drop is related to the resistance of the cables and the current to the X-ray unit.

In practice, with static X-ray units, the resistance of the mains cables is fairly constant so it is possible to compensate for this volt drop using a *static mains resistance compensator*. For mains-dependent mobile units the volt drop can vary for different parts of the hospital – obviously, the mains cables that reach the tenth floor are longer than the cables to the ground floor. This means that this type of mobile unit has an *adjustable mains resistance compensator*. Usually, the plug for the unit in the ward is coded in some way so that we know the correct setting for the compensator.

INSIGHT

Many modern mobile X-ray units overcome this problem by being 'mains-independent'. Such units remove power from the mains in small amounts *between exposures* (they require to be plugged into the mains when not in use) and then release this power through the X-ray tube during the exposure. The electrical power may be stored in special batteries or in capacitors (see Ch. 16).

SUMMARY

In this chapter you should have learnt the following:

- Simple electron theory of conduction (see Sect. 10.3)
- The requirements for a flow of electric current (see Sect. 10.4)
- The relationships between mA, mAs and millicoulombs (see Sect. 10.5)
- The meaning of potential difference and EMF (see Sect. 10.6)
- The meaning of electrical resistance (see Sect. 10.7)
- The factors affecting electrical resistance (see Sect. 10.7.1)
- Ohm's law (see Sect. 10.8)
- The effect of connecting resistors in series (see Sect. 10.8.1)
- The effect of connecting resistors in parallel (see Sect. 10.8.2)
- How to undertake calculations using Ohm's law (see Sect. 10.8.3)
- The meaning of electrical energy and power (see Sect. 10.9)
- The meaning of the joule (see Sect. 10.9.1)
- The meaning of the watt (see Sect. 10.9.2)
- Power in a resistor (see Sect. 10.9.3)
- Power loss in cables (see Sect. 10.10)
- Mains cable resistance and X-ray exposures (see Sect. 10.10.1).

SELF-TEST

a. Explain what is meant by the terms *electrical conductor* and *electrical insulator* and show how their electrical behaviour may be described by the simple electron theory of conduction.

b. List the factors upon which the resistance of a conductor depends.

c. 1 metre of wire of a given cross-sectional area is found to have the same resistance as a length of wire of the same material but with double the cross-sectional area. How long is the second wire?

d. Define Ohm's law and the unit of resistance.

e. Resistors are connected as shown in the diagram below:

Calculate the total resistance of the unit, I, I_1, I_2, V_1 and V_2.

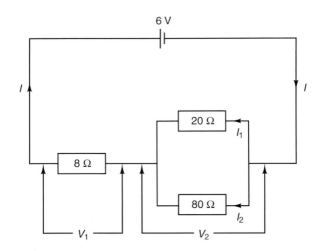

f. A current of 5 A flows through a 10 Ω resistor for 2 min. Calculate the energy used in the resistor and the power used.

g. The EMF from the mains supply to an X-ray set is 400 V. The resistance of the mains cables is 0.5 Ω. When a certain exposure is made, a current of 40 A is drawn from the mains. Calculate the volt drop in the cables and the potential difference available across the X-ray set during the exposure.

FURTHER READING

Ball J L, Moore A D 1997 Essential physics for radiographers, 3rd edn. Blackwell Scientific Publications, London, ch 7

Dowsett D J, Kenny P A, Johnston R E 1998 The physics of diagnostic imaging, Chapman & Hall Medical, London, ch 2

Chapter 11

Magnetism and Magnetic Resonance

CHAPTER CONTENTS

11.1 Aim 93

11.2 Magnetic Poles 93
       11.2.1 Force Between Two Magnetic
               Poles 94

11.3 Magnetic Fields 94

11.4 Magnetic Flux and Flux Density 95

11.5 Magnetic Induction 95
       11.5.1 Intensity of Magnetism 96

11.6 Types of Magnetic Materials 97
       11.6.1 Diamagnetism 97
       11.6.2 Paramagnetism 97
       11.6.3 Ferromagnetism 98

11.7 Hysteresis 99

11.8 Magnetic Resonance Imaging 99
       11.8.1 Nuclear Spins 100
       11.8.2 Producing an MRI Signal 101
       11.8.3 Image Weighting – Proton Density
               and the T_1 and T_2 Processes 102

Self-Test 105

Further Reading 105

11.1 AIM

The aim of this chapter is to explore the phenomenon of magnetism and to consider briefly its application to radiographic science. The key principles of magnetic resonance imaging (MRI) are also considered.

11.2 MAGNETIC POLES

If a magnetic compass is suspended freely, it will align itself in a north–south direction. Such a compass contains a *permanent* magnet (i.e. a magnet which is not easily demagnetised). Such a magnet contains two *poles*: the end pointing to the north is called the north pole of the magnet and the end pointing to the south, the south pole. Thus we see that there are two types of magnetic pole (north and south) in the same way as there are two types of electrical charge (positive and negative).

Many of the properties of magnetism are similar to those of electrical charges, as may be seen by comparing this chapter with Chapter 9. However, there is one fundamental difference between magnetic poles and electrical charges: electrical charges may exist in isolation (e.g. a single electron) whereas poles always exist in *pairs*. Consider the situation shown in Figure 11.1.

If we take a permanent magnet and cut it in half, when the two halves are separated we get two magnets with both north and south poles. Further subdivisions of the magnet will produce

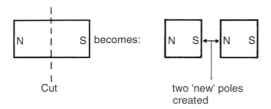

Figure 11.1 The effects of cutting a bar magnet in two. Magnetic poles always exist in pairs so there are now two bar magnets.

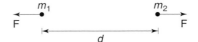

Figure 11.2 The mutual force of repulsion between two like poles, m_1 and m_2, separated by a distance, d. Note the similarities between this and Figure 9.1.

further smaller bar magnets, each with a north and a south pole. This would lead us to suspect that individual *atoms* of the material behave like small bar magnets with a north and a south pole; there is evidence that this is the case. As we shall see in Chapter 12, magnetism is caused by moving electrical charges, so magnetic atoms are produced by the circulation in their orbitals of the charged electrons of the atoms. When the orbitals of the electrons of an atom tend to be in the same direction, then the total effect is to produce a very magnetic atom (e.g. iron), whereas if the orbitals are in opposite directions they tend to cancel out each other's effect and so a very weak magnetic atom exists.

11.2.1 Force Between Two Magnetic Poles

The effect of two magnetic poles on each other is very similar to the effect of electrical charges on each other (see Sect. 9.3) and may be stated as:

Like poles repel while unlike poles attract.

Calculating the magnitude of the force between two poles in a vacuum is likewise a similar argument to that between two charges. For the purpose of such calculations, a north pole is considered to be positive and a south pole is considered to be negative. Thus if poles of strength m_1 and m_2 are separated by a distance d (Figure 11.2) then a mutual force F exists between them,

$$F \propto \frac{m_1 \times m_2}{d^2} \qquad \text{Equation 11.1}$$

In the International System of Units (SI) system the constant of proportionality in this equation

is $\frac{1}{4}\pi\mu_0$ so that Equation 11.1 can now be rewritten:

$$F = \frac{m_1 m_2}{4\pi\mu_0 d^2} \qquad \text{Equation 11.2}$$

where F is in newtons, d is in meters and m_1 and m_2 are in webers (Wb). μ_0 is the 'permeability of free space' and has a value of $4\pi \times 10^{-7}$ henry per meter (H.m^{-1}). The henry is further discussed in Chapter 13.

Again the similarities between Equations 11.2 and 9.2 emphasise the close link that exists between magnetism and electricity. This similarity is further extended if the poles are embedded in a medium:

$$F = \frac{m_1 m_2}{4\pi\mu d^2} \qquad \text{Equation 11.3}$$

where μ is the 'permeability' of the medium. The term d^2 in the equations shows that the force between magnetic poles (like that between electrical charges) obeys the inverse-square law (see Ch. 3).

11.3 MAGNETIC FIELDS

A magnetic field is said to exist at a point if a force would be experienced by a magnetic pole placed at that point. Thus the term *magnetic field* is used to indicate the extent of the magnetic effect around (and within) a magnetised body.

Figure 11.3 illustrates the concept of magnetic lines of force around a bar magnet. The arrows on the lines of force indicate the direction of the force exerted on a north pole placed at that point. If this north pole were free to move it would thus travel along the line of force. The total number of lines of force is referred to as the *magnetic flux* and this will be considered in more detail in the following section.

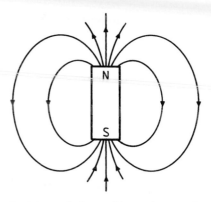

Figure 11.3 Magnetic lines of force due to a bar magnet. The arrows point in the direction a north pole would move if placed in that position.

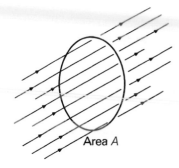

Figure 11.4 Lines of magnetic flux through an area *A*.

INSIGHT

Although there are many similarities between electrical and magnetic lines of force, there are some fundamental differences. One such difference is that magnetic lines of force are *continuous*, as can be seen in Figure 11.3. In contrast, electrical lines of force always begin on a positive charge and end on a negative charge.

11.4 MAGNETIC FLUX AND FLUX DENSITY

Consider Figure 11.4. The total number of lines of force passing through the area *A* is defined as the *magnetic flux (N)* passing through (or linked with) *A*. The *magnetic flux density (B)* is the number of lines of flux in a unit area placed at right angles to the lines of flux. If we assume that the area *A* in Figure 11.4 is at right angles to the parallel lines of magnetic flux, then the relationship can be stated thus:

$$B = \frac{N}{A} \qquad \qquad Equation\ 11.4$$

As already mentioned, the unit of magnetic flux is the weber (Wb) and the unit of flux density is the tesla (T), so:

$$1\ T = 1\ Wb \cdot m^{-2}$$

The definition within the SI system relates the electrical units and the units of magnetic flux density through the motor principle.

We shall use the concepts of magnetic flux and magnetic flux density in Chapter 13 when we consider electromagnetic induction and in Chapter 15 when we consider the motor principle.

11.5 MAGNETIC INDUCTION

When discussing electrostatics we saw that a charge could be induced in a material and we now find that a similar situation exists for magnetism, i.e. magnetism may be induced in a suitable material. This is achieved by placing the substance within a magnetic field and so subjecting it to a *magnetising force (H)*. If the substance contains magnetic atoms, these will tend to rotate to align with the direction of the magnetising force.

Figure 11.5 illustrates this principle where an unmagnetised sample (Figure 11.5A) initially has its atoms pointing in random directions. When it is subjected to a magnetising force (Figure 11.5B) then these tend to line up with the direction of the force. This process produces a north pole at one end of the sample and a south pole at the other and so magnetism is said to have been induced in the sample. *Note* the similarity between magnetic induction and the induction of charge in a sample caused by the rotation of polar molecules (see Sect. 9.7.2.2).

The effect of aligning atoms is to produce a total flux density, *B*, within the sample which is greater than that in the air alone, such that:

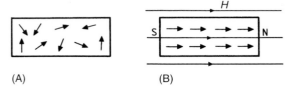

(A)   (B)

Figure 11.5   Inducing magnetism in a sample (the arrows represent the north end of a molecular magnet). (A) The randomised distribution of molecular magnets when no magnetic field is applied; (B) the molecular magnets align with a magnetic field.

$$B = \mu H \qquad \qquad \textit{Equation 11.5}$$

where μ is the permeability of the medium (see Sect. 11.2.1). Here the magnetising force, H, is regarded as the *cause* of the magnetic flux density, B, in a medium of permeability μ.

Different substances respond to different extents. A sample containing very magnetic atoms has a large value of μ so that, once the whole sample is magnetised, a correspondingly large magnetic flux density results.

Table 11.1 shows the *relative permeability* of some common materials – the relative permeability (μ_r) is found by comparing the permeability of the substance (μ) with that of a vacuum (μ_0). This is stated mathematically thus:

$$\mu_r = \frac{\mu}{\mu_0} \qquad \qquad \textit{Equation 11.6}$$

As can be seen from Table 11.1, there is a wide variety of relative permeability in different substances, ranging from just under unity for

bismuth (difficult to magnetise) to 80 000 for mumetal (easily and strongly magnetised).

11.5.1   Intensity of Magnetism

The total magnetic flux density, B, obtained by applying a magnetising force, H, to a substance is composed of two factors:

1.   the magnetic flux density due to the air around the sample ($\mu_0 H$)
2.   the magnetic flux density due to the induced magnetism in the material.

The total flux density is given by the equation $B = \mu H$ (see Equation 11.5). However, it is sometimes desirable to separate these two factors so that the magnetism induced in the sample may be considered separately. This is known as the *intensity of magnetism, I*, of the sample and measures the extent to which the sample itself has become magnetised.

INSIGHT

The intensity of magnetism is defined as *the magnetic moment per unit volume of the magnetised sample*. This is the turning force which will be applied to a field perpendicular to its axis. If a pole strength p per unit area is induced in a sample of cross-sectional area A and length L, then the magnetic moment is pAL.

Thus the intensity of magnetism $= \dfrac{\text{magnetic moment}}{\text{volume}} = \dfrac{pAL}{AL} = p$ (in $Wb \cdot m^{-2}$).

The tesla (T) is the unit of magnetic flux density, employed in MRI to describe the magnetic field strength of the magnet, whether low, medium or high field. Clinical MRI systems operate at about 0.02–0.3 T, 0.5–1 T and 1.5–2+ T respectively. The gauss (G) is not an SI unit, but an older CGS (centimetre-gram-second) unit. It is still in popular usage as a unit of measurement for the magnetic fields surrounding MRI systems. Note that 1 T = 10 000 G (1 G = 1×10^{-4} T). The 5 G line encloses an area of restricted access, particularly to avoid affecting cardiac pacemakers. It is

Table 11.1	Relative permeability of materials	
Material	Relative permeability (μ_r)	Comments
Vacuum	1.0	By definition
Air	1.000004	Usually taken as 1.0
Water	0.99999	Diamagnetic
Bismuth	0.999985	Diamagnetic
Platinum	1.0001	Paramagnetic
Cobalt	240	Ferromagnetic
Nickel	660	Ferromagnetic
Iron	5500	Ferromagnetic
Stalloy	6700	Ferromagnetic alloy
Mumetal	80 000	Ferromagnetic alloy

interesting to note that the earth's magnetic field is only about 0.5 G, some 20 000 times less powerful than a 1 T magnet. The powerful fields obtained in MRI use the phenomenon of superconductivity (see Sect. 10.3.1.1).

11.6 TYPES OF MAGNETIC MATERIALS

We are all probably aware that some materials are easily and strongly magnetised while others appear to be unaffected by the presence of an external magnetic field. Thus we may confidently expect to pick up some steel pins using a bar magnet but would not expect to pick up wooden matches using the same magnet. Such differences in magnetic behaviour of different materials result in there being three basic types of magnetic substance. These are called *diamagnetic, paramagnetic* and *ferromagnetic*. Radiography uses ferromagnetic materials in the construction of transformers (see Ch. 17). They are also used in permanent MRI magnets. Ferromagnetic implants in patients can be of concern in MRI, as they may show up as image artifacts or even move within the powerful magnetic field. External ferromagnetic objects such as scissors or even oxygen cylinders can be pulled into the MRI magnet at high speed, creating a projectile hazard. Diamagnetic and paramagnetic materials are also relevant to MRI and will be considered below.

11.6.1 Diamagnetism

Diamagnetism is the term given to the influence of the applied magnetic field on the electrons orbiting the nuclei within any substance. As we shall see in Chapter 13, Lenz's law of electromagnetic induction describes the opposing effect between the induced currents and the varying magnetic fields applied to a conductor. Electrons orbiting a nucleus may be considered as conductors with zero electrical resistance. They thus suffer changes in their orbitals when an external magnetic field is applied. These changes in the orbitals of the electrons caused by the magnetic field interacting with them result in the orbitals opposing the external magnetic field (similar to Lenz's law for a conductor). They remain in this condition until the magnetic field is removed and then they revert to their original orbitals. Two conclusions follow:

1. All materials contain some diamagnetic properties
2. Magnetic induction is produced within the sample which *opposes* the direction of the applied magnetic field, so the relative permeability is always less than unity. Bismuth (Table 11.1) has a relative permeability of 0.999985 and is an example of a diamagnetic material.

Diamagnetism is normally a very weak phenomenon and is usually completely obscured by paramagnetism and ferromagnetism when these exist in a material. Diamagnetism is not affected by the temperature of the material. Most body tissues are diamagnetic, weakly opposing the magnetic field in MRI.

11.6.2 Paramagnetism

The cause of magnetism in individual atoms is the spinning and orbiting of electrons around their nuclei. If the effect of each electron is cancelled out by the effect of another electron, as outlined above, then the material is diamagnetic. If the resultant effect, however, allows us to consider the atom as an elementary bar magnet then the material is *paramagnetic*. In such materials the atoms will align with an external magnetic field, as shown in Figure 11.5.

Temperature is a measure of the kinetic energy of the atoms of a material (see Sect. 8.3) and so is a factor that tends to destroy the ordered alignment of atoms within the sample. For this reason, a paramagnetic sample rapidly becomes demagnetised at room temperature after the external magnetic field has been removed – the demagnetisation is caused by the disruption that results from collisions between the atoms. As the temperature is increased, it becomes more difficult to magnetise a paramagnetic sample and there is a point at which it may not be possible to magnetise the material at all. At this point it is solely a diamagnetic since this effect is not influenced by the temperature.

Platinum (Table 11.1) has a relative permeability of 1.0001 and is an example of a paramagnetic material. Note that the figure of the relative permeability is composed of a *positive* effect due to paramagnetism and a negative effect due to diamagnetism.

Gadolinium-based contrast agents used in MRI are paramagnetic, weakly reinforcing the magnetic field and giving an increase in signal on T_1-weighted imaging sequences (see Appendix D). Certain body substances, such as methaemoglobin, deoxyhaemoglobin and melanin, are paramagnetic. There is also a group of so-called superparamagnetic substances – materials which exhibit a large positive magnetic susceptibility. But they differ from ferromagnetic materials by consisting of small particles which do not display bulk ferromagnetic properties. They become transiently magnetised within a magnetic field. An example is particles of iron oxide, used as a negative contrast agent in MRI in T_2-weighted imaging sequences (see Appendix D). Some blood products such as haemosiderin are also superparamagnetic.

11.6.3 Ferromagnetism

Diamagnetism and paramagnetism are extremely weak magnetic phenomena compared to *ferromagnetism*. Ferromagnetic materials (Table 11.1) have relative permeabilities which are measured in hundreds or thousands. Because of this the magnetic flux density of magnetised ferromagnetic materials may be sufficiently large to allow us to put it to practical uses – ferromagnetic materials are used in transformer cores.

The reason for the strong magnetic induction of ferromagnetic materials lies in the behaviour of so-called *magnetic domains* within them. Such a domain is a small volume within the material where all the atoms are pointing in the same direction. The random alignment of these domains in an unmagnetised sample is shown in Figure 11.6A.

If an external magnetic field is applied to this material, it will apply a rotating force to each

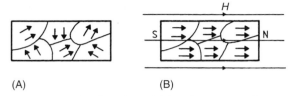

(A)   (B)

Figure 11.6 The 'domains' within a ferromagnetic material (the arrows represent the north end of each molecular magnet). (A) The material in its unmagnetised state; (B) how the domains align with the external magnetic field in a magnetised sample.

domain, causing the atoms in the domain to turn. If the force is sufficiently strong, all the domains will align with the magnetic field. In this condition the sample is said to have reached *magnetic saturation* since no further magnetisation is possible.

It is because of the alignment of the atoms within each domain that a ferromagnetic material shows such a strong induced magnetisation to an applied magnetic field: each domain behaves like a team of atomic magnets working together. In a paramagnetic material the atoms behave as individual magnets and so it is much more difficult to align them to an applied magnetic field because of the disruptive effect of interatomic collisions.

Ferromagnetic materials change their properties with temperature. At a particular temperature, known as the *Curie temperature*, the atoms can no longer overcome the disrupting effect of the increased interatomic collisions and so the domains disappear. Thus, below the Curie temperature the material is ferromagnetic and above the Curie temperature the material is paramagnetic. Because of the resulting atomic disorder, the relative permeability is greatly reduced.

Examples of ferromagnetic materials and their relative permeabilities are given in Table 11.1. We are probably most familiar with the magnetic properties of iron, but stalloy, because of its use in transformer cores, is also important in radiographic science. The Curie temperature for iron is 1043 K (770°C).

An important phenomenon in the magnetisation of a ferromagnetic material is the effect known as *hysteresis* and this will now be considered briefly. Because hysteresis is of great importance in the choice of materials for a transformer core, it will be discussed fully in Chapter 17, which deals with the AC transformer.

11.7 HYSTERESIS

For diamagnetic and paramagnetic materials, the intensity of magnetisation within the sample, I, is proportional to the magnetising force, H. Thus if H is doubled then I is also doubled. However, this is not the case with ferromagnetic materials due to the effect of the domains on each other. Two types of forces exist between the domains:

1. An *elastic* or *reversible* force caused by the movement of the domain boundaries – some domains get larger at the expense of others when an external magnetic field is applied. This is reversible when the field H is removed
2. A *frictional* or *irreversible* force corresponding to the rotation of the domains as they attempt to align themselves with the external magnetic field in a series of minute jerks.

This jerking movement between the domains means that the applied magnetic field increases before some of the domains respond to it by rotating. Thus the orientation of the domains and hence the induced magnetism (I) *lags behind* the magnetising force (H). If the magnetising force is now removed, some magnetism will remain in the sample and require a magnetising force in the opposite direction to remove it. This effect of the magnetism lagging behind the magnetising force is known as *hysteresis* and will be discussed further in Chapter 17, where its effect on the efficiency of an AC transformer will be considered.

INSIGHT

The effect described for hysteresis is exactly the same as the situation which exists if you try to rotate a book on a table top. The rotational force applied must increase to a point where it is greater than the frictional forces between the book and the table top before the book will rotate. If the book is to be returned to its original orientation, a rotational force in the opposite direction, larger than the frictional forces, must now be applied.

11.8 MAGNETIC RESONANCE IMAGING

The technique of MRI evolved from nuclear magnetic resonance (NMR), which was discovered by Bloch and Purcell in 1946. NMR is still used to obtain spectra, giving us information about the presence of chemical molecules and their concentrations, a technique known clinically as magnetic resonance spectroscopy (MRS). The term NMR fell out of favour in clinical imaging as patients may have misunderstood the term 'nuclear'. The technique of MRI uses magnetic fields and radiowaves and does not in fact involve any radioactivity or other ionising radiation.

The term NMR tells us that:

- The atomic *nucleus* is involved
- A *magnetic* field is applied
- *Resonance* occurs.

Resonance takes place when energy is applied to a physical system at that system's natural or resonant frequency (Table 11.2). The magnetic properties of MR-sensitive nuclei, including the single proton of the hydrogen nucleus, rotate or precess within a powerful magnetic field, as shown by Figure 11.7. The speed of this rotation is proportional to the strength of the magnetic field. Energy is efficiently transferred at this particular frequency and the amplitude of the system's energy increases. In the case of MRI, the system consists of hydrogen nuclei whose magnetic fields are oscillating at a particular frequency. The energy is transferred into the patient's hydrogen nuclei by a radiofrequency (RF) antenna. Shortly afterwards, 'relaxation' of the nuclei occurs,

Table 11.2 Frequency of hydrogen proton precession (Lamor frequency) in differing magnetic field strengths	
Field strength (tesla)	Frequency of precession (MHz) (Lamor frequency)
0.5	21.3
1.0	42.6
1.5	63.9
2.0	85.2
3	127.8

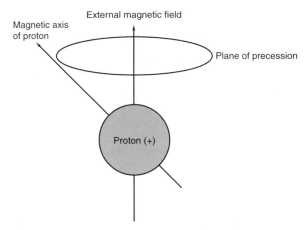

Figure 11.7 A spinning proton has a distinct magnetic axis. If this proton is placed in an external magnetic field, the proton will align with the field so that its axis of rotation sweeps out a cone, rather like a spinning top as it is about to fall over. This movement is called precession.

returning a measurable radio signal. Clinical NMR gives us a chemical spectrum, based on other nuclei such as phosphorus as well as hydrogen, whereas clinical MRI gives us a two-dimensional or three-dimensional image based on the magnetic properties of hydrogen.

11.8.1 Nuclear Spins

All atomic particles, including protons, neutrons and electrons, possess a property known as spin. This can be assigned to discrete possible energy levels at set values, such as 'spin up' and 'spin down' with a fixed energy difference between them (Figure 11.8). It can be seen that it is possible for an atomic particle to acquire energy from an external source (such as an RF emission) and move from the low-energy to the high-energy state. However, this higher-energy situation may not be stable and so the particle will lose its energy ('relax' back) over time.

There are fixed energy differences between many energy levels in the atom, for example between electron orbitals and (less obviously) in the nucleus. When particles move between these levels, they gain or lose fixed amounts of energy. Now particles such as electrons prefer to be paired up. This pairing consists of a spin-up electron and a spin-down electron and results in a stable state, with cancelling of the overall spin property. It occurs in chemical bonds. A similar situation occurs with particles in the atomic nucleus. If these are also paired up, no overall nuclear spin property will result. Nuclei with an odd number of total protons and neutrons (i.e. nucleons) will have an overall spin state. As mentioned above, both protons and neutrons have spins. It is also interesting to note that both protons and neutrons have magnetic fields. So nuclei with an odd number of contained particles will have useful magnetic properties which we can manipulate in MRI. Examples include hydrogen-1 (also written as ^{1}H), oxygen-17, carbon-13 and fluorine-19. The numbers refer to the mass number of the isotope.

As can be seen from Table 11.3, ^{1}H is very common within the body, found in water, fats, carbohydrates, proteins and so on. It also has a very high relative sensitivity in MRI (i.e. it produces a lot of signal). It would be nice to be able to use carbon or oxygen for clinical MRI as these are common biological elements. Unfortunately their most common isotopes are ^{12}C and ^{16}O, both

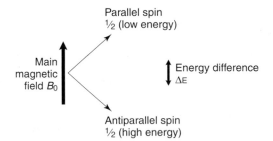

Figure 11.8 A simple representation of the spin states of a hydrogen nucleus.

Table 11.3 Concentrations and magnetic sensitivity of isotopes found in the body		
Isotope	Body concentration (mol.l^{-1})	Relative sensitivity
^{1}H	99	1.0
^{13}C	0.1	0.016
^{17}O	0.31	0.29
^{19}F	0.0066	0.83
^{31}P	0.35	0.066

of which do not have a useful spin property. ^{31}P is the most common isotope of phosphorus and does have a useful spin property – it is used in MRS to study metabolic processes (adenosine triphosphate, adenosine diphosphate and phosphocreatine) but is not present in very high concentrations within the body.

Figure 11.8 shows us that a hydrogen nucleus can be considered to have two spin states, one low-energy and the other high-energy. Resonant radio energy can move some spins to the higher-energy state. The MR process does *not* mean that nuclei themselves are physically made to flip over. It is their magnetic fields that are manipulated in MRI.

11.8.2 Producing an MRI Signal

Although the actual process is more complex and subtle, we can assume for the sake of simplicity that the ^{1}H nucleus (which is a proton) exists in two spin states within the influence of a strong static magnetic field B_0, namely 'spin up' and 'spin down'. We are talking about millions of protons within tissues. There is a slight excess of spins within the spin-up condition (aligned with the main or static magnetic field) and thus the overall magnetisation of the tissue is parallel to the static field. This orientation is referred to as $0°$.

Figure 11.9 shows that the directions of the magnetic fields of individual protons (typically referred to as nuclear spins or just spins) are

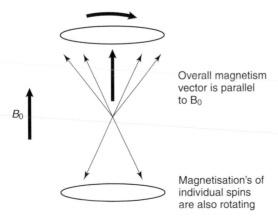

Overall magnetism vector is parallel to B$_0$

B_0

Magnetisation's of individual spins are also rotating

Figure 11.9 A simplified representation of how spins behave in a magnetic field.

actually rotating. This occurs when the protons are placed within a strong magnetic field. The spins can be thought of as having angular momentum, rotating around the axis of B_0 and at an angle to it.

When tissue is placed in a strong magnetic field, two things happen. The magnetic orientations of the spins previously aligned randomly in every direction:

- line up either parallel or antiparallel with the main or static magnetic field B_0
- rotate at the resonant frequency, which is called the Larmor frequency.

The Larmor frequency (ω) at which the spins rotate is influenced by the gyromagnetic ratio (γ) which is a constant for a particular MR-sensitive isotope, such as ^{1}H or ^{31}P. The gyromagnetic ratio of ^{1}H is 42.6 MHz per tesla. Larmor frequency is also determined by the field strength B_0 of the magnet.

The Larmor equation states that:

$$\omega = \gamma B_0 \qquad \qquad Equation\ 11.7$$

This means that, if resonance is to occur, we have to apply an RF electromagnetic field B_1 to a patient at a greater frequency using a high field magnet than when using a low field magnet (Table 11.2).

Many physical systems, such as guitar strings, tuning forks and bridges – the Millennium Bridge in London demonstrated this spectacularly – have a natural or resonant frequency. At that frequency energy can be readily transferred from outside, increasing the system's amplitude, provided that the energy is applied at the resonant frequency. If the frequency is too high or low (i.e. off resonance), energy exchange will not occur.

INSIGHT

The Larmor equation is very important in MRI, since:

- Local changes in field strength within a patient, perhaps from poor magnet design or metallic implants within the body, will mean that effective resonance does not occur and drop-off in signal results
- Variations in resonant frequency can be applied

deliberately by applying *gradients*, which are linearly varying magnetic fields, across the body. This is how the RF pulse can be targeted to resonate a particular tissue and thus produce slices through the body in three planes.

An RF electromagnetic field is applied to tissue at the Larmor frequency and at $90°$ to B_0. This is produced from a current-carrying loop of wire known as a transmit coil. An electromagnetic field is generated by a current in a coil. This field has two components at right angles, one electrical and one magnetic.

The RF waves transfer some energy to the nuclear spins in the patient, promoting some from the lower-energy parallel spin state to the higher-energy antiparallel spin state.

This process 'flips' the overall magnetisation towards the transverse plane, at $90°$ from B_0 and in the direction of the receiver coil. The size of the flip angle α depends on the strength and duration of the RF transmit pulse.

The effect of an RF pulse on the 'flip angle' of the tissue magnetisation is illustrated in Figure 11.10.

The absorption of RF energy in the patient: (1) changes spin levels and (2) causes the rotating spins briefly to get into phase (i.e. they all point in the same direction as they rotate, rather than being aligned randomly). This is rather like the

spins all pointing together towards say 3 o'clock on a clock face as they rotate, rather than facing to every point on the clock.

The signal in the receiver coil is alternating and falls off in amplitude with time once the RF pulse is turned off. This is referred to as a free induction decay and shown in Figure 11.11. If all the spins are in phase they will rotate around together at the Larmor frequency, rather like a rotating beam from a lighthouse, as shown by Figure 11.12. Every time the direction of the in phase spins is towards the receiver coil, a strong electrical signal will be induced in that coil. This is according to the laws of electromagnetic induction, where a changing magnetic field induces a current in a conductor.

The reduction in amplitude with time occurs because the spins dephase over time once the RF pulse is turned off. As the spins no longer all produce current in the receiver coil at the same instant, the amplitude of the signal decreases until a new RF pulse is applied.

11.8.3 Image Weighting – Proton Density and The T_1 and T_2 Processes

The most basic tissue characteristic in MRI is the *proton density*. This is the closest analogy that we have to the processes of X-ray attenuation in

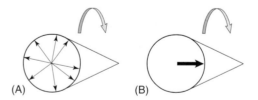

Figure 11.11 The effect of a radiofrequency (RF) pulse on spin phase, looking along the long axis of B_0. (A) No RF pulse, rotating spins out of phase. (B) RF pulse on, rotating spins in phase.

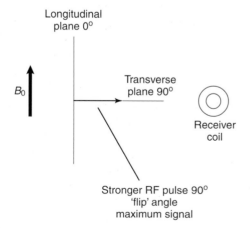

Figure 11.10 Diagram to show the influence of radiofrequency (RF) pulse on flip angle.

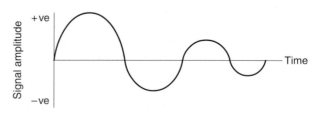

Figure 11.12 Diagram showing the decay of a magnetic resonance signal with time.

computed tomography (which depend on tissue and electron density). Therefore, tissues with a high number of protons per cubic millimetre have the potential to give us a good strong signal. In addition, a large voxel (volume element) will always give us more signal than a small one, assuming that they both contain the same type of tissue.

The T_1 and T_2 processes, which are discussed in more detail below, are fundamental to the way that MRI works. Unlike computed tomography, which really only deals with one tissue characteristic – the linear attenuation coefficient μ in X-ray absorption – in MRI we can image lots of tissue characteristics. This is often what gives MRI its sensitivity and specificity when assessing pathology. It was the hope that different tissues, including malignant or benign tumours, would have very different T1 and T_2 times that drove forward early clinical MRI development. It is important to note that fat appears bright on a T1-weighted image, while fluid appears bright on a T2-weighted image.

Once the RF field B_0 is turned off at the end of an RF pulse, *the T1 and T2 processes occur simultaneously*. The T1 process occurs relatively slowly, over several hundred milliseconds to a few seconds, while the T2 process occurs more quickly, over several tens to a few hundred milliseconds.

Therefore the basic MRI image is made up of the T_1 signal characteristics, T_2 signal characteristics and the proton density of tissues. It normally contains a mixture of all of these. By manipulating the operator parameters in MRI we can weight the images so that the collection of signal from one process predominates over the others.

The T_1 process is variously referred to as T_1 recovery or relaxation, longitudinal recovery or relaxation and spin-lattice relaxation.

The effect of applying an RF pulse is to cause the overall magnetisation vector of the tissue to move from 0° (i.e. from the longitudinal plane, parallel to B_0) to any other angle with respect to it. If the vector is tipped into the transverse plane (i.e. to 90° from the longitudinal plane), then maximum signal will result in a receiver coil. When the RF pulse is turned off, the vector will gradually relax or recover back towards the longitudinal plane. Thus the component of the magnetisation in the transverse plane will reduce

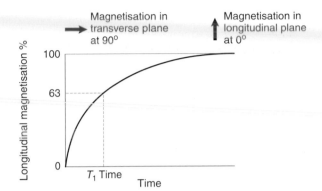

Figure 11.13 Diagram showing longitudinal relaxation, illustrating the T_1 time.

or relax with time. Relaxation generally refers to a releasing of energy back to the local environment. The component of the magnetisation in the longitudinal plane will increase or recover with time, as shown by Figure 11.13.

The T_2 process is called T_2 relaxation, transverse relaxation or spin-spin relaxation. As mentioned previously, before the RF pulse is applied to a tissue the spins are oriented randomly in all directions around the 360° circle of the transverse plane. The RF pulse briefly causes the precessing out-of-phase spins to line up with one another in phase until the RF is turned off. Then the spins gradually dephase in the transverse plane, with a resultant fall-off in signal which is known as free induction decay. This is shown by Figure 11.14.

Explaining how T_1- and T_2-weighted scans are obtained is a complex topic that is beyond the scope of this chapter. However, T_1 images are sampled early on in the longitudinal recovery and transverse recovery processes. This emphasises longitudinal recovery time differences between fat and water. T_1 scans are relatively quick to obtain. T_2 images are sampled late on in the longitudinal and transverse recovery processes. This emphasises transverse recovery differences between fat and water. T_2 scans used to be relatively slow to obtain and patient motion artefact was more likely. On modern scanners T_2-weighted images can be obtained very rapidly using fast spin echo or single-shot imaging in under 1 s and do not suffer from motion artefact. The type of image weighting is obtained by adjusting various key parameters in pulse sequences (see Appendix D) which are series

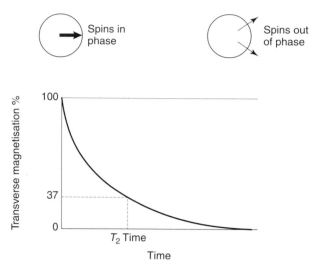

Figure 11.14 Diagram showing transverse relaxation, to illustrate the T_2 time.

of RF pulses (in spin echo imaging) and RF pulses plus applied magnetic gradients (in gradient echo imaging). In this context a gradient is an extra magnetic field which varies in amplitude in a regular linear way, rather like a constant slope or gradient.

SUMMARY

In this chapter you should have learnt:

- Magnetic poles always exist in *pairs* because the atoms of a magnetic substance behave like small bar magnets (see Sect. 11.2)
- The force between two magnetic poles is given by the equation $F = (m_1 \times m_2)/(4\pi\mu_0 d^2)$ where F is in newtons, m_1 and m_2 are in webers, d is in meters and μ is in henry per meter (see Sect. 11.2.1)
- If μ_0 is the permeability of a vacuum, and μ is the permeability of a substance, then the *relative permeability*, μ_r is given by $\mu_r = \mu/\mu_0$ (see Sect. 11.2.1)
- A *magnetic field* exists at a point if a force would be experienced by a magnetic pole placed at that point (see Sect. 11.3)
- The *magnetic force*, H, is the magnitude of the magnetic field (or field strength) (see Sect. 11.3)

- The *magnetic flux density*, B, is a measure of the amount of magnetic flux per unit area (Wb.m^{-2}) and has the special unit the tesla (T), where 1 T = 1 Wb.m^{-2}. It is dependent on the medium through which it passes (see Sect. 11.4)
- The relationship between the magnetising force, H, and the magnetic flux density, B, is given by the equation $B = \mu H$, where μ is the permeability of the medium (see Sect. 11.5)
- If:
  - μ_r is less than unity then the material is *diamagnetic*
  - μ_r is just greater than unity then the material is *paramagnetic*
  - μ_r is much greater than unity then the material is *ferromagnetic* (see Sect. 11.6)
- All materials are *diamagnetic*, but the effect is usually negligible compared to the *paramagnetism* or *ferromagnetism* in the same sample (see Sect. 11.6.1)
- At high temperatures, paramagnetic materials become diamagnetic. Ferromagnetics become paramagnetics above the *Curie temperature* (see Sects 11.6.2 and 11.6.3)
- The reason for the relatively high permeabilities of ferromagnetic materials is the internal ordered arrangement of atoms into *magnetic domains*. Within each domain the atoms point in the same direction but the direction of the domains is randomised in the non-magnetised material (see Sect. 11.6.3)
- The application of a magnetising force, H, to a ferromagnetic material results in two types of forces within the material:
  - one that allows the expansion of some domains at the expense of others and which will disappear when the magnetising force, H, is removed
  - one that rotates the domains in the same direction as H but which will not disappear completely when H is removed (see Sect. 11.7)
- The fact that the domains are 'sticky' in their movement means that the

magnetisation of the sample (*I*) lags behind the magnetising force *H*. This is known as *hysteresis* (see Sect. 11.7)

- The fact that a strong external magnetic field can influence the protons in the nucleus and that this can be utilised in MRI (see Sect. 11.8). MRI employs the magnetic properties of hydrogen nuclei, often referred to as 'spins', which rotate or precess in a powerful magnetic field at the Larmor frequency. The Larmor frequency relates to the magnetic field strength (Sect. 11.8.2)
- If radiowave energy (the B_1 field) is applied at 90° to the spins and at the Larmor frequency, resonance occurs, with promotion of some of the spins to a higher energy state, aligned in the opposite direction from the main or static magnetic field (the B_0 field) of the magnet. The radiowave pulse also puts the rotating spins into phase in the transverse plane, producing a strong oscillating signal in a receiver coil (Sect. 11.8.2)

- Once the radiowave energy or pulse is removed the spins relax back to a lower-energy state with the release of a decaying signal which carries information on the type of body tissue occupied by the spins (Figure 11.14)
- There are two main ways in which the spins relax:
  - longitudinal relaxation, whereby the overall magnetisation returns to the plane of the main magnetic field
  - transverse relaxation, whereby the spins dephase in the transverse plane and lose signal coherence. These are also termed the T1 and T2 decay processes (Figure 11.12)
- The main types of MRI image include T_1 weighting (in which fat appears bright) and T_2 weighting (in which fluid appears bright) (Sect. 11.8.2)
- The technique of NMR or MRS produces a chemical spectrum rather than an image and may use other nuclei in addition to hydrogen.

SELF-TEST

a. Give the equation which can be used to calculate the force between two magnetic poles m_1 and m_2 separated by a distance *d* in a vacuum.

b. Draw the magnetic field around a bar magnet (for simplicity, the influence on this field by the earth's magnetic field can be ignored).

c. Materials may be diamagnetic, paramagnetic or ferromagnetic. Discuss the differences between the three types of materials.

d. Discuss the meaning of the term hysteresis.

e. Draw some basic diagrams to show what happens to the magnetic properties of hydrogen nuclei (spins) when a radio pulse is applied and then turned off in MRI.

f. Describe the main types of image appearance or weighting which can be found in MRI.

FURTHER READING

Ball J L, Moore A D 1997 Essential physics for radiographers, 3rd edn. Blackwell Scientific Publications, London, ch 8
Brown M A 1999 MRI: basic principles and applications, 2nd edn. Wiley-Liss, New York, chs 1 and 2
Dowsett D J, Kenny P A, Johnston R E 1998 The physics of diagnostic imaging. Chapman & Hall Medical, London, ch 19
Hashemi R H, Bradley W G 2003 MRI: the basics. Lippincott, Williams & Wilkins

Lufkin R B 1998 The MRI manual, 2nd edn. Mosby
McRobbie D W, Moore E A, Graves M J, Prince M R 2003 MRI: from picture to proton. Cambridge University Press, Cambridge
Ohanian H C 1994 Principles of physics. W W Norton, London, ch 21
Westbrook C, Talbot J, Kaut C K 2005 MRI in practice, 3rd edn. Blackwell, Oxford

Chapter 12

Electromagnetism

CHAPTER CONTENTS

12.1 Aim   106

12.2 Introduction   106

12.3 Electron Flow and 'Conventional' Current   106

12.4 Magnetic Field Due to a Straight Wire   107

12.5 Magnetic Field Due to a Circular Coil of Wire   107

12.6 Magnetic Field Due to a Solenoid   108

12.7 The Electromagnetic Relay   109
     12.7.1 Operation   110

Self-Test   110

Further Reading   111

12.1 AIM

The aim of this chapter is to consider the basic properties of magnetism discussed in Chapter 11 and show how these can be applied to a current-carrying conductor, thus giving an electromagnet.

12.2 INTRODUCTION

In Chapter 11 it was shown that magnetism is a phenomenon associated with atoms, and is due to the spinning and orbiting of electrons around those atoms. Electrons are negatively charged particles (Sect. 9.3), and so we may conclude that magnetism is caused by moving electric charges. It is thus reasonable to ask whether an electric current in a wire (for example) may also produce a magnetic field, since an electric current is just the flow of electrons in a conductor (Sects 10.3 and 10.4). This is found to be so in practice and the term *electromagnetism* is used to describe this effect (i.e. *electricity* producing *magnetism*).

12.3 ELECTRON FLOW AND 'CONVENTIONAL' CURRENT

When electricity was first discovered, it was assumed that it was the *positive* charges that flow in a conductor, and not the negative charges. This concept is now known as the 'conventional' current. However, it is now known that the positive charges in a solid material *do not have any net movement* (although they vibrate with heat energy; Ch. 8), since they form the protons in the nuclei of atoms (Ch. 26). Thus it is the electrons that move in a solid, as explained by the elementary electron theory of conduction (Sect. 10.3).

In gas or liquid, any positive and negative charges present may take part in current flow, since the positive charges are free to move, unlike in a solid. In radiography and many other subjects, however, it is the electron flow in conductors which is most frequently under consideration, and herein lies a difficulty, for many rules (or conventions) in electromagnetism and electromagnetic induction (Ch. 13) are based upon the totally erroneous assumption of the 'conventional' current, which in a mathematical sense is supposed to flow in the opposite direction to that of the electrons.

This and further chapters will therefore discuss both electromagnetism and electromagnetic induction on the basis of *electron flow only*, in an attempt to eliminate much of the confusion that undoubtedly exists at present in many people's minds. Some caution is therefore required when studying these subjects from other books, as they may invoke the 'conventional' current for their rules. Differences in the two approaches are explained in the Insights where appropriate.

12.4 MAGNETIC FIELD DUE TO A STRAIGHT WIRE

Historically, the presence of a magnetic field around a current-carrying conductor was first discovered by Oersted when passing a current through a straight wire placed near a magnetic compass, as illustrated in Figure 12.1.

If the wire is aligned in a north–south direction (i.e. along the direction of the compass needle), then an electric current through the wire causes deflections of the compass, as shown: *clockwise* when the wire is above the compass (A), and *anticlockwise* when the wire is below the compass (B). This is only possible if the lines of magnetic force (Sect. 11.3) are circular and in an anticlockwise direction when viewed along the same direction as the movement of the flowing electrons. We may therefore use the following convention:

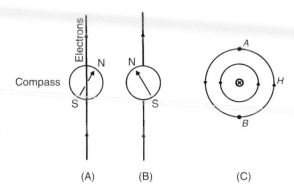

Figure 12.1 (A and B) The effect of the magnetic field produced by the electrons flowing in the wire upon a magnetic compass. (C) If we look along the wire in the direction of electron flow, then the field is an anticlockwise direction (⊗ means that the electrons are flowing away from the eye of the observer).

CONVENTION

Each moving electron produces an *anticlockwise* magnetic field about itself when viewed along the direction of its motion.

This convention is illustrated in Figure 12.1C, where the symbol ⊗ means that electron flow is away from the eye (⊙ is towards the eye). The arrows on the lines of force are in an anticlockwise direction, in accordance with our convention, and give the direction in which a north pole would move if placed in that position (Sect. 11.3). Thus, a weightless north pole would, if released, travel round and round the wire indefinitely in an anticlockwise circle.

12.5 MAGNETIC FIELD DUE TO A CIRCULAR COIL OF WIRE

Figure 12.2A shows a circular coil of wire in which an electric current is made to flow. Now, each individual moving electron produces anticlockwise magnetic lines of force about itself (Sect. 12.4), as illustrated in Figure 12.2A. The closeness of the lines of force to each other represents the total magnetic effect (i.e. the magnetic flux density, as described in Sect. 11.4). The addition at a point of all the magnetic flux densities represented by the lines of force produces the total magnetic flux density at that point. Note that, within the coil, the lines of force all tend to be in the direction C to D, while outside the coil, they are from D to C. A top view of the coil (Figure 12.2B) shows the pattern of the overall lines of force so obtained. It is interesting to note the similarity of these lines of force to those of a short bar magnet (see Figure 11.3), where they emerge from the north-pole end and travel around the magnet to the south-pole end and back again. Here we have the reason for the 'atomic magnets', where (on a tiny scale) the coil would be equivalent to the net flow of electrons around a particular atomic nucleus,

producing lines of force as in Figure 12.2B and hence the magnetised atom.

12.6 MAGNETIC FIELD DUE TO A SOLENOID

A solenoid consists of several coils joined together, and so produces magnetic lines of force, as shown in Figure 12.3A, similar to a bar magnet. The effect of a piece of soft iron within the solenoid is to increase the magnetic flux density many times because of the induced magnetism within the soft iron (Sects 11.5 and 11.6.3). This effect is reflected by an increase in the number of lines of force in Figure 12.3B compared to Figure 12.3A. The combination of solenoid and soft iron in this manner is known as an electromagnet.

INSIGHT

A general method of calculating the magnetic flux from any general shape of current-carrying conductor is due to Biot and Savart. The formula shown in Figure 12.4 may be used to calculate the magnetic flux density from any general shape of wire. (Table 12.1 shows some of these examples.)

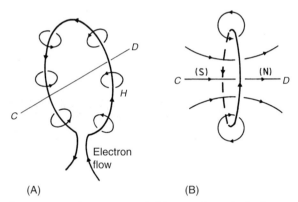

(A)   (B)

Figure 12.2   The magnetic field around a coil of wire carrying a current. Note the similarity to the field around a small bar magnet.

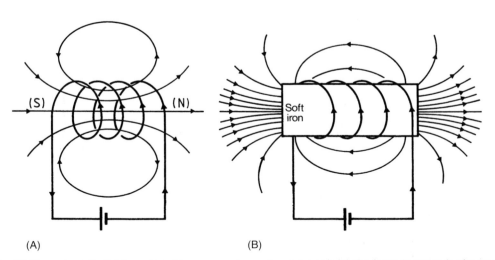

(A)   (B)

Figure 12.3   (A) The magnetic field produced by a current-carrying solenoid; (B) the large increase in the magnetic field produced when using a soft-iron core in the solenoid.

Now $\beta = \mu H$ *(see Equation 11.5)*

$H = \dfrac{B}{\mu} = \text{constant} \times \dfrac{Il}{r^2}$ (from rearranging the equation in Figure 12.4)

so that the units of the magnetic field strength (or magnetising force) H are in amperes per metre.

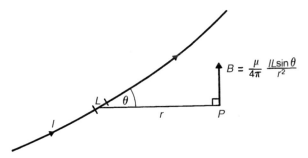

$$B = \dfrac{\mu}{4\pi}\,\dfrac{IL\sin\theta}{r^2}$$

Figure 12.4 Biot and Savart's law for determining the magnetic flux density due to any shape of current-carrying conductor.

12.7 THE ELECTROMAGNETIC RELAY

The electromagnetic relay is a very useful electrical device for switching electrical circuits on and off by remote control. It makes possible the switching of large currents and/or voltages to remote devices (e.g. an X-ray tube) by the application of a small current to the solenoid of the electromagnetic relay. The great advantage of the use of an electromagnetic relay for this purpose lies in the increased safety factor to the operator, since no large voltages or currents need to be connected to any of the controls on the operating console. Such controls on the X-ray panel (e.g. X-ray tube changeover switch) supply power to electromagnets which switch on the appropriate part of the X-ray electrical circuit. This may be verified by hearing the 'clonking' noise which occurs at the high-tension transformer when a different tube is

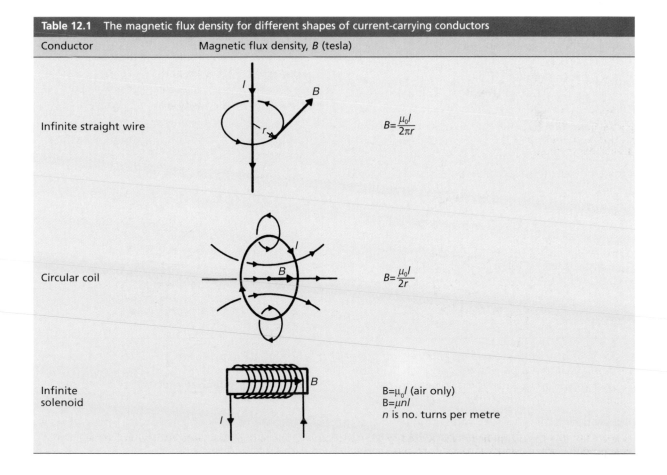

Table 12.1 The magnetic flux density for different shapes of current-carrying conductors

Conductor	Magnetic flux density, B (tesla)
Infinite straight wire	$B = \dfrac{\mu_0 I}{2\pi r}$
Circular coil	$B = \dfrac{\mu_0 I}{2r}$
Infinite solenoid	$B = \mu_0 I$ (air only) $B = \mu n I$ n is no. turns per metre

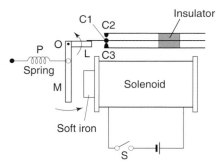

Figure 12.5 The electromagnetic relay (see text for details of operation).

selected. Many of the functions that were formerly carried out by relays are now carried out by solid-state switches.

The general structure of the electromagnetic relay is as shown in Figure 12.5.

12.7.1 Operation

When switch S is open, no current flows through the solenoid and so the soft iron piece M is held in the position shown by the spring P. Contacts C_1 and C_3 are in contact, while C_1 and C_2 are open. When S is closed, the current passing through the solenoid magnetises the soft iron core (Sect. 11.5), which attracts M by induced magnetism. M pivots about O so that the arm L lifts C_1 away from C_3 and into contact with C_2. Thus, if the external circuit is joined, current will flow between C_1 and C_2 but no current will flow between C_1 and C_3. Opening S reduces the current in the solenoid to zero and hence restores the system to its original condition, since M loses its magnetism and is quickly pulled away under the action of the spring P (C_1 and C_3 are closed and C_1 and C_2 are open).

SUMMARY

In this chapter you should have learnt:

- Atomic magnetism is caused by electrons orbiting atomic nuclei. Electromagnetism is caused by isolated moving particles (e.g. free electrons) (see Sect. 12.3)
- Negative and positive charges may flow in a vacuum, gas or liquid, but only negative charges (electrons) may flow in a solid. This is because the atomic nuclei (which contain the positively charged protons) are not free to move in a solid (see Sect. 12.4)
- Circular magnetic fields exist around moving charges: anticlockwise around negative charges and clockwise around positive charges when viewed along the direction of motion (see Sect. 12.5)
- The magnetic flux density due to a current-carrying solenoid may be increased many times by inserting within it a material of high permeability, e.g. soft iron, since $B = \mu H$ (see Table 11.1). The magnetic domains become aligned with the direction of H, so adding to the overall magnetic flux density (see Sect. 12.6)
- The electromagnetic relay is a device used for switching a circuit on and off under remote control, depending upon whether a solenoid is energised or not. The advantage of such a system is that a low current may be used to switch a high current or voltage at a remote location, thus increasing the safety factor against electrical shock for the operators of the equipment (see Sect. 12.7).

SELF-TEST

a. Compare the similarities between the atomic magnets within a bar magnet and the magnetic field produced by an electric current in a coil of wire.

b. Why does a piece of soft iron within a solenoid increase the magnetic effect of the solenoid when an electric current is passed

through it? Explain why this increase does not continue indefinitely as the current through the solenoid is increased. (*Hint*: see Sect. 11.6.3.)

c. What is an electromagnetic relay? Draw a simple diagram of its construction and hence explain how it operates.

FURTHER READING

Ball J L, Moore A D 1997 Essential physics for
    radiographers, 3rd edn. Blackwell Scientific Publications,
    London, ch 8
Bushong S C 2004 Radiologic science for technologists:
    physics, biology and protection. Mosby, New York, ch 8

Dowsett D J, Kenny P A, Johnston R E 1998 The physics of
    diagnostic imaging. Chapman & Hall Medical, London,
    ch 2

Chapter 13

Electromagnetic Induction

CHAPTER CONTENTS

13.1 Aim   112

13.2 Introduction   112

13.3 Conditions Necessary for Electromagnetic Induction   113

13.4 Faraday's Laws of Electromagnetic Induction   113

13.5 Lenz's Law   114

13.6 Sign Convention for the Induced Current   114

13.7 Mutual Induction   115

13.8 Self-Induction   116

13.9 The AC Generator   117

Self-Test   118

Further Reading   119

13.1 AIM

The aim of this chapter is to consider the laws of electromagnetic induction. The direction of the induced current will be identified. The concepts of mutual induction and self-induction will be discussed in preparation for Chapter 17, where the application of these will be considered in transformer design.

13.2 INTRODUCTION

In Chapter 12 we covered the topic of electromagnetism and in this chapter we will deal with the topic of *electromagnetic induction*. As can be seen from the definitions below, one is just the reverse of the other. They may each be defined as follows:

DEFINITIONS

Electromagnetism is the production of a magnetic field by the passage of an electrical current (see Ch. 12).

Electromagnetic induction is the production of electricity by the interlinking of a conductor with a changing magnetic field, or moving a conductor relative to a stationary magnetic field (also known as the generator effect).

13.3 CONDITIONS NECESSARY FOR ELECTROMAGNETIC INDUCTION

Consider the simple experiment depicted in Figure 13.1. A solenoid *L* is joined to a meter which can measure both the magnitude and the direction of the current flowing through the solenoid. The following effects are observed:

- No current flow is observed on the meter if the magnet is *stationary* with respect to the solenoid (Figure 13.1A and C)
- A current flows through the meter whenever the magnet is *moved* towards or away from the solenoid (Figure 13.1B and D)
- The *magnitude* of the induced current is *greater* if the magnet is moved faster
- Reversing the direction of the movement of the magnet reverses the direction of the induced current (Figure 13.1B and D)
- Reversing the pole of the magnet which is closer to the solenoid reverses the direction of the induced current for a given movement.

From this simple experiment we can conclude that *only a changing magnetic field relative to the conductor* is able to induce electricity in the conductor. Also we can see that the amount of electricity produced is in some way related to the *rate of change of the magnetic field* relative to the conductor. Finally we can conclude that the *direction of movement of the magnetic field* influences the direction of the induced current. These concepts will be discussed in more detail in the following sections of this chapter.

13.4 FARADAY'S LAWS OF ELECTROMAGNETIC INDUCTION

Faraday produced two laws of electromagnetic induction which cover some of the observations we made in the previous section. These may be defined as follows:

1. A change in the magnetic flux linked with a conductor induces an electromotive force (EMF) in the conductor
2. The magnitude of the induced EMF is proportional to the rate of change of the magnetic flux linkage.

In order to understand Faraday's laws we need to have a clear understanding of *EMF* and *magnetic flux linkage*.

EMF was considered in Section 10.6 and can be considered as the force which is capable of causing electrons to flow (i.e. EMF will cause a current to flow in a complete circuit). It is important to note that Faraday's laws do not specify whether or not the conductor is connected to an external circuit but, in either case, an EMF will be induced in it.

In Section 11.4 *magnetic flux* and *magnetic flux density* were discussed. The magnetic flux through a volume *V* may be visualised as being proportional to the number of lines of flux passing through that volume (Figure 13.2). Thus, if a magnetic flux of 10 weber (Sect. 11.4) passes through *V*, then the magnetic flux linkage with

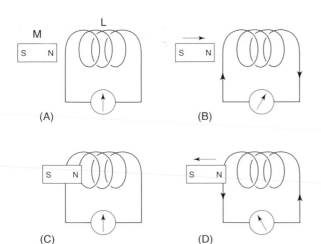

(A)   (B)

(C)   (D)

Figure 13.1 An example of electromagnetic induction. A current flows only when there is relative movement between the bar magnet (*M*) and the solenoid (*L*).

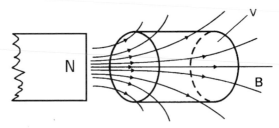

Figure 13.2 The magnetic flux linkage associated with a volume *V*.

V is also said to be 10 weber. If the magnet in Figure 13.2 is moved to the left of the page, then the number of lines of flux (or the flux linkage) in the volume *V* will be reduced.

We now see that moving the magnet relative to the solenoid will alter the flux linkage between the magnet and the solenoid and so an EMF will be induced – Faraday's first law. Also, a rapid movement of the magnet increases the rate of change of flux linkage and so increases the size of the induced EMF – Faraday's second law.

Changing the magnetic flux linkage associated with a particular conductor may be achieved in two ways:

1. By moving the conductor relative to a stationary magnet – this principle is used in the alternating current (AC) generator or dynamo (Sect. 13.9)
2. By varying the magnitude of the magnetic flux while the conductor is stationary – this principle is used in the AC transformer (see Ch. 17).

13.5 LENZ'S LAW

In our initial observations regarding the induced current (Sect. 13.3) we noted the direction as well as the size of the current. Faraday's laws apply to open or closed circuits but, as Lenz's law concerns the direction of the induced current, it can only be applied to *closed* circuits. The law can be stated as follows:

> The *direction* of the induced *current* in a conductor caused by a changing magnetic flux is such that its own magnetic field *opposes* the changing magnetic flux.

INSIGHT

Lenz's law is an example of the application of the law of conservation of energy (Sect. 5.3). If the direction of the induced current was such that its magnetic field helped the changing magnetic field, then we would be getting something for nothing so we could establish perpetual motion of the conductor and the magnetic field. This would

be in defiance of the law of conservation of energy.

When the north pole of a bar magnet is moved towards a solenoid (Figure 13.1B), the current will flow in the solenoid in such a direction that it produces a north pole at the end closest to the magnet. This has the effect of producing a force of repulsion between the bar magnet and the solenoid and so *work* must be done against this force in order to keep the magnet moving towards the solenoid. Thus *mechanical energy* is transformed to *electrical energy* and the law of conservation of energy is maintained. The reverse occurs when the magnet is withdrawn.

13.6 SIGN CONVENTION FOR THE INDUCED CURRENT

When current flow was considered as the flow of positive charge, this was determined using Fleming's right-hand rule. As we now know that current flow is a flow of electrons, Fleming's hand rules are liable to cause confusion and so the direction of current flow will be determined using the convention shown below:

CONVENTION

Consider a situation similar to that shown in Figure 13.3A where a conductor is moved at right angles to a magnetic field (Figure 13.3B) – the direction of the movement and the direction of the magnetic field are as shown in the diagram. We wish to determine whether the induced electron flow along the conductor will be either into the page or out of the page. This can be determined as follows:

1. Mark the position of the conductor and draw a line to indicate the direction of movement
2. Draw a second line (*B*) to represent the permanent magnetic field direction to intersect the first line at the point *P* (Figure 13.3B)
3. Now draw a circle with the conductor at its centre such that its circumference passes through the point *P*

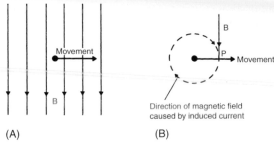

Figure 13.3   An example of the use of the convention described in the text for establishing the direction of the induced current.

4. This circle represents the magnetic field which will be caused by the current induced in the conductor. The direction of this magnetic field is the same as the direction of the permanent magnetic field at the point *P* – the field is in a clockwise direction

5. As we learnt in Section 12.4, *the magnetic field around a current-carrying conductor is anticlockwise when the electrons are travelling away from us.* Thus, because of the clockwise magnetic field we can conclude that the electrons (of the induced current) are travelling towards us.

13.7 MUTUAL INDUCTION

If a changing current is passed through one conductor, then this will produce a changing magnetic field around this conductor (see Ch. 12). If a second conductor is placed within this changing magnetic field, then (by Faraday's laws) an EMF will be generated in the conductor and a current will flow in it if the conducting loop is complete (Figure 13.4). By Lenz's law this current will be in the opposite direction to the original current. The size of this secondary current will vary with the magnetic field – it will be a current of changing magnitude as there is a changing magnetic field. This changing secondary current will produce its own changing magnetic field which will induce an EMF and current in the first conductor. Thus *each conductor induces electricity in the other* and the effect is known as *mutual induction.*

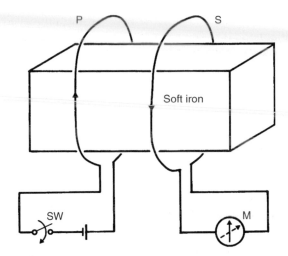

Figure 13.4   Principles of mutual induction. A changing current in coil *P* (the primary coil) induces a current in coil *S* (the secondary coil) and vice versa. The soft iron core magnifies the effect by improving the magnetic flux linkage between the coils. *SW*, switch; *M*, ammeter.

Consider Figure 13.4. When the switch *SW* is closed, electrons will flow from the negative pole of the battery to its positive pole via the coil *P*. During the time while the rate of flow of electrons builds up, there is a changing magnetic field around *P*. This is linked to *S* via the iron core (the iron core greatly enhances the flux linkage) and so an EMF and current flow will occur in *S*. The direction of the pointer on the ammeter *M* indicates that this flow of electrons in *S* is in the opposite direction to that in *P*, thus verifying Lenz's law. After a short time, the current in *P* is constant and so *S* is no longer influenced by a *changing* magnetic field. As a result no EMF is generated in *S* (Faraday's first law). If the switch *SW* is now opened, the magnetic field around *P* collapses and so an EMF is again generated in *P*, but this time it is in the opposite direction. If a more powerful battery is now used, this will produce a greater current in *P*, thus a greater magnetic field and consequently a greater EMF in *S* (the magnitude of the induced EMF is proportional to the rate of change of the magnetic flux). Finally, if we undertake the experiment with the iron bar present, and then with the iron bar removed, we find that the EMF produced in the coil *S* is greatest when the iron bar is present. This is because of improved magnetic flux linkage (Faraday's second law).

From this experiment we can show that the EMF induced in the secondary winding E_s is:

- proportional to the rate of change of the current in P (the primary)
- dependent on the detailed design of the two conductors and the flux linkage between them. This is called the *mutual inductance* (M).

Thus:

$$E_s = M \times \text{rate of change of primary current}$$
Equation 13.1

The greater the mutual inductance, M, the greater the mutual effect between the two conductors. M is measured in henrys and may be defined as:

DEFINITION

A mutual inductance of 1 *henry* exists between two conductors if 1 volt is induced in one conductor where there is a current change of 1 ampere per second in the other.

As will be explained in Chapter 17, an AC transformer works on the principle of mutual induction.

13.8 SELF-INDUCTION

Consider the solenoid in Figure 13.5A. If the switch SW is closed, current flow starts to build up in the solenoid. As this current increases, each turn of the solenoid produces a changing magnetic flux which is linked to the other turns of the solenoid (the flux from one turn is shown in Figure 13.5A). Thus, from Faraday's and Lenz's laws, an EMF in the opposite direction to the EMF from the battery will be induced in the solenoid. This is known as a back-EMF. This effect is known as *self-induction* and, if the self-induction is large, the current in the coil will take an appreciable time to build up to its maximum

value. The self-induction in an electrical system is defined in a very similar manner to the mutual induction and is given by the equation:

$$E_B = L \times \text{rate of change of current}$$
Equation 13.2

Here E_B is the back-EMF and L is the self-inductance, measured in henrys. Thus we can say that:

DEFINITION

A conductor has a *self-inductance* of 1 *henry* if a back-EMF of 1 volt is induced when the current flowing through it changes at 1 ampere per second.

A graph of the current flowing through the solenoid is shown in Figure 13.5B. As can be seen, the induced back-EMF slows down the rate of growth of the current and so it takes an appreciable time to reach its maximum value, determined by Ohm's law (see Sect. 10.8). If the wire of the solenoid were unwound to become a straight conductor, then there would be no magnetic flux linkage and consequently no back-EMF. Thus the current would rise to its maximum value very quickly.

As in the case of mutual induction, a soft iron bar placed in the solenoid will enhance the self-induction as the magnetic flux linkage between the coils is improved.

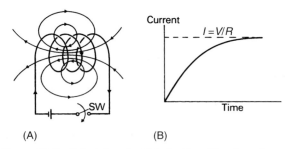

Figure 13.5   Principles of self-induction. The changing magnetic flux produced by the current flow through the solenoid when the switch SW is closed links with all the turns of the coil. This produces a back-electromotive force which slows down the rate of growth of current in the coil.

As will be explained in Chapter 17, an autotransformer works on the principle of self-induction.

13.9 THE AC GENERATOR

Electric power is produced from an AC generator. This is an example of a situation where mechanical energy is converted to electrical energy. The basic components of such a generator are shown in Figure 13.6A. A permanent magnetic field exists between the poles of the magnet, and coils of copper wire are made to rotate through this field. For simplicity, only one coil is shown in the diagram. The EMF generated in the device is collected at brushes positioned at A and B.

Consider the situation where the coil shown is rotated in a clockwise direction. Thus, from the initial position, side X of the coil will move upwards through the magnetic field and side Y will move downwards (Figure 13.6B). At this point in its movement, the coil is cutting the maximum number of lines of flux as it is moving at right angles to the flux lines, and so the maximum EMF will be generated. If we use the convention discussed earlier (see Sect. 13.6) to establish the direction of electron flow, we can see that electrons will travel towards us on side X and away from us on side Y. Thus an excess of electrons will exist at brush A and a shortage of electrons will exist at brush B: brush A is negative and brush B is positive. This situation is shown as position 1 on the graph in Figure 13.6C. Now consider the situation when the coil has turned in a clockwise direction from its initial position through 90°: this is the second position of the coil shown in Figure 13.6B. In this position both side X and side Y of the coil are moving parallel with the lines of magnetic flux and so no current is generated – this is again shown as position 2 in Figure 13.6C. In position 3 the coil has rotated through 180° from its original position. Side X of the coil is now moving downwards through the magnetic field and side Y is moving upwards. As in position 1, a maximum number of lines of flux are being cut as the conductor is moving at right angles to the flux, and so, again, the maximum

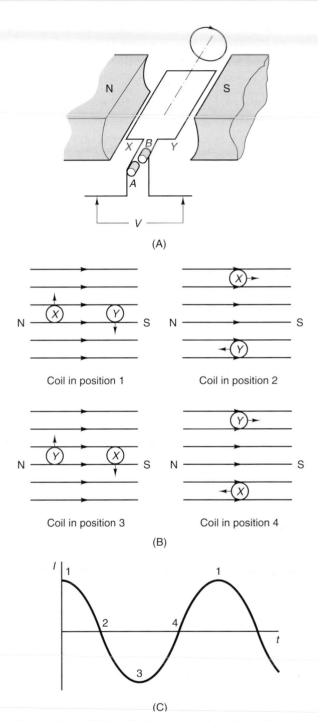

(A)

Coil in position 1   Coil in position 2

Coil in position 3   Coil in position 4

(B)

(C)

Figure 13.6 (A) Simplified diagram of an alternating current generator; (B) four positions of the coil relative to the magnetic field; (C) the current waveform produced when the coil moves through positions 1, 2, 3, 4 and returns to 1. A complete turn of the coil will produce one cycle of current. See text for further details.

EMF will be generated. The polarity of *A* and *B* is now the reverse of position 1. In position 4 the conductor is again moving parallel to the lines of flux so no EMF is generated. The conductor then returns to position 1 and so one cycle is complete. The process is then repeated. The type of current shown in Figure 13.6C is known as an AC and will be the subject of Chapter 14.

In cases where there is no external circuit connected, then no current is able to flow and only sufficient work to overcome the frictional resistance is necessary to keep the rotational movement at the same speed. As soon as an external circuit is connected, then a current is able to flow in the circuit and in the winding. It should come as no surprise to discover that this current will flow in such a direction as to oppose the motion of the coil (remember Lenz's law). This means that mechanical work must be performed to overcome this resisting force, i.e. mechanical energy is converted into electrical energy.

The effect of suddenly increasing the electrical load demanded from the generator (e.g. when making an X-ray exposure) is suddenly to increase the opposition to its rotation. Hence, the generator slows down momentarily and the induced EMF (which depends on the speed of rotation) is reduced. Thus we find that, in times of increased demand on the generators, there is a drop in the voltage they supply. In X-ray units this is taken into account by the inclusion of a *mains voltage compensator* on the unit.

SUMMARY

In this chapter you should have learnt:

- That an EMF is induced in a conductor if it is linked with a changing magnetic field (see Sect. 13.3)
- Faraday's first and second law of electromagnetic induction (see Sect. 13.4)
- Lenz's law, which determines the direction of the current flowing as the result of the induced EMF (see Sect. 13.5)
- The sign convention for the direction of the induced current (see Sect. 13.6)
- The meaning and a simple application of mutual induction (see Sect. 13.7)
- The meaning and a simple application of self-induction (see Sect. 13.8)
- The mode of operation of an AC generator (see Sect. 13.9).

SELF-TEST

a. What is meant by the term *electromagnetic induction* and how does it differ from the term *electromagnetism*?

b. State and explain Faraday's and Lenz's laws of electromagnetic induction. List the factors on which the magnitude of the induced EMF depends.

c. In what circumstances is it possible to have an induced EMF without an induced current?

d. If a wire is moved as indicated by the arrow across a magnetic field, *B*, what will be the direction of the EMF induced in the wire? In what direction would the wire be moved relative to the magnetic field to produce:

(i)   the maximum EMF

(ii) zero EMF?

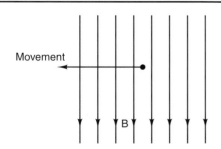

Movement

B

e. A bar magnet having its north pole pointing downwards is dropped through a horizontal loop of wire. What is the direction of the induced current in the wire when the magnet is moving downwards:

(i)   above the wire

(ii) below the wire?

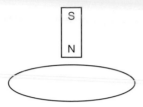

f. What is meant by *mutual induction* and *self-induction*? Define the unit in which each is measured.

g. Explain the generation of an EMF in an AC generator. What is the effect on this generator of a sudden increase in the load drawn from it? Explain how this affects the output from the generator.

FURTHER READING

Ball J L, Moore A D 1997 Essential physics for radiographers, 3rd edn. Blackwell Scientific Publications, London, ch 9

Dowsett D J, Kenny P A, Johnston R E 1998 The physics of diagnostic imaging, Chapman & Hall Medical, London, ch 1

Ohanian H C 1994 Principles of physics. W W Norton, London, ch 22

Thompson M A, Hattaway R T, Hall J D, Dowd S B 1994 Principles of imaging science and protection. W B Saunders, London, ch 5

Chapter 14

Alternating Current Flow

CHAPTER CONTENTS

14.1 Aim   120

14.2 Introduction   120

14.3 Types of DC and AC   120

14.4 Sinusoidal AC   121
    14.4.1 Peak Current (or Voltage)   122
    14.4.2 Average Current (or Voltage)   122
    14.4.3 Effective (or RMS) Current
        or Voltage   123

14.5 AC and the X-ray Tube   124
    14.5.1 Voltage Across the X-ray
        Tube (kVp)   124
    14.5.2 Current Through the
        Tube (mA)   124
    14.5.3 The Mains Voltage and
        Current   124

14.6 Basics of AC Circuits   124
    14.6.1 Phase Difference   125
    14.6.2 Reactance and Impedance   125
    14.6.3 Power in AC Circuits   126

14.7 Simple AC Circuits   126
    14.7.1 Resistors in AC Circuits   126
    14.7.2 Capacitors in AC Circuits   127
    14.7.3 Inductors in AC Circuits   127
    14.7.4 RLC in Series–Resonance
        Circuits   128

14.8 Three-Phase AC   129
    14.8.1 Star and Delta Connections   130
    14.8.2 Three-Phase Circuits in
        Radiography   131

Self-Test   133

Further Reading   133

14.1 AIM

The aim of this chapter is to introduce the reader to alternating current (AC) flow. The various parameters used to measure such a current will be discussed. Simple AC circuits will be considered, as will three-phase power supplies.

14.2 INTRODUCTION

Direct current (DC) electricity (Ch. 10) is representative of a flow of electrons in one direction only. This chapter deals with the situation where electrons flow through a circuit first in one direction and then in the other – this is known as an AC flow.

14.3 TYPES OF DC AND AC

Figure 14.1 shows different types of DC and AC in graphical form – the magnitude of the current is plotted against time.

Figure 14.1A is a case where the number of electrons passing a point per second in the circuit is constant and so we get a horizontal straight line. This is an example of the type of DC described in Chapter 10.

Figure 14.1B is a case where the electrons always move in the same direction but the number of electrons passing a point varies with time – the electrons move as a series of

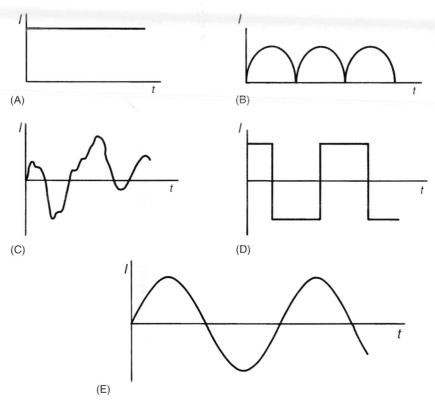

Figure 14.1 Types of direct current (DC) and alternating current (AC). (A) Constant DC; (B) pulsatile DC; (C) irregular AC; (D) square-wave AC; (E) sinusoidal AC.

(A)

(B)

(C)

(D)

(E)

pulses and so this is known as a pulsatile or pulsating DC.

In Figure 14.1C there is no discernible pattern in the flow of the electrons except to say that they flow in both directions at different times. This is an example of an irregular AC waveform.

Figure 14.1D shows a situation where the number of electrons travelling in one direction is constant for a short period of time and then the same number of electrons travel in the opposite direction for the same period of time. This is an example of a square-wave AC waveform.

Lastly, Figure 14.1E shows an example of a sinusoidal AC waveform. This is the most common type of AC waveform and will be discussed in detail in the rest of this chapter.

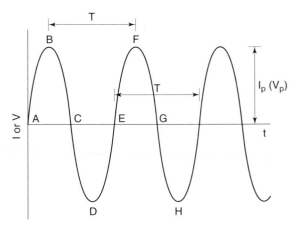

Figure 14.2 A sinusoidal current or voltage waveform.

14.4 SINUSOIDAL AC

The sinusoidal AC waveform is illustrated in more detail in Figure 14.2, together with some of the quantities used to measure it. These are defined below:

DEFINITIONS

One cycle One complete waveform, starting at any point and continuing until we reach the same point on the pattern. This is usually measured from zero to zero (*ABCDE*) or from peak to peak (*BCDEF*).

Period (T) The time taken to complete one cycle, measured in seconds.

Frequency (f) The number of cycles which occur in 1 second, measured in cycles per second or hertz (Hz).

Amplitude The maximum value of positive or negative current (or voltage) on the waveform. This may be referred to as the peak value.

There is a simple relationship between the period (*T*) and the frequency (*f*), which can be seen if we consider the following situation. Suppose we have a frequency of 10 Hz (10 cycles per second). Since the waveform is regular, each cycle must last for 0.1 second. Thus we can say:

$$f = \frac{1}{T} \qquad\qquad Equation\ 14.1$$

For a sinusoidal current this equation may be rewritten as:

$$I_t = I_p \sin 2\pi ft$$

where I_t is the current at a time *t* and I_p is the amplitude or the peak value of the current. A similar equation can be produced for the voltage.

14.4.1 Peak Current (or Voltage)

The peak current is the same as the amplitude, i.e. it is the *maximum positive or negative value of the current*. Similarly, the peak voltage is the maximum value of the voltage. In radiography, the peak voltage across the tube, when the anode is positive and the cathode is negative, is usually quoted. If an X-ray tube is operating at 75 kVp then the peak potential difference between the anode and the cathode is 75 kV. The reasons for quoting the tube voltage as kVp will be considered later in this chapter.

14.4.2 Average Current (or Voltage)

As we can see from Figure 14.2, the average current flowing in one cycle of a sinusoidal waveform is zero, as the current flowing in one direction during the positive half-cycle has the

same overall value (but opposite sign) as the current flowing in the opposite direction during the negative half-cycle. The same conclusion applies to any number of complete cycles. A similar argument suggests that the average voltage for a sinusoidal waveform is also zero. Thus for a sinusoidal waveform:

$$I_{AV} = 0$$
$$V_{AV} = 0 \qquad\qquad Equation\ 14.2$$

However, if the waveform is *rectified* (or made unidirectional; Ch. 19), then a value of the average current (or voltage) is obtained. The voltage waveform produced for *half-wave rectification* is shown in Figure 14.3A. This results in a pulsating voltage which (assuming a complete external circuit) results in a net electron flow in one direction – this allows us to consider average values of voltage and current which are not zero.

The voltage waveform for a *full-wave rectified* circuit is shown on the same scale in Figure 14.3B. Again a pulsating voltage is produced where the average value is twice that for the half-wave rectified circuit as there are twice as many peaks in unit time.

Thus we can say for half-wave rectification:

$$I_{AV} = 0.318I_p$$
$$V_{AV} = 0.318V_p \qquad\qquad Equation\ 14.3$$

and for full-wave rectification:

$$I_{AV} = 0.636I_p$$
$$V_{AV} = 0.636V_p \qquad\qquad Equation\ 14.4$$

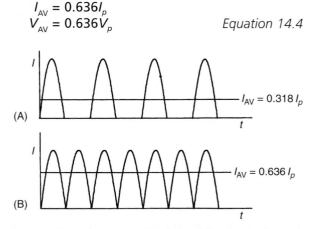

Figure 14.3 Forms of rectified sinusoidal alternating current (AC). (A) Half-wave rectification; (B) full-wave rectification.

14.4.3 Effective (or RMS) Current or Voltage

If an AC supply is connected across a resistor, then electrons will flow in one direction during the first half-cycle and in the opposite direction during the second half-cycle. As there is no net movement of electrons for any given number of complete cycles, the average current is zero. This does not mean, however, that the net heating effect is zero. Electrons will produce heat within a resistor irrespective of their direction of travel. The average current is therefore a quantity which is not suitable for determining the energy or power expended in a circuit which is connected to an AC supply. The quantity of importance is the effective or root mean square (RMS) value of the current and may be defined as:

DEFINITION

The *effective current* is that value of constant current which, flowing for the same time, would produce the same expenditure of electrical energy in a circuit as the AC.

The effective value of the current is also known as the RMS value, for reasons which we will consider below.

The effective or RMS voltage is defined in a very similar manner:

DEFINITION

The *effective voltage* is that value of constant voltage which, being present for the same time, would produce the same expenditure of electrical energy in a circuit as the alternating voltage.

INSIGHT

Consider the graphs shown in Figure 14.4. The AC I has an average value of zero because each positive value is matched with an equal and opposite negative value.

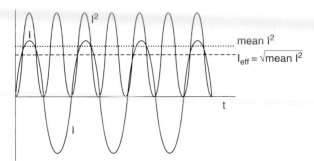

Figure 14.4 Graphic representation of an effective (root main square or RMS) value of current.

Thus the peak positive value is matched with a peak negative value. If we take these peak values and square them, this allows us to get rid of the negative sign and so it is possible to get an average value of the peak current squared. If we now take the square root of this value we have the root of the mean of the square of the peak value of the current. This is the effective value of the current, i.e.:

$$I_{RMS} = \frac{I_p}{\sqrt{2}}$$

In Section 10.9.3 it was shown that the general equation for DC electrical power was $W = V \times I$, where W is expressed in watts, V in volts and I in amperes. In an AC circuit both V and I are continually changing and so it is the effective or RMS value of each which must be taken into account when using the above equation:

$$W = V_{RMS} \times I_{RMS} \qquad \textit{Equation 14.5}$$

Here W is the *average* power generated in the circuit, taking into account at least one half-cycle of AC.

We can manipulate Equation 14.5 in a similar way to Equation 10.16 to get:

$$W = I_{RMS}^{2} \times R$$

$$W = \frac{V_{RMS}^{2}}{R} \qquad \textit{Equation 14.6}$$

Note that we can apply Ohm's law (Ch. 10) to AC circuits provided the same types of units for voltage or current (e.g. RMS) are used throughout the equation.

The RMS values of current or voltage can be related to the peak relationships by the following equations:

$$I_{RMS} = 0.707I_p$$
$$V_{RMS} = 0.707V_p \qquad \text{Equation 14.7}$$

and:

$$I_p = 1.414I_{RMS}$$
$$V_p = 1.414V_{RMS} \qquad \text{Equation 14.8}$$

Thus, for an AC, the effective value is just over 70% of the peak value.

14.5 AC AND THE X-RAY TUBE

In order to produce X-rays, an X-ray tube requires a high potential difference (voltage) across it and a current flowing through it. The voltage available from the mains supply is far too low for use directly across the X-ray tube so a means of increasing it to the high values of thousands of volts is required. This is relatively easy to accomplish using an AC transformer (Ch. 17). Because this transformer increases the voltage, it is known as a step-up transformer. The filament of the X-ray tube requires a fairly low voltage supply so that it can produce the electrons which form the mA through the tube, and so the mains voltage passes through a step-down transformer before being applied to the filament. Thus an alternating voltage may either be increased using a step-up transformer or decreased using a step-down transformer.

In AC circuits the voltages or currents are usually expressed in terms of their effective values unless otherwise stated. When considering the X-ray circuit, the following convention applies:

- The voltage across the tube (kV) is expressed in terms of the peak voltage, i.e. kVp
- The current flowing through the tube (mA) is expressed in terms of the average current
- The mains voltage and current to the X-ray set are expressed as effective or RMS values.

14.5.1 Voltage Across the X-ray Tube (kVp)

The potential difference across the X-ray tube is expressed in terms of the peak value for the following reasons:

- The maximum energy of X-ray photons emitted by the anode is the same value in keV, i.e. an X-ray tube operated at 100 kVp will emit X-ray photons with a maximum energy of 100 keV. (This will be explained in more detail in Ch. 28)
- The voltage rating of the high-tension cables must be able to withstand the maximum voltage applied to them. This occurs during the peak value of the voltage.

If the voltage applied to the X-ray tube is a constant potential (Ch. 19), then this is effectively a DC supply so the peak and the effective values are the same.

14.5.2 Current Through the Tube (mA)

The mA meter is designed to measure the *average* current flowing through the X-ray tube during an exposure. The intensity of the radiation beam is proportional to the average current. If we take the average current (mA) and multiply this by the exposure time in seconds we get the mAs for that exposure. This represents the total charge which has passed through the X-ray tube during the exposure. The quantity of X-rays produced during the exposure is proportional to the mAs.

14.5.3 The Mains Voltage and Current

The electrical mains is the source of power and so it makes sense to quote the mains supply in terms which make the calculations of power most convenient – the effective or RMS values. The mains voltage in the UK has a nominal value of 230 volts$_{RMS}$ and so this gives us a peak value for this voltage of approximately 325 volts (from Equation 14.8).

14.6 BASICS OF AC CIRCUITS

Having considered the different measures that can be made of an AC or voltage, we are now ready to look at the consequences of passing this current through some basic circuits.

14.6.1 Phase Difference

So far in this chapter we have only considered the case where the peak voltage occurs at the same time as the peak current. The current and voltage are then said to be *in phase*. This is not necessary for all types of AC circuits and we can get situations where a *phase difference* exists between the current and the voltage. Examples of such phase differences are shown in graphical form in Figure 14.5. In Figure 14.5A the current (*I*) lags behind the voltage (*V*) – a waveform displaced to the right occurs later than, and therefore lags behind, the waveform with which it is being compared. Also in Figure 14.5B we have a situation where *I* leads *V*.

The angle between the two waveforms is expressed as the *phase angle*, where 360° is equivalent to one cycle. This situation is often represented using a *vector diagram* (Figure 14.6A). (If you are not familiar with vector diagrams and vector addition, refer to Appendix A.) A phase angle of θ exists between the current and the voltage, where *OC* is the current vector and *OA* is the voltage vector, both of which rotate anticlockwise at a rate of *f* revolutions per second, where *f* is the frequency of the AC supply. In this example the voltage vector leads the current vector by θ. The magnitude of the voltage and the current at any stage during the cycle can be given by the vertical distance of the tip of each vector – the length *OB* for the voltage vector *OA*, as shown in the figure.

The angle θ between the vectors is maintained throughout the rotation of both vectors.

14.6.2 Reactance and Impedance

When we considered the opposition to the flow of DC in a circuit we found that this opposition consisted of *resistance* and was measured in ohms (see Ch. 10). There are two additional measures of AC resistance in a circuit – the *reactance* and the *impedance*. Both are measured in ohms as in DC resistance but measure different quantities, as explained below.

Consider Figure 14.7, where a phase difference of θ exists between the voltage across the circuit and the current flowing through it.

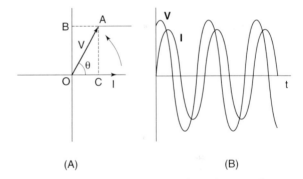

(A)   (B)

Figure 14.6   (A) A vector diagram for voltage and current. The vectors *V* and *I* rotate anticlockwise and the vertical height of each gives the instantaneous values of voltage and current. The angle θ is maintained throughout the rotation. *I* lags behind *V* on this diagram. (B) Plot of the voltage and the current against time for the vector diagram shown in (A).

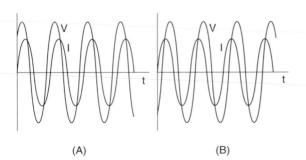

(A)   (B)

Figure 14.5   Phase differences between current and voltage waveforms. (A) *I* lags behind *V*; (B) *I* leads *V*.

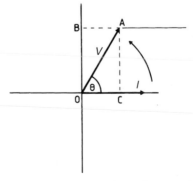

Figure 14.7   A vector diagram for voltage and current separated by a phase angle of θ.

The *reactance, X,* is defined as the ratio OB/OC where OB is measured in volts and OC in amperes. The important point to note is that the measurements of the voltage and of the current taken are at right angles to each other. As will be shown later in this chapter, reactance is produced by capacitors and inductors, but not by resistors.

The *impedance, Z,* is defined as the ratio OA/OC where OA is measured in volts and OC is measured in amperes.

To summarise, resistance, reactance and impedance all represent opposition to the flow of current and are all measured in ohms. They are expressed by the ratio of volts to amperes but the voltage vector is different in each case – it is *in phase* with the current *for resistance,* at *right angles* to the current *for reactance* and at the *phase angle* to the current *for impedance.* Impedance is thus the general term for opposition to current flow, and reactance and resistance form separate components of this. The examples shown in Section 14.7 will help to clarify these concepts.

14.6.3 Power in AC Circuits

If an instantaneous voltage V causes an instantaneous current I to flow through a circuit, then the power W at that instant can be calculated from the equation $W = VI$ (see Sect. 10.9.3). However, in most cases we are not concerned with the instantaneous power during a point in the cycle but with the average power over one or more cycles. To get this value we use the effective (or RMS) values of the voltage and current (see Equation 14.5):

$$W = V_{RMS} \times I_{RMS}$$

This formula only holds true when there is no phase difference between V and I, i.e. $\theta = 0°$. It will be shown in the next section that reactance does not contribute to the power drawn from a supply – hence only the power produced in the resistance in the AC circuit needs to be considered. The latter is obtained by resolving V along I (i.e. $V \cos \theta$) so that the final expression of the power in an AC circuit is:

$$W = V_{RMS} \times I_{RMS} \times \cos \theta \qquad \text{Equation 14.9}$$

The *power factor* is the value of $\cos \theta$. This is unity for a circuit containing only resistors as there is no phase difference between voltage and current. If the circuit contains components which cause a phase difference between current and voltage, the value of the power factor will be less than unity.

The *wattless component* of the voltage V is $V \sin \theta$ and represents the component of V which produces no average power because it is in phase with the reactance. Likewise, the current flowing through a reactance is termed *wattless current.*

The power rating of high-tension transformers used in radiographic equipment is often quoted in kVA – kilovolts times amperes. This specifies the maximum output of the transformer when running continuously into a resistive load, i.e. V and I are in phase. The RMS values of the kV and current are used to calculate the values of kVA.

14.7 SIMPLE AC CIRCUITS

In Section 14.6 we considered a general account of *phase, reactance* and *impedance* and how they apply in general to AC circuits. In this section these concepts are applied to individual circuit components and their combined effect in a simple circuit is considered.

14.7.1 Resistors in AC Circuits

Figure 14.8 shows the connection of an AC supply across a resistor. In this case there is no phase difference between the voltage and the current and so the vector diagram shows both pointing in the same direction. They both rotate together, giving sinusoidal voltage and current waveforms which peak at the same times and cross the axis at the same times.

As already explained, the average power generated in the resistor is given by the equation:

$$W = V_{RMS} \times I_{RMS}$$

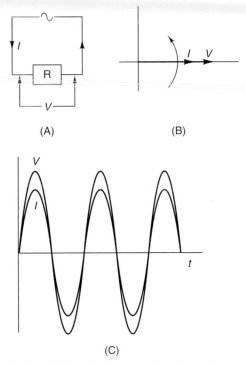

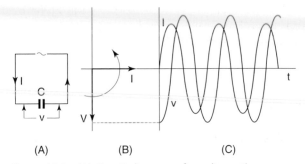

Figure 14.9 (A) Circuit diagram of an alternating current passing through a pure capacitance (C); (B) voltage and current vector diagram; (C) voltage and current plotted against time for the vector diagram in (B). Note that I leads V by 90°.

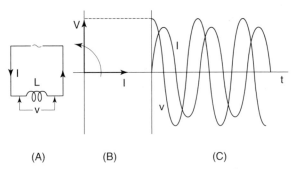

Figure 14.10 (A) Circuit diagram of an alternating current passing through a pure inductor (L); (B) voltage and current vector diagram; (C) voltage and current plotted against time for the vector diagram in (B). Note that I lags behind V by 90°.

Figure 14.8 (A) Circuit diagram of an alternating current passing through a pure resistance (R); (B) voltage and current vector diagram; (C) voltage and current plotted against time for the vector diagram in (B). Note that V and I are in phase.

14.7.2 Capacitors in AC Circuits

The detailed construction of capacitors and their functions in radiography will be discussed in Chapter 16. In this section we are purely interested in the effect caused when a capacitor is introduced into an AC circuit.

As can be seen from Figure 14.9, this results in a phase difference between the voltage and the current. The vector diagram indicates that the voltage across the capacitor lags behind the current flowing in and out of the capacitor by 90°. Thus a perfect capacitor in an AC circuit is considered as having reactance but no resistance.

The value of the *capacitance reactance* (X_C) is given by:

$$X_C = \frac{1}{2\pi f C} \qquad \textit{Equation 14.10}$$

where f is the frequency of the AC supply (in hertz) and C is the capacitance of the capacitor in farads (see Ch. 16 for definitions of *capacitance*

and the *farad*). Thus the capacitance reactance is inversely proportional to the frequency of the supply and the capacitance of the capacitor.

If we apply Equation 14.9 to the capacitor we can calculate that the average power generated in the capacitor is *zero* (cos 90° = 0). This is because in one half-cycle power is being supplied to the capacitor and in the other half-cycle the capacitor is giving the power back to the circuit.

14.7.3 Inductors in AC Circuits

If we consider Figure 14.10, we can see that, when an inductor is placed in an AC circuit, the current and voltage are again out of phase. In this case the voltage leads the current by 90°. Thus a perfect inductor in an AC circuit is considered as having reactance but no resistance.

The reactance of an inductor (X_L) is given by the equation:

$$X_L = 2\pi f L \qquad \text{Equation 14.11}$$

where f is the frequency of the AC supply and L is the value of the inductance in henrys. Thus the inductive reactance is directly proportional to the frequency (opposite to the capacitor; see Equation 14.10).

Because the current and voltage are 90° out of phase, the net power drawn from the circuit is *zero*.

We have now seen that both capacitors and inductors which have only reactance consume zero power and so we can say that reactance consumes no power. Resistance, as mentioned earlier (see Equation 14.5), does consume power.

14.7.4 RLC in Series: Resonance Circuits

Consider Figure 14.11A, where a resistor (R), an inductor (L) and a capacitor (C) are connected in series with an AC supply. From the previous sections where we considered the effect of each on the circuit we can now draw a vector diagram of the inductive reactance (X_L), the capacitance reactance (X_C) and the resistance (R). Such a vector diagram is shown in Figure 14.11B. (*Note* that the vectors for the reactance and the resistance are separated by the same phase angle as the voltages across each of the components.) We can now do vector addition to calculate the impedance (Z). As the capacitance reactance and the inductive reactance are in opposite directions, the net reactance is $(X_L - X_C)$. The diagram for the vector addition is shown in Figure 14.11C. This shows that the impedance Z will have a phase difference of θ with respect to the current. (*Note* that the voltage and impedance vectors will be coincident and so the voltage and current will also have a phase difference of θ between them.)

We can now use Pythagoras' theorem, as applied to Figure 14.11C, to calculate the impedance thus:

$$Z^2 = R^2 + (X_L - X_C)^2$$
$$Z = \sqrt{[R^2 + (X_L - X_C)^2]} \qquad \text{Equation 14.12}$$

We can also calculate the phase angle as follows:

$$\tan\theta = \frac{(X_L - X_C)}{R}$$
$$\therefore \theta = \tan^{-1}\frac{(X_L - X_C)}{R} \qquad \text{Equation 14.13}$$

Finally, if we know the supply voltage, we can calculate the current flowing through the circuit:

$$Z = \frac{V}{I}$$
$$\therefore I = \frac{V}{Z} = \frac{V}{\sqrt{[R^2 + (X_L - X_C)^2]}}$$

$$\text{Equation 14.14}$$

It is important to remember that, if V is expressed in terms of peak voltage, then the current calculated will be the peak current; if V is in RMS units, so will be I.

A sample calculation may help to consolidate your understanding.

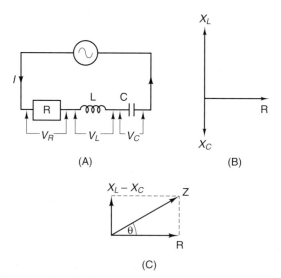

(A)   (B)

(C)

Figure 14.11 (A) Circuit diagram of an alternating current passing through a resistor (R), an inductor (L) and a capacitor (C). A vector diagram (B) shows the vectors of each of the components and (C) shows the net reactance and the overall impedance (Z) of the *RLC* circuit.

EXAMPLE

A resistor of resistance 26 Ω is connected in series with an inductor of inductance 100 mH and a capacitor of capacitance 50 μF in an AC circuit with a frequency of 100 Hz. If the voltage has a peak value of 400 V, calculate the *impedance*, the *phase angle* and the *peak current*.

$$X_L = 2\pi f L \qquad \text{(from Equation 14.11)}$$
$$= 2\pi \times 100 \times 10^{-3}$$
$$= 2\pi \times 10$$
$$= 62.8\ \Omega \qquad \text{(from Equation 14.10)}$$

$$X_C = \frac{1}{2\pi f C}$$

$$= \frac{1}{2\pi \times 100 \times 50 \times 10^{-6}}$$

$$= \frac{10}{2\pi \times 100 \times 50}$$

$$= 31.8\ \Omega$$
$$= \text{net reactance} = (X_L - X_C)$$
$$= (62.8 - 31.8)\Omega$$
$$= 31\ \Omega$$

We can now calculate the impedance (Z):

$$Z = \sqrt{[R^2 + (X_L - X_C)^2]} \qquad \text{(from Equation 14.12)}$$
$$= \sqrt{[(26)^2 + (31)^2]}$$
$$= \sqrt{[676 + 961]}$$
$$= \sqrt{1637}$$
$$= 40.5\ \Omega$$

The phase angle can now be calculated:

$$\theta = \tan^{-1}\frac{(X_L - X_C)}{R} \qquad \text{(from Equation 14.13)}$$
$$= \tan^{-1}(31/26)$$
$$= \tan^{-1} 1.19$$
$$= 50°$$

Finally the peak current may be calculated thus:

$$I = \frac{V}{Z}$$

$$= \frac{400}{40.5}$$

$$= 9.9\ A$$

14.7.4.1 Resonance

In Figure 14.11C, Z is always greater than R because it is the hypotenuse of the triangle. Since $I = V/Z$ the current becomes greater as Z decreases or smaller as Z increases. The smallest possible value of Z is when $XL = XC$, so that $\theta = 0°$ and the impedance is composed solely of the resistance R. The current is then at a maximum for the circuit. This effect is called resonance and depends on the values of L, C and f, as shown below.

Resonance occurs when:

$$X_L = X_C$$

$$2\pi f L = \frac{1}{2\pi f C} \qquad \text{(by cross-multiplication)}$$

$$\therefore f^2 = \frac{1}{4\pi^2 LC}$$

$$\therefore f = \frac{1}{2\pi\sqrt{LC}} \qquad Equation\ 14.15$$

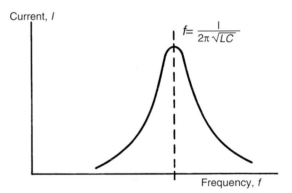

Figure 14.12   Resonance in a resistor, inductor, capacitor (*RLC*) circuit. The current is at a maximum at the resonance frequency.

For given values of L and C, the value of f obtained from this equation is that frequency at which *resonance* or maximum current occurs. Higher or lower frequencies than this *resonance frequency* produce lower currents so that a resonance curve similar to Figure 14.12 is obtained. This principle of resonance in AC circuits is used in the receiver section of the magnetic resonance scanner (see Appendix D) where a capacitor is used in series with an inductor to produce a resonant frequency of the same value as the signal from the patient which we wish to record. Thus the receiver is relatively insensitive to other frequencies. This allows us to collect the signal from a specific area within the patient. (A similar principle is also used to allow us to tune a radio to a specific station frequency.)

14.8 THREE-PHASE AC

The basis of the generation of electricity was explained in Section 13.9. The requirements for electrical power vary widely depending on the piece of machinery used. Thus any national electrical supply must be able to cope with a wide variation in the demand for electrical power. This is done by making available one or more phases of AC. This is made possible by the winding geometry of three-phase AC generators. These have three symmetrical windings (W_1, W_2 and W_3 in Figure 14.13A) on a rotor. These windings are separated by an angle of 120° and, when the rotor is rotated, each in turn moves through a magnetic field.

Each set of windings has a sinusoidal alternating voltage induced in it (see Sect. 13.9) but these voltages are out of phase with each other because of the different times they encounter the strongest regions of the magnetic field within the generator. These voltages (V_1, V_2 and V_3 from the windings W_1, W_2 and W_3) are known as *phase voltages* and are separated by 120° from each other, as shown in Figure 14.13B. Thus a phase difference of 120° exists between each phase voltage. These voltages are now stepped up for transmission over long distances and are then stepped down for use in homes and hospitals. This is accomplished using star and delta connections of the phase voltages, as outlined below.

14.8.1 Star and Delta Connections

Star and delta connections of the phase voltages are shown in Figure 14.14. If we assume that an RMS voltage of 230 volts is induced in each winding of the generator, then three sets of 230 volts supply are available from the delta connection. The centre of the star connection is called the neutral and is kept as near earth potential as possible by equalising the power outputs from the three phases. This allows the possibility of six voltages from the star connection:

- three phase voltages of 230 volts are possible if a connection is made to the neutral and to one end of a winding
- three line voltages of 398 volts are possible by making connections to the ends of two of the windings – one such connection is shown between W_1 and W_3.

Note that the line voltage is 398 volts and not 460 volts, as would be expected, as each phase voltage is 230 volts. This is because of the phase difference between the phase voltages. It may be shown (see Insight below) that the line voltage is also sinusoidal and has a magnitude which is a factor of $\sqrt{3}$ greater than the phase voltage.

INSIGHT

The voltage across L_1 and L_3 in Figure 14.14 is the difference between the voltages across

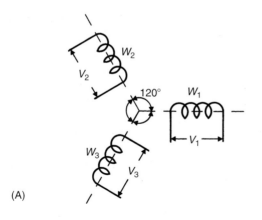

(A)

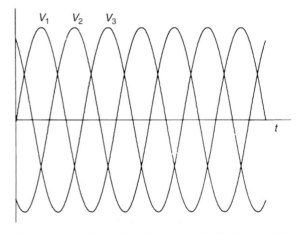

(B)

Figure 14.13 Three-phase electrical generation. (A) Diagrammatic representation of the three sets of windings in the alternating current generator; (B) graphical representation of the three voltage phases against time, showing the 120° separation between each phase.

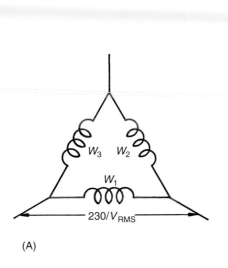

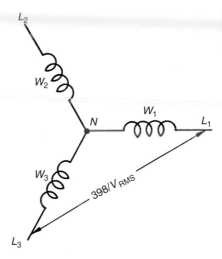

(A)

(B)

L_1–N and L_3–N. If we consider a situation where the potential of N is zero, L_1–N is 10 volts and L_3–N is 4 volts, then the potential difference between L_1 and L_3 is 10 – 4 = 6 volts. Thus we may use the vector diagram shown in the figure below to calculate the line voltage (L) across V_1–V_3.

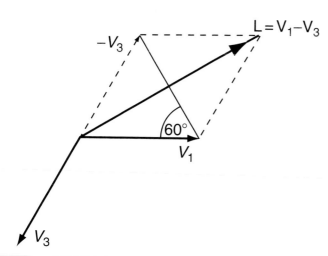

Now sin 60° = $\sqrt{(3)}/2$

$$= \frac{(L/2)}{V_1} \text{ from the figure}$$

$$\therefore L = \sqrt{(3)}V_1$$

Thus the *line voltage* is $\sqrt{3}$ times the *phase voltage*. In the UK the phase voltage is 230 volts (RMS) and so the line voltage is 398 volts (RMS).

The transfer of power from the generating station to a city is shown diagrammatically in Figure 14.15. The four wires L_1, L_2, L_3 and N are distributed to domestic, hospital and industrial users and the appropriate voltages (phase or line) are available, i.e. phase voltages for domestic use and both phase and line voltages for hospital and industrial use. The star connection is often referred to as a *three-phase four-wire supply*, for obvious reasons.

14.8.2 Three-Phase Circuits in Radiography

Three-phase supplies are used in radiography for three main purposes:

1. The line voltage from a three-phase supply is used to ensure that a 398-volt supply is available for most static X-ray sets. This means that the turns ratio (see Ch. 17) required in step-up transformers is less than that required for a 230-volt supply

2. The three-phase X-ray generator uses all three phases to produce an almost constant voltage across the X-ray tube during an X-ray exposure. This will be further discussed in Chapter 19

3. The induction motor used to rotate the anode of the X-ray tube uses three phases. This is further discussed in Chapter 21.

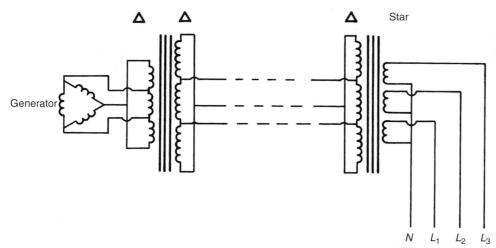

Figure 14.15 Generation and distribution of three-phase supplies. The consumer has a choice of three phase voltages (e.g. L_1–N) or three line voltages (e.g. $L_1 - L_2$).

SUMMARY

In this chapter you should have learnt:

- Sinusoidal AC is described mathematically by the formula $I = I_p \sin 2\pi ft$ and $V = V_p \sin 2\pi ft$ where I_p, V_p are the peak current and voltage and f is the frequency of the AC supply in hertz (see Sect. 14.4)
- One *cycle* is one complete waveform; the *period* is the time for one cycle; the *frequency* is the number of cycles per second; and the *amplitude* is the maximum value of voltage or current (see Sect. 14.4)
- The *frequency* (f) and the *period* (T) are related by the following equation $f = 1/T$ (see Sect. 14.4)
- For *sinusoidal waveform* the average current (or voltage) = 0. For *half-wave rectified AC* the average current (or voltage) = 0.318 × peak current (voltage). For *full-wave rectified AC* the average current (or voltage) = 0.636 × peak current (voltage) (see Sect. 14.4.2)
- The definition of the RMS current is that value of constant current which, acting over the same time, would produce the same expenditure of electrical energy in a circuit as the AC. All AC voltages and currents are quoted in RMS values unless otherwise stated. $I_{RMS} = 0.707 \times I_p$; $V_{RMS} = 0.707 \times V_p$ (see Sect. 14.4.3)

- Voltages across the X-ray tube are expressed in peak voltages (kVp); current through the tube is expressed in average value (mA), and mains supply is expressed in RMS values (see Sect. 14.5)
- The power used in a circuit is given by the equation $W = V_{RMS} \times I_{RMS} \times \cos \theta$ where $\cos \theta$ is the *power factor*. $V \sin \theta$ is the *wattless voltage* and $I \sin \theta$ is the *wattless current* (see Sect. 14.6)
- AC circuits involving the use of capacitors and/or inductors produce a *phase difference* between the current and voltage waveforms. This may be represented by rotating vectors (see Sect. 14.6.1)
- *Resistance, reactance* and *impedance* are all measured in ohms and are the ratio of voltage to amperes (both peak or RMS) at 0°, 90° and θ to the current respectively. θ is the phase difference between the current and voltage waveforms (see Sect. 14.6.2)
- *Inductors* have reactance of $2\pi fL$ which *leads* the current by 90°. *Capacitors* have reactance of $1/2\pi fC$ which *lags behind* the current by 90° (see Sect. 14.7)
- Reactance consumes no net power from an AC supply (see Sect. 14.7.3)
- *Resonance* occurs in an AC circuit when the current is greatest at a particular frequency.

For a series *RLC* circuit the resonance frequency (*f*) is given by the equation $f = 1/2\pi LC$ (see Sect. 14.7.4)

- Three-phase circuits consist of three sinusoidal waveforms 120° apart. These may be connected by *star* or *delta* configurations (see Sect. 14.8)

- The *phase voltage* is that across individual windings; the *line voltage* is that obtained across each of the three connections of the star and delta connections. For a delta connection, the line and phase voltages are equal; for a star connection, the line voltage is √3× the phase voltage (see Sect. 14.8.1).

SELF-TEST

a. What is meant by sinusoidal AC? Illustrate your answer with a graph of current against time.

b. Explain what is meant by peak, average and RMS (or effective) values of a sinusoidal AC. What is the relationship between these values of the current? How will these relationships change if the current is full-wave rectified?

c. A 10-V RMS supply is connected across a 100-Ω resistor. What is:

   (i)   the RMS current in the circuit

   (ii) the peak current in the circuit

   (iii) the average current in the circuit

   (iv) the average power produced in the resistor?

d. If a resistor of resistance 40 Ω, an inductor of inductance 200 mH and a capacitor of capacitance 80 μF are connected in series to an AC supply of frequency 50 Hz and peak voltage 300 V, what are the net impedance in the circuit, the phase angle and the peak current through the circuit?

e. What is meant by the resonance frequency of an *RLC* circuit? What will be the resonance frequency of a circuit that contains an inductor of inductance 200 mH and a capacitor of capacitance 80 μF connected in series?

f. A UK hospital is connected to a three-phase four-wire mains supply. What are the RMS values of the line voltages and phase voltages available?

FURTHER READING

Ball J L, Moore A D 1997 Essential physics for radiographers, 3rd edn. Blackwell Scientific Publications, London, ch 10

Chapter 15

The Motor Principle

CHAPTER CONTENTS

15.1 Aim   134

15.2 Introduction and Definition of the Motor Principle   134

15.3 Direction and Magnitude of the Force on the Conductor   135

15.4 Convention for the Direction of the Force   135

15.5 Interaction of Two Electromagnetic Fields   137
   15.5.1 Two Parallel Wires of Infinite Length   137

15.6 The DC Electric Motor   137

15.7 The AC Induction Motor   138

15.8 Magnetic Deflection of an Electron Beam   139

15.9 The Motor Principle in Radiography   140

Self-Test   140

Further Reading   140

15.1 AIM

The aim of this chapter is to consider the motor principle. The application of this principle to the direct current (DC) motor and the alternating current (AC) induction motor will be considered, as will the magnetic deflection of electrons. Finally, the relevance of these to radiography will be discussed.

15.2 INTRODUCTION AND DEFINITION OF THE MOTOR PRINCIPLE

In Chapter 12 we considered the topic of electromagnetism where a magnetic field was produced by an electric current. This chapter considers what happens when an electromagnetic field is created *in the presence of* another magnetic field. If we consider two bar magnets lying in close proximity one to another, then (depending on their orientation) a force of repulsion or attraction will exist between them (see Ch. 11). If one of the bar magnets is now replaced by a *solenoid* (see Sect. 12.6), we would expect a force between the solenoid and the bar magnet when an electric current is passed through the solenoid, since it behaves like a bar magnet under these circumstances. This force will cause the solenoid to move if it is free to do so. When the current is switched off, the magnetic field due to the solenoid disappears and so does the force between it and the magnet. This interaction between electromagnetism and another magnetic field is known as the *motor principle* (or motor effect) and may be formally defined:

DEFINITION

A current-carrying conductor will experience a force when placed within a magnetic field.

The principle of the electric motor is that it converts electrical energy into kinetic energy (mechanical energy) through the interaction of the two magnetic fields.

15.3 DIRECTION AND MAGNITUDE OF THE FORCE ON THE CONDUCTOR

Consider a length L of straight wire which is carrying an electric current I, the whole wire being placed in a uniform magnetic flux density B, as shown in Figure 15.1. In this diagram it is assumed that the direction of B and of the wire are both in the plane of the paper. Experimentally the following results are observed:

- The *direction* of the force on the wire is always into or out of the paper, i.e. at *right angles* to the direction of B and I
- The *direction* of the force on the wire is *reversed if the current is reversed*
- The *magnitude* of the force is proportional to:
  - the magnetic flux density, B
  - the magnitude of the electric current, I
  - the length of the wire, L

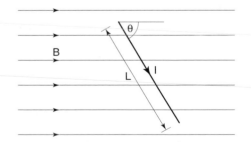

Figure 15.1 The interaction of the permanent magnetic field, *B*, with the magnetic field caused by the current flowing through the wire causes a force to act on the wire – the motor principle.

- the sine of the angle between the direction of B and I, i.e. sin θ in Figure 15.1. Thus the force on the wire is at its maximum when the wire is at right angles to the field (sin 90° = 1) and zero when the wire is parallel to the field (sin 0° = 0).

Combining the factors in the last bullet point above we have:

$$F = BIL \sin θ \qquad \text{Equation 15.1}$$

where F is in newtons, B in teslas, I in amperes and L in metres.

The findings discussed above may be used to define the *tesla* as follows:

DEFINITION

A magnetic flux density of *1 tesla (T)* exists if the force on a straight wire of length *1 metre* is *1 newton* when the wire carries a current of *1 ampere* and is placed at *right angles* to the direction of magnetic flux.

The direction of the force on the current-carrying conductor may be obtained using the appropriate rule or convention. As we saw before, in Chapter 13, Fleming's right- and left-hand rules were produced to deal with 'conventional current' and not electron flow. To avoid confusion, a different convention will be presented to calculate the direction of the force on the current-carrying conductor.

15.4 CONVENTION FOR THE DIRECTION OF THE FORCE

Consider the situation shown in Figure 15.2A, where a wire is carrying an electric current such that the electrons are flowing away from the eye of the observer into the paper. The magnetic field, H, produced by this current is in an anticlockwise direction, as shown. If an external magnetic field, B, is applied to the wire as shown, it is found that the wire experiences a force which pushes it to the right. Figure 15.2B shows the

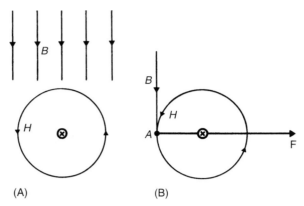

(A)   **(B)**

Figure 15.2 Convention for establishing the force acting on a current-carrying conductor placed in a magnetic field. For an explanation of how to use the convention, see the text.

convention which will be used to determine the direction of the force – this is similar in many ways to the convention used in Section 13.6 to determine the direction of the induced current. The direction of the force can be determined as follows:

1. Mark the position of the wire, and draw the direction of electron flow and the magnetic field around it. In Figure 15.2B this is an anticlockwise magnetic field as the electrons are flowing away from us
2. Align one of the lines of force from the external magnetic field (B) so that it touches the field around the wire at the point where both fields are in the same direction. This occurs at point A in Figure 15.2B
3. Now draw a line from this point through the wire (AF). The direction in which you draw this line indicates the direction of the force acting on the wire. This line is drawn from left to right in this case, agreeing with the previous findings.

This procedure can be applied to any direction of current and any orientation of the wire and the magnetic field. In some cases, however, the applied magnetic field is not exactly perpendicular to the wire and so cannot be made to line up to the field produced by it, as described so far. In this situation, the applied magnetic field may be split into two components: one parallel to the wire (which produces no force on the wire) and one perpendicular to the wire (which will produce a force on the wire according to the

above convention). The following examples should help to clarify the above points.

EXAMPLES

a. The situation of the wire and the external magnetic field is shown in the left-hand diagram below. In the right-hand diagram the observer is looking along the wire (as if looking from the bottom of the page). The convention described previously can now be applied, giving an upward direction of force.

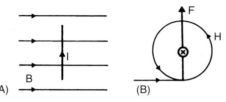

(A)   (B)

b. In this case, when we draw the right-hand diagram, the electrons will be flowing towards the observer and so the magnetic field around the wire will be in a clockwise direction. By applying the convention it can be found that the force is downwards into the paper (the opposite of the previous situation).

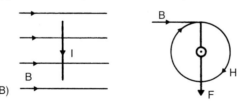

(B)

c. In diagram C the wire and the lines of flux are parallel and so no force will be experienced by the wire when current flows through it.

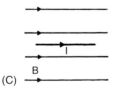

(C)

d. In the situation shown in diagram D the wire is not at 90° to the lines of flux and so these must be split into two components, B_0 which is parallel to the wire and B_{90} which is at right angles to it. This is shown in the right-hand diagram. As described in the previous example, the field which is parallel to the wire (B_0) will have no effect on it and so can be ignored.

Application of the convention now shows that the force acting on the wire will be in an upwards direction, as in the first example.

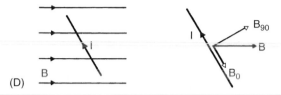

(D)

15.5 INTERACTION OF TWO ELECTROMAGNETIC FIELDS

So far in this chapter we have seen that a force exists on a current-carrying conductor when it is in the presence of a magnetic field and that this is known as the motor principle. It is immaterial whether the magnetic field interacting with the conductor is from a permanent magnet or whether it is produced electromagnetically. In this way, if two current-carrying solenoids are held close together, they behave in the same way as two bar magnets with a north pole at one end of the solenoid and a south pole at the other. Thus the solenoids will attract or repel each other depending on the orientation in which they are placed: like poles repel and unlike poles attract (see Sect. 11.2.1).

15.5.1 Two Parallel Wires of Infinite Length

This rather improbable situation is used in the International System of Units (SI) system to define the ampere and so will be considered here.

Figure 15.3 shows two parallel wires C and D carrying currents I_C and I_D respectively. Figure 15.3A shows the plan view of the wires while Figure 15.3B is the view obtained by looking along the wires towards C and D where the electron flow is into the paper for both wires. The magnetic field around each wire will consist of a series of concentric circles with the field being in an anticlockwise direction. We will now consider how the magnetic field of one wire will interact with the magnetic field of the other. The magnetic field from wire C (B_C) is 'upwards' at wire D while the field from wire D (B_D) is 'down-

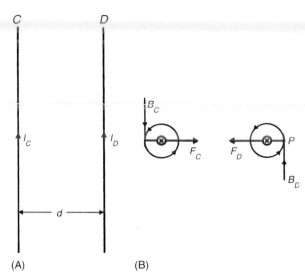

Figure 15.3 (A) The mutual force between two parallel current-carrying wires of infinite length. (B) The same wires rotated through 90° so that the flow of electrons is into the paper. This arrangement is used for the definition of the ampere.

wards' at wire C. If we now apply our convention to this situation we can see that we get forces F_C and F_D, as shown in Figure 15.3B. Thus there is a mutual force of attraction between the wires. This situation is used as the basis of the definition of the ampere in the SI system:

DEFINITION

A current of 1 *ampere* flows in one infinite straight wire if an equal current in a similar wire placed 1 metre away in a vacuum produces a mutual force of 2×10^{-7} newton per metre.

15.6 THE DC ELECTRIC MOTOR

The electric motor is, of course, the prime example of the motor principle in that it converts electrical energy into mechanical energy. To understand the workings of the electric motor we need to understand the motor principle and also electromagnetic induction (see Ch. 13). A simplified DC electric motor is shown in Figure 15.4, where a battery is connected to a coil of wire *KLMN* via brushes B at a commutator C. The coil

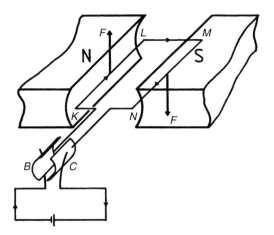

Figure 15.4   The direct current electric motor. See text for details.

of wire is in the magnetic field of a permanent magnet, the direction of whose field is from left to right in the figure.

When the current is switched on, the electron flow is in the direction indicated in the diagram, and the coil is affected by a clockwise force due to the motor principle (i.e. an *upward* force on *KL* and a *downward* force on *MN*, as may be verified using the convention in Sect. 15.4). The commutator *C* turns with the coil *KLMN* so that the current always flows in the same direction relative to the permanent magnet. Hence the coil always experiences a clockwise force and keeps turning. Without the commutator, *KLMN* would eventually stop at right angles to the permanent magnetic field.

Since a clockwise force is being continuously applied to the coil, it would seem logical to assume that the speed of rotation would continuously increase. This does not, in fact, happen. The speed of rotation increases up to a certain rate and then remains constant. To understand why this happens we need to look at electromagnetic induction. We have a conductor *KLMN* which is moving relative to a magnetic field, i.e. undergoing a change of magnetic flux, so an electromotive force (EMF) and current must be induced according to Faraday's and Lenz's laws (see Sects 13.4 and 13.5). The faster the coil rotates, the greater is the induced EMF and current because the rate of change of flux linkage increases (Faraday's second law). The direction

of the induced EMF is in the opposite direction to the applied EMF so this opposes the motion of electrons along *KLMN*. Thus the faster the coil rotates, the smaller is the net current which flows. Thus for a free-moving frictionless motor the rotational speed becomes such that no current at all flows because the forward- and back-EMFs cancel each other out. It is for this reason that an electric motor does not rotate more and more quickly; it achieves a steady speed of rotation due to the back-EMF induced in the windings.

When the motor is under load – performing mechanical work – then the rotational speed reduces so that a net current may flow and electrical energy may be transformed into mechanical and other types of energy.

15.7 THE AC INDUCTION MOTOR

The type of motor commonly used in an AC circuit is an AC induction motor, so called because it works on the principle of electromagnetic induction (particularly Lenz's law). The principle of such a motor may be understood by considering the simple experiment depicted in Figure 15.5A where a bar magnet is moved around the rim of a supported copper disc. It is found that the disc follows the movement of the magnet. The sequence of events is as follows:

- A moving magnetic flux from the magnet is linked with the conductor – the copper disc
- From Faraday's laws we know that an EMF will be induced in the disc. From Lenz's law we can deduce that a current will be induced in the disc in such a way as to oppose the change producing it.

The disc thus moves in the same direction as the magnet in order to reduce the relative motion between them, so opposing the change producing the current, as required by Lenz's law. In a frictionless system, the disc would eventually move at the same speed as the magnet so that there would be no relative motion and no induced currents.

A rather more efficient system is shown in Figure 15.5B where more magnets are used and

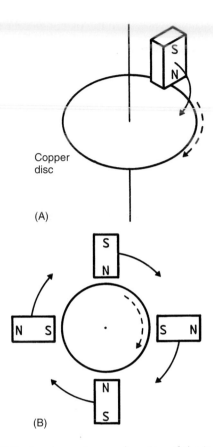

(A)

(B)

Figure 15.5 An elementary explanation of the induction motor. Rotating the magnets in (A) and (B) will cause the disc to rotate in the same direction because of eddy current formation in the copper.

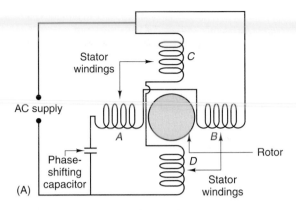

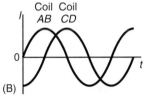

(A)

(B)

Figure 15.6 (A) Cross-section showing the typical arrangement of stator coils and rotor in an induction motor; (B) current waveform produced by the two pairs of coils because of the influence of the phase-shifting capacitor. Note that the current from one pair of coils is at its maximum when the current from the other pair is at zero.

so a higher magnetic flux linkage is obtained. The copper disc follows the direction of rotation of the magnets for the reasons outlined above. It is not necessary to use permanent magnets since current-carrying solenoids will act as magnets.

The arrangement of the coils for such a motor is shown in Figure 15.6. The current through AB will be 90° out of phase with the current through CD. This produces a magnetic field which appears to rotate at the same frequency as the AC mains supply (50 Hz) and so the disc will also rotate at the same speed (50 revs per second (r.p.s.) = 3000 revs per minute (r.p.m.)).

INSIGHT

An AC induction motor is used to cause the rotation of the anode in the rotating anode X-ray tube. The anode assembly is attached to a rotor and these devices are contained within the glass envelope. The stator coils (which produce the rotating magnetic field) are fixed around the outside of this envelope, but the magnetic fields can penetrate the glass and cause the anode to rotate. This will be discussed further in Chapter 21.

15.8 MAGNETIC DEFLECTION OF AN ELECTRON BEAM

There are a number of situations in radiography where we wish to deflect a beam of electrons, e.g. a beam of electrons is made to scan the face of a television monitor to produce an image. Figure 15.7 shows an electron beam travelling in a vacuum and passing through such a magnetic field. It can be seen that the path taken by the electron beam when it passes through the magnetic field is circular since the direction of the deflecting force is always at right angles to

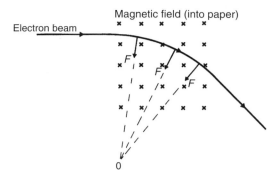

Figure 15.7 The deflection of an electron beam due to a magnetic field. The electrons enter the magnetic field from the left and are deflected on a circular path with 0 as the centre of the circle. The electrons continue on a straight path when they leave the influence of the magnetic field.

the direction of travel. Thus the electrons are deflected when they pass through the magnetic field. After leaving the magnetic field, the beam again travels in a straight line.

The angle of deflection increases as the magnetic flux density increases, so that the direction of the beam can be controlled by varying the magnetic flux density. Thus by placing magnetic deflection coils on either side of a television monitor we can scan the electron beam in a pattern (known as a *raster*) across the face of the monitor.

15.9 THE MOTOR PRINCIPLE IN RADIOGRAPHY

The motor principle is relevant to radiography whenever electrical energy is transformed into mechanical energy via magnetic energy. Obvious examples of this include the use of electric motors to drive mobile X-ray machines and the use of motors to tilt or elevate X-ray tables. The motor principle is also utilised in rotating the anode of the rotating anode X-ray tube. Finally, the motor principle is applied to allow scanning of the electron beam in television cameras and monitors.

SUMMARY

In this chapter you should have learnt:

- The definition of the motor principle (see Sect. 15.2)
- The factors affecting the direction and magnitude of the force acting on a current-carrying conductor in a magnetic field (see Sect. 15.3)
- A convention to establish the direction of the force on a current-carrying conductor in a magnetic field (see Sect. 15.4)
- The interaction between two electromagnetic fields and how this is applied to two parallel wires (see Sect. 15.5)
- The operation of the DC motor (see Sect. 15.6)
- The operation of the AC induction motor (see Sect. 15.7)
- The factors influencing the magnetic deflection of an electron beam (see Sect. 15.8)
- The applications of the motor principle in radiography (see Sect. 15.9).

SELF-TEST

a. Define the motor principle.

b. List the factors which determine the magnitude of the force experienced by a current-carrying conductor placed in a magnetic field and give an equation to calculate this force.

c. Describe the operation of a DC induction motor.

d. List three uses of the motor principle in radiography.

FURTHER READING

Ball J L, Moore A D 1997 Essential physics for radiographers, 3rd edn. Blackwell Scientific Publications, London, ch 8
Ohanian H C 1994 Principles of physics. W W Norton, London, ch 21

Thompson M A, Hattaway R T, Hall J D, Dowd S B 1994 Principles of imaging science and protection. W B Saunders, London, ch 5

Chapter 16

Capacitors

CHAPTER CONTENTS

16.1 Aim 141

16.2 Introduction 141

16.3 Electrical Capacity (Capacitance) 141
16.3.1 Definitions and unit of capacitance (farad) 142

16.4 Capacitance of a Parallel-Plate Capacitor 143
16.4.1 Area of the Plates 143
16.4.2 Separation of the Plates 143
16.4.3 Dielectric Constant of Material Between the Plates 143

16.5 Capacitors in Parallel 144

16.6 Capacitors in Series 144

16.7 Charging a Capacitor Through a Resistor from a DC Supply 145

16.8 The Time-Constant for a Capacitor Resistor Circuit 145

16.9 Discharging a Capacitor Through a Resistor 146

16.10 Capacitors and Alternating Current 146

16.11 Capacitors in Radiography 146
16.11.1 Capacitor Discharge Mobile Units 147
16.11.2 Voltage Smoothing 147
16.11.3 Phase Splitting for AC Induction Motors 148
16.11.4 Electronic Timers 148

Self-Test 148

Further Reading 149

16.1 AIM

The aim of this chapter is to introduce the reader to the subject of capacitors and capacitance. The chapter then considers the factors that influence the performance of a capacitor, how capacitors can be linked to other components and how capacitors are used in radiography.

16.2 INTRODUCTION

In Chapter 14 we considered the influence of a capacitor on the current and the voltage in an alternating current (AC) circuit. We were able to do this without an understanding of the construction or the operation of a capacitor. However, there are circumstances where capacitors are used where we need to understand either the construction and/or the operation of the capacitor to understand its function within the piece of equipment. This chapter deals with the physics of the capacitor and its principal applications in radiography.

16.3 ELECTRICAL CAPACITY (CAPACITANCE)

We have previously shown in Chapter 9 that when a body has a net positive or negative charge it also possesses an electrical potential, because work must be done in moving a unit positive charge from infinity to the body. This

141

potential is positive if the charge on the body is positive and negative if the charge on the body is negative.

The *electrical capacity* or *capacitance* of the body is the relationship between the charge put on the body and its potential:

$$\text{capacitance} = \frac{\text{charge}}{\text{potential}}$$

$$\text{or } C = \frac{Q}{V} \qquad \textit{Equation 16.1}$$

16.3.1 Definitions and Unit of Capacitance (Farad)

The definition of capacitance varies slightly depending on the type of body holding the charge. When a body consists of *one surface* only (e.g. a sphere) the following definition applies:

DEFINITION

The *capacitance* of a body is the ratio of the total charge on the body to its potential.

If the body consists of *two surfaces* close together we must consider the *potential differences* between the surfaces rather than the potential on each. This leads to the following alternative definition of capacitance:

DEFINITION

The *capacitance* of a body is the ratio of the total charge of one sign on the body to the potential difference between its surfaces.

It is important to remember that capacitance involves both charge and potential and so it is not correct to think of capacitance as 'the amount of charge a body can hold' unless we add the phrase 'per unit potential difference'.

The International System of Units (SI) unit of capacitance is the *farad* and may be defined as:

DEFINITION

An electrical system has a capacitance of 1 *farad* if a charge of 1 coulomb held by the body results in a potential (or potential difference) of 1 volt.

Thus Equation 16.1 may be expressed as:

$$\text{farads} - \frac{\text{coulombs}}{\text{volts}} \qquad \textit{Equation 16.2}$$

INSIGHT

An alternative definition of capacity, and one that is often more useful in radiography, is to consider capacity in terms of the *change* of charge divided by the corresponding *change* in potential.

If a capacitor starts with a charge Q and a potential difference then by definition:

$$C = \frac{Q}{V} \qquad \textit{Equation A}$$

If an extra charge, ΔQ, is added to the plates and an extra potential difference ΔV, results, then:

$$C = \frac{(Q + \Delta Q)}{(V + \Delta V)}$$

i.e. *capacitance is the total charge divided by the total potential difference.*

By cross-multiplying the above equation we get:

$$CV + C\Delta V = Q + \Delta Q \qquad \textit{Equation B}$$

But we can say from Equation A that:

$$CV = Q$$

Thus Equation B can be rewritten:

$$C\Delta V = \Delta Q$$

$$\therefore C = \frac{\Delta Q}{\Delta V}$$

This gives the alternative definition of capacitance which can be used in radiography for calculations involving capacitor discharge circuits, etc.

For practical purposes, the farad (F) is rather a large unit in which to measure capacitance and so it is more commonly expressed in units of *microfarads* (μF) or *picofarads* (pF), where:

$$1\ \mu F = 10^{-6}\ F$$

and

$$1\ pF = 10^{-12}\ F$$

16.4 CAPACITANCE OF A PARALLEL-PLATE CAPACITOR

Figure 16.1 shows a parallel-plate capacitor with two plates of equal area (A_1), separated by a distance, d. The plates are made of electrical conductors so that charge may flow in and out of each plate. If the capacitor is *charged* – e.g. by connecting it across a battery as shown – then a charge of $+Q$ will exist on one plate and a charge of $-Q$ on the other. If the battery is disconnected, the charge will continue to be stored on the plates of the capacitor as the positive charge on one plate attracts the negative charge on the other. This is why a capacitor is often described as a device for storing charge. (A large capacitor will retain this charge for a long period of time after it has been disconnected from the source of electromotive force (EMF). For this reason it should be treated *with extreme care* as *severe electric shock* may result from touching the plates or the electrical connections to the capacitor.)

When the capacitor is fully charged, a potential difference equal to that of the battery exists across the plates. Thus, the capacitance of the parallel-plate capacitor is given by the equation $C = Q/V$ where Q is the charge of one sign on one of the plates and V is the potential difference between the plates.

Certain characteristics of the capacitor will affect its capacitance and these will now be considered.

16.4.1 Area of the Plates

If the area of the plates (A) is increased, then more charge will be able to flow on to the plates from the battery until the charge per unit area is the same as before. It can be seen that if the area of the plates is doubled then the amount of charge which they will hold, to give the same charge per unit area, will also be doubled. In this situation V remains unaltered as it is the same as the potential difference from the battery and $Q \propto A$. Since $C = Q/V$ we can say that:

$$C \propto A$$

Note: If the plates are not directly opposite each other, then the area taken for this calculation of capacitance is the effective area, i.e. the area of the plates which are in direct opposition to each other.

16.4.2 Separation of the Plates

If the rest of the capacitor remains unaltered but the plates are brought closer together, then the charges on opposite plates will experience a greater force of attraction so that the battery will be able to 'push' more charge on to the plates. Once again V is constant, but $Q \propto 1/d$. Since $C = Q/V$ we can then say that:

$$C \propto \frac{1}{d}$$

16.4.3 Dielectric Constant of Material Between the Plates

A material with a high dielectric constant is an insulator where it is relatively easy to induce a charge on its surface (see Sect. 9.7.2). The effect of placing such a material between the plates of a charged capacitor is shown in Figure 16.2. The

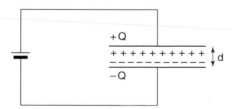

Figure 16.1   A parallel-plate capacitor charged by a battery.

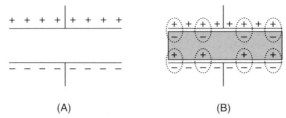

(A)   (B)

Figure 16.2   (A) Parallel-plate capacitor with no dielectric between the plates. (B) Capacitor after a dielectric has been introduced between the plates. The induction of charge in the dielectric 'cancels' some of the charges stored on the plates (shown as ringed charges). This means that the battery can now place more charge on the plates of the capacitor.

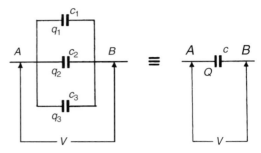

Figure 16.3   Capacitors in parallel. The capacitor C is equivalent to the effect of C_1, C_2 and C_3 connected together in parallel.

close proximity of the charges on the plates and on the dielectric results in some 'cancellation' of charges (as shown ringed in Figure 16.2B). If this capacitor is now reconnected to the battery, it will be seen that more charge will flow on to the capacitor. Thus, once again, V is the same value but Q has increased and so the capacitance of the capacitor increases with the dielectric constant (K), so we can say:

$$C \propto K$$

This leads to the definition of the *dielectric constant*.

DEFINITION

The *dielectric constant* of a material is the ratio of the capacitance of the capacitor with the dielectric to the capacitance without the dielectric (i.e. with a vacuum between the plates of the capacitor).

From this it can be seen that the dielectric constant of a vacuum is unity. If we take the above three components together we get:

$$C \propto \frac{KA}{d}$$

By the addition of a constant of proportionality (ε_0) this now becomes:

$$C = \frac{\varepsilon_0 KA}{d} \qquad \text{Equation 16.3}$$

16.5 CAPACITORS IN PARALLEL

If capacitors are connected in parallel (Figure 16.3), then they behave together like one capacitor of a particular value. The value of this *total* or *equivalent* capacitance may be calculated as follows.

The total capacitance, C, is defined as $C = Q/V$. The total charge, Q, is the sum of all the charges on the individual capacitors (q_1, q_2, etc.), while the potential difference across each capacitor is the same value, V. Thus:

$$C = Q/V$$
$$= \frac{(q_1 + q_2 + q_3)}{V}$$
$$= \frac{q_1}{V} + \frac{q_2}{V} + \frac{q_3}{V}$$
$$C_1 = \frac{q_1}{V} \; ; \; C_2 = \frac{q_2}{V} \; ; \; C_3 = \frac{q_3}{V}$$
$$\therefore C = C_1 + C_2 + C_3 \qquad \text{Equation 16.4}$$

Thus the total capacitance is obtained by summing the individual capacitances. *Note* that the total capacitance must always be larger than the largest value of individual capacitance.

16.6 CAPACITORS IN SERIES

When capacitors are connected in series (Figure 16.4), the total or equivalent capacitance can be established as follows.

If a potential difference, V, is connected across the three capacitors, this results in charges of $+q$ and $-q$ on the plates of each individual capacitor.

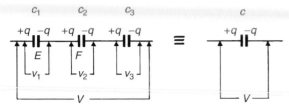

Figure 16.4 Capacitors in series. The capacitor C is equivalent to the effect of C_1, C_2 and C_3 connected together in series.

Thus the capacitors are now fully charged and the following relationships can be established:

$$\frac{1}{C} = \frac{V}{Q}$$

$$= \frac{(V_1 + V_2 + V_3)}{Q}$$

$$= \frac{V_1}{Q} + \frac{V_2}{Q} + \frac{V_3}{Q}$$

$$\frac{V_1}{Q} = \frac{1}{C_1}; \frac{V_2}{Q} = \frac{1}{C_2}; \frac{V_3}{Q} = \frac{1}{C_3}$$

$$\therefore \frac{1}{C} = \frac{1}{C_1} + \frac{1}{C_2} + \frac{1}{C_3} \qquad \textit{Equation 16.5}$$

Note that in this case the total capacitance is less than the value of any of the individual capacitances.

16.7 CHARGING A CAPACITOR THROUGH A RESISTOR FROM A DC SUPPLY

Consider the situation illustrated in Figure 16.5A where a battery is connected across a resistor R and a capacitor C in series. When the switch S_1 is

closed, electrons will flow on to one of the plates of the capacitor and away from the other plate, as shown in the illustration. The potential difference across the capacitor, V_C, therefore increases due to the charge on the plates. However, it does not increase indefinitely, but settles to a value that is the same as (but of opposite polarity to) that of the battery. To understand why this is the case, consider the forces acting on an electron at the point P. When the switch S_1 is initially closed, a complete circuit is made and, due to the EMF from the battery, a force is exerted on the electron, pushing it towards the capacitor. However, as soon as the plate starts to build up electric charge, it in turn exerts a force on the electron at P in the opposite direction, which slows down the rate of flow of charge on to the plate. Eventually the two opposing forces on the electron will become equal and there is no further flow of electrons through the circuit. At this stage the potential across the capacitor is equal and opposite to the potential across the battery. This situation is shown in Figure 16.5B where there is an initial rapid rise in potential (V_C) when S_1 is closed, but this slows down and approaches V_B relatively slowly.

The effect of the resistance R is to limit the electron flow rate so that V_B is approached more slowly for large values of R than for small values of R, as shown in Figure 16.5B.

From this it can be seen that a *capacitor does not pass direct current (DC)*, for, after the short time required to charge the capacitor, all further electron movement (flow of current) ceases.

16.8 THE TIME-CONSTANT FOR A CAPACITOR RESISTOR CIRCUIT

The above experiment is an example of the exponential law (see Ch. 4). This can be seen by comparing the graph in Figure 16.5 with those in Chapter 4. The potential difference between the plates of a discharging capacitor can be calculated from the equation:

$$V_C = V_0 e^{-t/RC} \qquad \textit{Equation 16.6}$$

where V_0 is the potential difference between the plates before discharging the capacitor, t is the time

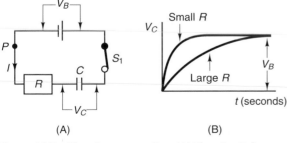

(A)   (B)

Figure 16.5 Charging a capacitor. (A) The circuit for charging a capacitor (C) though resistor (R). (B) Graph showing the effect of using different resistors on the rate of charge.

of the discharge (in seconds), R is the resistance in ohms and C is the capacitance in farads. The quantity RC is called the *time-constant* of the circuit. If R is in ohms and C is in farads then RC is in seconds. After a discharge time of 1 time-constant, i.e. $t = RC$, then the potential difference across a discharging capacitor has dropped to $1/e$ of its initial value, i.e. 0.37 of its initial value. Thus if the original potential difference is 6 V, the value after 1 time-constant is $0.37 \times 6 = 2.2$ V. After 2 time-constants the value will be reduced to a further 0.37, i.e. $0.37 \times 2.2 = 0.8$ V. Note that this is very similar to the concept of half-life discussed in Chapter 4 since both are examples of exponential decay.

If we consider a capacitor being charged then the equation for the potential across it is:

$$V_C = V_0 (1 - e^{-t/RC}) \qquad \textit{Equation 16.7}$$

V_0 is the charging source EMF. Again RC is the time-constant. After 1 time-constant the potential across the capacitor will be $1 - 1/e$, which is 0.63. Thus, for a charging capacitor after 1 time-constant the potential across its plates will be 0.63 of its final value (the final value will be the same as the charging source EMF).

16.9 DISCHARGING A CAPACITOR THROUGH A RESISTOR

In Figure 16.6A a charged capacitor with a potential V_C between its plates is allowed to discharge through the resistor R when the switch S_2 is closed. When this happens, electrons travel from the negative plate of the capacitor, through the resistor

R and on to the positive plate. Hence the charge on the plates and the potential between them (V_C) is reduced. The reduction in V_C means that there will be less 'push' on the electrons through the resistor so less will flow in the next time interval, resulting in a smaller drop in V_C. The situation continues, as shown in Figure 16.6B, until the capacitor is completely discharged and the potential difference is zero. Again, the effect of R is to slow down the current and so the rate of fall of V_C.

16.10 CAPACITORS AND ALTERNATING CURRENT

We have already shown in this chapter that a capacitor will eventually possess the same potential difference as the electrical supply connected across it. If the potential difference of the supply is changed, a new equilibrium will become established where, once again, the two values of potential difference are equal. Thus, if an alternating supply is connected across the capacitor, the potential of the capacitor 'follows' the potential of the supply. Thus it can be said that *a capacitor passes AC* since the potential difference (PD) on the capacitor changes continually, in sympathy with the PD of the supply.

As we have already seen in Chapter 14, when a capacitor is introduced to an AC circuit, the PD across the plates lags 90° behind the current. The effect of this phase difference must be taken into account for many of the uses of capacitors in AC circuits.

16.11 CAPACITORS IN RADIOGRAPHY

The ability to store electrical charge on the plates of a capacitor has important practical consequences in radiography. Some of the practical uses of capacitors in radiography are listed below:

- capacitor discharge mobile units
- voltage smoothing
- phase splitting for AC induction motor
- electronic timers.

There is insufficient space in this text to describe all these uses in detail and so only a brief

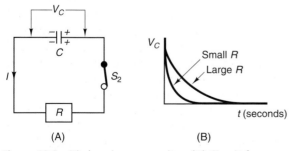

(A) (B)

Figure 16.6 Discharging a capacitor. (A) Circuit for discharging capacitor (C) through resistor (R). (B) Graph showing the effect of different resistors on the rate of discharge.

overview of each will be given. The applications of capacitors in electronic timers will be studied in more detail in Chapter 20.

16.11.1 Capacitor Discharge Mobile Units

When an exposure is made on a mains-dependent mobile unit, a large current (around 30 A) is drawn from the mains during the exposure. This large current can cause large power losses in the mains cables (remember, $P = I^2R$). The capacitor discharge mobile works on the principle that a small current is drawn from the mains to charge a capacitor before the X-ray exposure, and this capacitor is allowed to discharge through the X-ray tube during the exposure. Since the electrical energy to the tube comes from the capacitor, no significant stress is applied to the mains supply during the exposure.

Figure 16.7 shows the basic principles of such a circuit. With the switch open, the capacitor is initially charged until the required potential (V_C is the same value as the kV which will be applied to the tube) is established across its plates. On closing the switch electrons flow from the negative plate of the capacitor to the positive plate via the X-ray tube. This means that a potential difference (kV) is applied across the tube and charge (mAs) flows through it, comprising a radiographic exposure. At the end of the exposure the switch is opened. As a result of the exposure, the capacitor loses some of the charge on its

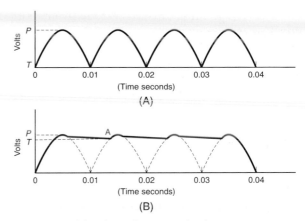

Figure 16.8   (A) Voltage from a single-phase transformer after it has been rectified. (B) The same voltage after capacitor smoothing, where P represents the peak and T the trough. The difference between the peak and the trough is known as the ripple. Note how capacitor smoothing reduces the voltage ripple.

plates and so the potential difference at the end of the exposure is less than the initial potential difference. This must be taken into account when selecting exposure factors on such a unit.

16.11.2 Voltage Smoothing

When an alternating voltage is full-wave rectified (see Ch. 19) and applied to a component, the voltage waveform will be as shown in Figure 16.8A. Thus, during each half-cycle a potential difference ranging from the peak voltage to 0 V is applied across the component. This difference between the peak and the trough in the voltage is known as the *voltage ripple*. In this case the ripple is 100%. There are some situations where it is beneficial to reduce this ripple. This is done by connecting a capacitor (or sometimes two capacitors) in parallel with the component so that the voltage supply is smoothed by the capacitor before it is applied to the component. The result of capacitor smoothing of the voltage is shown in Figure 16.8B. The broken line shows the voltage waveform from the rectification circuit. Initially the capacitor charges so that the potential between its plates is the same as the peak potential from the rectification circuit. As this supply voltage drops, the capacitor discharges through the component so that the potential difference between its plates slowly drops. When this potential has dropped by

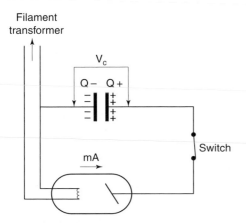

Figure 16.7   Simplified diagram of the principles of a capacitor discharge X-ray circuit.

a small amount the potential from the supply 'catches up' with it (point *A* on the graph) and charge will once again flow on to the capacitor so that it reaches its peak potential difference at the same time as the supply voltage.

This application is important in medium-frequency rectification systems as, by using capacitors that are suitably matched to the components being supplied with electrical energy, the voltage ripple can be reduced to less than 1%.

16.11.3 Phase Splitting for AC Induction Motors

As was discussed in Section 14.7.2, when a capacitor is introduced into an AC supply, it causes a phase shift between the current and voltage. This is utilised in the AC induction motor. The detail of the operation of this motor is given in Section 15.7. The role of the capacitor is to produce a current in one pair of coils which is 90° out of phase with the current in the other pair. This produces a magnetic field which *appears* to rotate at the same speed as the mains frequency and so produces rotation of the motor rotor.

16.11.4 Electronic Timers

The ability to store electrical charge on the plates of a capacitor has important practical consequences in radiography. These will be discussed in Chapter 20.

SUMMARY

In this chapter you should have learnt:

- The meaning of the term *electrical capacitance* (see Sect. 16.3)
- The definition of the farad – the unit of capacitance (see Sect. 16.3)
- The factors affecting the capacitance of a parallel-plate capacitor (see Sect. 16.4)
- The definition of the term *dielectric constant* (see Sect. 16.4)
- The fact that capacitors connected in parallel have a total capacitance, C, given by the equation $C = C_1 + C_2 + C. . ._x$ (see Sect. 16.5)
- The fact that capacitors connected in series have a total capacitance, C, given by the equation $1/C = 1/C_1 + 1/C_2 + 1/C. . ._x$ (see Sect. 16.6)
- The consequences of charging a capacitor from a DC source through a resistor (see Sect. 16.7)
- The definition and the uses of the *time-constant* for a capacitor/resistor circuit (see Sect. 16.8)
- The consequences of discharging a capacitor through a resistor (see Sect. 16.9)
- The effect on the voltage and the current in an AC circuit when a capacitor is introduced to the circuit (see Sect. 16.10)
- Some of the applications of capacitors in radiography.

SELF-TEST

a. What is meant by the term *capacitance?* Define the unit in which capacitance is measured.

b. A 1 μF capacitor is charged until the PD between its plates is 80 kV. What is the charge on the capacitor? The capacitor is then connected across an X-ray tube and an exposure of 10 mAs is made. (*Remember*: 1 mAs = 10^{-3} C.) What is the PD across the capacitor at the end of the exposure?

c. List the factors that affect the capacitance of a parallel-plate capacitor and give the equation that interlinks these factors.

d. How would you connect three capacitors to give:

(i) the maximum capacitance

(ii) the minimum capacitance?

e. What is the total capacitance produced by the following arrangement of individual capacitors?

(*Hint*: first calculate the total capacitance of the capacitors in parallel.)

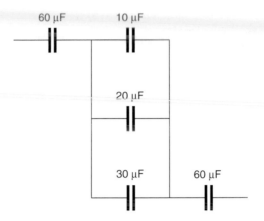

f. A capacitor of 10 µF has a potential difference of 200 V between its plates. It is connected to a resistor of 100 kΩ for a time of 2 s. What will be the potential difference between the plates of the capacitor at the end of that period and how much charge will then be stored by the capacitor?

FURTHER READING

Ball J L, Moore A D 1997 Essential physics for radiographers, 3rd edn. Blackwell Scientific Publications, London, ch 7

Chapter 17

The AC Transformer

CHAPTER CONTENTS

17.1 Aim   150

17.2 Introduction   150

17.3 The Ideal Transformer   151

17.4 Faraday's Laws and Lenz's Law Applied to Transformers   152

17.5 Transformers in Practice   153

17.6 Transformer Losses   153
    17.6.1 Copper Losses   153
    17.6.2 Iron Losses   154
    17.6.3 Regulation   157

17.7 The Autotransformer   158
    17.7.1 Losses and Regulation in the
            Autotransformer   159
    17.7.2 Functions of the
            Autotransformer   159

17.8 The Constant-Voltage Transformer   160

17.9 Transformer Rating   160

Self-Test   161

Further Reading   162

17.1 AIM

The aim of this chapter is to discuss the main concepts that govern the operation of the step-up or the step-down alternating current (AC) transformer. In addition to this, two forms of specialist transformers are discussed, namely the autotransformer and the constant-voltage transformer. Finally there is an overview of the factors that affect transformer rating and how these factors relate to radiographic exposures.

17.2 INTRODUCTION

An AC transformer has an electrical input and an electrical output. For the transformer to function the input is an AC supply. The electrical output potential difference may either be greater or smaller than the electrical input voltage. If the output voltage is greater than the input voltage, then the transformer is a *step-up* transformer; if it is less, then the transformer is a *step-down* transformer. A transformer is thus a device that changes ACs or voltages from one level to another.

The transformer has a wide range of applications in radiography. For example, the mains voltage is too low to be applied directly across the X-ray tube and so it is increased using a step-up transformer (the high-tension transformer). On the other hand, the mains voltage is too high to be connected directly across the filament and so it is reduced in the filament transformer – an example of a step-down transformer.

Two other types of transformer are encountered in radiography and so will also be discussed in this chapter. These are the *autotransformer* and the *saturated core* or *constant-voltage* transformer.

17.3 THE IDEAL TRANSFORMER

Let us start by defining this device:

DEFINITION

An *ideal transformer* is one whose output electrical power is equal to its input electrical power – there is no power 'lost' in the transformer itself.

There is, of course, no such thing as the ideal (or perfect) transformer, although real transformers with efficiencies of 98% or more are not uncommon. Although it is not a practical reality, the concept of the ideal transformer is a useful one in that it simplifies the mathematics which can be used to describe the behaviour of transformers.

Consider such an ideal transformer, shown in Figure 17.1, where two isolated sets of windings share a common core – there are a number of other configurations of core and windings but the one shown in Figure 17.1 is the simplest. The input or *primary* side of the transformer consists of n_p turns around the core and has an alternating voltage V_p across it. The output or *secondary* side of the transformer consists of n_s turns and has

a voltage V_s induced in it. This is a case of mutual induction, as discussed in Section 13.7. The sequence of events is as follows:

- The alternating voltage in the primary winding V_p causes an AC to flow through the winding
- This AC, I_p, produces a *changing magnetic flux density (B)* in the soft iron *core*
- The *changing magnetic flux density* is linked to the secondary winding so that an electromotive force (EMF), V_s, is induced in it according to Faraday's and Lenz's laws of electromagnetic induction (see Sects 13.4 and 13.5).

As already mentioned in the introduction to this chapter, an AC supply is essential for the operation of the transformer since no EMF will be generated in the secondary if the magnetic flux is constant (Faraday's first law).

The purpose of the soft iron core is to contain all the magnetic flux within it so that the magnetic flux linkage between the primary and the secondary is as near perfect as possible. The core is able to do this because of its strong induced magnetism, resulting from its high magnetic permeability (see Table 11.1).

The mathematics of the ideal transformer are relatively simple if we first consider the effect of the magnetic flux on a single turn of wire around the core. Since we are assuming that the transformer is ideal, there is no magnetic flux loss and the EMF induced is independent of the position of the wire. Thus the same voltage will be

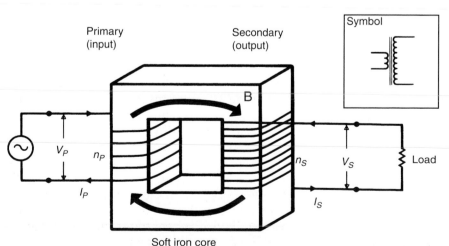

Primary (input)   Secondary (output)

B

V_P n_P n_S V_S Load

I_P

I_S

Soft iron core

Figure 17.1 An 'ideal' transformer showing the core and the primary and secondary windings. In practice the core is laminated, as shown in Figure 17.2. As there are more turns on the secondary winding than on the primary winding, this is a step-up transformer. The symbol for a step-up transformer is also shown. See text for details.

Symbol

induced in each turn of the primary and in each turn of the secondary. If we call this voltage v, then we can say that the total primary voltage is the voltage in each turn multiplied by the number of turns. Thus:

$$V_p = v \times n_p \text{ or } \frac{V_p}{n_p} = v$$

Similarly, for the secondary:

$$V_s = v \times n_s \text{ or } \frac{V_s}{n_s} = v$$

Thus we can combine the two equations above to get:

$$\frac{V_p}{n_p} = \frac{V_s}{n_s}$$

By cross-multiplying this equation we get the formula:

$$\frac{V_s}{V_p} = \frac{n_s}{n_p} \qquad \text{Equation 17.1}$$

This equation is true for either peak or root mean square (RMS) values of the voltage, provided V_s and V_p are both expressed in the same units.

The ratio V_s/V_p is known as the *voltage gain* of the transformer. This is greater than unity for a step-up transformer and less than unity for a step-down transformer.

The ratio n_s/n_p is known as the *turns ratio* of the transformer. Again, if this is greater than unity we have a step-up transformer and if it is less than unity we have a step-down transformer. If we have a transformer with a turns ratio of 200:1, we know that there are 200 times as many turns on the secondary as on the primary and that the voltage across the secondary is 200 times that of the primary.

The *current* flowing in the secondary of the transformer may be calculated from the power in the primary winding and secondary winding (for simplicity, in the following discussion, RMS values are assumed). In the ideal transformer the power in the primary and the power in the secondary are equal. Thus:

$$V_p \times I_p = V_s \times I_s$$

$$\therefore \frac{I_p}{I_s} = \frac{V_s}{V_p}$$

From Equation 17.1 we know:

$$\frac{V_s}{V_p} = \frac{n_s}{n_p}$$

Thus, for an ideal transformer, we can say:

$$\frac{I_p}{I_s} = \frac{n_s}{n_p} \qquad \text{Equation 17.2}$$

If we consider Equations 17.1 and 17.2 we can see that, if the voltage is increased by a factor of n_s/n_p, then the current is reduced by the same factor. Thus a step-up transformer will increase the voltage but will decrease the current by the same factor.

17.4 FARADAY'S LAWS AND LENZ'S LAW APPLIED TO TRANSFORMERS

We have already considered Faraday's laws of electromagnetic induction (Sect. 13.4) and Lenz's law (Sect. 13.5) and we can now look at how these are applied to transformers.

As discussed in the previous section, there is a changing magnetic flux produced by the alternating supply connected to the primary and, since this is linked to both the primary and secondary windings, by Faraday's laws, an EMF is produced in each of the windings. Assuming we have an ideal transformer, the magnitude of the EMF in each turn of the primary winding is equal to the magnitude of the EMF in each turn of the secondary.

Lenz's law may be used to determine the direction of the induced current in the secondary. As it acts to oppose the changing magnetic flux, it will be in the opposite direction to (180° out of phase with) the current in the primary. The eddy currents induced in the core (these will be discussed later in this chapter as they are part of the transformer 'losses') will also be in the opposite direction to the primary current.

INSIGHT

Some students find it surprising that it is the current drawn from the secondary of a transformer that determines the primary current, especially as the secondary voltage for a given transformer is determined by the primary voltage. The explanation of this fact is as follows.

Consider a situation when the secondary winding is open circuit – it is not connected to anything – so no current can flow through it, although an EMF is induced across it. If we assume that we have an ideal transformer, then the same EMF will be induced by this magnetic flux in the primary winding and by Lenz's law this will be in the opposite direction to the forward-EMF. Thus no current flows in the primary winding when the secondary current is zero.

If the secondary is now connected across an external circuit so that some current flows through it, this current, by Lenz's law, will oppose the magnetic flux in the core. The core flux is thus reduced and so the back-EMF in the primary is reduced. The forward-EMF in the primary is now greater than the back-EMF and so a current flows. Thus a current in the secondary has caused a current to flow in the primary, the relative magnitudes of each being given by Equation 17.2.

17.5 TRANSFORMERS IN PRACTICE

It is not possible to construct an ideal transformer, as there are always power 'losses' within the transformer itself. This means that the power in the secondary is always less than the power in the primary by an amount equal to the transformer losses. The efficiency of a transformer may be defined as follows:

DEFINITION

The *efficiency* of a transformer is the ratio of the output power to the input power.

Note: It is often convenient to express the transformer efficiency as a percentage. For example, if a transformer is 95% efficient and 100 watts of power is supplied to the primary of that transformer, then 95 watts is produced in the secondary. In this case 5% of the power is 'lost' because of power loss in the windings and core, i.e. this 5% is not available as useful electrical power.

Equation 17.1 gives a reasonable estimate of the voltage change in practical transformers but Equation 17.2 no longer applies because of the power losses in practical transformers. This may be illustrated by the following example.

EXAMPLE

A transformer has a turns ratio of 100:1 and an efficiency of 95%. If a current of 5 A_{RMS} flows in the primary when a voltage of 10 V_{RMS} is applied across it, what is the output RMS voltage and output RMS current?

From Equation 17.1 we get:

$$\frac{V_s}{V_p} = \frac{n_s}{n_p}$$

$$\therefore \frac{V_s}{10} = \frac{100}{1}$$

$$V_s = 1000 \ V_{RMS}$$

We also know that efficiency is the ratio of the output power to the input power. Thus:

$$\text{efficiency} = \frac{(V_s \times I_s)}{(V_p \times I_p)}$$

$$\therefore \frac{95}{100} = \frac{(1000 \times I_s)}{(10 \times 5)}$$

$$\therefore I_s = \frac{(50 \times 95)}{(100 \times 1000)} \ \text{(by cross-multiplication)}$$

$$= 47.5 \ \text{mA}_{RMS}$$

Note that an ideal transformer would have produced the same secondary voltage but the secondary current would be 50 mA_{RMS}.

17.6 TRANSFORMER LOSSES

A detailed analysis of the sources of transformer losses is considered in this section. These are summarised in Table 17.1 and discussed below.

17.6.1 Copper Losses

The term *copper* refers to the copper wire of the windings of the transformer which has a small

Table 17.1 A summary of the losses associated with a practical transformer

Transformer loss	Comments
Copper losses	Caused by the resistance of the copper windings. Also known as I^2R losses
Iron losses	Losses produced in the transformer core
Imperfect magnetic flux linkage	Very small loss
Eddy currents	Caused by electromagnetic induction within the core of the transformer – reduced by core lamination
Hysteresis	Caused by the work required to move the magnetic domains – reduced by the appropriate choice of core material (e.g. stalloy)
Regulation (a consequence of all the above losses)	Output voltage decreases with increased current load because of the increased transformer losses due to the resistance of the windings

but finite resistance. If we consider a current I_{RMS} flowing through a resistance R, then there is a power of $(I_{RMS})^2R$ watts produced within the resistor. (The copper loss is often referred to as the I^2R loss of the transformer.) The copper loss produces a small heating within the coils of the transformer.

We wish to keep the copper loss as low as possible and, as it is related to I^2R, it makes sense to keep R low when I is large. As we saw in Chapter 10, the resistance of a conductor is inversely proportional to its cross-sectional area. For this reason the winding of the transformer which carries the larger current is made of the thicker wire. In the step-up transformer this is the primary winding and in the step-down transformer it is the secondary winding.

17.6.2 Iron Losses

The term *iron losses* refers to the losses that occur in the soft iron core of the transformer. These take three forms, as outlined below.

17.6.2.1 Magnetic Flux Losses

If the iron core is magnetically saturated, then all of the magnetic flux will not be contained within the core. This means that magnetic flux will be produced by the primary which is not linked with the secondary. The EMF induced in the secondary and the output electrical power will be lower than if the flux linkage were perfect. By the appropriate design of the transformer core, this loss is made very small indeed and so can be neglected for most practical purposes.

17.6.2.2 Eddy Currents

From Faraday's and Lenz's laws we know that when a changing magnetic flux is linked with a continuous conductor an EMF and current are induced in the conductor. Also, the direction of the induced current opposes the effect of the changing magnetic flux linkage. The iron core of the transformer is a continuous electrical conductor and so the varying flux passing through the core will induce electric currents within the core itself in such a direction as to oppose the changing magnetic flux within the core. This principle is shown in Figure 17.2A where the direction of the eddy currents in the core is in the opposite direction to the current in the winding. The effect of these currents is twofold:

1. The flow of electrical current through the core causes heating of the core due to the electrical resistance of the core
2. The magnetic flux associated with the eddy currents is in the opposite direction to the flux from the winding and so there is a reduction in the flux interlinking with the secondary – flux which interlinks with the secondary is the flux produced at the primary minus the eddy current flux. This constitutes a power loss within the transformer core.

Eddy currents may be reduced but not entirely eliminated by *lamination* of the core, as shown in Figure 17.2B and C. The laminated sheets of soft iron are bolted together to produce the required cross-sectional area. Each lamination is insulated from its neighbours by the application of a thin layer of insulation (e.g. shellac varnish) to its surface. This means that the eddy currents produced

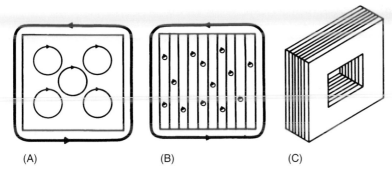

Figure 17.2 (A) Flow of eddy currents in an unlaminated transformer core. If the core is laminated as shown in (B) and (C), then the eddy current flow is restricted and so the eddy current losses are limited.

(A)   (B)   (C)

in the core are now confined to the small cross-sectional area of each lamination. As resistance is inversely proportional to cross-sectional area, lamination produces an increase in resistance and a consequent reduction in the size of the eddy current. There is, however, some eddy current present and this causes heating of the transformer core. Because of this, the transformer core requires to be cooled either by air or by immersing the transformer in oil, the latter acting as both a coolant and an insulator.

17.6.2.3 Hysteresis Losses

We introduced the topic of hysteresis in Section 11.7 and we are now ready to look at this in more detail and also to look at its implication for transformer losses.

Hysteresis is the lagging-behind of the induced magnetism in a ferromagnetic material when the applied magnetic field changes. Consider the changes which will occur in a transformer core during $1\frac{1}{2}$ cycles of AC. The magnetising force H changes with the current (see Figure 17.3A) and this produces changes in the magnetic intensity I as shown in Figure 17.3B. This graph is referred to as a *hysteresis loop* and the shape and size of this loop are important in the function of the transformer. The shape of this loop is explained as follows.

Consider a situation where the core is initially unmagnetised. As the magnetic domains are in randomised directions there is no magnetic intensity within the core. This represents the origin O on both of the graphs. The current increases until it reaches its peak value at point A. The magnetising force increases with the current and so initially does the magnetic intensity. This, however, flattens as magnetic saturation of the sample occurs so that

the line is horizontal at point A on the hysteresis graph. The current now follows the curve AB and, as the magnetising force decreases, so the magnetic intensity reduces along the curve AB on the hysteresis graph. Note that at point B the magnetising force is zero but there is still some magnetic intensity left in the ferromagnetic core sample. This magnetic intensity is known as the *remanence* in the core. To get rid of this remanence – so completely demagnetising the core – a *coercive force*, represented by OC, must be used. Because the current has been reversed, the magnetising force is also reversed and this continues until magnetic saturation is again produced at D. This occurs at the negative peak value of the current. As the current is reduced, the magnetising force is again reduced and it is zero when the current is at point E on the graph of current. At this point on the hysteresis graph there is again a remanence represented by OE (equal and opposite to OB) and this must be destroyed by the coercive force OF. The magnetising force now continues to its positive peak, A, and the magnetic intensity follows the curve FA. The hysteresis loop is now complete.

The *area of the hysteresis loop* is important as it represents the work done in taking the sample round a complete hysteresis cycle. In considering the transformer core, the smaller the amount of work done, the smaller the iron loss from hysteresis. This should become clearer if we consider the hysteresis loops for soft iron and for steel.

Figure 17.4 shows the differences in the hysteresis loops for soft iron and steel. These differences may be summarised as follows:

- The saturation of soft iron occurs at much lower values of magnetising force than the saturation of steel

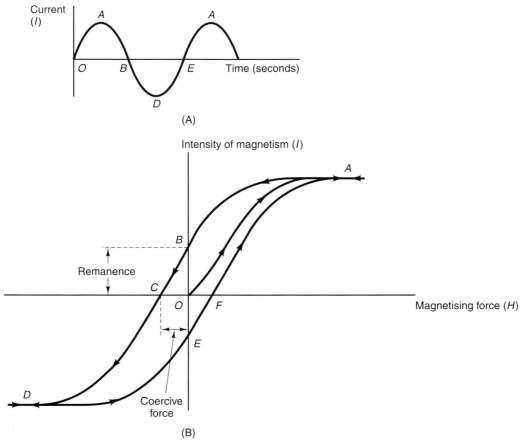

Figure 17.3 (A) Typical alternating current supply for a transformer winding; (B) hysteresis loop for a ferromagnetic sample. For an explanation of the connection between the two, see the text.

- The value of the coercive force is much greater for steel than for soft iron
- The area of the hysteresis loop is much greater for steel than for soft iron.

Soft iron is therefore suitable for situations where a strong induced magnetism is required with the minimum expenditure of energy, and where the induced magnetism may be switched off at will. Note that, although the remanence is greater for soft iron than for steel, the coercive force is so small that a slight agitation of the sample will cause it to demagnetise. Suitable applications for soft iron are electromagnetic relays (see Sect. 12.7) and transformer cores (used as an alloy – stalloy).

Steel is a more suitable material for permanent magnets since it has a higher coercive force than soft iron and is thus more difficult to demagnetise.

The high coercive force and the large area of the hysteresis loop make it unsuitable for use in the transformer core.

Subsidiary hysteresis loops. It is not necessary to take a ferromagnetic sample around a complete hysteresis loop, i.e. from magnetic saturation one way to magnetic saturation the other. In such cases *subsidiary hysteresis loops* result, as shown in Figure 17.5. This is the type of hysteresis loop produced in most transformers – the exception being the saturated core transformer which produces a complete hysteresis loop. The material with the hysteresis loop with the smallest area is still the most appropriate core material for a transformer.

The material usually selected for transformer cores is *stalloy* or *permalloy* as their small hysteresis

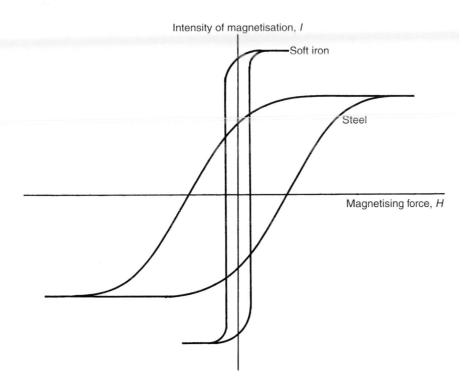

Intensity of magnetisation, I

Soft iron

Steel

Magnetising force, H

Figure 17.4   A comparison of the hysteresis loops for soft iron and steel.

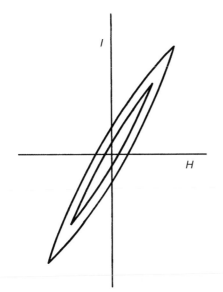

I

H

Figure 17.5   Subsidiary hysteresis loops where the ferromagnetic sample is not taken to full magnetic saturation.

loops limit the hysteresis 'loss'. The power loss due to hysteresis in the core increases the kinetic energy of the atoms of the core and so manifests itself in the form of heat.

17.6.3 Regulation

Regulation in a transformer is a consequence of the resistance of the windings. If the electrical load drawn from the secondary is *increased* – a higher current is made to flow in the secondary – it is found that the potential difference across the secondary is *decreased*. This effect is known as the transformer regulation.

Regulation occurs in any source of electricity which contains an internal resistance. In the case of the transformer, the internal resistance is taken as the resistance of the secondary winding. Figure 17.6 shows a graph of the voltage output from a given transformer for differing secondary currents. The output current is zero when the secondary is open-circuit and this corresponds to the open-circuit voltage (V_0 in Figure 17.6). In this condition the transformer has zero regulation – it behaves as an ideal transformer and so Equation 17.1 may be used to calculate the secondary voltage. When the secondary of the transformer is connected to a load, current will flow in the secondary winding and the output voltage falls linearly with the secondary current.

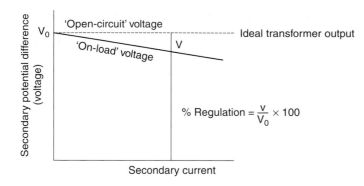

Figure 17.6 The greater the current drawn from the secondary winding of the transformer, the smaller becomes the potential difference across it. This effect is caused by the resistance of the windings and is known as transformer regulation.

The transformer regulation therefore varies with the transformer load and so the output current is usually quoted with the regulation, e.g. *a transformer has a regulation of 2% when the secondary current is 400 mA*. The regulation is often expressed as a percentage and may be defined as follows:

DEFINITION

The *percentage regulation* at a given load can be calculated by:

$$100 \times \frac{\text{(open-circuit voltage – on-load voltage)}}{\text{open-circuit voltage}}$$

In Figure 17.6:

$$\text{percentage regulation} = 100 \times \frac{V}{V_0}$$

Most transformers used in radiography have a low percentage regulation and so the on-load voltage is close to the open-circuit voltage. In the case of the high-tension transformer, however, there must be a correction for this regulation otherwise there would be a fall in the kVp if the tube mA was increased. Such corrections are made by compensating circuits, which are beyond the scope of this text.

INSIGHT

The primary winding of a step-up transformer has such a low resistance that its effect on regulation may be ignored. If an EMF of V_0 is induced in the secondary and the secondary resistance is r, then a current I will produce a voltage drop of Ir (Ohm's law: $V = IR$) across the internal resistance r. This means that the potential difference which is available to the external circuit has been reduced by an amount Ir. Thus:

$$V = V_0 - Ir$$

This formula should explain why the regulation is linear with the current, as shown in Figure 17.6. It should also be noted that when the secondary is open-circuit then the secondary current is zero and so the voltage drop because of the internal resistance is zero. In such a situation $V = V_0$.

17.7 THE AUTOTRANSFORMER

The autotransformer is a useful device for selecting a range of output voltages whose values are not very different from the input voltages (usually differing by a factor of between 0.5 and 2.0). It is constructed in such a way that the number of turns across which the primary voltage is applied can be varied (by moving S_1 in Figure 17.7). It is also possible by moving the switch S_2 to alter the number of turns on the secondary or output side of the transformer – S_1 selects the number of primary turns, n_p, while S_2 selects the number of secondary turns, n_s.

The principle of operation of this transformer is illustrated in Figure 17.7. The transformer consists of a *single winding* (with a primary and a secondary side) round a soft iron core. This transformer therefore operates on the principle of self-induction (see Sect. 13.8). If we consider

17.7.2 Functions of the Autotransformer

In X-ray units, the autotransformer is positioned between the mains supply and the input to the high-tension transformer. The autotransformer had a number of functions but only two of these are pertinent to this discussion. They are:

1. mains voltage compensation
2. kV selection.

17.7.2.1 Mains Voltage Compensation

In Figure 17.7 the mains voltage is connected to the autotransformer across n_p primary turns, selectable by switch S_1. To understand the workings of the mains voltage compensation at S_1 it is best to consider a numerical example. Let us assume that there are normally 200 turns across n_p and that the normal mains voltage to the transformer is 400 volts. If we assume that this is an ideal transformer, we have a normal volt-drop of 2 volts per turn in the transformer. To ensure the correct output from the transformer across n_s, this volt-drop must be maintained at this level irrespective of the mains voltage input to the transformer. If the mains voltage falls to 380 volts (because of increased demand), then the volt-drop per turn within the transformer will be less than 2 volts per turn (in fact, it will be 1.9 volts per turn). To get back to the 2 volts per turn and thus the correct operation of the transformer, the switch S_1 must be adjusted to spread this voltage across 190 turns. This gets the autotransformer back to its normal operating voltage of 2 volts per turn. For this reason the switch S_1 is usually referred to as the *mains voltage compensator*.

17.7.2.2 kV Selection

Again, this is probably easiest to understand if we consider a numerical example. As already mentioned, the output from the autotransformer forms the input to the high-tension transformer in the X-ray circuit. Suppose we have an ideal high-tension transformer with a turns ratio of 250:1. If we wish an output voltage from this transformer of 100 kV, then we need an input voltage of 400 V, and if we want an output voltage of 50 kV, then we need an input voltage

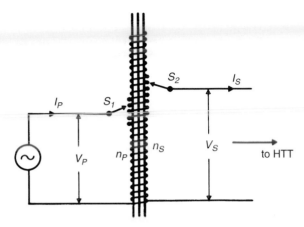

Figure 17.7 A circuit diagram for an autotransformer. This works on the principle of self-induction. The number of primary turns n_p can be varied at S_1 and the number of secondary turns n_s can be varied at S_2. Thus the output from the transformer can be varied. HTT, high-tension transformer.

this as an ideal transformer, we can argue that the same magnetic flux links each turn of the winding and so the induced EMF in each turn is constant. Thus Equations 17.1 and 17.2 can also be applied to the autotransformer, the only difference being that the primary and secondary turns are selected from the same winding. As mentioned earlier, the differences between the input and output voltages at the autotransformer are restricted and so the ratio of n_s/n_p is usually in the range between 0.5 and 2.0.

17.7.1 Losses and Regulation in the Autotransformer

All the sources of power loss discussed in Section 17.6 also apply to the autotransformer. However, the less severe design constraints required for the autotransformer make it possible to use a thick winding of copper wire with a consequent reduction in winding resistance. Thus the copper losses and the regulation are lower for the autotransformer than for the conventional transformer as both these losses are dependent on the resistance of the windings. One practical consequence of this is that there is not a great deal of heat generated in the autotransformer and so it is air-cooled.

of 200 V. The input voltages for the high-tension transformer are determined at the autotransformer. If we consider the autotransformer used in the previous example, it has a voltage difference of 2 volts per turn. Thus, if we wish to get 100 kV from the high-tension transformer, we move the switch S_2 until n_s is 200 turns. Similarly, if we wish to get 50 kV, S_2 is adjusted so that n_s is 100 turns. For this reason S_2 is referred to as the *kV selector*.

17.8 THE CONSTANT-VOLTAGE TRANSFORMER

The constant-voltage transformer is designed in such a way that there can be considerable variations in the input voltage to the transformer but the output voltage remains relatively constant. For reasons which will be discussed in Chapter 21, the output from the X-ray tube is sensitive to the temperature of the tube filament and so some units use a constant-voltage transformer to ensure a well-stabilised voltage supply to the filament. Figure 17.8A gives a diagrammatic representation of the construction of such a transformer and Figure 17.8B shows a graph of the input and output voltages.

This transformer operates on the principle that the secondary limb of the core, B, is magnetically saturated during normal operation. The magnetic flux produced at the primary core, A, passes through two other magnetic circuits, the much thinner secondary core, B, and a central path of high magnetic resistance in core C – this high magnetic resistance is caused by the fact that there is an air gap between one end of C and the rest of the core (remember, air is less permeable than iron; see Table 11.1). The thinner core, B, is rapidly brought to magnetic saturation and the excess magnetic flux then passes through C. As can be seen from the graph, once B is saturated then an increase in input voltage does not produce any more magnetic flux in B and so the output voltage from the transformer remains fairly constant. Magnetic saturation occurs at an input voltage of X, and Y represents the normal operating input voltage of the transformer. Note that a large fall in the input voltage (say to Z on

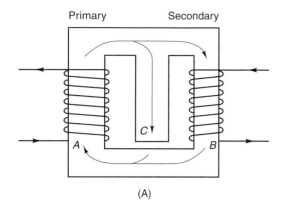

(A)

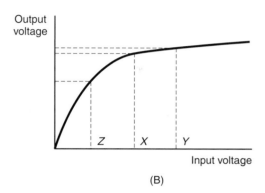

(B)

Figure 17.8   (A) Construction of a typical constant-voltage transformer; (B) graph of the input and the output voltage for such a transformer.

the graph) can result in the limb B becoming unsaturated with a resultant fall in the output voltage.

17.9 TRANSFORMER RATING

Transformer rating was briefly discussed in Section 14.6. The term *rating* means the maximum combination of factors which a system can withstand without damage. If the rating is exceeded for a transformer, this may cause damage to the electrical insulation of the windings because of overheating or it may cause electrical breakdown.

The transformers in an X-ray unit are energised when the X-ray exposure is made. There are basically two types of exposure in radiography:

1. fluoroscopy – this uses a low amount of power for a relatively long time

2. radiographic exposures – these use a relatively large amount of power for a short time.

Each of the above produces heat in the high-tension transformer and this transformer thus requires oil cooling. In particular, a long exposure must be made at a relatively low current (and therefore low power), otherwise the heat generated in the transformer will not be convected away sufficiently quickly by the oil and the transformer will overheat. Short exposures may use higher current values since the total energy deposited in the windings will still be low enough to cause no damage.

The detailed specification of the rating of any one transformer may be complicated, dealing with all the conceivable situations in which the transformer may be used. There are three main factors that must be considered:

1. the maximum kVp which the secondary winding may produce
2. the maximum continuous current the transformer may supply – this would be used in fluoroscopy
3. the maximum current supplied for short exposures – this would be used during radiographic exposures.

SUMMARY

In this chapter you should have learnt:

- The concept of an ideal transformer and the equations for voltage and current produced from such a transformer (see Sect. 17.3)
- How Faraday's laws and Lenz's law apply to transformers (see Sect. 17.4)
- The types of losses that occur in a practical transformer and how these are minimised (see Sect. 17.6)
- Transformer regulation and its effect on the output voltage from a transformer (see Sect. 17.6.3)
- The operating principles and main functions of an autotransformer in an X-ray set (see Sect. 17.7)
- The operating principles of a constant-voltage transformer (see Sect. 17.8)
- The factors to be considered for transformer rating in radiography (see Sect. 17.9).

SELF-TEST

a. If 110 V_{RMS} is applied to the primary of an ideal transformer with a turns ratio of 500:1, what is the RMS voltage output from the secondary? What is the peak voltage output from the secondary?

b. What is meant by the efficiency of a transformer? A transformer has a primary winding consisting of 500 turns and a secondary winding consisting of 50 000 turns. This transformer has an efficiency of 95%. The voltage applied to the primary is 240 V_{RMS} and the secondary current is 1.9 mA_{RMS}. What is the primary current?

c. Explain why the potential difference across the secondary of a high-tension transformer is reduced when the electric current drawn from it is increased.

d. A step-up transformer has a turns ratio of 500:1 and a regulation of 2% when the secondary output current is 400 mA. What is the secondary output voltage that accompanies this current if the primary input voltage is 200 V?

e. An ideal autotransformer normally has an input voltage of 200 V across a primary side consisting of 800 turns.

(i) How many turns must be engaged on the secondary side to achieve an output voltage of 150 V?

(ii) If the input voltage were now to fall to 160V, what would be the secondary output voltage from the transformer, assuming that the switches were in the same position as in (i)?

(iii) How many turns should now be engaged at the input of the transformer to restore the output voltage to 150 V?

f. What is meant by the term *transformer rating*? Explain two ways in which damage may occur to a transformer if the rating is exceeded. Why is it necessary to contain some transformers (e.g. the high-tension transformer in the X-ray circuit) in an oil bath?

FURTHER READING

Ball J L, Moore A D 1997 Essential physics for radiographers, 3rd edn. Blackwell Scientific Publications, London, ch 10

Chapter 18

Semiconductor Materials

CHAPTER CONTENTS

18.1 Aim   163

18.2 Introduction   163

18.3 Intrinsic Semiconductors   164
    18.3.1 Positive Holes   164
    18.3.2 Silicon   165

18.4 Extrinsic Semiconductors   166
    18.4.1 *N*-type Semiconductors   166
    18.4.2 *P*-type Semiconductors   167
    18.4.3 Diagrammatic Representation of N- and P-types   168

18.5 The *PN* Junction   168
    18.5.1 Minority Carriers at the *PN* Junction   169
    18.5.2 Forward Bias   169
    18.5.3 Reverse Bias   170
    18.5.4 The *PN* Junction as a Diode   170
    18.5.5 *PN* Junction Characteristics   171

18.6 The Transistor   171
    18.6.1 The *NPN* Junction Transistor   171
    18.6.2 The Field-Effect Transistor   172

18.7 The Thyristor   173

18.8 Semiconductor Devices in Radiography   174

Self-Test   175

Further Reading   176

18.1 AIM

The aim of this chapter is to introduce the reader to semiconductors and semiconducting devices which are important to radiography. While this is a very large field, the chapter concentrates on the barrier layer rectifier, the transistor and the thyristor, all of which have made a major impact on radiographic science. Finally, there is an overview of the uses of semiconductor devices in radiography.

18.2 INTRODUCTION

The use of semiconductor materials and the associated technology play an increasingly important part in our everyday lives as well as in radiographic science. It is possible to produce many thousands of electronic circuits on a small silicon chip using very-large-scale integration (VLSI) techniques. This enables the production of microprocessors which are capable of being programmed to perform specific tasks. Such devices are cheap and easy to program, can perform a wide range of functions and are very reliable. Because of this, microprocessors are found in devices from wristwatches to aircraft flight systems and it is not surprising to learn that they are used in many devices in diagnostic imaging and radiotherapy departments.

However, the microprocessor is a complicated solid-state device and a detailed description of its operation is beyond the scope of this text. Other, simpler, solid-state devices are widely used in X-ray circuitry and hence are suitable for inclusion in this chapter after a general description of the properties of semiconductor materials.

18.3 INTRINSIC SEMICONDUCTORS

An intrinsic semiconductor is a chemically pure semiconductor which is also assumed to have perfect regularity of atoms within its crystal lattice. The concept of semiconducting materials was briefly introduced in Section 10.3.2 where the properties of conductors, insulators and semiconductors were compared in terms of the energy band model for the orbiting electrons. This was illustrated in Figure 10.3 and this diagram is reproduced here as Figure 18.1. As shown in Figure 18.1B, one of the characteristics of semiconductors is that there is a small energy gap (up to a few eV) between the top of the valence band and the bottom of the conduction band. At very low temperatures all the outer electrons have energies near the bottom of the valence band. Thus no electrons are able to take part in electrical conduction, as there are no free electrons in the conduction band. As mentioned in Chapter 10, increasing the temperature of a semiconductor increases its conductivity. Thus at normal room temperatures many electrons are able to gain sufficient energy (because of the increased kinetic energy of the atoms) to jump up to the conduction band and so take part in electrical conduction.

18.3.1 Positive Holes

Associated with each electron which is able to jump up to the conduction band is a 'vacancy' in the valence band, referred to as a positive hole or just hole. This hole may be filled by an electron from the valence band of a neighbouring atom, but in doing so the electron leaves a hole in the valence band of that atom. In this way a hole may appear to move around the crystal lattice of a semiconductor (behaving like a positive charge) until eventually an electron drops down from the conduction band to fill the hole and remove it from the valence band. This process is referred to as recombination. At any one moment all three of the above processes are occurring:

1. Electrons are being excited into the conduction band creating holes in the valence band
2. There is movement of electrons in the conduction band and holes in the valence band
3. There is a recombination of electrons in the conduction band with holes in the valence band
4. The overall conductivity of such an intrinsic semiconductor is the sum of the effects of the movements of the electrons in the conduction band and the holes in the valence band.

INSIGHT

Consider the situation depicted in part A of the diagram below, where there is a row of ball bearings at the base of a box, with no available space between them for sideways movement to take place. If we now lift ball bearing C on to the lid of the box, it is possible for ball bearing D to move to the left to fill the space once occupied by C. In doing so, D has now created a space to its right, i.e. the hole may be considered as moving in the opposite direction to the ball.

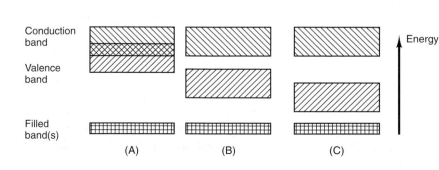

Conduction band	
Valence band	
Filled band(s)	
(A) (B) (C)	↑ Energy

Figure 18.1 Energy level bands for (A) a conductor, (B) a semiconductor and (C) an insulator.

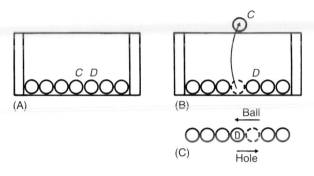

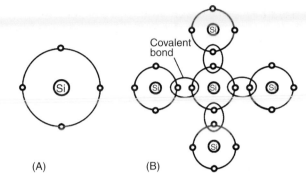

Figure 18.2 Pure silicon as an example of an intrinsic semiconductor. (A) A silicon atom showing the four electrons in its valence shell; (B) the covalent bonds formed in a pure silicon crystal by each silicon atom sharing electrons with four neighbouring silicon atoms.

Now consider the above situation as it refers to the valence and conduction bands of a semiconductor. No net movement is initially possible in the valence band because it is full of electrons. When an electron is raised to the conduction band, movement within the valence band is possible. Thus if an electron moves from right to left within the band, it leaves a hole in its starting position, i.e. the hole appears to move from left to right. If an electron is removed from the valence band of an atom, then the atom is positively charged since the protons in the nucleus now outnumber the orbiting electrons; the hole is referred to as a positive hole. Thus if a semiconductor is passing a current such that the electron flow in the conduction band is from left to right, there will also be an effective flow of positive charge associated with the movement of positive holes in the valence band in the opposite direction.

18.3.2 Silicon

Silicon is currently the most widely used general semiconductor material. Silicon has an atomic number of 14 and hence has 14 protons in its nucleus and 14 electrons orbiting that nucleus (see Ch. 26). This means that the two inner shells (K- and L-shells) are completely full and contain two and eight electrons respectively. The next shell out from the nucleus is the M-shell and this exhibits a stable configuration when it contains either eight or 18 electrons (see Ch. 26). In this case, it contains four electrons and so may be regarded as an incomplete shell in the solitary silicon atom. However, in the silicon crystal there

is a regular arrangement of atoms in which each silicon atom shares its outer electrons with four neighbouring atoms so that each atom appears to have eight electrons in its M-shell and thus stability (Figure 18.2). Such electron bonds are known as *covalent bonds* and the electrons are termed *valence electrons* and inhabit the valence energy band of the atom. The covalent bonds give the crystal its regularity by inhibiting the movement of any particular atom. At room temperature, these bonds are being continuously broken and reformed as some of the valence electrons are gaining sufficient energy to reach the conduction band (bond broken) and electrons from the conduction band fall back into the valence band (bond reformed). The eight-electron configuration of the M-shell behaves like a full shell and so the valence band is effectively full until an electron moves up to the conduction band. As previously explained, when this happens, electron flow in the conduction band and positive-hole flow in the valence band are both possible.

Intrinsic semiconductors, such as the silicon we have just considered, have very limited practical use. If small amounts of specific impurities are added to them (this process is called *doping*), then they exhibit properties which allow us to use them as rectifiers, transistors, thyristors and integrated circuits (ICs), all of which are found in most X-ray generators. Intrinsic semiconductors which have impurities added to them in this way are known as *extrinsic semiconductors* and will now be discussed.

18.4 EXTRINSIC SEMICONDUCTORS

The addition of small amounts of specific impurities to silicon or germanium is the basis on which most extrinsic semiconductors are produced. The doping may be heavy or light, depending on the component being produced. A typical concentration is one part of impurity to 10 million parts of pure silicon. The electrical conductivity of the extrinsic semiconductor is much greater than that of an intrinsic semiconductor and the level of conductivity can be controlled by altering the ratio of doping material to pure material. The impurity atoms within the silicon crystal lattice are therefore the source of this greatly increased electrical conductivity. This is because the type of impurity is chosen either to enhance electron flow in the conduction band (this gives an *N-type* semiconductor) or to enhance the flow of positive holes in the valence band (this gives a *P-type* semiconductor). These two types of extrinsic semiconductor will now be considered.

18.4.1 *N*-type Semiconductors

As we have already seen, single atoms of intrinsic semiconductors have four valence electrons. To produce an *N*-type extrinsic semiconductor, a *pentavalent impurity* (one with five valence electrons) is used as the doping material. Arsenic, antimony and phosphorus are examples of pentavalent elements which are suitable. Figure 18.3 illustrates the effect of introducing an atom of phosphorus, for example, into the crystalline structure of silicon. Four of the valence electrons in the phosphorus form covalent bonds and the fifth electron is unbonded. This electron has an energy level which is just below the bottom of the conduction band (see Figure 18.3B). At normal room temperatures it is therefore virtually a free electron since it is easily lifted into the conduction band and can therefore take part in electrical conduction if a potential difference is applied across the crystal.

Since such pentavalent atoms provide a 'spare' electron, they are known as *donor impurities*. However, it must be remembered that some electrons from the valence band will also be able to jump into the conduction band due to the normal vibrational energy within the atom at

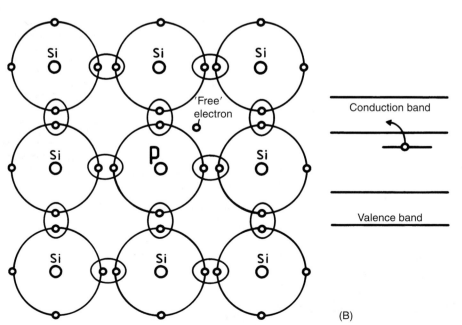

(A)   (B)

Figure 18.3 An example of an *N*-type extrinsic semiconductor. (A) The addition of a pentavalent impurity produces a 'free' electron which does not take part in the covalent bond formation; (B) the energy of such free electrons is close to the conduction band so that they can readily be enabled to take part in electrical conduction.

room temperature (this is similar to the intrinsic semiconductor; see Sect. 18.3). Positive holes will also be produced in the valence band and add to the conductivity. At normal room temperatures, this effect is much less than the effect produced by the donor atoms. Thus, in the case of an *N*-type semiconductor, the *majority carriers* are the electrons in the conduction band and the *minority carriers* are the holes in the valence band.

18.4.2 *P*-type Semiconductors

As discussed in the previous section, the *N*-type semiconductor has enhanced conductivity because of the movement of electrons (negative, hence the *N*) and so it seems logical to assume that the *P*-type semiconductor functions because of the movement of positive holes. In the case of intrinsic semiconductors, we saw that holes were in the valence band, and that this allowed the movement of electrons within this band, thus giving the appearance of positive-hole movement (see previous Insight). In the *P*-type semiconductor the movement of electrons within the valence band is encouraged by the creation of more positive holes within this band.

Figure 18.4 illustrates the result of introducing a trivalent material (one with three valence electrons) into a silicon crystal lattice. The material used in this case is aluminium, and it results in a broken covalent bond between it and the silicon atoms as there are not sufficient electrons in its outer shell to form the four covalent bonds. The energy level of this broken bond is only just above the valence band (Figure 18.4B) and so, at normal room temperatures, electrons have sufficient energy to leap this small gap. Thus the electrons which have left the valence band of the silicon leave positive holes behind them and so there is an increase in the number of positive holes in the valence band because of the trivalent impurity. This type of impurity is known as an *acceptor impurity* since it accepts electrons from the silicon atoms, thus creating holes in the valence band.

The *majority carriers* in the *P*-type material are positive holes in the valence band and the *minority carriers* are electrons which have sufficient energy to rise to the conduction band at room temperature, as in pure silicon (see Sect. 18.3.2).

Table 18.1 summarises the main points we have considered so far regarding intrinsic semiconductors and the *N*-type and *P*-type of extrinsic semiconductor. *Note* that an increase in temperature does not affect the conductivity due to the majority carriers, but only that due to

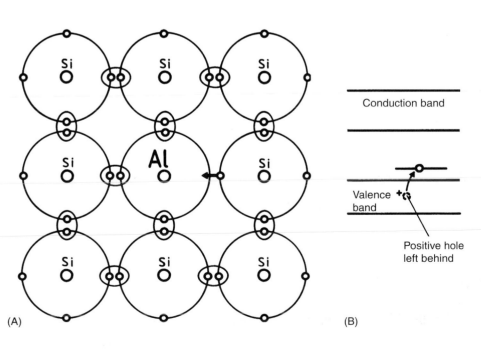

Conduction band

Valence band

Positive hole left behind

Figure 18.4 An example of a *P*-type extrinsic semiconductor. (A) The addition of a trivalent impurity produces a 'hole' in the outside electron shell; (B) such acceptor atoms take an electron from the valence band, leaving a positive hole capable of flowing through this band.

(A)

(B)

Table 18.1 Summary of the properties of semiconductors

	Intrinsic semiconductor	Extrinsic semiconductor	
		N-type	P-type
Typical material	Pure silicon or germanium	Silicon or germanium with added impurities	
Type of impurity	None	Pentavalent	Trivalent
Term for impurity	–	Donor	Acceptor
Conductivity	Low	High	High
Majority carrier	Electrons and positive holes in equal numbers	Electrons in conduction band	Positive holes in valence band
Minority carrier		Positive holes in valence band	Electrons in conduction band
Effect of temperature	Increases both the number of electrons and the number of positive holes	Increases number of minority carriers (positive holes) only	Increases number of minority carriers (electrons) only

Figure 18.5 A diagrammatic representation of N- and P-type semiconductors. In both illustrations the ringed charges represent the fixed charges while the unringed charges represent the free charges which form the majority carriers (electrons for the N-types and positive holes for the P-type).

minority carriers. This is due to the increased number of electrons able to reach the conduction band from the valence band as the temperature increases.

18.4.3 Diagrammatic Representation of N- and P-types

When we discuss the PN junction in the next section we need to form a mental picture of what occurs when an N-type and a P-type semiconductor are fused together. This is made easier if we have a simple symbolic representation of each, as shown in Figure 18.5. In the N-type the majority carriers are the free donor electrons, represented by the minus (–) sign. Each nucleus of the donor impurity has an excess positive charge because of the loss of its outer electron. These fixed positive charges are represented by the circle enclosing the + sign. In the P-type, the positive holes are free and so are shown as a plus (+) sign while the

electrons captured by acceptor atoms give these an overall negative charge. Since these atoms form part of the crystal lattice they are not free to move and so the minus sign is shown ringed (⊖). Thus in both the diagrams the ringed charges are fixed and the unringed charges are free or mobile.

Note that in both the diagrams there are minority carriers caused by the elevation of electrons from the valence band to the conduction band. Since these play little part in the electrical properties of the material they have been omitted from the diagrams for simplicity.

18.5 THE *PN* JUNCTION

When *P*- and *N*-types are heat-fused together to form *PN* junctions, interesting effects appear. Examples of the *PN* junction include the *PN* junction diode, the transistor and the thyristor, which have one, two and three *PN* junctions respectively.

If we use the diagrammatic representation which we have just discussed, then the *PN* junction may be shown as in Figure 18.6. When *P*- and *N*-types are brought together and heat-fused in intimate contact, then free electrons from the *N*-type and free positive holes from the *P*-type are able to penetrate across the boundary between them. This diffusion of charge across the barrier results in recombination of the positive holes and the free electrons (the free electrons

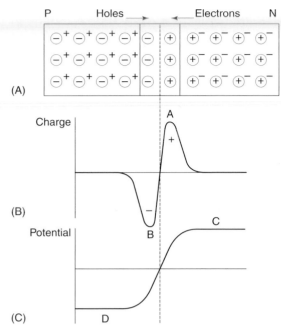

Figure 18.6 The *PN* junction. (A) The diffusion of electrons across the *PN* junction in one direction and positive holes in the other forms a charge barrier which prevents further flow. (B) Gain in charge across the junction and (C) potential difference established across the barrier.

drop into the positive holes so that their charges are cancelled; see Sect. 18.3.1). Thus for a short distance on either side of the *PN* junction (about 0.5×10^{-6} m) no free carriers exist – this is therefore known as a *depletion layer*. However, a net charge exists on either side of the junction because the *N*-type has lost electrons and the *P*-type has lost positive holes (Figure 18.6B). Thus there is a negatively charged area just within the *P*-type region and a positively charged area just within the *N*-type region. The two peaks of charge shown in Figure 18.6B increase in size until no further net flow of majority carriers takes place. For example, a free electron from the *N*-type will only be able to pass over to the *P*-type if it has sufficient energy to overcome the repulsion of the negative peak at the *PN* junction.

The charge distribution produces its own potential difference, as depicted in Figure 18.6C. The height of *CD* is known as the potential barrier since it acts in opposition to the flow of majority carriers from either side of the barrier.

For a silicon *PN* junction this potential barrier is about 0.4 V, so free carriers of energy lower than 0.4 eV cannot overcome this barrier.

18.5.1 Minority Carriers at the *PN* Junction

The above discussion concerned only the effect of the *PN* junction on the majority carriers. For majority carriers a potential barrier is formed which prevents any further flow.

However, this barrier actually aids the transport of *minority* carriers between the materials. Consider the potential gradient between *D* and *C* (Figure 18.6C). If a free electron (the minority carrier in a *P*-type material) is in position *D* it is strongly attracted by the positive potential of the *N*-type material and rapidly moves to *C*. At equilibrium, of course, there are equal numbers of minority carriers moving in both directions.

Minority carriers are dependent on temperature, since an increase in temperature increases the number of electrons which can jump from the valence to the conduction band. *Thus the flow of minority carriers across a PN junction increases with temperature.* This affects the behaviour of the *PN* junction under conditions of reverse bias, as will be explained later in this chapter.

18.5.2 Forward Bias

If a source of potential difference (e.g. a battery) is connected across a *PN* junction, as shown in Figure 18.7A, then a current will flow across the junction because the potential barrier is lowered. This is shown graphically in Figure 18.7B. The negative side of the battery reduces the positive potential of the *N*-type and the positive side of the battery reduces the negative potential of the *P*-type. Thus the original height of the barrier is lowered and energetic free carriers from either side are able to surmount the barrier. A steady electrical current is therefore set up as long as the battery is connected. This type of connection, which produces current flow across the *PN* junction, is called *forward bias*. The removal of the battery results in the full height of the barrier being re-established and so no further current can flow.

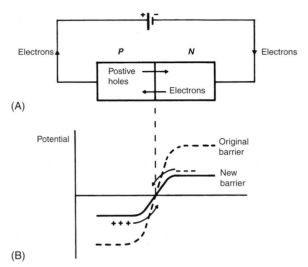

(A)

(B)

Figure 18.7 (A) The *PN* junction connected in forward bias. The potential from the battery lowers the potential barrier and allows current to flow across the junction. (B) The position of the barrier before connection into the circuit and after the device is connected, as shown in (A).

18.5.3 Reverse Bias

If the source of potential difference is now connected in the opposite orientation, as shown in Figure 18.8A, then this is known as *reverse bias*. No current flows through this circuit due to the increase in the potential barrier at the *PN* junction. The graph in Figure 18.8B shows that the negative side of the battery increases the negative potential of the *P*-type and the positive side of the battery increases the positive potential of the *N*-type. Thus no current flows, as none of the majority carriers have sufficient energy to surmount this higher barrier. In fact, when a *PN* junction is connected in reverse bias, the depletion layer extends further into each semiconductor on either side of the *PN* junction.

The discussion so far has been regarding majority carriers. However, as discussed earlier, a small electrical current due to the thermally generated minority carriers is able to flow.

18.5.4 The *PN* Junction as a Diode

In our discussion in the last two sections we have shown that current will readily flow through a *PN* junction when it is forward-biased, but very little

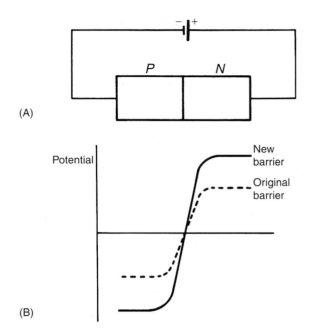

(A)

(B)

Figure 18.8 (A) The *PN* junction connected in reverse bias. The potential from the battery raises the potential barrier, as shown in (B), and further prevents electrical conduction.

current will flow through the junction when it is reverse-biased. Thus the *PN* junction can act as a one-way valve (a diode) which allows current only to flow in one direction. For this reason *PN* junctions are used to create *solid-state rectifiers* or *PN junction diodes*. The symbol for such a device is shown below.

Note that electrons may only flow through the diode against the direction of the arrow of the symbol. Such devices have replaced thermionic diodes for the following reasons:

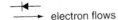

• they contain no filament and thus have a longer life, consume less power and produce less heat
• they are smaller in size than thermionic diodes, thus enabling the production of a more compact X-ray unit
• they have a smaller forward voltage drop, thus enabling a higher kVp to be applied to the X-ray tube (see Ch. 21)

- the reverse current is less than a vacuum diode and so they are more efficient rectifiers.

18.5.5 *PN* Junction Characteristics

If the current flowing through a *PN* junction is plotted against the potential difference across it, then the graph produced is referred to as the characteristic curve for the device. Such a graph is shown in Figure 18.9.

As the potential difference across the diode is increased in a forward direction, so the current through it increases, as shown by *OA* on the figure. If we compare this with the forward-bias characteristic for the vacuum diode we can note that, in this case, there is no saturation current. However, passing too high a current through a *PN*-junction diode can cause irreparable damage.

A normal reverse bias produces only a very low reverse current due to the flow of minority carriers which happen to move into the vicinity of the *PN* junction and so get swept across it. As we have already discussed, this reverse current is very sensitive to temperature as this alters the production of minority carriers due to thermal

excitation. If the reverse bias is further increased, then the reverse current increases dramatically (see *BC* in Figure 18.9). This is called the *zener voltage* or *breakdown voltage* and at this value of reverse bias the diode ceases to act effectively as a rectifier. At this negative bias the minority carriers which cross the potential barrier gain enough energy to ionise atoms with which they collide. This results in the liberation of additional electrons and hence the large current. This phenomenon is also referred to as *solid-state multiplication* or *electron avalanching*.

18.6 THE TRANSISTOR

The transistor has replaced the triode valve in most electronic circuits. The transistor itself as a single item has been replaced by large numbers of transistors and other components produced in a silicon chip. Large-scale integration of this sort was mentioned in the introduction to this chapter and the silicon chip so produced is referred to as an *integrated circuit* or IC. The transistors in such an IC are the *field-effect type* and will be discussed later in this chapter. First, however, the junction transistor is considered.

18.6.1 The *NPN* Junction Transistor

The junction transistor is composed of three alternating layers of semiconductor materials, so both *NPN* junction transistors and *PNP* junction transistors exist, although only the *NPN* transistor is considered in this section. An *NPN* transistor is shown in Figure 18.10A together with its electrical symbol (Figure 18.10B) – the symbol for a *PNP* transistor is shown in Figure 18.10C. The central *P*-type semiconductor is known as the base and the *N*-types on either side of it are known as the emitter and the collector. Note that the direction of the arrow on the emitter in the transistor symbol indicates the direction of positive-hole flow – electron flow will be in the opposite direction.

The factors that determine which is the emitter and which is the collector are the geometry of the device and the amount of doping in each. Typically, the emitter contains 1000 times more

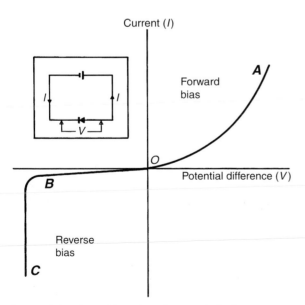

Figure 18.9 The *PN* junction characteristic. For explanation, see text.

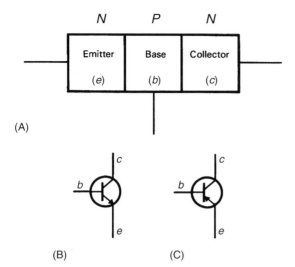

Figure 18.10 (A) The *NPN* junction transistor and (B) its symbol. The symbol for the *PNP* transistor is shown in (C).

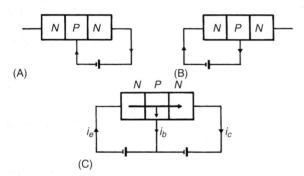

Figure 18.11 The principle of operation of the *NPN* junction transistor (see text for explanation).

doping than the collector and 100 times more than the base. The emitter thus contains a ready supply of free electrons (from the N-type doping) which are available to flow through the transistor as a whole.

Figure 18.11 shows the separate actions of the transistor in terms of its two *PN* junctions. In Figure 18.11A the base and the collector are connected to a battery in reverse-bias conditions. Thus only the very small current, due to the thermally generated minority carriers, flows. Figure 18.11B shows the junction between the emitter and the base connected in forward bias. This time a larger current than in the previous section is able to flow.

However, if these two circuits are connected simultaneously (Figure 18.11C), it is found that almost the same current flows through the emitter and the collector, while the current through the base is much smaller. At first sight this suggests that the base to collector *PN* junction has been destroyed, thus allowing a larger current to flow than was previously possible. In fact, this is not the case. It should be remembered that reverse bias applies to majority carriers – positive holes in the base. Thus, when electrons are injected into the base from the emitter, they become minority carriers within the base and so readily cross the collector-to-base *PN* junction. This process is so efficient that approximately 98% of the electrons injected into the base from the emitter are able to diffuse across the base and form the collector current. The remaining 2% form the base current. This ratio of approximately 50:1 for the collector current and the base current remains constant for a particular transistor. Thus the base current may be used to control the collector current, as an increase in the base current will allow a subsequent increase in the collector current. A small signal current to the base will produce an amplified signal current (amplification 50:1) between the emitter and the collector.

18.6.2 The Field-Effect Transistor

The field-effect transistor (FET) varies the current flowing through the semiconductor by varying the electrical field. In this way it can be used to rapidly alter the current in a circuit in a similar way to the function of the triode valve, which it has largely replaced. A simple cross-sectional diagram of the FET is shown in Figure 18.12, where a central rod of N-type material has a collar of P-type material around it. When the transistor is in a circuit, current flows along the central rod (from left to right in the diagram), one end of which is referred to as the *source* and the other as the *drain* – electrons flow from source to drain. If a negative potential is put on the P-type collar (the gate), then the *PN* junction is under reverse bias, and this extends the depletion layer further into the N-type material, as shown by the dashed line in Figure 18.12. This means that the

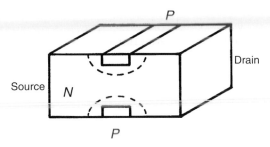

Figure 18.12 A section through a field-effect transistor (FET). The connection of a reverse bias between *P*- and *N*-type semiconductors extends the depletion layer and inhibits electron flow.

majority carriers have been removed from this area and so the electrical conductivity of the area is reduced, with a consequent reduction in the current flowing through the *N*-type. Hence the current through the FET can be reduced by increasing the negative voltage bias on the gate. At a particular pinch-off potential no current is able to flow.

The FET has a high input impedance compared to a junction transistor and that means that a lower current is needed to control the device. A typical value of input impedance for such a device is 10^8 Ω, compared to 10^5 Ω for a junction transistor. This is an important consideration when trying to amplify very low signals. However, the FET is a more delicate device and is easily damaged by voltage surges or by static electricity (e.g. touching it may supply sufficient static to cause damage).

18.7 THE THYRISTOR

The thyristor is a silicon-controlled rectifier (SCR) and can be made to act as an *electronic switch*. Its behaviour is similar to that of the thyratron valve, which it has virtually replaced. Its structure is shown in Figure 18.13A: it is composed of four alternating *N* and *P* semiconductor layers (both *NPNP* and *PNPN* thyristors are available but in this case only the operation of the *NPNP* type is described). Junctions J_1 and J_3 are forward-biased but junction J_2 is reverse-biased. Consequently, if the thyristor is connected into a circuit, only a small leakage current flows through it – it behaves as an open switch. If a positive pulse is applied to the *P*-type layer (the *gate*) at junction J_1 then positive holes are injected into the *P*-type material and flow across the junction J_1 so that the potential barrier at that junction is greatly reduced. The reduced potential difference across J_1 means that a higher reverse potential difference than before exists across J_2 and, if high enough, will cause electrical breakdown to occur at this junction due to the avalanche effect (see Sect. 18.5.5). Once this breakdown occurs, a large current may flow through the thyristor – it behaves as a closed switch. It is not possible to switch the thyristor off by applying a negative pulse to the gate, but it will switch off when the potential difference across it is zero or if potential applied across the device is reversed – the avalanching effect can no longer be maintained under such conditions. This makes the thyristor very suitable for switching alternating currents as

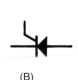

(B)

(C)

Figure 18.13 (A) An example of an *NPNP* thyristor. A gate signal as shown makes the thyristor conduct until the potential across the device is reduced to zero. (B and C) Symbols for the thyristor and the triac respectively.

(A)

the potential difference across it drops to zero every 0.01 seconds.

The thyristor does have a slight disadvantage when used with alternating currents in that it will only allow current to flow when the N end is negative and the P end is positive. This is overcome by connecting two thyristors in parallel but facing in opposite directions – this is known as a *flip-flop circuit*. A *triac* is, however, able to switch alternating currents. The symbol for this is shown in Figure 18.13C. It behaves in the same way as the two thyristors, connected in parallel but facing in opposite directions. Triacs or flip-flop circuits are often used to switch the X-ray exposure on and off.

18.8 SEMICONDUCTOR DEVICES IN RADIOGRAPHY

Semiconductor devices are used extensively in radiography. This chapter has given a brief overview of some of the types that are used. The development of integrated circuits in the 1960s resulted in the production of complete miniaturised circuits containing transistors, capacitors, resistors and diodes. Such circuits were produced on a single chip of silicon about 1 mm^2 and about 0.1 mm thick. This process, using VLSI, is able to produce circuits containing in excess of 7000 logic gates per chip.

This technology offers components of very high reliability at very low production costs. There is also significant space-saving over electromechanical devices. Both of the above have resulted in many of the circuits in X-ray generators containing significant amounts of 'chip technology'.

The microprocessor is another development based on silicon chip and VLSI technology. Using Boolean logic and inbuilt programs, microprocessors are used to monitor and control many pieces of equipment used in radiography.

The description of the function of such circuits is the subject of a book in its own right and is beyond the scope of this text. Table 18.2 gives an indication of some of the areas where semiconductor devices are used.

Table 18.2 Applications of semiconductor devices	
Semiconductor device	Applications
Solid-state diode	Rectification of the high-tension supply to the X-ray tube using multiple *PN* junctions connected in series to form stick rectifiers
	Rectification of the supply to devices that require a unidirectional supply, e.g. certain types of meter
Transistors	Electronic timing circuits
	Safety interlocks that avoid exceeding the rating of the X-ray tube
	Amplifying circuits, e.g. in the closed-circuit television chain
Thyristors/triacs	Primary switching of the X-ray exposure, i.e. the triac switches the exposure on and off – following the signal from the timer
Logic circuits	These can check that a number of functions have taken place in sequence, e.g. they can check that the anode is rotating at the correct speed before an exposure is made
Microprocessors	These have many applications in more sophisticated measurement and controls, e.g. microprocessors can check a certain set of exposure factors to ensure that they are not outside the rating of the selected tube focus

SUMMARY

In this chapter you should have learnt:

- A semiconductor has a conductivity between that of an insulator and a conductor, reflecting the small energy gap between the conduction and the valence bands (see Sect. 18.3)
- An intrinsic semiconductor, such as silicon, is a chemically pure semiconductor with a regular arrangement of atoms within its crystal lattice (see Sects 18.3 and 18.3.2)
- Extrinsic semiconductors have carefully measured quantities of impurity added to the intrinsic semiconductor by a process known as doping (see Sect. 18.4)
- An N-type semiconductor is produced when a pentavalent or donor impurity is added to the silicon. This gives a supply of free electrons in the semiconductor (see Sect. 18.4.1)
- A P-type semiconductor is produced when a trivalent or acceptor impurity is added to the silicon. This gives a supply of positive holes within the semiconductor (see Sect. 18.4.2)
- The majority carrier in the N-type material is the free electron and the majority carrier in the P-type is the free positive hole (see Sects 18.4.1 and 18.4.2)
- Minority carriers are thermally produced and are present in all types of

semiconductor at room temperature. Minority carriers in the N-type are positive holes and in the P-type are free electrons (see Sects 18.4.1 and 18.4.2)
- A PN junction produces a potential barrier to the flow of electrons and holes. The height of this barrier grows when the junction is reverse-biased and diminishes when the junction is forward-biased. Thus the PN junction will allow current to flow in one direction only – electrons can flow from N to P (see Sects 18.5 to 18.5.5)
- A transistor is a solid-state device consisting of two PN junctions. A small base current is used to control a larger collector current so that signal amplification using a transistor is possible (see Sects 18.6–18.6.2)
- A thyristor is a solid-state device that acts as an electronic switch. A gate signal switches the device on and it can be switched off by allowing the potential difference across the thyristor to drop to zero. Triacs are similar to thyristors but will switch alternating current (see Sect. 18.7)
- Semiconductor devices have many uses in radiography, including rectification, signal amplification, switching and microprocessor control (see Sect. 18.8).

SELF-TEST

a. What is meant by the term intrinsic semiconductor?

b. How is the conductivity of an intrinsic semiconductor altered by the addition of trivalent or pentavalent impurities? What is meant by the terms:

(i)   extrinsic semiconductor

(ii) P-type semiconductor

(iii) N-type semiconductor?

c. What are the majority carriers and the minority carriers in the P-type and the N-type semiconductors?

d. What is meant by the term PN junction? Explain the meaning of the terms:

(i)   depletion layer

(ii) potential barrier

as applied to a PN junction. Explain why the PN junction conducts current when it is forward-biased but will not normally conduct current when it is reverse-biased.

e. What are the advantages of a solid-state rectifier over a diode valve?

f. Describe the action of a junction *NPN* transistor.

g. Describe the action of a thyristor.

FURTHER READING

Ball J L, Moore A D 1997 Essential physics for radiographers, 3rd edn. Blackwell Scientific Publications, London, ch 13

Chapter 19

Rectification

CHAPTER CONTENTS

19.1 Aim   177

19.2 Introduction   177

19.3 Half-Wave Rectification   178

19.4 Four-Diode Full-Wave Rectification   178
    19.4.1 Comparison of X-ray Tube Current
        for Half- and Full-Wave
        Rectification   179

19.5 Three-Phase Rectification   180
    19.5.1 The Six-Pulse Generator   180

19.6 Constant-Potential Circuits   180
    19.6.1 Capacitor Smoothing   181

19.7 Medium-Frequency Generators   182

Self-Test   184

Further Reading   184

19.1 AIM

The aim of this chapter is to consider the various aspects of rectification as it applies to the X-ray generator. There is some initial discussion regarding the need for rectification and the ideal voltage waveform to apply to the X-ray tube. There is then a description of systems of rectification of increasing complexity, which move towards this ideal voltage.

19.2 INTRODUCTION

In Chapters 13 and 17 it was seen that it is convenient to use an alternating current (AC) supply for diagnostic and therapeutic X-ray generators and linear accelerators because of the ease with which the potential can be stepped up or down. Both X-ray tubes and linear accelerators require a high potential difference across them in order to produce X-rays of the required energy. The voltage is therefore stepped up using the high-tension transformer. On the other hand the filament requires a potential of about 10 volts and a current of several amperes to heat it to a temperature sufficient for thermionic emission to occur, so the filament transformer (a step-down transformer) is used. As shown in Chapters 21 and 28, the X-ray tube is designed to emit radiation when the cathode is negative and the anode is positive. The nearer the voltage across the tube is to a constant voltage, the more efficient the production of X-rays from the tube. This means that ideally we would like to change the alternating voltage supplied from the high-tension transformer to be turned into a *constant unidirectional voltage*. This process of converting an AC supply into a constant unidirectional supply, or a pulsating unidirectional supply, is called *rectification*. We will now consider different types of rectification, many of these are no longer in common use, but that serve to show how rectification systems have developed.

19.3 HALF-WAVE RECTIFICATION

As the name suggests, half-wave rectification utilises only half of the available cycles during an exposure; the other half-cycle is suppressed. The X-ray tube is a diode valve and, like the *PN* junction (Ch. 18.5.4), will only permit current flow through it when the cathode is negative. When the anode has a negative potential on it, normally no current flows and no X-rays are produced. This means that X-ray photons are only produced for 50% of the exposure time and the maximum energy of the photos will vary with the potential across the tube at the time of their production. In addition, the load that can be applied to the X-ray tube is severely restricted (see Insight below). For these reasons this type of rectification, also called single-phase, single-pulse rectification, is seldom encountered in medical radiology today, although they may be found in crystallography and industrial X-ray units (Figure 19.1).

___

INSIGHT

The target of the X-ray tube is made of tungsten and so readily emits electrons by thermionic emission. If the anode is allowed to rise in temperature to a point where significant thermionic emission occurs (about 1500 °C), electrons will be able to travel from the anode to the cathode during the inverse part of the cycle. This will cause irreparable damage to the cathode assembly. Thus, the target temperature must be maintained below this value, so restricting the loading that can be applied to the tube.

___

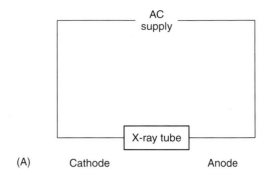

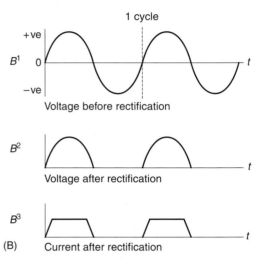

Figure 19.1 (A) Simplified diagram of a single-phase self-rectified circuit. (B) Voltage and current flow before and after rectification.

19.4 FOUR-DIODE FULL-WAVE RECTIFICATION

The circuit described in the previous section on half-wave rectification has the disadvantage that only alternate half-cycles are used to produce X-rays. Thus, we can consider the tube as being 'switched off' for half of the exposure time. In order to utilise both halves of the AC cycle, *full-wave* rectification making use of four diodes arranged in a *Gratz bridge circuit* (Figure 19.2), are used.

Note that the diodes are arranged in two pairs and that the bar (or arrow) in the diode symbol *always* points away from the negative side of the output. D_1 and D_2 rectify one half-cycle, while diodes D_3 and D_4 rectify the other half-cycle. The

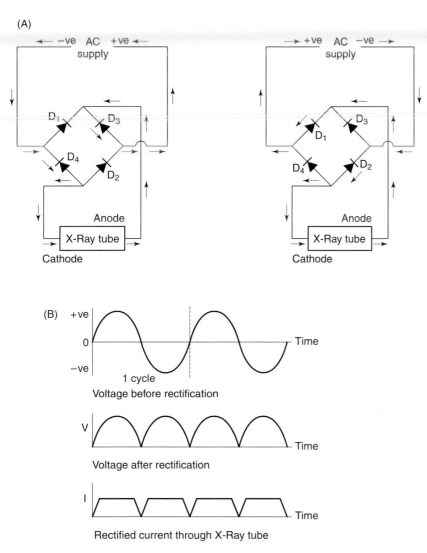

Figure 19.2 (A) Full-wave rectification circuit showing electron movement in both halves of the alternating current cycle. (B) Voltage waveforms before and after rectification and current flow through the X-ray tube after rectification.

arrows in Figure 19.2A show the direction of electron movement. It can be seen that electron movement through the tube is in the same direction in both half-cycles and that, although the potential varies, it never becomes negative.

19.4.1 Comparison of X-ray Tube Current for Half- and Full-Wave Rectification

Figure 19.3 shows the current waveforms for half- and full-wave rectification for the same mA selector setting. *Note* the current waveforms for half-wave rectification are twice the height of those for the full-wave rectification. The reason for this is that the mA selected is the average current through the X-ray tube (see Sect. 14.2.2). Since every other current waveform is missing, the height of each of the remaining waveforms must be doubled to achieve the same average current. This is an important consideration for short exposure times, as the half-wave circuit deposits twice as much energy to the anode during the 'on' half-phase. Thus, at the same mA the anode reaches a higher temperature than it would do in a full wave circuit, so restricting the loading. For longer exposures the effect of individual half-cycles is less and as a result both units will have similar ratings. These differences will be further discussed in Chapter 22.

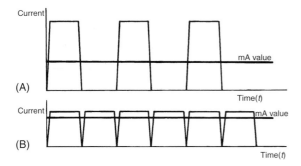

Figure 19.3 The current and mA (average current) for (A) half-wave and (B) full-wave rectification for the same mA selection.

19.5 THREE-PHASE RECTIFICATION

In Chapter 14, we considered three-phase electrical supplies. If all three phases are used to supply an X-ray generator, the resultant voltage across the X-ray tube is not a constant potential but the ripple is very small. The circuit in these generators may or may not have capacitor smoothing (as described in Sect. 19.6.1). However, in this case, to allow greater clarity in the diagrams, capacitor smoothing has not been considered.

19.5.1 The Six-Pulse Generator

This generator is depicted in Figure 19.4. The movement of electrons through this circuit is slightly more complicated because of the three phases. Figure 19.4B shows the voltage waveforms from the three secondaries of the high-tension transformers. Consider the point in time when phase 1 is at peak negative and phases 2 and 3 are at half their positive peaks (this point is shown by a bold vertical line through the figure). At this stage all the electrons flow is through rectifier D_1 which is forward-biased. They then flow through the X-ray tube from cathode to anode. After this, electrons from the anode will flow through D_4 and D_6 to transformers 2 and 3 respectively. Thus, no electrons are gained or lost in the circuit. (You may wish to test your understanding of the circuit by checking that you can identify the electron movement at some other stage of the voltage cycle shown in Figure 19.4B.) *Note*: The primary of the high-tension transformer is delta-wound and the secondary is star-wound (see Sect. 14.8.1). The delta winding of the primary allows a higher primary current to flow. The star winding of the secondary means that the centre of the star is at earth potential, thus giving electrical symmetry around the X-ray tube.

There were also three-phase 12-pulse rectification systems available. However, generators using these systems were very uncommon due to the cost of the units.

19.6 CONSTANT-POTENTIAL CIRCUITS

None of the circuits described so far conforms to the ideal situation described in the introduction to this chapter where a *constant potential* (or *voltage*) is applied to the X-ray tube. In all of the circuits described so far, the voltage has been pulsating and not constant.

This has three practical disadvantages:

1. The anode of the X-ray tube receives rapidly varying amounts of energy
2. The intensity of the X-ray beam varies over each half-cycle, as will be explained in Chapter 29
3. The effective energy of the X-ray beam varies over each half-cycle – again, as will be explained in Chapter 29, the effective energy (or quality) of the X-ray beam is related to the voltage across the X-ray tube.

19.6.1 Capacitor Smoothing

Capacitor smoothing of a pulsating unidirectional voltage has already been discussed in Section 16.11.3. This is illustrated in Figure 19.5. The similarities between the resultant waveform and that in Figure 16.8 should be noted.

The capacitors charge up quickly when the exposure starts but discharge more slowly

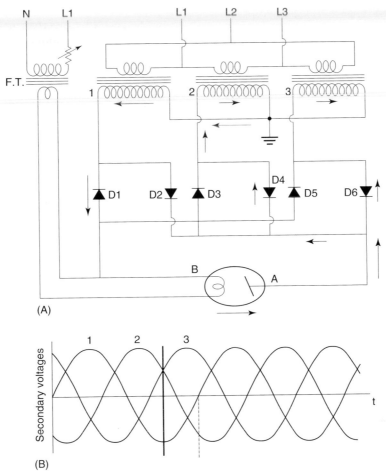

Figure 19.4   (A) Simplified diagram of a three-phase six-pulse circuit (arrows indicate electron movement at time t, as shown by the bold vertical line in (B). (B) Voltage waveforms at secondary side of circuit before rectification.

through the X-ray tube. There is therefore a reduction in the voltage ripple across the X-ray tube compared to a full-wave circuit. *Note* that the amount of smoothing depends on the capacitance of the capacitor selected and the value of mA selected. A larger capacitor will store more charge (at a given voltage) than a smaller one. If the current through the X-ray tube is large, the capacitor will be able to discharge more quickly and its potential will fall more rapidly. The high-tension cables used to connect the high-

tension transformer to the X-ray tube also possess capacitance but it is quite small, so it only has a significant smoothing effect when the current is very small, e.g. during fluoroscopy. The result is that, although this voltage is smoother, with less ripple it is still not a constant potential. A constant potential can be produced if this voltage is now 'clipped' by the use of triode valves. However, triode smoothed circuits are complex and are no longer used in X-ray generators.

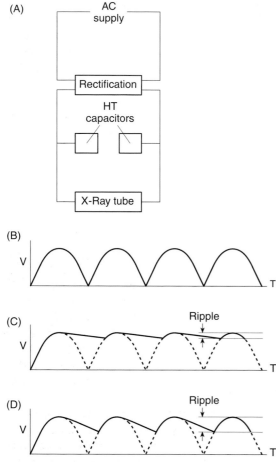

Figure 19.5 (A) Box diagram of a circuit with capacitor smoothing. (B) Voltage waveform to X-ray tube with no smoothing. (C) Voltage waveform to X-ray tube with different values of mA selected (C low mA and D high mA)

19.7 MEDIUM-FREQUENCY GENERATORS

The improvement of semiconductor devices in solid-state rectification has led to the development of the medium-frequency generator (Figure 19.6). With the exception of intraoral dental units, which use solid-state single-phase full-wave rectification, this technology has superseded the older systems and is now found in almost all X-ray generators, including battery-powered mobile units. The rectification system in the generator can

be thought of as consisting of a number of subcircuits:

- initial rectification and smoothing of the incoming AC supply, if used
- a frequency multiplication circuit
- the high-tension transformer
- rectification
- and finally smoothing circuit.

Note the input supply may be from a battery, single-phase or three-phase mains supply. If the supply is a single-phase AC supply, then it is first necessary to rectify this and smooth it to a near-constant potential. This is achieved by the use of a large-capacitance smoothing capacitor (see Sect. 19.5.1). When a three-phase supply is used, this is rectified (see Sect. 19.5.1) and then capacitor-smoothed again, producing a near-constant potential. In most modern mobile units the power source for the exposure is drawn from a nickel-cadmium battery (charged from a single-phase

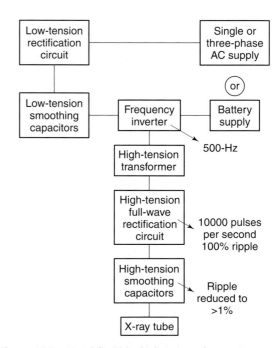

Figure 19.6 Simplified block diagram of a medium-frequency rectification system.

mains supply). This battery supply requires no smoothing as it is a direct current supply. The supply is then passed through a frequency inverter which uses an oscillator and silicon-controlled rectifiers to convert this to an alternating voltage with a frequency of 5000 Hz. This high-frequency, low-tension alternating voltage is now passed through the high-tension transformer. Here the voltage is increased to the desired kV for the exposure and the high-tension output passes to a Gratz bridge rectification circuit. The rectification produces a unidirectional voltage with 10 000 voltage pulses per second.

Finally the ripple present is smoothed out using high-tension smoothing capacitors before the power is applied to the X-ray tube. Because the frequency is so high, the interval the capacitor is discharging as the voltage drops is very short and the ripple present after smoothing is less than 1%, and so can be regarded as an almost constant potential. These generators have an additional advantage, because the increased frequency results in improved transformer efficiency. This means that the high-tension transformer can be made less bulky, leading to improvements in the overall design of the unit.

SUMMARY

In this chapter you should have learnt:

- The reasons an AC supply is required for an X-ray generator and why this needs to be rectified before it is applied to the X-ray tube (see Sect. 19.2)
- The advantages and disadvantages of half-wave rectification and how the X-ray tube can be used as a diode valve to attain this (see Sect. 19.3)
- The rectification used in a single-phase full-wave unit and the voltage waveform it produces (see Sect. 19.4)

- A comparison between the current waveforms produced by a half-wave and a full-wave rectified unit (see Sect. 19.4.1)
- How capacitors may be used to smooth a full-wave rectified waveform (see Sect. 19.5.1)
- How a three-phase AC supply is rectified using a three-phase, six-pulse rectification circuit (see Sect. 19.6.1)
- How rectification is attained in a modem generator using a medium-frequency rectification system and why the advantages of this system have made other rectification circuits obsolete (see Sect. 19.7).

SELF-TEST

a. Explain why an AC supply is desirable for the operation of an X-ray generator and a unidirectional supply is desired for the operation of the X-ray tube. How are these contradictory requirements achieved?

b. Compare the advantages and disadvantages of a self-rectified unit with those of a full-wave rectified unit.

c. Draw a diagram showing electron movement in a full-wave rectification circuit and the voltage

waveforms before and after passing across such a circuit.

d. Explain the effect of voltage 'ripple' on the energy of the X-ray beam and describe how capacitor smoothing may be used to reduce ripple.

e. State the advantages of modern medium-frequency rectification systems over those of earlier systems.

FURTHER READING

Ball J L, Moore A D 1997 Essential physics for
    radiographers, 3rd edn. Blackwell Scientific Publications,
    London, ch 13
Curry T S III, Dowdey J E, Murry R C Jr 1990 Christensen's
    physics of diagnostic radiography, 4th edn. Lee & Febiger,
    London, ch 3
Dowsett D J, Kenny P A, Johnston R E 1998 The physics
    of diagnostic imaging. Chapman & Hall Medical,
    London, ch 4

Johns H E, Cunningham J R 1983 The physics of radiology,
    4th edn. Charles C Thomas, Illinois, USA, ch 30
Thompson M A, Hattaway R T, Hall J D, Dowd S B 1994
    Principles of imaging science and protection.
    W B Saunders, London, ch 7

Chapter 20

Exposure and Timing Circuits

CHAPTER CONTENTS

20.1 Aim   185

20.2 Preparation for Exposure   185

20.3 The Switching Section   186
    20.3.1 Primary Switching   186
    20.3.2 Secondary Switching   186

20.4 The Timing Section   188
    20.4.1 Time-Based Timers   188
    20.4.2 The mAs Timer   188
    20.4.3 Automatic Timers   190

Self-Test   192

Further Reading   192

20.1 AIM

The aim of this chapter is to introduce the reader to the principles involved in switching the X-ray exposure on and off. The chapter will also consider the physics involved in timing the X-ray exposure.

20.2 PREPARATION FOR EXPOSURE

Before the X-ray tube can deliver an exposure for a predetermined time interval, it must first be prepared for exposure. This is done during the 'prep' stage of the exposure sequence and during this time two major things happen:

1. The appropriate filament of the X-ray tube is raised to its working temperature so that it emits the required number of electrons by thermionic emission (see Sect. 21.7.1) to allow the tube current (mA) to flow during the exposure
2. The anode is made to rotate at the required speed prior to the exposure being made.

If an exposure is made before these processes are completed, there is a risk that the incorrect mA will be delivered or that the target of the anode may be subjected to localised overheating, resulting in damage to the anode. In Section 16.7 and 16.9 it was shown that selection of a suitable resistance would determine the time taken to charge or discharge a capacitor. This principle is used to provide a delay function prior to the X-ray

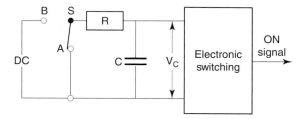

Figure 20.1 Simplified circuit diagram of a typical stator delay circuit. See text for details.

exposure, using a circuit similar to that shown in Figure 20.1.

Initiating the prepare sequence causes the switch to move to position A, 'shorting' the capacitor to removing any residual charge present. It then moves into position B, which permits a direct current (DC) supply to charge the capacitor through the resistor R. When the capacitor is charged it operates a relay which closes a switch in the exposure circuits, permitting the exposure to commence.

There are two circuit sections responsible for this event:

1. the switching section
2. the timing section.

20.3 THE SWITCHING SECTION

The function of the switching section is to connect the high voltage (kVp) to the X-ray tube during the exposure and to disconnect this supply from the tube at the end of the exposure. Such switching commonly occurs between the autotransformer and the high-tension transformer, where it is known as *primary switching*, or between the high-tension transformer and the X-ray tube, where it is known as *secondary switching*.

20.3.1 Primary Switching

All modern X-ray units make use of solid-state switching. This type of switching has the advantage that there are no moving parts, overcoming the problems of inertia and arcing that were experienced with mechanical switching. A simple

circuit containing a solid-state switching system is shown in Figure 20.2. Silicon-controlled rectifiers (SCRs), a type of thyristor, are used for this purpose. As you may remember from Section 18.7, two thyristors are required to switch an alternating current (AC) as each conducts the half-cycle when that SCR is forward-biased. At the end of each half-cycle each SCR will cease to conduct as the potential difference across it drops to zero and so a voltage pulse must be applied to its gate if it is required to conduct during the next half-cycle.

As an alternative to the SCR, a triac may be used. This device acts as two SCRs connected in inverse parallel and, if pulsed with an alternating supply, will conduct in both phases of the AC cycle. Like the SCR, the device will only conduct when the voltage is not at 0 volt and the device has been pulsed.

Thus, during the exposure the timer is simply required to apply a sequence of synchronised pulses to the gate of the device at a time slightly later than the mains zero to switch them back on and ensure their continued conduction. At the end of the exposure these pulses stop and conduction through the device stops at the end of the next half-cycle. The system allows accuracy of one voltage pulse (i.e. an exposure time of 0.01 second in the case of a two-pulse unit, or 0.002 seconds in the case of a medium-frequency unit: see Sect. 19.4).

20.3.2 Secondary Switching

Solid-state devices such as SCRs cannot withstand the very high voltages present in the high-tension circuit; therefore, high-tension valves must be used. In the past, triode valves

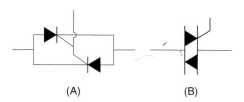

(A)   (B)

Figure 20.2 Simplified circuit diagram of primary switching using (A) two silicon-controlled rectifiers and (B) a triac.

were used; modern generators make use of a grid-controlled X-ray tube.

As will be seen in Chapters 21 and 28, X-rays are produced when electrons flow from the cathode to the anode of the X-ray tube. These electrons are normally focused on to the target of the tube by a focusing cup, which is at a negative potential equal to that of the filament. If a separate additional bias is applied to the focusing cup, then it is possible to make it more negative than the filament. X-ray tubes offering this facility are known as grid-controlled tubes.

If the focusing cup is made about 3 kV more negative than the filament, it will produce a sufficiently large electrostatic field to prevent any electrons from crossing the X-ray tube; this additional negative potential is termed *grid bias*. At the start of the exposure this bias is removed, electrons may cross from the cathode to the anode and X-radiation is produced. At end of the exposure the high negative bias is re-established on the focusing cup, thus stopping electron flow. The grid-controlled tube acts as an electronic exposure switch as well as a producer of X-rays.

Secondary switching is used in capacitor discharge units to control the passage of the charge from the capacitor through the X-ray tube during the exposure time. It was also used in cine-radiography and pulsed fluoroscopy, where the system is capable of giving up to 500 exposures per second. In such cases the switch shown in Figure 16.7 does not exist as the X-ray tube will act as the high-tension switch.

INSIGHT

A similar form of grid-controlled switching is now used in a number of dental units. In such units the current through the tube is switched off when the voltage falls below a certain percentage of the peak kV. The principles of the process are shown in Figure 20.3.

As we can see from Figure 20.3A, in a conventional X-ray unit, X-rays are produced during each of the voltage pulses but only the X-rays produced at the centre of each voltage pulse (near the peak kV) are of diagnostic value. X-rays produced when the tube voltage is significantly lower than the peak kV have very low photon energies and so will be absorbed by the patient and contribute nothing to the diagnostic image. If we can prevent production of these low-energy X-rays, we can limit the patient radiation dose and also help to prolong the life of the X-ray tube. This is achieved by applying a strong negative bias to the focusing cup if the tube voltage is below a certain value: no current will flow through the tube and no X-rays are produced. This is shown in Figure 20.3B.

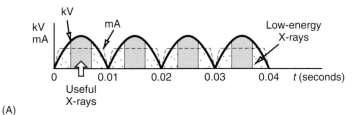

(A)

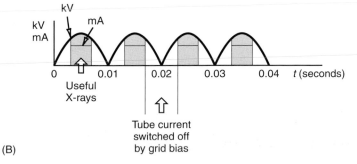

(B)

Figure 20.3 The use of a grid-controlled X-ray tube to limit patient dose. (A) Low-energy X-rays are produced which contribute to patient dose but do not contribute to the image. (B) By applying the necessary bias to the cathode, current is prevented from flowing when the tube voltage is below a predetermined limit, thus preventing production of much of the low-energy radiation.

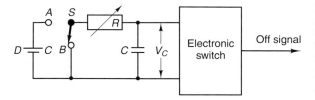

(A)

Figure 20.4   Simplified circuit diagram (A) and output graph (B) for a capacitor-controlled timer. Note that when the switch (S) is in position A the timer is switched off and the capacitor is 'shorted', ensuring it cannot retain any electrical charge. To switch on, the switch should be moved to position B. This will allow the capacitor (C) to receive charge through the variable resistor (R).

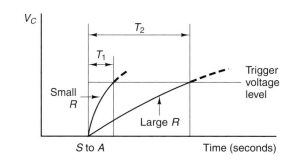

(B)

20.4 THE TIMING SECTION

The function of the timing section is to ensure that the appropriate signals are passed to the switching section to allow X-ray production to be switched on and off at the appropriate times. As we can see from Figure 20.4, the fixed resistor shown in Figure 20.1 has been replaced by a variable resistance; thus the time taken to charge to a predetermined potential across its plates is determined by value of this resistance. When this trigger voltage is achieved, a signal is sent to the switching system, which terminates the X-ray exposure by stopping current flow through the X-ray tube. If we consider the situation for thyristor switching (see Sect. 20.3.1), then it can be seen that the exposure can be terminated by simply removing the triggering voltage pulses from the gates of the thyristors. Thus, at the end of the next half-cycle, the thyristors will cease to conduct and the exposure will terminate.

20.4.1 Time-Based Timers

If the circuit in Figure 20.4 is arranged in such a way that the capacitor receives charge from a fixed single source (e.g. a rectified supply from the autotransformer), then the time it takes to charge the capacitor will be influenced only by the value of resistance selected by the radiographer. This is the basis of a time-based timer, i.e. a timer where the radiographer manually selects the exposure time (along with the kVp and the mA). The X-ray output at a given value of kVp is a function of the tube current (mA) and the exposure time (see Ch. 29). As the time-based timer only controls the exposure time, it cannot compensate for any fluctuations in the tube current that would influence the X-ray output from the tube. This problem is overcome by the mAs timer, which will be discussed in the next section.

20.4.2 The mAs Timer

A simplified diagram to show the operating principles of an mAs timer is shown in Figure 20.5. *Note* that on this occasion the capacitor is charged from two sources, V_1 and V_2. V_1 is a stable source of voltage (e.g. a rectified supply from the autotransformer). The amount of charge which the capacitor receives from V_1 is controlled by the variable resistor, R. This supply is connected to the capacitor (C) when the switch S moves from position B to position A at the start of the exposure. V_2 is a rectified supply from the midpoint of the

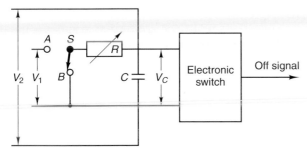

Figure 20.5 Simplified diagram showing the operating principles of an mAs timer. When the timer is switched on, the capacitor (C) receives charge from V_1 and V_2. For further explanation of the operating principles, see text.

high-tension transformer, so that the amount of charge from this source is directly related to the amount of charge passing through the X-ray tube (the mAs). This supply is again switched on with the exposure. (In the discussion below it is assumed, for simplicity, that the charge from V_2 is the same as the charge through the X-ray tube. This is not always the case, but the principle of operation of the timer is still the same.)

Suppose the capacitor requires 500 millicoulombs of charge to raise its potential (V_C) to the trigger voltage of the electronic switch. Consider the situation where the variable resistor, R, is set in such a position that the capacitor will receive 400 millicoulombs from V_1. Then the capacitor must receive 100 millicoulombs (or 100 mAs) from V_2 to reach its trigger voltage and terminate the exposure. If we assume that the charge to the capacitor from V_2 is the same as the charge passing through the X-ray tube, then the exposure will be terminated when 100 mAs has passed through the tube.

From the above discussion it can be seen that the radiographer will position the variable resistor, R, to determine the charge from V_2 and hence the charge passing through the X-ray tube during the exposure – the radiographer therefore selects the required mAs. This has the advantage over the time-based timer that fluctuations in the tube current (mA) will be accommodated by the timer so as to achieve the selected mAs. As the output from the tube at a given kV is proportional to the mAs, the above timer can be used with generators such as the capacitor

discharge and the falling-load generators, where the mA across the X-ray tube will change during the exposure.

Both the time-based timer and the mAs timer are manually controlled timers. We have the fundamental problem that they control the output from the X-ray tube according to the skill and judgement of the radiographer, who needs to estimate correctly the amount of radiation that will be absorbed by the patient. The density (or blackening) of the image is related to the amount of radiation striking the image-recording device. In the situations described so far, the radiographer judges how much radiation should leave the tube so that when this beam passes through the patient the correct amount will strike the image-recording device.

The principles of this process are shown in Figure 20.6. If R units of radiation leave the X-ray tube and A units are absorbed by the patient, then (R–A) units will strike the imaging device. Thus, ensuring the correct exposure to the film depends on the radiographer's skill in judging how much radiation the patient will absorb and selecting the duration of the exposure accordingly.

Automatic timers, which we will now consider, measure the amount of radiation to a small sample of the recording device and terminate the

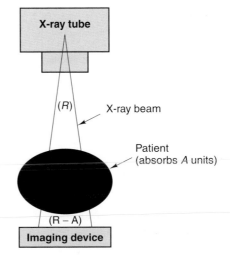

Figure 20.6 Diagram showing the X-ray absorption involved in image production. If R units of radiation leave the X-ray tube and the patient absorbs A units, then (R–A) units of radiation will reach the imaging device.

exposure when this radiation has reached a predetermined value. The radiographer has control of the kV selected, but has no direct control over the *duration* of the exposure.

20.4.3 Automatic Timers

There are three basic types of automatic timer. The first two – the ionisation timer and the phototimer – operate on similar principles, controlling the *duration* of the exposure but permitting the radiographer to select the kV used. The main difference between these two timers is the method by which the X-radiation is detected and converted into an electrical current.

20.4.3.1 Ionisation Timers

The ionisation timer makes use of the fact that X-radiation will cause ionisation in air. A radiolucent chamber is placed between the patient and the image-recording device and as radiation passes through this chamber it ionises the air within it. The ionised air molecules are attracted to the electrodes in the chamber by a potential difference between them, and as a result a small electrical current directly proportional to the amount of X-radiation flows between the electrodes. This small current is then amplified and used to charge the capacitor.

20.4.3.2 Phototimers

Phototimers make use of a photo cell, which is placed between the patient and image-recording device. The cell consists of a phosphor screen which emits light as radiation passes through it. The amount of light emitted is directly proportional to the amount of radiation passing through the phosphor screen. The light emission is then carried by light guides to a photodetector, a solid-state device such as a photodiode or a photo resistor which converts the light into an electrical current directly proportional to the light intensity. These devices are radiopaque and are placed in an area which is outside the field of the radiation beam. The photo cell, light guides and photodetector are encased in a light-proof covering to prevent external light affecting the current produced. As with the ionisation chamber, the current produced is then amplified and used to charge the capacitor.

With both timers, as in the case of the mAs timer, the capacitor is charged from two sources. V_1 is a stable source of voltage (e.g. a rectified supply from the autotransformer). This is shown in the simplified diagram of the ionisation timer in Figure 20.7. The amount of charge which the capacitor receives from V_1 is controlled by the variable resistor, R. V_2 is an amplified supply from an ionisation chamber (or photo cell) which can measure the amount of radiation that has passed through the patient. If we assume that the amount of charge from V_1 is determined by the position of the variable resistor, R, then the remainder of the charge required to raise the potential of the capacitor to the trigger voltage of the switching device must be from the source V_2. As this is directly related to the amount of radiation passing through the patient to the imaging device, this will be constant irrespective of the amount of radiation absorbed by the patient. The timer, in this case, terminates the exposure when the correct amount of radiation has passed through the ionisation chamber or photo cell. Thus, if the ionisation chamber or photo cell is positioned over the correct part of the patient, the radiograph should always receive the correct exposure. If we vary the resistance of the variable resistor, R, we can vary the amount of charge required from V_2, thus allowing imaging devices of differing sensitivities (speeds) to be used.

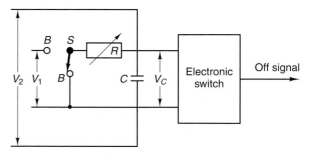

Figure 20.7 Simplified diagram to show the operating principles of an autotimer. When the timer is switched on, switch (S) is in position B and so the capacitor (C) receives charge from two sources – V_1, a stable voltage supply, and V_2, from an ionisation chamber or a photo cell.

20.4.3.3 Anatomically Programmed Timers

With the ionisation timer and phototimer, although the timers control the duration of the exposure, the radiographer has control over the selection of the exposure variables, such as the kV, focus used, the image-recording medium, and, with some units, the mA used.

With anatomically programmed timers, the radiographer selects the exposure, by body part and projection from a number of pre-installed options. These options will determine the kV, mA, type of image-recording medium (the film/screen combination), focus to film distance and ionisation chamber (or photo cell) to be used to detect the radiation that has passed through the patient.

This range of exposures, which is stored in the memory of a microprocessor, is programmed into the X-ray unit by the manufacturer of the X-ray generator. On installation of the unit a senior radiographer programs the final selection of exposure factors for each permitted exposure in the range into the computer memory, which is then 'locked' to prevent unauthorised access.

A simplified diagram of this type of timer is shown in Figure 20.8. Full details of its operation are beyond the scope of this text. On exposure, interlocks are used to check that the X-ray tube is at the correct focus to film distance and the recording medium is in place. The radiation detection device is then selected and exposure commences. When sufficient radiation has passed through the detector the microprocessor terminates the exposure through the exposure switching circuit.

Since the radiation dose received by the patient and the amount of scattered radiation produced are dependent on the quality and amount of radiation delivered during the exposure, this type of timer ensures that the optimum quantity of radiation delivered and kV are used for each exposure, minimising both the dose to the patient and the amount of scattered radiation produced.

Autotimers are usually used in conjunction with a guard timer. This is a pre-set time-based timer (see Sect. 20.4.1) which will terminate the X-ray exposure if the autotimer fails.

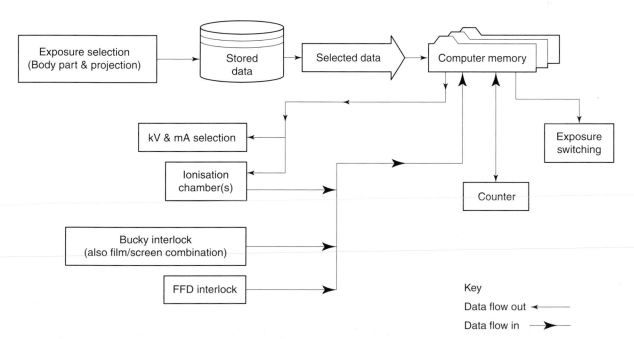

Figure 20.8 Simplified diagram showing the principles of an anatomically programmed timer. FFD, focus to film distance.

SUMMARY

In this chapter you should have learnt:

- The role of the circuits which prepare the X-ray unit for exposure (see Sect. 20.2)
- The role of the switching section in the X-ray generator (see Sect. 20.3)
- The function and operation of primary exposure switching (see Sect. 20.3.1)
- The function and operation of secondary exposure switching using a grid-controlled X-ray tube (see Sect. 20.3.2)
- The principles of the timing section of the X-ray generator (see Sect. 20.4)

- The principles and mode of operation of time-based timers (see Sect. 20.4.1)
- The principles and mode of operation of the mAs-based timer (see Sect. 20.4.2)
- The principles and mode of operation of autotimers utilising ionisation chambers or photo cells (see Sect. 20.4.3.1 and 20.4.3.2)
- The principles and an outline of the operation of the anatomically programmed timer (see Sect. 20.4.3.3).

SELF-TEST

a. Discuss the role of the 'prep' circuits in preparing a rotating anode X-ray tube for exposure.

b. Describe the role of primary exposure switching using thyristors in the X-ray circuit.

c. Describe how the X-ray exposure can be switched on and off using a grid-controlled X-ray tube, giving two uses of such an arrangement.

d. Describe the operation of a time-based timer in an X-ray circuit.

e. Describe the operation of an mAs-based timer in an X-ray circuit.

f. List three types of autotimer and describe the operation of an autotimer in an X-ray circuit.

g. Outline the principal differences between manual-controlled and automatic timers.

h. Discuss how automatic timers contribute to the reduction of the radiation dose absorbed by the patient.

FURTHER READING

Carter P H 1994 Chesney's equipment for student radiographers, 4th edn. Blackwell Publishing, London, ch 4
Curry T S III, Dowdey J E, Murry R C Jr 1990 Christensen's physics of diagnostic radiography, 4th edn. Lee & Febiger, London, ch 2

Webb S (ed) 2000 The physics of medical imaging, 2nd edn. Institute of Physics Publishing, Bristol, ch 2

Part 3

Construction and Operation of X-ray Tubes

PART CONTENTS

21. Diagnostic X-ray Tubes   195

22. Monitoring and Protection of X-ray Tubes   207

23. Orthovoltage Generators and Linear Accelerators   214

Chapter 21

Diagnostic X-ray Tubes

CHAPTER CONTENTS

21.1 Aim 195

21.2 Introduction 195

21.3 Construction of X-ray Tubes 196

21.4 Construction of the Tube Shield (Housing) 196
21.4.1 Electrical Safety 197
21.4.2 Radiation Safety 198

21.5 Construction of the Rotating Anode Tube Insert 198
21.5.1 Insert Envelope 198
21.5.2 The Anode Assembly 199
21.5.3 The Anode Heel Effect 200
21.5.4 The Cathode Assembly 201

21.6 Construction of the Stationary Anode Tube Insert 202
21.6.1 The Anode 202
21.6.2 Cathode and Filament(s) 202

21.7 Principles of Operation of the X-ray Tube 202
21.7.1 Thermionic Emission 202
21.7.2 The Space Charge Effect 203
21.7.3 Tube Current (mA) and Filament Current 204
21.7.4 Electron Focusing 204
21.7.5 Tube Voltage (kVp) 204
21.7.6 X-ray Production 205

21.8 Modern Trends in X-ray Tube Design 205

Self-Test 206

Further Reading 206

21.1 AIM

The aim of this chapter is to discuss the factors involved in the construction of diagnostic X-ray tubes.

21.2 INTRODUCTION

The rotating anode X-ray tube is the most common type of X-ray tube found in diagnostic imaging departments. The reason for this is that it is able to produce higher intensities of X-rays than the stationary anode tube. This is due to two factors:

1. The heat deposited in the anode during an X-ray exposure is spread over a larger area and so there is a smaller temperature rise at the anode surface
2. The cooling characteristics of the rotating anode are superior to those of the stationary anode and this effective dissipation of heat means that larger loads can be applied without causing thermal damage to the target.

The stationary anode tube has a very low rating (see Ch. 22) and is only found in dental and some portable X-ray units. These units are connected to a 13-amperes mains supply. This limits the amount of electrical power which can be applied to it, preventing overloading of the tube.

21.3 CONSTRUCTION OF X-RAY TUBES

The X-ray tube consists of two main components: the *insert*, which is usually mounted inside the *shield*.

These components and the light-beam diaphragm (we will discuss its role later in this chapter) are shown in Figure 21.1. The components of this tube are discussed individually in Section 21.5. Although the inserts for the rotating anode tube and the stationary anode tube differ substantially, the shields for both types of tube are very similar in design and function.

21.4 CONSTRUCTION OF THE TUBE SHIELD (HOUSING)

It is necessary to protect the patient and the radiographer from the electrical and radiation hazards posed by the X-ray tube insert while in operation. The insert is therefore incorporated within a suitable container – the shield – which must satisfy the following criteria:

- There must be no danger of electrical shock if the shield is touched during operation of the X-ray tube
- No significant amounts of radiation should escape from the shield other than the radiation necessary for taking the radiograph

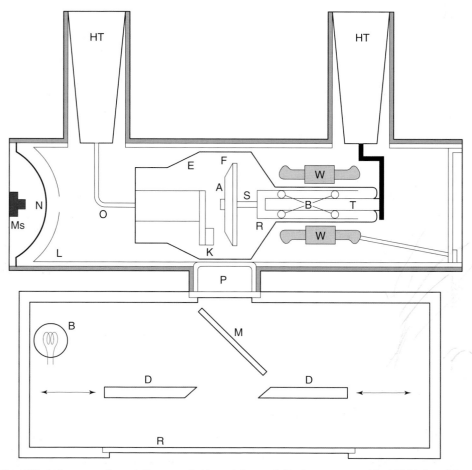

Figure 21.1 Simplified diagram of a rotating anode X-ray tube and diaphragm assembly. HT, high-tension socket; Ms, microswitch; N, bellows; L, lead lining; A, anode disc; S, anode stem; R, rotor assembly; T, rotor support; Br, bearings; W, stator windings; E, glass envelope; K, cathode assembly; O, oil; P, tube port and aluminium filter; F, focal track; B, light bulb; M, mirror; D, moveable diaphragms (only one pair shown); R, plastic diaphragm front.

- The shield must give secure support to the X-ray tube insert, the high-tension cables and the connecting cables within the shield
- Adequate insulation must be provided between the insert and the tube shield to avoid electrical breakdown
- There must be adequate cooling of the insert and facilities to allow expansion of the cooling oil
- There must be facilities at the tube port to allow adequate filtration of the emergent beam so that low-energy radiations may be removed from the beam.

As can be seen from this list, the shield must satisfy many requirements. A schematic diagram of the shield for a rotating anode X-ray tube is shown in Figure 21.1. Note that the insert is held in position by a support at the anode end.

The metal casing surrounding the insert is made of either aluminium or steel and is lined with about 3 mm of lead to provide sufficient radiation protection. This housing is filled with pure oil which acts as an electrical insulator and as a coolant. A neoprene diaphragm at one end of the shield allows for expansion of the oil when the oil is heated. The assembly is usually fitted with a microswitch which will prevent further exposures if the oil is very hot. Within the casing there is a radiolucent window – the tube port – which will allow the useful beam of radiation to leave the tube via the light-beam diaphragm.

21.4.1 Electrical Safety

Electrical safety is designed around four basic principles:

1. insulation of live components
2. earthing of component housings
3. restricted access to live components
4. isolation of the circuits from the mains supply when not in use.

All of the above are utilised in the design of the X-ray tube. Insulation exists between the live components and the housing in the form of the oil in the housing. As we saw in Section 10.3.3, the resistance of an insulator (and so its insulating properties) diminishes as the temperature of the insulator increases and so the role of the oil in

heat dissipation is also important from the point of view of electrical safety.

The tube shield is connected to earth via the outer braiding of the high-tension cables (Figure 21.2) and so the casing will always remain at earth potential. If a live wire within the casing becomes disconnected and touches the shield, then the current will readily flow to earth and the casing will present minimal electrical hazard to someone touching it at the time.

The live components in the X-ray tube are secured inside the tube shield and the ends and the high-tension cable connectors are securely

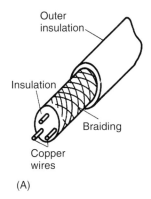

(A)

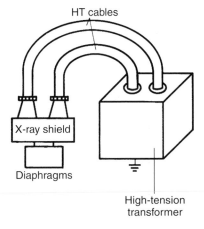

(B)

Figure 21.2 (A) Structure of a high-tension cable. Note the thickness of the insulation surrounding the central conductors. LT, low tension. (B) The X-ray tube shield is made electrically safe by connecting the copper braiding of the high-tension (HT) cables to both the shield and the casing of the high-tension transformer tank. The latter is securely earthed.

fixed. This means that, under normal circumstances, the operator has no easy access to the live components.

In addition, the circuits may be isolated from the mains by switches, fuses or circuit breakers.

21.4.2 Radiation Safety

Radiation safety is important for the operators of X-ray equipment and for patients and others who may be in the vicinity at the time of making an X-ray exposure. The lead lining of the tube housing (Figure 21.1) limits the radiation leakage from the tube and so provides protection to both the operator and the patient. It should be borne in mind that X-rays are emitted *in all directions* from the focus on the anode but only those which pass through the tube port are allowed to leave the housing. The anode itself has a high absorption and so the lead lining at the anode end of the shield is often absent or thinner than at the cathode end.

The radiation leakage rate from the tube is normally measured at a distance of 1 metre from the housing and should not exceed an air kerma of 1.00 milligray per hour, measured at a distance of 1 metre from the focus (for definitions of the kerma and the gray, see Ch. 33). Any break in the lead lining will result in radiation leakage from the tube, so the leakage levels should be checked at regular intervals as part of the quality checks on the X-ray unit.

Radiation safety means exposing the patient only to the minimum dose necessary to produce a radiograph of acceptable quality. As we will see in Chapter 28, the spectrum of X-rays produced at the target is a continuous spectrum containing a mix of low-, medium- and high-energy photons. Some of the photons have very low energy and will not be able to pass through the patient to reach the image receptor. These photons would contribute to the patient dose but not to the image production. Some of these are removed by the glass envelope of the insert and the oil as the beam passes to the tube port. This is known as the *inherent filtration* of the tube. Further filtration takes place through the aluminium filters placed at the tube port (Figure 21.1). These are known as

added filtration. Thus the *total filtration* of the beam is determined by the *inherent filtration* plus the *added filtration*. Details of this information are frequently marked on the end of the shield.

Scattered radiation contributes to the patient dose and the operator dose and causes degradation in the radiographic image quality. As we will see in Chapter 30, the amount of scatter produced at a given set of exposure factors is dependent on the volume of tissue irradiated. The volume can be reduced by reducing the area irradiated using a *light-beam diaphragm* (Figure 21.1). This also means that parts of the body not required on the radiograph can be protected from radiation. In this way, adequate collimation using a light-beam diaphragm (or cones) will reduce the patient dose and the operator dose and produce an improvement in the image quality.

21.5 CONSTRUCTION OF THE ROTATING ANODE TUBE INSERT

21.5.1 Insert Envelope

X-ray production is at its most efficient when a vacuum exists between the cathode and the anode of the X-ray tube, so these structures are enclosed within an evacuated metal or heatproof glass envelope which must be sufficiently strong to preserve this vacuum. Where a glass envelope is used it is joined to the anode spindle at one end and to the nickel cathode support at the other end by *re-entrant seals* – so called because the glass is shaped to point inwards at the area of contact. Slightly different glass seals are used at each end so that the thermal expansion of the glass is similar to that of the metal used in the construction of the anode spindle and cathode. This reduces the stress on the glass when the insert is hot and so limits the chance of cracking. The glass must be a good electrical insulator or a substantial current will flow through it when the high potential difference is applied between the anode and the cathode. However, electrical charges are built up on the inside of the glass during operation and so the glass must have sufficient electrical conductivity to allow these to leak away, usually between exposures, avoiding the build-up of high amounts of static charge. The glass is gently rounded so that there are no sharp corners which would allow the build-up of high amounts of static charge (see Sect. 9.9).

During operation of the X-ray tube, a thin film of tungsten will be deposited on the inside of the envelope as a result of the release of tungsten vapour from the filament and the target. This film acts as a filter to emergent radiation and where a glass envelope is used may eventually cause electrical breakdown within the tube as it can act as an electrical conductor around the inside wall of the glass envelope. If this happens, the tube is classed as 'gassy' and is of no further use. The rate of tungsten vaporisation can be reduced by not keeping the tube in the 'prep' mode (see Sect. 20.2) any longer than is required and by keeping exposures well within the rating of the tube (see Ch. 22).

As shown in Figure 21.3, metal envelopes do not completely surround the insert. The cathode end of the envelope is formed from a ceramic material to provide the necessary electrical insulation between the anode and the cathode. The metal component of the envelope is earthed, and as a result there is no build-up of static charges on the metal envelope. This improves the focusing of the electron beam within the insert and also reduces the effect of the build-up of vaporised tungsten on the inner walls of the envelope.

21.5.2 The Anode Assembly

The simplest anode configuration is shown in Figure 21.1, where the anode consists of a disc

Material	Use	Reason for use
Molybdenum	Disc	Half the density and twice the specific heat capacity of tungsten
Tungsten	Focal track (90%)	High atomic number. High melting point. Low vapour pressure. Suitable mechanical properties
Rhenium	Focal track (10%)	High atomic number. More elastic than tungsten, therefore less pitting of the focal track
Graphite	Disc backing	Low density. Acts as 'heat sink'. Radiates heat by black-body radiation

Table 21.1 Materials used in the design of the modern rotating anode disc

with an accurately bevelled edge on which is deposited a target track. A number of different materials are used in the design of the anode disc, as shown in Table 21.1.

A small amount of rhenium, which has an atomic number and melting point similar to that of tungsten, is alloyed with the tungsten of the target track. This improves the thermal expansion of the target track, making it more resistant to pitting. Tungsten is used as the main component in the target track for the following reasons:

- Tungsten has a high atomic number ($Z = 74$) and so is an efficient producer of X-rays (see Ch. 28)
- Tungsten has a high melting point (3387°C), so it can withstand the heat generated during the X-ray exposure without melting
- Tungsten has a low vapour pressure so it does not readily vaporise at its normal working temperature
- Tungsten can be readily machined to give the smooth surface required for X-ray production.

The bevelled edge permits the use of the *line focus principle*. As already discussed in Section 2.3, this results in an effective focus which is smaller than the real focus. The real focus can be longer than the effective focus. Thus the filament may be relatively long without giving rise to excessive geometric unsharpness. Thermionic emission from the filament is proportional to its surface

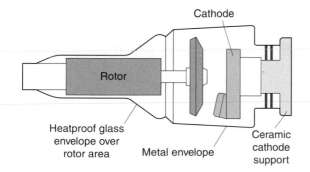

Figure 21.3 Simplified diagram of an X-ray insert with a metal envelope.

area and so a long filament will provide the high values of mA required by many exposures.

The area over which the heat is deposited is the larger area of the real focus (Figure 21.4), which is smaller than the apparent focus. The advantage of the line focus principle is that the temperature rise experienced by a large area for a given amount of heat is less than that experienced by a small area, since more atoms are able to take part in the heat dissipation processes. The line focus principle enables the anode to be designed so that the area of the real focus is about three times the area of the apparent focus. This enables a reasonable compromise between the need to minimise the temperature rise at the target (thus requiring a large focal area) and the need for minimising the geometric unsharpness (thus requiring a small focal area). The anode face is usually set at an angle between 7° and 15° to the central axis of the X-ray beam. This is called the *target angle*.

The disc has a central hole in it through which it is connected to a molybdenum anode stem and hence to the rotor of the induction motor (Figure 21.1). The rotor, stem and anode disc are accurately balanced so that no appreciable wobble occurs when the whole assembly rotates. The rotor is made to spin by the 'rotating' magnetic fields produced by the stator coils situated externally to the insert, using a similar process to the alternating current (AC) induction motor described in Section 15.7. The rotor moves smoothly on steel ball bearings coated in a soft metal, such as tin or silver, which acts as a lubricant but does not destroy the vacuum inside the envelope; a lubricant such as oil would evaporate

and compromise the vacuum. The rotating magnetic field produced by the stator coils causes the rotor (and thus the anode disc) to rotate at the same frequency as the applied voltage.

The rotation of the anode during the exposure has the effect of elongating the area bombarded by the electron beam in a lateral direction, reducing the amount of heat generated per unit area even further. The positive terminal from the high-tension supply is connected to the rotor support and through this there is a continuous electrical connection to the anode disc.

The conduction of heat from the anode disc to the ball bearings is inhibited by the fact that the anode stem has a small cross-sectional area (see Sect. 8.4.1) and is made of molybdenum (a relatively poor thermal conductor). However, some heat will inevitably reach the ball bearings and could cause sufficient expansion to produce a risk of seizure. This risk is reduced by applying a black coating to the outer surface of the rotor so that it loses heat efficiently by black-body radiation (see Sect. 8.4.4).

Many modern X-ray tubes also have graphite backing on the anode disc. This has a greater thermal capacity than molybdenum and draws heat from the anode and then dissipates it by black-body radiation. This results in the possibility of greater loads being applied to the anode and also in reduced heat dissipation to the ball bearings.

21.5.3 The Anode Heel Effect

Consider Figure 21.5. X-rays are produced slightly below the surface of the target material. X-rays passing along path 1 will therefore pass through a smaller section of the target than those passing along path 2. There is absorption of the X-rays as they pass through the target and so the rays which pass through the greatest thickness of target are the more heavily absorbed – there will be a lower intensity of X-rays along path 2 than along path 1. This means that the X-ray intensity at the anode end of the beam will be less than at the central axis, while the intensity at the cathode end will be greater than at the central axis. This is known as the *anode heel effect*. The effect increases as the target angle is reduced and also increases

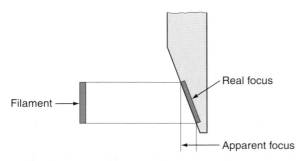

Figure 21.4 The line focus principle. Due to the angulation of the anode, apparent focus is much smaller than the real focus.

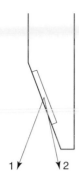

Figure 21.5 The anode heel effect. Ray 2 is more attenuated than ray 1, owing to its longer path through the tungsten target.

- Tungsten has a low thermionic work function and so will readily emit electrons by thermionic emission
- Tungsten has a low vapour pressure and so does not easily evaporate. This helps prolong the life of the filament, as evaporation would cause the wire to become thin. It also prolongs the life of the tube as it prevents the formation of a tungsten film on the inner wall of the glass envelope
- Tungsten is a strong metal which can be drawn into a thin wire which will not easily distort. This helps to maintain the shape of the filament helix over a period of time.

with the age of the X-ray tube. This latter increase is caused by the fact that the target becomes pitted with use.

21.5.4 The Cathode Assembly

The terms *cathode* and *filament* are often interchanged when discussing the X-ray tube. However, the correct usage of the term 'cathode' implies the whole cathode assembly, including the filament, focusing cup, supporting wires and cathode support. The filament is therefore part of the cathode but the cathode is not part of the filament.

The focusing cup, which supports the filaments, is offset from the central axis of the tube so that the electrons emitted from the filaments are aligned with the bevelled edge of the anode disc. It is made of either nickel or stainless steel, each of which has a high melting point, and is a relatively poor thermionic emitter – each has a high thermionic work function. In addition, the thermal expansion of these materials is close to that of certain types of glass, thus reducing the stress on the seals during operation of the tube. When the filaments produce electrons by thermionic emission these would repel each other by electrostatic repulsion – like charges repel – and so would strike a large area of focal spot. The area of the focal spot is reduced by the negative bias on the focusing cup which 'squeezes' the electrons together.

The filaments are made of a thin tungsten wire for the following reasons:

A rotating anode X-ray tube usually has two filaments. They may be positioned side by side, as shown in Figure 21.6: this is known as a dual-focus tube. Alternatively they may be positioned end to end, which means that the electron beams fall on different parts of the bevelled surface of the anode disc, which can be set at differing angles. This in-line configuration with different anode angles is referred to as a *biangular tube*.

In both instances the differing sizes of filament result in differing sizes of electron foci on the anode. The larger is known as the *broad focus* and would be used in situations where a high radiation

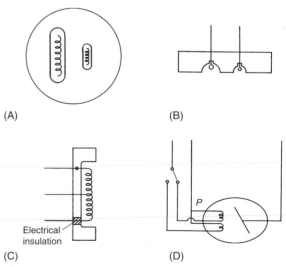

Figure 21.6 Details of cathode filament assemblies. (A) Face-on view of dual filaments; (B) dual filaments viewed from above; (C) in-line filaments viewed from the side; (D) electrical connections.

output was required from the tube, while the smaller – the *fine* focus – would be used in situations where it is desirable to keep geometric unsharpness (see Sect. 2.6) to a minimum.

One side of each filament is connected to the focusing cup while the other is insulated from it (Figure 21.6C). This connection between both filaments also forms the common connection between the filament circuit and the high-tension circuit. This is represented by point P in Figure 21.6D. From this diagram it can be seen that three conductors are required in the high-tension cable coming to the cathode end of the X-ray tube.

The secondary side of the filament transformer is also connected to one side of the high-tension circuit and this transformer could be a source of electrical hazard to the operator of the X-ray unit. For this reason and for reasons of ensuring good electrical insulation and heat dissipation, the filament transformer is contained in the same oil-filled tank as the high-tension transformer.

All high-tension cables for X-ray units contain at least three conducting wires, even though only one is required at the anode end of the tube. This means that manufacturers only need to make (and X-ray departments only need to stock) one type of cable. Only one of the three wires at the anode end is used to make an electrical connection to the tube.

21.6 CONSTRUCTION OF THE STATIONARY ANODE TUBE INSERT

21.6.1 The Anode

The anode of the stationary anode tube is constructed of two materials, copper and tungsten, and so is known as a *compound anode*. The main part of the anode assembly is made of copper because of its good thermal conductivity. (*Note* that the cooling of the target of the stationary anode tube is discussed in detail in Sect. 8.7.1.) The face of the anode is inclined at an angle of about 15° to the central axis of the insert and has an inset of a thin (about 2–3 mm) tungsten plate known as the *target* on which the electrons are focused.

21.6.2 Cathode and Filament

The basic construction of the cathode is the same as that of the cathode of a rotating anode tube. The main differences in construction are that the focusing cup is aligned along the central axis of the insert and there is only a single filament present.

21.7 PRINCIPLES OF OPERATION OF THE X-RAY TUBE

As we will see in Chapter 28, X-rays are produced by electrons which are accelerated from the cathode to the anode of the X-ray tube. The number of electrons crossing the tube is controlled at the mA selector while the kinetic energy of the electrons – and thus the photon energy of the X-ray beam – is indicated by the kV selector.

21.7.1 Thermionic Emission

The electrons are emitted by the heated filament by a process termed thermionic emission. In atoms, the outer-shell electrons are more loosely bound than the inner electrons because they are further away from the nucleus (remember $F \propto 1/d^2$). The application of heat to a body increases the kinetic energy of its atoms and so increases the violence of their collisions. As a result of these collisions, the outer electrons may be dislodged from the atom. Electrons so released near the centre of a body travel only a relatively short distance but if they are released near the surface of the material they may have sufficient kinetic energy to leave the body.

The higher the temperature of a body, the greater the kinetic energy of the atoms, and the greater number of electrons with sufficient energy to break free from the influence of the surface atoms of the body. We have also stated that the electrons, which are released by thermionic emission, are released from the surface atomic layers of the body. It follows that any alteration to these outer layers will alter the ability of a body to perform as a thermionic emitter. This has two practical consequences in radiography:

1. All the surfaces involved in thermionic emission (e.g. the tube filament) must be manufactured to a high degree of purity and must be kept scrupulously clean during assembly
2. The thermionic emission characteristics of a body may be altered by the deliberate addition of 'impurities' either to the whole body or just to the body surface.

The efficiency of thermionic emitters may be compared by comparing their work function, which is normally expressed in electron-volts (eV; see Sect. 6.4.3). The work function is the amount of work which must be performed by an electron in escaping from the body. Alternatively, it can be considered as the amount of work which must be performed on an electron to enable it to escape from the body. Substances which are good thermionic emitters have a lower work function than those that are poor thermionic emitters since, in the former, less work is required to allow the electrons to escape.

From the above discussion it should be apparent that the amount of thermionic emission from a body is controlled by:

- the temperature of the body
- the material of the body
- the surface area of the body.

The relationship between the temperature of a tungsten filament and the number of electrons liberated in unit time is shown in Figure 21.7.

21.7.2 The Space Charge Effect

If we assume that a body is electrically neutral before the application of heat, then each electron which leaves the body by thermionic emission will cause the body to have a net positive charge. After a very short time a state of equilibrium is set up where electrons leave the body and enter a 'cloud' of electrons near its surface and are then attracted back to the body, i.e. electrons are attracted back to the body as fast as they are emitted. The number of electrons in this cloud remains fairly constant since electrons are entering and leaving the cloud at equal rates. This cloud of electrons is known as the *space charge*. If the temperature of the body

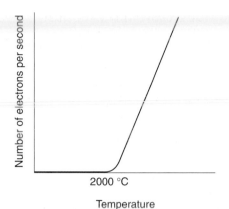

Figure 21.7 Graph of thermionic emission against temperature for a tungsten filament. Note that a small change in temperature produces a large change in emission.

is increased, then the number of electrons in the space charge will also increase due to the increased electron emission from the body. If the body is left to cool, it will reduce the space charge to zero by attracting electrons from it back to the body.

INSIGHT

If we take a normal tungsten filament light bulb and switch it on, then the filament of this bulb is producing significant numbers of electrons by thermionic emission. These electrons form a space charge around the filament and return to it in the process described above. If we bring a large positive charge close to this light bulb, we can cause these electrons to 'flash over' to this positively charged body. If we switch off the power supply to the bulb, the filament cools down almost immediately, thermionic emission ceases and no further flash-over occurs until the bulb is switched on again.

If a positively charged body is placed close to the space charge, then some of the electrons within the space charge will be attracted towards that body and so an electrical current flows between the heated body and the positive body via the space charge. This property is explored further in Section 21.7.3.

21.7.3 Tube Current (mA) and Filament Current

Figure 21.8 shows a circuit diagram of the X-ray tube and high-tension circuit which has been greatly simplified to illustrate the difference between the tube current (mA) and the filament current (I_f). The relationship between the temperature of the tungsten filament and the number of electrons released by thermionic emission has already been discussed in Section 21.7.2. This section will look at the application of this information to the X-ray tube. In Figure 21.8, B_1 represents the power supply across the X-ray tube and B_2 represents the power supply across the filament. Suppose B_2 causes a current I_f to flow through the filament circuit. The passage of this current through the filament causes the filament to heat and the subsequent temperature rise will cause electrons to be emitted by thermionic emission. These electrons are drawn towards the positive anode and constitute the tube current (mA). When all the electrons in the space charge are 'in use' it is said to be operating under saturation conditions. This is the normal operating condition of the X-ray tube. The only method of increasing the tube current is to increase the number of electrons in the space charge by increasing the temperature of the filament, causing more electrons to be released. Thus the selection of a given mA by the radiographer determines the filament heating current required to produce that mA. A typical set of filament currents for an X-ray tube is shown in Table 21.2.

Table 21.2 Filament heating currents for different tube currents for a typical X-ray tube

Filament heating current (A)	Tube current (mA)
5	200
7.5	400
9	800

21.7.4 Electron Focusing

During X-ray exposure, the anode of the X-ray tube is positively charged and the cathode is negatively charged. As a result of this, the electron space charge emitted from the filament is repelled from the negative cathode and attracted to the positive anode. The situation which would arise if both the cathode and the anode were flat plates is shown in Figure 21.9A. The electric force field (see Sect. 9.4) consists of parallel lines starting at the anode and finishing at the cathode. Electrons are emitted from the filament, F, and are attracted to the positive anode. However, the electrons repel each other, so the beam of electrons will increase in size as it travels across the X-ray tube. The area, W, on the anode represents an unacceptably large focal area as this would produce a large geometric unsharpness (see Sect. 2.6) on the resultant radiograph. This problem is overcome by the use of a focusing cup (see Sect. 21.5.4), as shown in Figure 21.9B. The thermionic electrons from F now experience two forces – one towards the anode and the other towards the central axis of the beam. The force towards the central axis of the beam is greater than the force of electrostatic repulsion between the electrons and so the beam of electrons is focused on to a small area of the anode – W in Figure 21.9B. The interactions between the electron beam and the anode are discussed in more detail in Sections 28.4–28.6.

21.7.5 Tube Voltage (kVp)

The kVp selected by the radiographer controls the peak potential difference across the X-ray tube. The higher the kVp, the higher the peak potential difference and so the greater the force of attraction

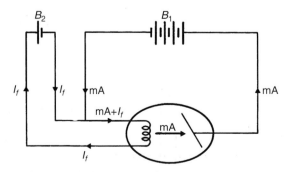

Figure 21.8 Simplified diagram to show the difference between tube current (mA) and filament heating current (I_f).

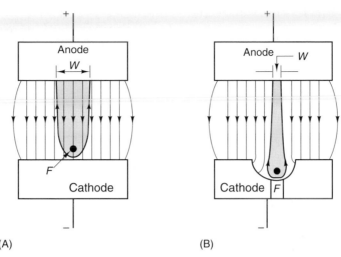

Figure 21.9 Simplified explanation of the focusing of electrons in the X-ray tube. (A) The result of no focusing cup on the cathode; (B) the electrostatic charge around the concave focusing cup directs the electrons from the thermionic emitter, *F*, towards the central axis so they strike a smaller area, *W*, on the anode.

between the anode and the cathode. Because of this, the electrons will strike the anode with greater kinetic energies and so will produce more energetic X-ray photons. This will be discussed in more detail in Chapter 28 when we consider X-ray production in detail. In this chapter we will finish with a brief synopsis of the process so that the construction of various parts of the X-ray tube may be more clearly understood.

21.7.6 X-ray Production

In the X-ray tube, electrons are produced at the cathode by thermionic emission. These electrons are then accelerated towards the anode and are made to give up their energy when they collide with the atoms of the target material. The main mechanism of X-ray production is when the electron is made to lose kinetic energy because of the pull of the positive nucleus of the target atoms. This is known as *Bremsstrahlung radiation*. The intensity (*I*) of the Bremsstrahlung radiation varies with both the energy (*E*) of the electrons striking the target and with the atomic number (*Z*) of the target material, as shown in the equations below:

$$I \propto Z \times E \qquad \text{Equation 21.1}$$
$$\text{or } I \propto Z \times \text{kVp}^2 \qquad \text{Equation 21.2}$$

The process of X-ray production is very inefficient and up to 99% of the energy of the electrons may be converted into heat which must rapidly be transferred from the focal area to avoid damage to the target of the tube (see Sect. 8.7.2).

21.8 MODERN TRENDS IN X-RAY TUBE DESIGN

There are a number of modern trends in the design of specialist X-ray tubes which are not within the scope of this text. The reader should consult either more specialist texts on tube design or manufacturers' literature. Specialist designs include:

- the metal/ceramic X-ray tube insert
- grid-biased X-ray tubes
- high-speed anode X-ray tubes
- stress-relieved anodes in rotating anode X-ray tubes
- X-ray tubes which allow automatic measurement of anode temperature
- alteration of the shape of the anode disc to allow improved loading (e.g. discus-shaped discs).

SUMMARY

In this chapter you should have learnt:

- The reasons why the stationary anode X-ray tube is of limited use in the modern X-ray department and why it has largely been replaced by the rotating anode X-ray tube (see Sect. 21.2)
- The fact that X-ray tubes consist of two major components – the insert and the shield (see Sect. 21.3)
- The construction of the X-ray tube shield (see Sect. 21.4)
- The methods of ensuring the electrical safety of the X-ray tube shield (see Sect. 21.4.1)
- The methods of ensuring the radiation safety of the X-ray tube shield (see Sect. 21.4.2)
- The construction of the rotating anode tube insert (see Sect. 21.5)
- The construction of the anode assembly of the rotating anode X-ray tube (see Sect. 21.5.2)
- The reason for and the result of the anode heel effect (see Sect. 21.5.3)
- The construction of the cathode assembly of the rotating anode X-ray tube (see Sect. 21.5.4)
- The construction of the stationary anode X-ray tube (see Sect. 21.6)
- The construction of the cathode and filaments of the stationary anode X-ray tube (see Sect. 21.6.1)
- The principles of operation of the X-ray tube (see Sect. 21.7)
- The interrelationships between the X-ray tube current (mA) and the filament heating current (see Sect. 21.7.3)
- The requirement for and the method of achieving focusing of the electron beam across the X-ray tube (see Sect. 21.7.4)
- The effect of the tube voltage (kVp) on the emergent X-ray beam (see Sect. 21.7.5)
- A basic description of X-ray production (see Sect. 21.7.6).

SELF-TEST

a. Indicate the functions of the components in the stationary anode tube insert and housing.

b. Draw a sketch diagram of a rotating anode X-ray tube to show the insert and housing. Indicate the function(s) of each of the major components.

c. List the reasons why tungsten is used in the construction of the filament and the reasons why tungsten is used in the construction of the target of the X-ray tube.

FURTHER READING

You will find further information on the rating of X-ray tubes in Chapter 22 of this text and more information on the factors affecting the X-ray spectrum in Chapter 28. In addition, you may find that sections from the following texts provide useful further reading:

Ball J L, Moore A D 1997 Essential physics for radiographers, 3rd edn. Blackwell Scientific Publications, London, ch 12

Bushong S C 2004 Radiological science for technologists: physics, biology and protection, 8th edn. Mosby, New York, ch 10

Curry T S III, Dowdey J E, Murry R C Jr 1990 Christensen's physics of diagnostic radiography, 4th edn. Lee & Febiger, London, ch 2

Dowsett D J, Kenny P A, Johnston R E 1998 The physics of diagnostic imaging. Chapman & Hall Medical, London, ch 3

Webb S (ed) 2000 The physics of medical imaging, 2nd edn. Institute of Physics Publishing, Bristol, ch 2

Chapter 22

Monitoring and Protection of X-ray Tubes

CHAPTER CONTENTS

22.1 Aim 207

22.2 Definition of Rating 207

22.3 Single Exposures 208
    22.3.1 Rating of Stationary Anode and
        Rotating Anode X-ray Tubes 210
    22.3.2 Effects of Anode Diameter and
        Speed of Rotation on Tube
        Rating 210

22.4 Multiple Exposures 210
    22.4.1 Anode Heating 211
    22.4.2 Anode Cooling 212

22.5 Automatic Monitoring of Rating 212

Self-Test 213

Further Reading 213

22.1 AIM

The aim of this chapter is to enable the reader to understand the concept of the rating of X-ray tubes and why it is monitored. The chapter will discuss factors which affect tube rating and the effects of single and multiple exposures on rating of the X-ray tube. An example of how a microprocessor is used to monitor these effects and prevent damage to the X-ray tube is illustrated.

22.2 DEFINITION OF RATING

The general term *rating* is used to describe the practical limits which are inherent in any device. An example of this is that a fuse rated at 5 amperes will tolerate currents up to 5 amperes. If a current above 5 amperes passes through the fuse, then the fuse will melt, causing a break in the circuit. A high-tension transformer is a more complicated device than a fuse and so has a more complicated set of rating conditions (see Sect. 17.9). Similarly, the rating of an X-ray unit – the X-ray tube and the associated equipment – depends both on how it is constructed and how it is being used. The rating may be defined as follows:

DEFINITION

The *rating* of an X-ray unit is the combination of exposure settings which the unit can withstand without incurring unacceptable damage.

All radiographic exposures cause slight wear and tear on the X-ray tube, since the anode becomes slightly pitted and the filament becomes slightly thinner as a result of any exposure. However, in this context 'unacceptable damage' means damage that would seriously impair the performance of the unit for further exposures or might indeed make it inoperative. In this context, a single short exposure where the mA was above the rating of the tube might damage the anode by melting the focal track. Alternatively, a long exposure at low mA may again damage the anode if the total amount of heat generated in the anode caused a sufficient temperature rise to melt the tungsten. It is also true that multiple exposures, each of which is individually within the tube rating, might damage the tube because of the total heat accumulated in the anode by the exposure series. As the anode takes a finite time to cool after an exposure, the closer the exposures follow each other, the more likely the anode is to suffer thermal damage. For this reason the rating for single and multiple exposures will be considered separately in this chapter.

22.3 SINGLE EXPOSURES

The rating for a single exposure is affected by a number of different factors; some of these are under the control of the operator while others are not, as shown in Table 22.1.

In any particular unit, the non-selectable factors are fixed and so a rating must be used which is applicable to that set of circumstances, e.g. a rating might be appropriate to an X-ray tube connected to a two-pulse unit. The rating can be plotted as a graph showing the effect on the rating of varying the quantities in the selectable group. A simplified form of such a graph is shown in Figure 22.1, where the rating curve corresponds to a 1.2-mm focus selection and a kVp selection of 80 kVp. The curve indicates the upper limit for all combinations of mA and time for this value of kVp. Thus, points below the line are safe, whereas points above the line are unsafe in that they would result in unacceptable damage to the X-ray tube. If we consider an exposure of 80 kVp, 100 mA and 0.2 seconds, then we can see that this exposure may

Table 22.1 Factors affecting the rating of a particular X-ray tube	
Selectable factors	Fixed factors
kVp	Rectification type
mA	Rating of high-tension cables and transformers
Exposure duration	Thermal capacity of anode
Focal spot size	Diameter of anode
Operating mode – fluoroscopy or radiography	Speed of anode rotation
	Anode angle
	Thermal capacity of tube shield
	Efficiency of heat loss from anode and tube shield

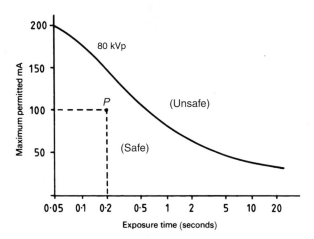

Figure 22.1 Graph of rating at a single kVp.

be safely made, as the point P is below the 80-kVp line. Note that because of the wide range of exposure times possible, it is usual to use a logarithmic scale on the x-axis.

It can also be seen from the graph that higher values of mA will be tolerated for short exposure times – 150 mA at a time of 0.1 second is within the rating – whereas, at long exposure times, only lower values of mA are within the rating – for an exposure time of 2 seconds the maximum mA permissible within the rating is 50 mA. In each case the limiting factor is the anode temperature. For longer exposure times there can be significant cooling of the anode during the exposure. This is shown by the flattening-off of the curve at longer exposure times.

In clinical practice, a range of kVp values is applied to the X-ray tube. Rating calculations take this and the focus size into account, producing separate rating graphs for broad and fine focus. Examples of such graphs are shown in Figure 22.2, where part A is the rating chart for the broad focus and part B for the fine focus. As can be seen from these graphs, the rating of the tube is lower for the fine focus than for the broad focus. This is caused by the fact that for a fine focus the electron beam is concentrated on to a smaller area, thus producing a higher temperature rise for the same value of mA.

Figure 22.2 also shows that larger values of mA are permitted as the kVp is reduced; the difference between the curves is most marked for the shorter exposure times. As was discussed in Chapter 21, electrons are produced at the filament of the X-ray tube and are accelerated towards the anode. The higher the kVp across the tube, the more kinetic energy each electron possesses when it interacts with the anode target. Thus, the same number of electrons per second (mA) will deliver more energy per second to the target and so will increase the possibility of thermal damage. The graph shows this inverse relationship between the kVp and the mA.

INSIGHT

Consider a situation where for a given exposure time (t) the anode may be given a total energy E without causing thermal damage. The energy of a single electron crossing the X-ray tube is proportional to the kVp across the tube. The total number of electrons is related to the current (mA) and the exposure time (t).

$$\therefore E \propto kVp \times mA \times t$$

Thus, for a given exposure time, halving the kVp should double the permissible mA.

Finally, the effect of different types of rectification when using the same X-ray tube needs to be considered. Figure 22.3 illustrates this effect for four different types of rectification, where the same focal spot and the same kVp have been selected. As can be seen from the graphs, the self-rectified circuit has the poorest rating, while the constant potential (or medium frequency) circuit has the best rating. Also note that the differences in rating are most marked at short exposure times. This is because the heating effect of individual pulses is most apparent in this situation. The more constant the heat production, the less the likelihood of thermal damage to the target – hence the best rating for constant potential.

For longer exposure times, the thermal capacity (see Sect. 8.3.2) of the anode disc is the dominating factor. This is independent of the type of rectification and so the curves all tend to come closer together as the exposure time increases. Also note that for longer exposure times the cooling of the tube shield and the heat dissipation within the high-tension transformer

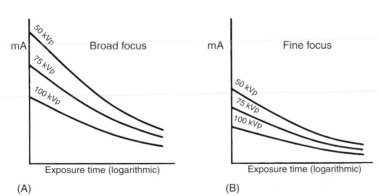

Figure 22.2 Graph showing the effect of tube focus on rating.

(A)   (B)

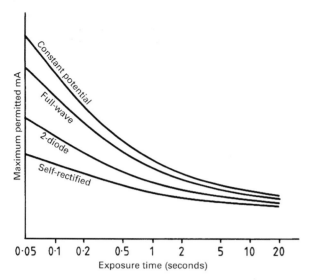

Figure 22.3   Graph showing effect of rectification system on rating.

are significant factors in determining the rating of the tube and X-ray unit.

22.3.1 Rating of Stationary Anode and Rotating Anode X-ray Tubes

In the stationary anode X-ray tube heat is lost by the process of conduction from the target through the copper anode and thence to the oil surrounding the insert in tube shield. The process is limited by the melting point of copper (1083°C) and the rate at which conduction occurs. As a result, the rating of stationary anode X-ray tubes is much lower than that of rotating anode X-ray tubes. Such X-ray tubes have a very limited application. In the rotating anode X-ray tube, heat loss by conduction is discouraged by the design of the anode stem (see Sect. 21.5.2) and the main method of heat loss from the anode is by radiation. Efficient heat loss by radiation is achieved by designing the anode disc so that it can tolerate high temperature rises (remember that the rate of heat loss by radiation is proportional to the fourth power of the kelvin temperature). During large exposures the anode disc often becomes incandescent and at such temperatures can lose heat effectively by radiation – hence the higher rating of the rotating anode tube.

22.3.2 Effects of Anode Diameter and Speed of Rotation on Tube Rating

When we consider the rating of the rotating anode tube we must consider not only the material used in its construction and its mass but also the effects of the anode diameter and the rate of anode rotation. In the rotating anode tube the electrons land on the focal track around the bevelled circumference of the disc. This means that the heat is deposited around the whole disc instead of in the same area, as in the case of the stationary anode tube. Because this heat energy is now deposited over a larger area, there is a smaller temperature rise per unit area and rating is improved.

If we increase the anode diameter we may increase its mass but this change also increases its circumference. This means that the heat energy is now deposited over a larger area and, as more atoms are involved in cooling, this leads to more efficient cooling, improving the rating. Doubling the diameter of the disc will increase its rating by 40–50%, but this has practical limitations because of the extra mechanical stress this imposes on the bearings. A simplified graph showing the improvement in rating is shown in Figure 22.4A.

If we double the speed of rotation of the anode, this means that only half the heat energy is deposited on to the anode for each rotation, although it makes twice as many rotations during a given exposure time. If there were no cooling between successive heatings of the same point, there would be no advantage of increasing the rotational speed.

The effect of increased anode rotation on the tube rating is shown in Figure 22.4B. Doubling the speed of rotation will again increase the rating by about 40–50%. It should also be noticed that the difference in rating diminishes with longer exposure times, since it is the overall thermal capacity of the anode that is the dominant factor.

22.4 MULTIPLE EXPOSURES

When single exposures are made there is a comparatively long interval between exposures.

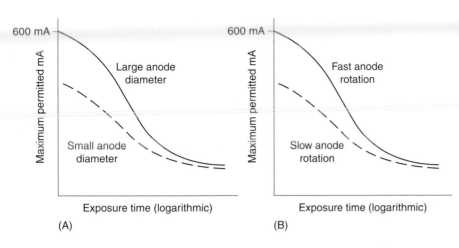

If a series of exposures is made there may be insufficient time for the anode disc to cool between exposures. While every single exposure in this series may be within the rating of the tube, the heating effect of subsequent exposures could raise the temperature of the anode above the permitted level, resulting in thermal damage to the focal track. In such cases it is necessary to consider additional factors to be able to predict the safety of any combination of exposures.

22.4.1 Anode Heating

The anode disc has a given mass and thermal capacity and so there is a given quantity of heat which will raise the whole anode disc to its maximum desirable operating temperature. This is known as the *heat storage capacity* of the anode and is expressed in kilojoules – in the example shown in Figure 22.5, this is 80 000 kilojoules.

For long exposures such as during fluoroscopy, the cooling which occurs during the exposure becomes important in calculating tube ratings. The anode initially heats up fairly quickly but then tends towards a thermal equilibrium, which occurs when the rate of heat generated in the anode by the electron beam is exactly balanced by the rate of heat loss from the anode. Examples of anode heating curves for a particular tube are shown in Figure 22.5, where the number of kilojoules stored by the anode at any moment is plotted against time. The maximum heat storage capacity of this anode is 80 000 kilojoules. Three different exposure rates are shown:

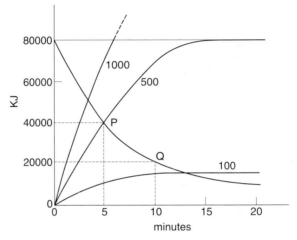

Figure 22.5 Graph showing anode heating and cooling curves.

1. The rate of 1000 kilojoules per second fairly rapidly exceeds the heat storage capacity of the anode and further exposure beyond this time would result in thermal damage
2. The rate of 500 kilojoules per second establishes thermal equilibrium at the maximum heat storage capacity of the anode
3. The exposure at 100 kilojoules per second – this would be the rate of heat production for a fluoroscopic kV of 100 kVp and a fluoroscopic current of 1 mA – produces thermal equilibrium with the anode at a fairly low temperature.

Note that in many cases it is convenient to show the heating and cooling curves on the same graphs.

22.4.2 Anode Cooling

The heat stored in the anode is lost at a finite rate and a cooling curve showing the rate at which this heat is lost plotted against time (assuming that the anode has received its maximum permitted number of kilojoules at $t = 0$) is shown in Figure 22.5. Suppose an exposure of 40 000 kilojoules is made: the point P shows this in the figure. The anode loses heat, as given by the curve below P, such that 5 minutes later, at point Q, only 20 000 kilojoules remains stored in the anode. An example of the use of such a graph is given below.

EXAMPLE

An exposure of 60 000 kilojoules is made on the X-ray tube for which Figure 22.5 is the cooling curve. The exposure requires to be repeated as soon as possible. How long must we wait between exposures to ensure that the anode does not exceed its maximum heat storage capacity?

Heat produced by the exposure = 60 000 kilojoules

The maximum heat storage capacity of the anode is 80 000 kilojoules and so it must cool down till it stores only 20 000 kilojoules before the exposure is repeated. By consulting the graph, it can be seen that this takes approximately 7 minutes.

In the cases discussed so far using cooling curves, it is assumed that no significant cooling of the anode takes place during the exposure. If this is not the case, e.g. during fluoroscopy, then anode heating curves are applied, as described above.

22.5 AUTOMATIC MONITORING OF RATING

With older X-ray generators it was necessary to use manufacturers' rating charts to ensure that exposures – particularly multiple exposures – were within the rating for the generator. This was a complex, error-prone process. Modern units are fitted with devices such as thermistors (temperature-sensitive resistors) and photo diodes which can be used to measure the temperature of the oil in the housing and of the anode disc. The electrical output from these is then passed to a microprocessor which can then calculate whether the proposed exposure is within the rating of the tube. The microprocessor takes into account not only the heat generated by the exposure but also any heat already stored by the anode disc and includes this in the calculation. This process is shown in flow chart form in Figure 22.6.

The first stage checks that the individual exposure is within the permitted loading for the selected focus, using stored data. The second stage checks that the exposure will not exceed the maximum rating for the X-ray tube. The heat lost between last exposure and current exposure is calculated and subtracted from the current temperature of the X-ray tube. The resultant figure is added to the heat generated by the exposure and this is then compared against the thermal capacity of the X-ray tube. If either of these tests results in an 'overload' condition, the computer activates an interlock which will prevent the exposure until 'safe' conditions exist.

SUMMARY

In this chapter you should have learnt:

- The definition of rating when applied to the X-ray tube and its associated equipment (see Sect. 22.2)
- The factors affecting single exposures (see Sect. 22.3)
- A comparison of the rating of stationary anode and rotating anode X-ray tubes (see Sect. 22.3.1)
- The effects of the anode diameter and the speed of rotation on the rating of the rotating anode tube (see Sect. 22.3.2)
- Additional factors which affect rating for multiple exposures (see Sect. 22.4)
- Automatic monitoring of rating (see Sect. 22.5).

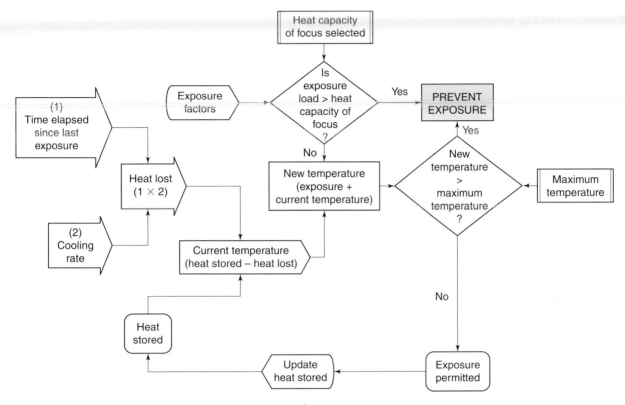

Figure 22.6 Flow chart showing computer monitoring of X-ray tube rating.

SELF-TEST

a. What is meant by the rating of an X-ray tube?

b. How does the rating of the X-ray tube depend on:

   (i)   the focal spot size

   (ii) the kVp

   (iii) the exposure time

   (iv) the rectification

   (v) the diameter of the anode disc

   (vi) the rate of anode rotation?

c. Why are the curves in a typical rating graph further apart for short exposure times than they are for long exposure times?

d. Under what circumstances can a single exposure, which is within the rating of the X-ray tube, nevertheless cause thermal damage to the anode? How is such damage avoided?

FURTHER READING

Dowsett D J, Kenny P A, Johnston R E 1998 The physics of diagnostic imaging, Chapman & Hall Medical, London, ch 3

Johns H E, Cunningham J R 1983 The physics of radiology. Charles C Thomas, Illinois, USA, ch 2

Chapter 23

Orthovoltage Generators and Linear Accelerators

CHAPTER CONTENTS

23.1 Aim 214

23.2 Introduction 214

23.3 The Orthovoltage Unit 215
    23.3.1 The X-ray Tube 215
    23.3.2 Beam Filtration 215
    23.3.3 Beam Collimation 216

23.4 The Linear Accelerator 216
    23.4.1 Introduction to the Linear
            Accelerator 216
    23.4.2 Construction of a Typical Linear
            Accelerator and its Principal
            Components 216
    23.4.3 The Magnetron 216
    23.4.4 The Waveguides and RF
            Circulator 217
    23.4.5 The Accelerating Waveguide
            and Accelerator 217
    23.4.6 The Bending Magnet and
            Treatment Head 218

Self-Test 219

Further Reading 220

23.1 AIMS

This chapter will review the main differences between diagnostic X-ray generators and the orthovolvoltage generator. It will also present an overview of the linear accelerator.

23.2 INTRODUCTION

X-rays at energies of up to 300 kV have been used to treat benign and malignant conditions since the early twentieth century. Historically this has been in two categories:

1. Superficial therapy using energies of up to 150 with beam filtration of 1–8 mm aluminium equivalent material at a focus to skin distance (FSD) of 10–30 cm
2. Orthovoltage or 'deep' therapy with energies of 150–500 kV with 0.5–3 mm copper filtration at a 50-cm FSD.

Superficial units are rarely found in clinical use today as many of the conditions they were used to treat are no longer common and other more efficient methods of treatment have been developed, many of which do not use ionising radiation. These units are unable to deliver a sufficient dose to areas of significant separation; they produce a high surface dose and a significant amount of scattered radiation is produced outside the beam as a result of Compton scatter. Orthovoltage units, with their increased higher energies and filtration, deliver less surface dose. Although the beam still produces large amounts of Compton scatter, the differential absorption of radiation by tissues of higher atomic number, such as bone, makes orthovoltage treatment suitable for use on patients with metastatic bone deposits and some primary bone lesions.

23.3 THE ORTHOVOLTAGE UNIT

There are a number of similarities and differences between these units and the general diagnostic unit. The orthovoltage unit uses a stationary anode X-ray tube, unlike the rotating anode used in diagnostic radiography. The circuit of a high-voltage generator is similar to that of modern microprocessor-controlled medium-frequency diagnostic generators (see Sect. 19.7). However the control panel differs in that a number of distinct stages must be followed in sequence before exposure can be initiated; these include the ability to select the additional filtration used – this automatically sets the kV and mA available. The radiographer must then select the dose to be delivered and the exposure time. This determines the setting of the back-up timer, which will terminate the exposure if the elapsed time exceeds the set time by 10%. Other differences are the beam filtration and the way in which the beam is collimated.

23.3.1 The X-ray Tube

Unlike the rotating anode design found in diagnostic units, the orthovoltage unit uses a hooded stationary anode insert (Figure 23.1). This is likely to have an insert with a metal–ceramic envelope, which overcomes the common cause of tube failure, which in these units is usually the breakdown of the glass envelope around the insert. As can be seen, the target is surrounded by shielding apart from two ports: the first is in line with the electron beam from the cathode and the second, covered by a beryllium window, is at 90° to this axis and in line with the tube exit port. This permits the beam of useful radiation to leave the anode and tube. The hood serves two functions: (1) it absorbs secondary electrons produced by electron interaction with the target; and (2) it attenuates unwanted

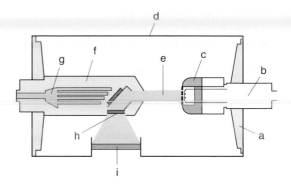

Figure 23.1 Simplified diagram of an orthovoltage metal–ceramic X-ray tube insert. a, ceramic insulator and support; b, cathode assembly; c, cathode block and filament; d, metal envelope; e, electron beam; f, hooded anode; g, oil coolant channels in anode; h, beryllium window; i, insert exit port.

radiation, reducing the thickness of the lead lining required in the tube housing, thus reducing the weight of the tube assembly. Note that the anode which loses heat through conduction to the oil surrounding the insert has, in addition to a large cross-sectional area, channels in it through which oil is circulated, thus improving the cooling process.

23.3.2 Beam Filtration

As with diagnostic X-ray tubes, the orthovoltage tube has both the inherent filtration that attenuates due to the components of the tube and additional filtration produced by filters placed in the beam path after it has left the tube. In most diagnostic units the filtration, which serves to 'harden' the beam by removing low-energy radiation from the beam, is in the form of a fixed thickness of an aluminium-equivalent material. With the orthovoltage tube this filtration can be changed to suit the energy spectrum used to treat the patient. At lower energies the filters are usually of a single material – aluminium, copper or tin. At higher energies a composite filter such as the Thoraeus filter, made of tin, copper and aluminium, is used. With these composite filters, it is important that the material of the highest atomic number is placed near the tube port. The function of the lower atomic number material is to remove the characteristic radiation produced by the filter material of higher atomic number.

23.3.3 Beam Collimation

Collimation in the diagnostic unit is provided by the adjustable diaphragms in the form of the light-beam diaphragm. The orthovoltage unit uses interchangeable cones or applicators of standard design. These are usually square or circular in shape and produce a beam field of up to 22 cm². The applicators are attached to the tube housing by a large lead plate with an aperture that determines the field size of the applicator. Specially shaped applicators are often used for specific treatment areas, e.g. the canthus of the eye.

23.4 THE LINEAR ACCELERATOR

23.4.1 Introduction to the Linear Accelerator

Linear electron accelerators, or linacs, as they are commonly known, accelerate electrons in a straight path and differ from the cyclotron (see Sect. 27.11.3), in which electrons follow a circular path. They have been used in radiotherapy since the 1950s to treat patients with malignant and benign disease. Since their introduction, they have virtually replaced earlier treatment systems such as cobalt units. The increasing complexity of treat-ment methods and improvements in technology have seen the unit develop from a relatively simple fixed-energy output unit to units with dual and multiple megavoltage output energies of up to 5 MeV, which are capable in some instances of techniques such as conformational therapy treatment. Improvements in electronics have resulted in increased unit reliability and stability of output. This is an important factor in radiotherapy treatment.

23.4.2 Construction of a Typical Linear Accelerator and its Principal Components

The construction of a typical linac and its principal components is shown in a simplified form in Figure 23.2. As can be seen from the figure, the linear accelerator can be divided into two large structures – a floor-mounted stand and a motor-driven gantry, which rotates about the treatment isocentre. These components are discussed individually in the following sections.

23.4.3 The Magnetron

The magnetron (Figure 23.3) is an evacuated cylindrical structure, consisting of a central

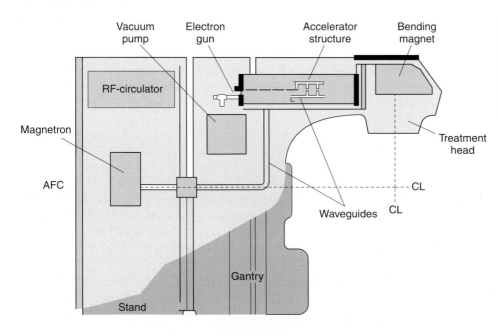

Figure 23.2 Simplified diagram of the principal components of a linear accelerator. RF, radiofrequency; AFC, automatic frequency control; CL, centre line.

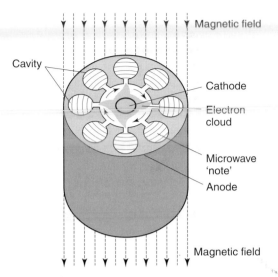

Figure 23.3 Section through a magnetron showing arrangement of anode, cavities, rotating electron field and electron field produced.

hollow, indirectly heated, oxide-coated cathode and surrounded by a copper anode containing a number of equidistant cavities that communicate with the space surrounding the cathode. The entire structure is enclosed in a magnetic field running parallel to the long axis of the magnetron. Both anode and cathode are supplied by a pulsed direct current supply from the modulator. The voltage of this supply is selected so that the electron cloud emitted by the cathode forms a rotating field with a number of spoke-like projections. As the 'spokes' pass over the entry to the anode cavities, they lose about 60% of their energy, inducing them to resonate at a radiofrequency, rather in the same way that a musical note is produced by a flute when a musician blows over it.

The resonance, at a frequency of 3000 MHz, corresponds to a wavelength of 10 cm. This results in the production of microwaves that are detected and transmitted into a waveguide. Stability of output is maintained by an automatic frequency control (AFC) which adjusts the size of the resonant cavity to maintain this frequency with an accuracy of ±20 kHz. The pulsed input means that, although the device operates at an average output of 2 kW, it has a peak output of 2–5 MW.

23.4.4 The Waveguides and Radiofrequency Circulator

Two types of waveguide are found in a linear accelerator: the first are simple hollow tubes that carry the radiofrequency waves from the magnetron to the accelerator section waveguides (at these frequencies the high impedance of solid conductors would result in significant power losses due to their impedance). The waveguides are sealed at both ends by a ceramic disc, which is transparent to microwave radiation and the first type of waveguide is filled with sulphur hexafluoride to improve its power-handling capabilities. A radiofrequency circulator is situated between the magnetron and the accelerator waveguide; its function is to act as a one-way valve permitting the radiofrequency radiation to pass through it but preventing any from passing back into the magnetron, which would be damaged if this occurred. The accelerator waveguide is evacuated and differs in structure and purpose. This will be discussed in more detail in Section 23.4.5.

23.4.5 The Accelerating Waveguide and Accelerator

The accelerating waveguide and accelerator are situated in the gantry of the linac. The waveguide uses the radiofrequency wave to accelerate electrons to very high velocities. The principle underlying this process is that an electrical field exerts a force on a charged particle placed in the field. It follows that, for the force to continue to act on the particle, it must move with it. The waveguide is divided into a buncher and a relativistic or accelerating section: this forms about two-thirds of the total length of the waveguide. The main difference between the two sections is that the washer-like annular inserts (shown in Figure 23.4) are closer together in the buncher section. The electrostatic fields slow the passage of the radiofrequency wave to approximately 0.4 C through this section. As already mentioned, this waveguide is evacuated. It is also a resonant structure. It is surrounded by a water jacket through which tempered cooling water

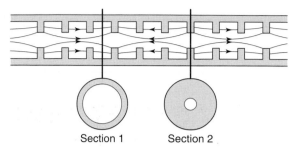

Figure 23.4 Section through an accelerating waveguide showing the annular inserts (sections 1 and 2). The electrostatic fields controlling the electron path are shown by the arrowed lines.

flows to minimise the thermal contraction and expansion of the guide which can change its resonance. An electron gun is attached to the buncher section and this injects electrons into the guide in pulses under the control of the modulator, in synchronisation with the radiofrequency wave. Typically only about one-third of the electrons are captured into the optimum part of the radiofrequency wave; however, because of the sinusoidal shape of the wave, the electrons which are in non-optimal locations will experience different degrees of acceleration and will decelerate and fall back until they are at the crest of the following wave. On reaching the accelerator section, the electrons gain velocity, reaching speeds of approximately 0.9 C. Because like charges repel one another, the electron beam tends to diverge. This is countered by steering coils positioned along the length of the cooling jacket that produce lines of magnetic force running parallel to the long axis of the guide. Focusing coils at the entrance and exit of the waveguide carry out a similar function and ensure that the electron beam is cantered to the centre of the guide and target.

23.4.6 The Bending Magnet and Treatment Head

The electron beam produced in the accelerator is travelling in a horizontal alignment with the gantry and must be deflected to assume an alignment which is perpendicular to it. This process is carried out by the bending magnet which deflects the electron beam through a 270° angle. The magnet is situated externally to the accelerator structure and, like the accelerating waveguide, is an evacuated structure. The radius of the bend depends on the velocity of the electrons; those with higher velocity are deflected in a turn with a larger radius, while lower-velocity electrons are deflected in a turn of smaller radius, effectively focusing the beam to a small area at 270° to its original path. The effect is similar to focusing light waves to a point by an achromic lens. For this reason the magnet is sometimes referred to as an achromic magnet (Figure 23.5). The effect of this is to produce a small electron beam that yields treatment fields that have well-defined edges, reducing the penumbra effect. Figure 23.6 shows the main components of the treatment head which is set for electron therapy. The electron applicator is attached to an external mounting on the treatment head. If X-ray treatment is required, the scattering foil which is designed to produce a 'flat' electron beam is rotated out of the electron beam and is replaced by a thin tungsten transmission target and a bell-shaped flattening filter. In both instances the radiation beam passes

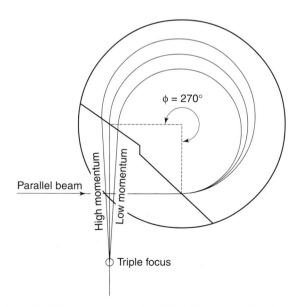

Figure 23.5 Diagram of a 270° bending magnet. Note that the electrons of differing speeds are focused to a point on the target (see text for more detail).

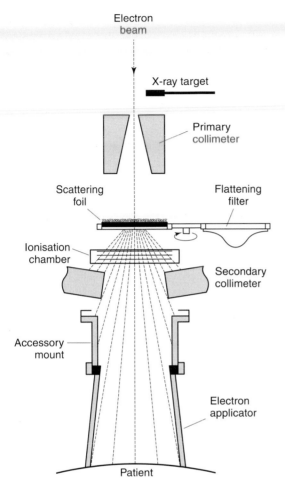

Figure 23.6 Treatment head set for electron therapy. For X-ray therapy the scattering filter is rotated out of the beam and replaced by the transmission target and flattening filter.

through a dual ionisation chamber. This monitors beam intensity and is also used to terminate the exposure when the desired amount of radiation has been produced.

SUMMARY

In this chapter you will have learnt:

- Why superficial therapy machines are no longer used for radiotherapy treatment (Sect. 23.2)
- How the orthovoltage X-ray tube insert differs in design from a diagnostic insert (Sect. 23.3.1)
- How the tube filtration differs between radiotherapy tubes and diagnostic tubes (Sect. 23.3.2)
- Why waveguides are used in preference to solid conductors (Sect. 23.4.4)
- The structures found in the treatment head of a linear accelerator (Sect. 23.6)

SELF-TEST

a. Describe the differences between an orthovoltage-ray tube and a general diagnostic-ray tube.

b. List the main components of a linear electron accelerator (linac).

c. State why solid conductors are not used for the transport of the radiofrequency wave.

d. Outline how a 'flat' beam is produced when using a linac for electron and X-ray therapy.

FURTHER READING

Bomford C K, Kunkler I H 2003 Walter's and Miller's textbook of radiotherapy, 2nd edn. Churchill Livingstone, Edinburgh, chs 9 and 10

Cherry P, Duxbury A 1998 Practical radiotherapy physics and equipment. Greenwich Medical Media, London, chs 9 and 10

Greene D, Williams P C 1997 Linear accelerators for radiation therapy, 2nd edn. Institute of Physics Publishing, Bristol

Morris S 2001 Radiotherapy physics and equipment, chs 5 and 7. Churchill Livingstone, London

Williams J R, Thwaites D I 2000 Radiotherapy physics in practice, 2nd edn. Oxford University Press, Oxford

Part 4

Atomic Physics

PART CONTENTS

24. Laws of Modern Physics   223
25. Electromagnetic Radiation   228
26. Elementary Structure of the Atom   237
27. Radioactivity   246

Chapter 24

Laws of Modern Physics

CHAPTER CONTENTS

24.1 Aim   223

24.2 Introduction   223

24.3 Classical Versus Modern Laws   223

24.4 Law of Conservation of Energy   224
      24.4.1 Mass–energy Equivalence   224

24.5 Law of Conservation of Momentum   225

24.6 Wave–particle Duality   225
      24.6.1 Waves as Particles   225
      24.6.2 Particles as Waves   226

24.7 Heisenberg's Uncertainty Principle   226

Self-Test   227

Further Reading   227

24.1 AIM

The aim of this chapter is to introduce the reader to the laws of modern physics. In many cases these are refinements or extensions to the laws of classical physics which were discussed in Chapter 5 and in this chapter reference will be made to the laws outlined in Chapter 5. In other areas there is disagreement between the classical and the modern laws and these will be identified and discussed.

24.2 INTRODUCTION

The laws of classical physics were discussed in Chapter 5 and these have been sufficient to explain the phenomena outlined in previous chapters of this text. However, in the following chapters on atomic and radiation physics, some important aspects of modern physics must be introduced in order to explain many of the phenomena discussed. The purpose of this chapter is to describe the laws of modern physics which are relevant to our need in the rest of the text.

24.3 CLASSICAL VERSUS MODERN LAWS

Modern physics started at the turn of the twentieth century with *Planck's quantum hypothesis* in 1900, in which he conjectured that radiation energy could only be absorbed or emitted by a body at discrete values of energy. Other dates of interest to the rest of this text include the *mass–energy relationship* postulated by Einstein in 1905, *the Bohr model of the atom* which was suggested in 1913 and *the de Broglie wavelength of particles*, which was introduced in 1924. Since these dates there have been major technical and theoretical strides, but these form part of the firm experimental foundation upon which modern physics is built.

One of the essential differences between classical and modern physics is the way in which matter is regarded. In classical physics matter and energy are completely separate entities and so we have *the Law of Conservation of Matter* (see Sect. 5.2) and *the Law of Conservation of Energy* (see Sect. 5.3), with no interconnection between the two laws. Also, in classical physics, *matter* is supposed to behave in one way – like matter! – and *waves* are supposed to behave like waves, and one cannot behave like the other; classical physics does not allow for the existence of a particle with a wavelength. However, there are no such rigid boundaries in modern physics. In particular, the work of Einstein showed that matter can be thought of as being interchangeable with energy if the conditions are right. This principle is known as *mass–energy equivalence* and will be discussed in more detail later in this chapter (see Sect. 24.4.1). In addition, it is found in modern physics that particles of matter do behave like waves and vice versa and this is known as the *wave–particle duality* principle (see Sect. 24.6).

With these concepts in mind, we will now consider the laws of modern physics in more detail in the remainder of this chapter.

24.4 LAW OF CONSERVATION OF ENERGY

This law now states that *the amount of energy in a system is constant*. In the context of modern physics this can be thought of as the sum of all the energies (rest energies + kinetic energies + potential energies) being a constant for any given system. The phrase *a system* can be used to define either a very small or a very large area, provided the influence of other bodies outside the system is negligibly small. In the context of modern physics, the use of the term *energy* in the above law embraces the contribution of matter to the total energy of a system under consideration. This concept of mass–energy equivalence will now be discussed.

24.4.1 Mass–energy Equivalence

Einstein showed that the mass of a body, m, and its energy, E (excluding potential energy), are related by the formula:

$$E = mc^2 \qquad \text{Equation 24.1}$$

where c is the velocity of electromagnetic radiation (often referred to as the velocity of light, as light is probably the best-known form of electromagnetic radiation). Thus the energy of a body is proportional to its mass (and vice versa), since c is a constant. If we consider a stationary body with a rest mass, m_0, then the rest energy of this body is given by $E_0 = m_0 c^2$. If we now consider this body travelling with a velocity, V, then its energy is now E_V and Einstein's equation is $E_V = m_V c^2$. Since the energy of the body when moving, E_V, is greater than the energy of the body when at rest, E_0, and since c is a constant, then m_V must be greater than m_0 – a body increases in mass as its velocity increases. The above statement seems to contradict our common experiences (because of the small values of velocity which we can normally produce) but if we take particles and accelerate them until they travel with a velocity close to the velocity of light (3×10^8 m.s^{-1}), then there is a measurable increase in the mass of the particles. The mass which they then possess is known as the *relativistic mass* of the particles.

The law of conservation of energy, stated earlier, is sometimes referred to as the law of conservation of *mass–energy* because of the concept of equivalence between mass and energy. It is also not uncommon to quote the *rest mass* of subatomic particles, either in units of mass or in units of energy – the rest mass of the electron can be stated as 9.1×10^{-31} kg (mass) or 0.511 MeV (energy).

As we can see from the above discussion, energy and mass can be considered as two manifestations of the same thing, and may be changed from one form to the other in appropriate circumstances, as the following examples show:

- The forces which hold the atomic nucleus together are obtained because some of the mass of the nuclear particles is converted into energy. Because of this the mass of the nucleus is less than the sum of the masses of the individual nuclear particles
- If a gamma-ray has an energy greater than 1.02 MeV and passes close to the nucleus of an atom, the ray may spontaneously disappear and create two particles of matter – an electron and a positron. This process is known as *pair production* and will be described in more detail in Chapter 30. The positron created in this interaction will interact with an electron and their mass will be converted into two photons of radiation, each photon having an energy of 0.51 MeV. The positron and the electron will now cease to exist and the radiation is referred to as *annihilation radiation*. This interaction shows that energy can be converted into mass and that mass can be converted into energy.

24.5 LAW OF CONSERVATION OF MOMENTUM

This law may be stated as *the total linear momentum in a system is constant*. The word *system* is used in the same context as for the law of conservation of energy. As we discussed in the section dealing with the laws of classical physics, the momentum of a body is the product of its mass and its velocity. Thus we can say:

sum of all (mass × velocity)
= constant for a system

Here, the mass referred to in the equation is the relativistic mass of the body, i.e. its mass when it is moving with the velocity, V. An example of the law of conservation of momentum being applied to modern physics is in Compton scattering (see Ch. 30) when some of the momentum of the incoming photon is given to an electron – the combined momentum of the scattered photon and the ejected electron is the same as the momentum of the incident photon.

24.6 WAVE–PARTICLE DUALITY

As we have just seen, modern physics regards mass and energy as being two manifestations of the same phenomenon. Similarly, modern physics blurs the distinction that exists in classical physics between a particle and a wave.

24.6.1 Waves as Particles

Classical physics was very successful in explaining many of the phenomena associated with electromagnetic radiation (e.g. diffraction and interference) by assuming that such radiation was made up of waves travelling at the velocity of light, c. In this case $c = v\lambda$, where v is the frequency of vibration of the radiation and λ is its wavelength. However, phenomena like the Compton effect and photoelectric absorption (both will be discussed in detail in Ch. 30) are not easy to explain using the wave theory. These effects are explained by considering that sometimes electromagnetic radiation behaves as 'packets' of energy which have an associated momentum. Such a packet of energy is called a photon or a quantum and the quantum theory predicts that:

- the quantum will have an energy, E, given by:

$$E = hv \qquad \qquad Equation\ 24.2$$

where h is a constant known as Planck's constant and v is the frequency of vibration of the associated wave. We will frequently use this formula in the chapters which follow on atomic physics!
- the quantum will have a momentum, p, given by:

$$p = \frac{hv}{c} \qquad \qquad Equation\ 24.3$$

Thus, the electromagnetic wave may also behave like a particle, possessing energy and momentum.

24.6.2 Particles as Waves

Moving particles of matter, whether these are large or very small, have both kinetic energy and momentum. Are there then occasions when they behave as waves? Perhaps the most dramatic example of particles behaving like waves is in the operation of the electron microscope. Here high-energy electrons are passed through or are scattered by a sample. A very highly magnified image of the sample is obtained so that individual large molecules may be seen in materials. The reason for the high degree of magnification is due to the very small wavelength of the electrons. Whether we consider an optical microscope or an electron microscope, the smaller the wavelength of the radiation used, the finer the detail it is possible to see.

De Broglie proposed that the following relationship exists between the momentum, p, of the particle and its associated wavelength, λ:

$$p = \frac{h}{\lambda} \qquad \textit{Equation 24.4}$$

In such cases λ is called the *de Broglie* wavelength and the existence of particles behaving like waves can be verified by a number of experiments.

Note the *inverse* relationship between the momentum of the particle and its associated wavelength. Thus the wavelength decreases as the momentum increases and vice versa. For example, the de Broglie wavelength associated with an electron moving at half the velocity of light is about 4×10^{-12} m, which is less than the diameter of the hydrogen atom (100×10^{-12} m). When the velocity of the electron is one-hundredth of that of light then the de Broglie wavelength is at the larger value of 240×10^{-12} m, which is now in the X-ray range of wavelengths (see Ch. 25) and so such electrons can be used for X-ray crystallography.

Within the context of radiographic science, it is more common to consider waves behaving as quanta rather than quanta behaving as waves. This is particularly true when we consider the production of X-rays (see Ch. 28) and the interactions of X-rays with matter (see Ch. 30).

24.7 HEISENBERG'S UNCERTAINTY PRINCIPLE

In classical physics it is possible *in principle* to measure exactly a number of quantities concerning the state of a body, e.g. the body's energy, position and momentum. Furthermore, if it were possible to build measuring apparatus which was infinitely precise, it would be possible to make *simultaneous exact measurements* of several of these quantities.

According to modern physics, it is not possible to treat quantities like mass and energy or matter and waves as being totally independent of each other. *Heisenberg's uncertainty principle* is an extension of the principle of wave–particle duality and concerns the maximum possible precision which may be obtained in ideal circumstances when measuring two quantities simultaneously. The central point of the principle is that *measuring one quantity affects another quantity*, so that it is never possible to measure both quantities simultaneously with complete accuracy – if we try to measure the momentum of a particle, this will automatically affect the position of the particle so that it is never possible to measure momentum and position *simultaneously* with complete accuracy. Effects due to this principle are too small to be observed in everyday life and concern atomic and nuclear systems. This principle is yet another difference between modern and classical physics – in classical physics it is assumed that perfect instruments produce perfect results.

If we now apply Heisenberg's uncertainty principle to the duality theory we can say that, although we can demonstrate that waves can behave like particles and that particles can behave like waves, it is not possible to set up a situation where both properties are demonstrated *simultaneously*.

SUMMARY

In this chapter you should have learnt:

- The differences which exist between the laws of classical physics and the laws of modern physics (see Sect. 24.3)
- The law of conservation of energy as applied to modern physics (see Sect. 24.4)
- The concept of mass–energy equivalence (see Sect. 24.4.1)
- The law of conservation of momentum as applied to modern physics (see Sect. 24.5)

- The concept of wave–particle duality (see Sect. 24.6)
- The concept that waves may behave as particles and that particles may behave as waves, with examples of each situation (see Sects 24.6.1 and 24.6.2)
- A brief outline of Heisenberg's uncertainty principle (see Sect. 24.7)

SELF-TEST

a. Discuss the concept of *mass–energy equivalence* and define the terms:

(i)   rest mass

(ii) relativistic mass.

b. Discuss the concept of wave–particle duality and identify a situation where a wave behaves as a particle and a situation where a particle behaves as a wave.

c. Outline Heisenberg's uncertainty principle.

FURTHER READING

You may find Chapter 25 of this text and chapters from the following texts provide useful further reading:

Beiser A 2003 Concepts of modern physics, 6th edn. McGraw-Hill, Boston

Johns H E, Cunningham J R 1983 The physics of radiology, 4th edn. Charles C Thomas, Illinois, USA, ch 1

Wheeler J, Zurek W H 1983 Quantum theory and measurement. Princetown University Press, USA

Chapter 25

Electromagnetic Radiation

CHAPTER CONTENTS

25.1 Aim   228

25.2 Introduction   228

25.3 Properties of Electromagnetic
Radiations   229
    25.3.1 Wave-Like Properties of
    Electromagnetic Radiation   229
    25.3.2 Particle-Like Properties   231

25.4 The Electromagnetic Spectrum   232

25.5 Light Amplification by Stimulated Emission
of Radiation (Laser)   232
    25.5.1 Basic Physics of Laser
    Production   232
    25.5.2 Potential Hazards of Lasers   234

25.6 Electromagnetic Radiations and
Radiography   234

Self-Test   236

Further Reading   236

25.1 AIM

The aim of this chapter is to discuss the properties of electromagnetic radiations. The wave–particle duality of such radiations will be further discussed. Having identified the contents of the electromagnetic spectrum, we will finally consider some parts of this spectrum in more detail as these are of particular relevance to radiography.

25.2 INTRODUCTION

As we will see from Figure 25.3 (p. 233), the electromagnetic spectrum encompasses a wide range of radiation types and we are only sensitive to a small section of these radiations. We can see the world around us because the retinas of our eyes are sensitive to a section of the electromagnetic spectrum which we know as light. Similarly, we can feel heat from the sun because our skin responds to the infrared part of the electromagnetic spectrum. However, we can accidentally walk through a beam of X-rays or we may handle an isotope which is producing gamma radiation but we cannot feel the presence of these radiations as none of our sense organs are able to detect them. It is important to remember, when we consider radiation protection, that although our sense organs are not immediately able to detect the presence of ionising radiations (X or gamma), they may still be damaged by them.

25.3 PROPERTIES OF ELECTROMAGNETIC RADIATIONS

All electromagnetic radiations exhibit a set of general properties which are listed below:

- The waves are composed of transverse vibrations of electric and magnetic fields
- The vibrations have a wide range of wavelengths and frequencies
- All electromagnetic radiations travel through a vacuum with the same velocity – 3×10^8 ms^{-1}
- All electromagnetic radiations travel in straight lines
- The radiations are unaffected by electric or magnetic fields
- The radiations may be polarised so that they vibrate in one plane only
- The radiations are able to produce constructive or destructive interference
- All the radiations obey the duality principle (see Sect. 24.6) and so can either be considered as waves or as quanta with energy and momentum.

From the above list it is obvious that all electromagnetic radiations have a lot in common, so how can they be used for such widely differing purposes? The answer to this lies in the differences which they exhibit in their interactions with matter. These are outlined in Table 25.1.

As discussed in Chapter 24, there is a wave–particle duality that exists when electromagnetic radiation interacts with matter. This will be discussed further in the following sections.

25.3.1 Wave-Like Properties of Electromagnetic Radiation

As the term *electromagnetic* suggests, electromagnetic radiation consists of both *electric* and *magnetic* fields. These fields are at right angles to each other and to the direction of propagation and are shown diagrammatically in Figure 25.1. As shown in E and B of the figure, both the electric and the magnetic vectors (see Sect. 6.3) vibrate *transversely* to the direction of propagation of the wave. In addition, the vectors vary in a sinusoidal manner, as shown in the figure. Thus, if we draw the variations of the electric vector (for example), a sine wave results, as shown in Figure 25.2. These periodic variations of the vectors are the reason why electromagnetic radiations are often referred to as *electromagnetic waves* and this was the sole method of explaining the behaviour of such radiations adopted by classical physics (see Sect. 24.6). The same parameters can be used to describe this type of wave

Table 25.1	Interactions of different electromagnetic radiations with matter
Interaction	**Notes**
Emission	All bodies will emit electromagnetic radiation in certain circumstances but the most efficient emission is from a 'black body' (see Sect. 8.4.4)
Reflection	Reflection of electromagnetic radiation is not possible for the higher-energy radiations (X and gamma radiation)
Refraction	Refraction of electromagnetic radiation is not possible for the higher-energy radiations (X and gamma radiation)
Transmission	Different materials are transparent to different wavelengths or photon energies
Attenuation	Different attenuation processes are possible depending on the photon energy of the radiation but, if the photons all have the same energy, the attenuation is always exponential. Photoelectric absorption can occur from ultraviolet to gamma radiations. Compton scattering is produced by X and gamma radiations. Pair production is an attenuation process which is possible if the photon energies are higher than 1.02 MeV
Luminescence – fluorescence and phosphorescence	Electron transitions within the material being irradiated cause the emission of photons which have less energy than the incident radiation. A single photon of incident radiation can produce many fluorescent photons

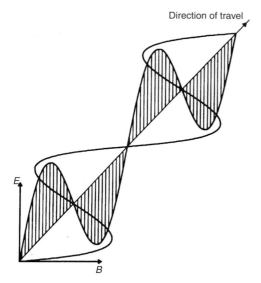

Figure 25.1 Electromagnetic radiation depicted as a wave consisting of alternating electrical and magnetic vectors vibrating at right angles to each other and to the direction of motion of the wave.

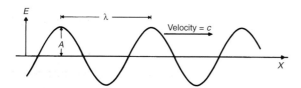

Figure 25.2 An electromagnetic sine wave produced by plotting energy (E) against distance (X). The wave has an amplitude of A and a wavelength λ and travels at the velocity of light, c (3×10^8 m.s^{-1}).

formation as can be used for any sinusoidal waves. These are:

- the *cycle* – one complete waveform (this can start from any point on the wave and end at the corresponding point on another wave)
- the *wavelength* – the distance travelled in completing one cycle (λ)
- the *frequency* – the number of cycles per second (Hz)
- the *amplitude* – the magnitude of the peak of the wave above the *x*-axis (A).

If we consider Figure 25.2, it should be apparent that we can calculate the distance travelled by the radiation in 1 second by multiplying the wavelength (λ) by the frequency (v). However,

the distance travelled in 1 second is simply the velocity of the radiation (c in a vacuum) and so we have:

$$c = v\lambda \qquad\qquad \textit{Equation 25.1}$$

in a vacuum.

As we mentioned earlier, one of the features of electromagnetic radiations is that they all travel with the same velocity (3×10^8 m.s^{-1}) in a vacuum. One ray is distinguished from another by the difference in wavelength and frequency – *blue light* has a wavelength of about 400 nm and a frequency of 7.5×10^{14} Hz while *red light* has a wavelength of about 800 nm and a frequency of 3.75×10^{14} Hz. From this it can be seen that *the greater the frequency, the smaller the wavelength* and vice versa.

In a transparent medium the waves travel at a velocity V given by the equation $c = nV$, where n is a constant for a given medium and a given incident wavelength and is known as the *refractive index*. The frequency of the radiation is unaltered as it passes through a transparent medium but the wavelength is reduced due to the reduction in the velocity of the wave. If the wavelength in the medium is λ', then Equation 25.1 becomes:

$$V = v\,\lambda'$$

Substituting the value of V for $c = nV$ we obtain:

$$c = nv\lambda' \qquad\qquad \textit{Equation 25.2}$$

in a medium of refractive index, n.

INSIGHT

Chapters 12 and 13 showed that it is possible to produce both a magnetic field from moving electrical charges (electromagnetism) and an electric field from a changing magnetic flux (electromagnetic induction). It can be shown mathematically that a changing electric field can sustain a changing magnetic field and vice versa, if they both travel at the velocity of light. This is the basis both for the linear propagation of electromagnetic radiations and for the fact that the wave does not gradually diminish in amplitude with time. Electromagnetic radiation can therefore be described as *a self-sustaining interaction of electric and magnetic fields travelling with the velocity of light.*

Two further properties of electromagnetic radiation which are a consequence of its wave-like nature are *polarisation* and *interference.*

25.3.1.1 Polarisation

A beam of light, from a bulb for instance, consists of many millions of waves whose electric vectors are pointing in random directions with respect to each other. If this light beam is passed through a polarising lens (similar to the one found in polarising sunglasses), then there is optimum transmission of the waves whose electric vectors are pointing in one direction and complete absorption of those at right angles to this direction (this is the mechanism by which polarising sunglasses limit the glare due to light reflection from water). The emergent light is said to be plane-polarised – all its vibrations are in the one plane.

25.3.1.2 Interference

Further evidence of the wave-like properties of electromagnetic radiations comes from the phenomenon of interference, where the amplitudes of two coherent beams (beams that are in phase with each other) can be added together. If the peaks of the waves coincide, then we get *constructive interference* and this produces bright areas. If the peak of the wave from one source coincides with the trough of the wave from the other source, then we get *destructive interference*, and this produces a dark area. Such interference patterns are used in radiographic science to produce holograms, but further discussion on this topic is well outside the scope of this text.

25.3.2 Particle-Like Properties

In Chapter 24 we discussed how consideration of electromagnetic radiations as quanta or photons having energy and momentum enabled us to explain a number of properties that are not explained by the wave theory. The energy of such a quantum, E, is proportional to the frequency of the associated wave such that:

$$E = h\nu \qquad \qquad \textit{Equation 25.3}$$

where h is a constant known as Planck's constant and ν is the frequency of vibration of the associated wave. The momentum, p, of the quantum is also proportional to the frequency, and is given by:

$$p = \frac{h\nu}{c} \qquad \qquad \textit{Equation 25.4}$$

where c is the velocity of electromagnetic radiation in a vacuum.

The photon energy and its wavelength can now be related. If we take Equation 25.3 and substitute $\nu = c/\lambda$ from Equation 25.1 we get:

$$E = \frac{hc}{\lambda} \qquad \qquad \textit{Equation 25.5}$$

In this equation h is Planck's constant (6.62×10^{-34} J.s^{-1}), c is the velocity of electromagnetic radiation in a vacuum (3×10^8 m.s^{-1}), λ is the wavelength measured in metres and E is the photon energy measured in joules. For practical purposes in radiography it is more convenient to measure the photon energy in keV (1 keV = 1.16 $\times$ 10^{-16} J) and the wavelength in nanometres (1 nm = 10^{-9} m). Because h and c are constants, Equation 25.5 can now be rewritten:

$$E = \frac{1.24}{\lambda} \qquad \qquad \textit{Equation 25.6}$$

This equation gives us an easy link between the energy of the photon in keV and the wavelength of the radiation in nanometres.

EXAMPLE

If the energy of the X-ray photon is 100 eV, what will be its wavelength in nanometres?

Using Equation 25.6:

$$E = \frac{1.24}{\lambda}$$

$$\therefore \lambda = \frac{1.24}{E}$$

$$= 1.24/100 \text{ nm}$$

$$= 0.0124 \text{ nm}$$

Lengths as small as 0.0124 nm or 1.24×10^{-11} m are difficult to imagine. This is less than the diameter of an atom of body tissue (about 10^{-10} m) but is greater than the diameter of the atomic nucleus (about 10^{-14} m).

25.4 THE ELECTROMAGNETIC SPECTRUM

The previous sections of this chapter have shown that electromagnetic radiation may have a very large range of wavelengths, i.e. a *spectrum* of wavelengths (and frequencies). It is convenient to split up such an electromagnetic spectrum into bands that are broadly categorised by their interaction with matter and hence the use to which the bands of radiation may be put. This is illustrated in Figure 25.3, which also shows the wavelengths, frequencies and energies corresponding to the approximate boundaries between the various bands. As we have previously discussed, the table of the electromagnetic spectrum shows that the smaller the wavelength of the radiation, the higher the frequency and the energy.

The common factor that links the interactions between different types of electromagnetic radiations is that *the value of the wavelength determines the size of object with which the radiation will directly interact*. This is illustrated in Table 25.2.

INSIGHT

At the beginning of this chapter (Table 25.1) are the types of interactions which are possible between electromagnetic radiations and matter, with brief comments. From this table you will note that refraction is associated with electromagnetic radiations which have wavelengths larger than X-rays. Refraction is a phenomenon associated with an interaction

Table 25.2 Common electromagnetic radiations and the type of body with which they will directly interact

Type of radiation	Body with which radiation directly interacts
Radiowaves	Transmitted and received by large metallic conductors – aerials
Infrared radiation	Interacts with whole molecules or atoms, giving them an increase in their kinetic energy in the form of heat
Visible light and ultraviolet radiation	Interact with the outer electrons (more loosely bound) of an atom
X-rays and gamma-rays	Interact with the inner electron shells or, if they have very high energy, interact with the tiny nucleus of the atom

between a photon and the outer electron orbitals of atoms. It is therefore associated with wavelengths which are able to interact with these electrons – ultraviolet and longer wavelengths. Smaller wavelengths become progressively less affected by the outer electron orbitals and so it is just possible to demonstrate refraction with very-large-wavelength X-rays, but it is not possible to refract X-rays which have shorter wavelengths.

The interactions between X-rays and matter, which are of great relevance to radiographic science, are discussed in detail in Chapter 30 of this book.

25.5 LIGHT AMPLIFICATION BY STIMULATED EMISSION OF RADIATION (LASER)

In the last few years, devices containing a laser source have increasingly become a part of our everyday life and are also increasingly used in radiographic imaging. For this reason a short section is included here describing the basic physics of laser production and also a section indicating the hazards of lasers if used carelessly.

25.5.1 Basic Physics of Laser Production

Laser is an acronym for light amplification by stimulated emission of radiation. The theory,

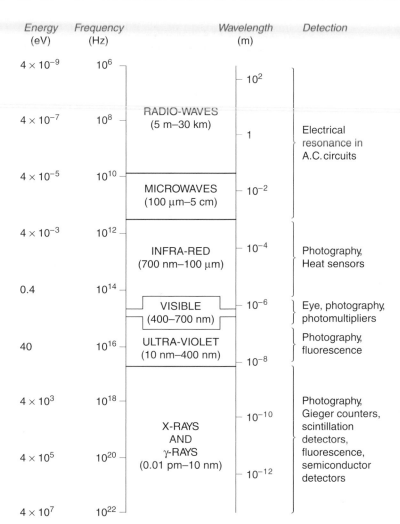

Energy (eV)	Frequency (Hz)		Wavelength (m)	Detection
4×10^{-9}	10^6		10^2	
4×10^{-7}	10^8	RADIO-WAVES (5 m–30 km)	1	Electrical resonance in A.C. circuits
4×10^{-5}	10^{10}	MICROWAVES (100 μm–5 cm)	10^{-2}	
4×10^{-3}	10^{12}	INFRA-RED (700 nm–100 μm)	10^{-4}	Photography, Heat sensors
0.4	10^{14}	VISIBLE (400–700 nm)	10^{-6}	Eye, photography, photomultipliers
40	10^{16}	ULTRA-VIOLET (10 nm–400 nm)	10^{-8}	Photography, fluorescence
4×10^3	10^{18}		10^{-10}	Photography, Gieger counters, scintillation detectors, fluorescence, semiconductor detectors
4×10^5	10^{20}	X-RAYS AND γ-RAYS (0.01 pm–10 nm)	10^{-12}	
4×10^7	10^{22}			

Figure 25.3 The electromagnetic spectrum (not drawn to scale). Typical values for wavelengths, frequencies and photon energies for different bands of the spectrum are shown, together with some of the methods used for their detection. (*Note:* 1 Hz = 1 cycle per second; 1 pm = 10^{-12}m, etc.) AC, alternating current.

which was first proposed by Albert Einstein in 1917, was further developed in the 1950s and the first laser was produced in 1960. We already know from Section 10.3 that in an atom electrons can exist at various energy levels depending on their position relative to the nucleus. We will also see in Chapters 26 and 31 that electrons can be temporarily raised to a higher energy level by the absorption of photons of energy. In many cases the electron remains in this excited state for only a few milliseconds and subsequently decays to its lower energy level by the emission of a photon of light (or other energy) – this process is known as fluorescence (see Ch. 31 for a more detailed description). If the light emitted from an atom is incident on another atom which is in an excited state, then the first photon can stimulate the emission of a second photon from this atom. The two photons will be identical in wavelength, phase and direction. This is the basis of laser.

The basic components of a simple laser are shown in Figure 25.4. The excitation of electrons to a higher energy level is achieved by illuminating the material with light of a frequency higher than that which the laser will emit. This light is produced from the flash lamp and is known as *optical pumping*. The two ends of the laser rod are polished flat and parallel. One end is coated with a completely silvered mirror and the other is coated with a semisilvered mirror. Pulsed light is

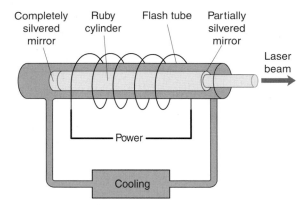

Figure 25.4 Main components of a laser.

flashed into the laser at high intensity from the flash lamp and this is reflected within the rods using the two mirrors, thus causing coherent photon emission from the atoms of the rod material. Eventually the high-intensity laser radiation will leave the rod through the semisilvered mirror. The wavelength of the light emitted depends on the design of the laser, so the beam may not be visible to the eye.

25.5.2 Potential Hazards of Lasers

Laser light has several properties which are important when we consider its safe use:

- the light is monochromatic, with its wavelength determined by the design of the laser
- the light is in the form of a tightly collimated parallel beam, often less than 1 mm in diameter
- because the light is in the form of a small, highly collimated area, even lasers of small power can deposit significant amounts of energy on a small area.

Assume that a 10-W laser beam is directed at a material. This does not sound much in terms of power in that many night lights are rated at 10 W or greater. However, the laser beam is a parallel, very narrow beam. If this beam is 1 mm in diameter, then the power deposited on the material is greater than 1000 $W.cm^{-2}$ – this can ignite paper or cause significant skin burns. If the laser beam enters the eye, the problem is further complicated by the fact that the lens of the eye

focuses the beam on to a small area of the retina. Thus the power deposited on this small area of retina can be increased by a factor of up to 10^5 because of lens focusing. If we consider the original 10-W laser, this will mean a power deposited on a small area of the retina of 10^8 $W.cm^{-2}$ – compare this to power to the retina of about 10 $W.cm^{-2}$ if we stare at the midday sun, and it is easy to appreciate how damaging this can be to the eye.

As mentioned earlier, the wavelength of the light from the laser is determined by the laser design. The retina of the eye can detect from about 400 nm to just over 700 nm. Thus if a laser is operating at, say, 900 nm we will not be able to see the beam from this laser. However the beam can still penetrate the lens system of the eye and cause damage to the retina of the eye. For this reason it is important to wear eye protection whenever lasers are in use, e.g. in an operating theatre, even if the laser beam is not visible.

25.6 ELECTROMAGNETIC RADIATIONS AND RADIOGRAPHY

The process of taking a radiograph (using film and intensifying screens) results in the emission of radiations whose wavelengths and energies are from three different parts of the electromagnetic spectrum, described in the previous section. These are summarised in Figure 25.5.

When the anode is bombarded by electrons it emits both *heat* and *light* as well as X-rays. The X-ray spectrum is composed of a continuous or Bremsstrahlung spectrum upon which may be superimposed a characteristic or line spectrum from the tungsten target (see Ch. 29). The absorption processes within the aluminium filter and the lead collimators also produce characteristic radiation from these elements, although these are of fairly low intensity. When the radiation beam passes through the patient, some of the photons are absorbed (A in Figure 25.5) and some are scattered (S in Figure 25.5). The above processes produce a minute amount of heat and other characteristic radiations from the elements which make up the body tissues. Some of the scattered radiation is absorbed by the grid. When the

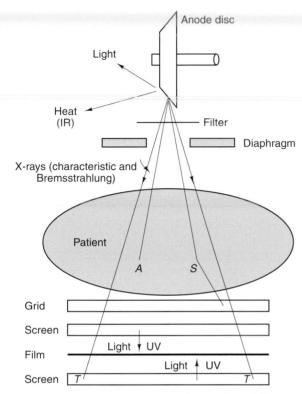

Figure 25.5 The production of radiation from different parts of the electromagnetic spectrum when a radiograph is taken. IR, infrared; UV, ultraviolet. See text for details.

transmitted X-ray beam (T) strikes the intensifying screens in the cassette, these produce fluorescent radiation in the ultraviolet and visible parts of the spectrum. These radiations are principally responsible for producing the image on the film.

Further examples of electromagnetic radiation relevant to radiography include:

- the emission of light from image intensifiers when bombarded with X-rays
- the emission of light from cathode-ray tubes and television monitors when the phosphors are bombarded by electrons
- the emission of light from fluorescent tubes to allow us to view radiographs

- the emission of gamma-rays from certain radioisotopes which allow imaging or treatment of organs
- the emission of light from sodium iodide crystals (in gamma cameras and computed tomography (CT) scanners) when bombarded with gamma-rays or X-rays
- the emission of light from photostimulable plates when scanned using a laser beam
- the use of a laser beam to 'write' information on to the film in a laser imager
- the use of low-intensity lasers to aid positioning of the radiation beam in radiotherapy.

SUMMARY

In this chapter you should have learnt:

- The properties that are common to all electromagnetic radiations (see Sect. 25.3)
- The different ways in which electromagnetic radiations can react with matter (see Sect. 25.3)
- How electromagnetic radiation can be described as having wave-like properties and how these properties can be used to explain polarisation and interference (see Sect. 25.3.1)
- How electromagnetic radiation can be described as having particle-like properties and the equation which links the photon energy and the wavelength of the radiation (see Sect. 25.3.2)
- The various components of the electromagnetic spectrum and the principal interactions of the radiations with matter (see Sect. 25.4)
- A brief description of the physics of laser production and a note of its potential dangers (see Sect. 25.5)
- The electromagnetic radiations which are of importance to radiography (see Sect. 25.6).

SELF-TEST

a. List the general properties of all electromagnetic radiations.

b. Define the following terms which may be used to describe electromagnetic radiations:

   (i)   cycle

   (ii) wavelength

   (iii) frequency

   (iv) amplitude.

c. Give two equations that link the photon energy and the wavelength of electromagnetic radiation. What is the wavelength of the radiation which has a photon energy of 50 keV? What is the photon energy of radiation which has a wavelength of 0.0124 nm?

d. List the main divisions of the electromagnetic spectrum in order of decreasing wavelength.

e. Describe the different types of electromagnetic radiations involved in the production of a radiograph.

f. List five examples other than those used in (e) above to show where electromagnetic radiations are used in radiography.

FURTHER READING

You will find further information on the methods of X-ray production in Ch. 28 and more information on the mechanisms by which X-rays interact with matter in Ch. 30 of this text. In addition you may find the chapters of the following texts useful:

Ball J L, Moore A D 1997 Essential physics for radiographers, 3rd edn. Blackwell Scientific Publications, London, ch 14

Curry T S III, Dowdey J E, Murry R C Jr 1990 Christensen's physics of diagnostic radiography, 4th edn. Lee & Febiger, London, ch 1

Dowsett D J, Kenny P A, Johnston R E 1998 The physics of diagnostic imaging, Chapman & Hall Medical, London, ch 2

Chapter 26

Elementary Structure of the Atom

CHAPTER CONTENTS

26.1 Aim   237

26.2 Introduction   237

26.3 The Atomic Nucleus   238
    26.3.1 The Stability of the Nucleus   240

26.4 Electron Orbitals   241

26.5 The Periodic Table of Elements   242

26.6 Electron Orbital Changes   243

26.7 Binding Energy of the Electron Shells   244

Self-Test   245

Further Reading   245

26.1 AIM

The aim of this chapter is to introduce the reader to the elementary structure of an atom. The principal particles which form the nucleus will be identified, as will the factors that determine whether or not the nucleus is stable. The differing electron orbitals and the influence of the electron orbitals on the chemical properties of the material will be discussed. The consequences of transitions of electrons between orbitals will also be identified.

26.2 INTRODUCTION

Any attempt to understand the universe around us must start with the fundamental question: *what is matter made of?* The atom as the fundamental building block of matter has therefore been the subject of a great deal of both theoretical debate and experimental study by physicists. Many of the modern theories concerning atomic and subatomic structures are extremely complex and are the subject of a number of textbooks in their own right. However, most of the phenomena which we encounter in radiography can be explained using a relatively simple *planetary model* of the atom. In this model there are solid electrons orbiting a solid nucleus – some phenomena can also be explained using the *quantum physics model* and where this is appropriate this model will be referred to in Insights.

The planetary model of the atom was first described by Rutherford in 1911. It describes an

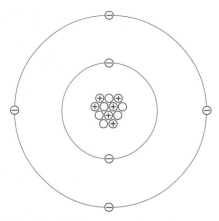

Figure 26.1   The basic structure of a carbon atom. At the centre of the atom is a nucleus which contains six protons (positively charged) and six neutrons (zero charge), i.e. the nucleus contains 12 nucleons. Six electrons (negatively charged) orbit the nucleus in defined orbitals. As the atom contains equal numbers of positive and negative charges, the whole atom is electrically neutral.

atom consisting of a small, positively charged central nucleus around which negatively charged electrons move in defined orbitals. This model can be used to illustrate the carbon atom, as shown in Figure 26.1. As we can see from this diagram, the nucleus of this atom consists of *12 elementary particles – six protons and six neutrons*. These particles are bound together in a small volume of extremely high density – about three thousand million, million times greater than the density of water. The protons in the nucleus carry a positive charge and the electrons carry an equal negative charge, so this atom is electrically neutral – the neutrons carry no charge. The electrons are arranged in orbitals or shells called *K, L, M* ... starting from the orbital closest to the nucleus. The *K*-shell can only contain two electrons and, in the case of the carbon atom, the *L*-shell contains the remaining four. Different atoms contain different numbers of protons and neutrons in the nucleus and different numbers of electron configurations, as will be discussed later in this chapter. As the particles which make up the atom are very tiny, the atom consists largely of empty space. For example, if an atom were to be enlarged until it was the size of a house, the size of the nucleus would be about the size of a pinhead, although it contains 99.95% of the total mass of the atom.

The masses and charges of the subatomic particles which will be considered in this and later chapters are summarised in Table 26.1.

INSIGHT

Rutherford carried out some elegant experimental work connected with the scattering of alpha-particles by atoms. From this he concluded that the only explanation for the wide scattering angles which he found experimentally was given by assuming that the atom consists of a very heavy positively charged nucleus with orbiting electrons. The alternative model, whereby all the subatomic particles were contained in a very small volume, was unacceptable because it would produce much smaller scattering angles for the alpha-particles.

Similar experiments have recently been carried out by physicists to try to establish whether protons and neutrons can be broken into smaller pieces. Unfortunately, if the energy of the projectile is large enough to break up the proton or neutron, then the energy is great enough to create new particles – remember $E = mc^2$ – and so it is difficult to tell which are fragments of the proton and which have been created as a result of energy being converted into matter. More subtle experiments use high-energy electrons to bombard the protons and neutrons and measure the angle of deflection of these particles. These angles are again over a wide range, suggesting that there are small solid structures within the protons and neutrons. These may be the basic building blocks of the universe; they are known as *quarks* and 18 different types of quark have been identified. Further discussion regarding this search to identify whether there is a smaller structure within the quark is well outside the scope of this text.

26.3 THE ATOMIC NUCLEUS

The number of protons and neutrons in the atomic nucleus determines both the mass and the charge of the nucleus and the configuration of

Table 26.1   Masses and charges of the main subatomic particles

Particle	Symbol	Rest mass		Rest energy	Charge[a]	Comments
		kg	amu[b]	(MeV)		
Proton	p	1.672×10^{-27}	1.007	938	+1	Nucleons, i.e. present in the atomic nucleus
Neutron	n	1.675×10^{-27}	1.009	939	0	
Alpha-particle	α	6.645×10^{-27}	4.003	3725	+2	Two protons and two neutrons. Ejected in α decay
Electron	e^- or β^-	9.109×10^{-31}	0.00055 or 1/1820	0.511	−1	Form stable discrete orbits around nuclei. Ejected from nucleus in β^- decay
Positron	e^- or β^+	9.109×10^{-31}	0.00055 or 1/1820	0.511	+1	Antiparticle of the electron – produces annihilation radiation when both meet
Pi meson	π^+	2.480×10^{-28}	0.150	139	+1	Keep the nucleus together (π^0 and π^- also exist)
Neutrino	ν	0	0	0	0	Emitted during β-decay and electron capture. Very weak attenuation by matter
Photon or quantum	h_ν	–	–	–	0	Travels at 3×10^8 m.s^{-1}. Forms part of the electromagnetic spectrum

[a]A charge of +1 is $+1.602 \times 10^{-19}$ coulomb.
[b]1 amu is 1 atomic mass unit, which is one-twelfth of the mass of a neutral $^{12}_{6}C$ atom.

electron orbitals of the atom. There are several important terms, which we will use in this and following chapters of this text, that require definition at this stage. These terms, which will help us to understand atomic structure, are defined in Table 26.2.

We can now consider the use of some of the terms in the table. The most common naturally occurring stable isotope of carbon has six protons and six neutrons, as shown previously in Figure 26.1. The *atomic number* (Z) of this isotope is therefore six and the *atomic mass number* is therefore 12. Thus the whole atom can be written as $^{12}_{6}C$. Thus $^{12}_{6}C$ is an example of a *nuclide* – one which contains six protons and six neutrons. In general, an element E is written as $^{A}_{Z}E$. An isotope of $^{12}_{6}C$, which is also naturally occurring but less abundant, has seven neutrons in its nucleus and may be written as $^{13}_{6}C$.

Note that it is not necessarily the case that isotopes of an element are radioactive, as is shown by this example; $^{12}_{6}C$ and $^{13}_{6}C$ are both isotopes of carbon but neither is radioactive.

Table 26.2   Terms used to describe a nucleus

Term	Symbol	Definition
Nucleon		A proton or neutron within a nucleus
Atomic number	Z	The number of protons in the nucleus
Atomic mass number	A	The total number of nucleons in the nucleus
Neutron number	N	The number of neutrons within the nucleus
Nuclide		A nucleus with a specific value of Z and A
Element	E	A nucleus with a given value of Z
Isotope (of an element)		Any nucleus that contains the same number of protons as the given nucleus but has a different mass number
Isobar		Any nucleus which has the same atomic mass number as another nucleus (i.e. has the same value of A)
Radionuclide or radioisotope		Any nuclide or isotope which is radioactive

An isotope of carbon which is radioactive is $^{14}_{6}$C – the well-known *carbon-14*. This again contains the six protons which identify it as a carbon nucleus, but this time it contains eight neutrons. $^{14}_{6}$C is an example of a *radionuclide* or a *radioactive isotope*. It decays, as we shall see in Chapter 27, by beta decay to form $^{14}_{7}$N (nitrogen) as the *daughter product*.

26.3.1 The Stability of the Nucleus

At first sight the atomic nucleus would appear to be inherently unstable as the neutrons are uncharged and the protons have a positive charge and so would electrostatically repel each other. This would suggest that the nucleus should fly apart because of the electrostatic forces between the protons.

In practice we find that some nuclei are so stable as to possess no measurable radioactivity ($^{12}_{6}$C is an example) while others decay with a half-life (see Sect. 4.5) of less than one-millionth of a second. The nucleus must therefore be visualised as a *dynamic* rather than a *static* structure where there are opposing forces acting – forces which tend to hold the nucleus together and forces which tend to disrupt the nucleus. Thus a *stable nucleus* is one where the disruptive forces never win and an *unstable nucleus* is one where they do succeed. This nucleus is said to undergo *radioactive decay*. It is not possible to predict the exact moment when any particular nucleus will decay, as it is a matter of probability rather than certainty. However, if there are a large number of unstable nuclei in a sample, the *law of radioactive decay* (see Sect. 4.3) is obeyed.

The forces which hold the nucleus together are quite unlike the other forces – e.g. gravity – with which we are familiar. They are known as *short-range nuclear forces* and act over distances of about 10^{-15} metres, over which range they are much more powerful than the electrostatic forces between the protons. These forces are shown diagrammatically in Figure 26.2. A strong force of attraction is evident below 10^{-15} m and this changes to a force of repulsion at about 10^{-16} m. The energy expended in keeping the nucleus together is known as the *nuclear-binding energy*

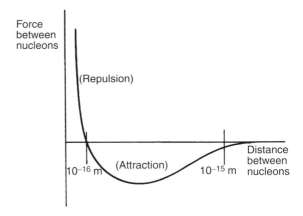

Figure 26.2 If the separation of the nucleons is between 10^{-15} and 10^{-16} metres, then a force of attraction exists between the nucleons which helps to hold the nucleus together. If the separation is greater or less than this distance, then the force is a repulsive force.

(NBE). If the NBE is divided by the number of nucleons within the nucleus, then a figure of about 8.4 MeV is obtained for most nuclei. This is known as the *binding energy per nucleon*. The binding energy between the nucleons is provided by the transformation of some of the nuclear mass into energy, as given by Einstein's equation $E = mc^2$. Each nucleon has a mass of approximately 931 MeV per atomic mass unit (amu), of which about 8.4 MeV is used for its NBE to nearby nucleons. Because of this, the mass of the nucleus is always less than the sum of the masses of the nucleons.

Considering the graph in Chapter 27 (Figure 27.1), it can be seen that, for low atomic numbers, equal numbers of protons and neutrons produce the greatest stability. This leads to the concept of nuclear shells, which suggests that there is a layering within the nucleus, with maximum stability being produced when a shell is complete. Further discussion of this concept is beyond the scope of this text.

INSIGHT

The π-meson is a particle with a mass between that of an electron and a nucleon and is thought to be responsible for the forces holding the nucleus together. The short-range forces are known as exchange forces and result in (for example) an adjacent proton and a neutron changing continually into a neutron and a proton and back again. This interchange may be written as:

$$p_1 + n_1 \rightarrow n_2 + \pi^+ + n_1 \rightarrow n_2 + p_2$$

The π^+-meson has left the original proton p_1, leaving it as a neutron n_2, and then forms a proton p_2 by combining with the original neutron n_1. The proton and the neutron are continuously exchanging their positions. Negative and neutral π-mesons also exist and are exchanged between nucleons.

26.4 ELECTRON ORBITALS

Consider an atom of hydrogen, as depicted in Figure 26.3. It is assumed in the planetary model of the atom that the solitary electron is on a circular path (path 1) around the nucleus. It may be shown that a body moving in a circle of radius r at a velocity V has an acceleration of V^2/r towards the centre of the circle. According to classical physics, such acceleration would result in the emission of electromagnetic radiation from the electron so that the electron is continuously losing energy and would eventually collide with the nucleus (see path 2). Electrons do not behave in this manner, or atoms as we know them would not exist. The electrons orbit in stable paths (path 1) – *discrete electron orbitals*. Further, these orbitals are grouped in 'shells' where there is a particular number of electrons of approximately the same energy in each orbital. (An explanation of the apparent contradiction of the predictions of classical physics (path 2 and path 1) is given in the Insight below.) The electrons fill up the inner shells first since the energies of the inner shells are less than the outer shells.

INSIGHT

The wave–particle duality of matter (see Sect. 24.6) may be used to explain the existence of discrete electron orbitals. Here it is assumed that an orbiting electron has a de Broglie wavelength which is able to fit around the circumference of an orbital an exact number of times (Figure 26.4). This fixes the size of each orbital. The condition necessary for this to occur is that $n\lambda = 2\pi r$ where n is a whole number and r is the mean radius of the orbital. Now λ is the de Broglie wavelength of the electron with momentum p and is given by $\lambda = h/p$.

$$\frac{nh}{p} = 2\pi r \text{ or } pr = \frac{nh}{2\pi}$$

But pr is the angular momentum of the electron and this must be a multiple of $h/2\pi$. There is now no question of electromagnetic radiation occurring from an orbital electron. This is an example of a situation where modern physics can be used to

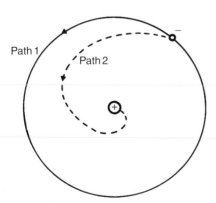

Figure 26.3 A stable, discrete electron orbital (path 1) compared to a decaying electron (path 2), as predicted by the laws of classical physics.

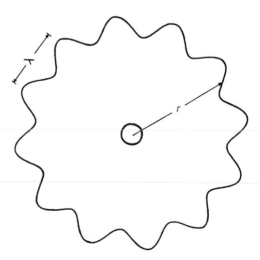

Figure 26.4 The use of the de Broglie wave concept to explain why electrons exist in discrete orbitals.

describe atomic phenomena which are not explicable by classical physics.

Table 26.3 shows the maximum number of electrons in each shell from the inner *K*-shell to the *N*-shell.

The shell number, *n*, starts from *n* = 1 for the *K*-shell and is known as the *principal quantum number*. The chemical properties of an element are controlled by the electron configuration of its atoms. Atoms with filled outer electron shells are chemically inert – neon ($^{20}_{10}$Ne) has full *K*- and *L*-shells, as illustrated in Figure 26.5, and so is an inert gas. Fluorine, where the *K*-shell contains two electrons and the *L*-shell contains seven, is a chemically active *electron acceptor* (the electron fills the vacancy in the *L*-shell) and sodium, where the *K*-shell contains two electrons, the *L*-shell contains eight electrons and the *M*-shell contains one, is a chemically active *electron donor*

Table 26.3 Numbers of electrons in atomic shells			
Principal quantum number or shell number (*n*)	Shell letter	Maximum number of electrons	$2n^2$
1	*K*	2	2
2	*L*	8	8
3	*M*	18	18
4	*N*	32	32

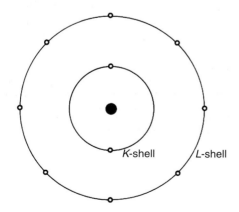

Figure 26.5   An atom of neon, showing both *K*- and *L*-shells containing their maximum number of permitted electrons. This means that the neon atom is chemically inert.

(the electron in the *M*-shell is donated, resulting in a filled *L*-shell).

The outer electron shells may contain sub-shells within them. Argon (*Z* = 18) has two electrons in its *K*-shell, eight electrons in its *L*-shell and eight electrons in the *M*-shell. The *M*-shell has a maximum complement of electrons of 18 and yet argon is chemically inert. An outer sub-shell of eight electrons is particularly chemically stable, a fact which is confirmed by the next inert gas, krypton, which has an electron configuration of 2, 8, 18, 8.

26.5 THE PERIODIC TABLE OF ELEMENTS

If the elements are arranged in order of increasing atomic number it may be shown that their chemical properties – such as valency – and their physical properties – such as specific heat – tend to occur in a periodic manner. Arranging these elements in these similar groups produces a *periodic table,* as shown in Table E on p. 403. The chemical similarities of the elements in each group may be explained by reference to their electron structure, as shown in Table F on p. 404-406. It has already been noted that the number of electrons increases with atomic number and that each electron takes an orbital of the lowest possible energy. This means that the inner shells are filled to stable or substable levels before the outer shells accommodate electrons.

There are two rules which determine the way in which the electron shells are gradually built up as the atomic number increases:

1. an electron shell *n* cannot contain more than $2n^2$ electrons where *n* is the shell number
2. the outer shell cannot contain more than eight electrons.

These rules are known as the *Bury–Bohr rules* after their co-discoverers and ensure that the orbital of minimum energy are filled first.

One additional constraint is required in order that electrons may fill orbitals in the correct manner. This is known as the *Pauli exclusion principle* and states that *no two electrons may have precisely the same orbital.*

The two K-shell electrons of an atom, for example, are not at precisely the same energy level because they orbit the nucleus in opposing directions and hence have slightly different orbitals. These two electrons complete the K-shell so that further electrons must start to fill up the L-shell (see lithium in Table F p. 404) at a greater distance from the nucleus and so at a higher energy. These L-shell electrons all have slightly different energies from each other and the shell is complete when it has eight electrons – neon satisfies these conditions where $n = 2$ and so $2n^2 = 8$.

The K- and L-shells are thus completed in sequence but the M-shell (which from the $2n^2$ formula can contain up to 18 electrons), when it reaches eight electrons (argon), then obeys the rule that the outer shell cannot contain more than eight electrons and so the ninth electron is placed in the N-shell (see potassium in Table F). This process is repeated each time there are eight electrons in the outer orbital (see rubidium, caesium, francium, etc.).

As mentioned above, the number of electrons in the outer orbital determines the chemical reactivity of the element. The ability of one atom to join another is called *valency* and the electron linkage between the atoms is called the *valency bond*. There are two basic types of valency bond:

1. *Ionic bonds* – see Figure 26.6A and B. This type of bond is created when one or more electrons are transferred from one atom to another, forming charged atoms (ions) which are attracted towards each other by electrostatic attraction, thus forming the bond. After the electron exchange the shells of each ion appear to be closed.
2. *Covalent bonds* – see Figure 2.6.6 C and D – are formed by the apparent sharing of electrons such that each atom appears to increase its number of electrons, thus forming an apparently closed shell.

26.6 ELECTRON ORBITAL CHANGES

The previous sections of this chapter have shown that electrons may only take up fixed or discrete orbitals around an atomic nucleus. We have also discussed the fact that the inner orbitals are filled before the outer orbitals, since this constitutes the lowest energy state of the whole atom. An atom in this state is said to be in its *ground state*, since it cannot have an electron configuration which will produce a lower energy. However, this is not to say that any particular atom at a given moment of time will be at its ground state, since interatomic collisions or interactions with electromagnetic radiations may have raised the energy of one of its electrons so that it is able to take up an orbital of higher energy – the electron will move further away from the nucleus. This process is called *excitation* of the atom. The excited electron is able to return to its original orbital and releases a quantum of electromagnetic radiation in the process. The energy of this quantum is equal to the energy difference between the excited state and the ground state. Alternatively, an orbiting

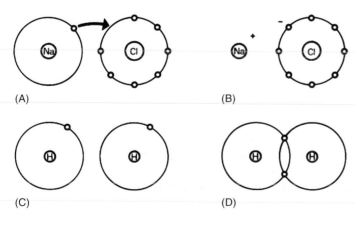

(A)   (B)   (C)   (D)

Figure 26.6 An ionic valency bond (or electron valency) is caused by the transfer of an electron from one atom to another – Na to Cl in (A) and (B). A covalent bond (covalency) is formed when two atoms share electrons in the same orbital, as shown between two hydrogen atoms in (C) and (D).

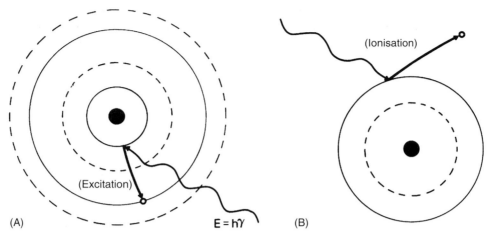

Figure 26.7   An incoming photon interacts with an orbiting electron of an atom. In (A) this photon has sufficient energy to cause excitation and in (B) the photon causes ionisation.

electron may receive sufficient energy to be able to escape from the atom completely – this might happen as a result of the interaction of a photon with the electron. This process is called *ionisation* since the remaining atom will now form a positive ion. Both processes are shown diagrammatically in Figure 26.7.

26.7 BINDING ENERGY OF THE ELECTRON SHELLS

Because the various electron shells are positioned at different distances from the atomic nucleus, they experience different forces of attraction from the nucleus. The K-shell is closest to the nucleus and so experiences the greatest force of attraction from the nucleus. It is therefore most difficult to remove an electron from the K-shell – the K-shell has the highest electron-binding energy. The electron-binding energy of a shell is the amount of work that must be done to remove an electron from that shell (normally stated in keV or eV). The L-shell is further away from the nucleus and so experiences less force of attraction. It also experiences some repulsion from the electrons in the K-shell. For this reason the binding energy of the electrons in the L-shell is less than the binding energy of the K-shell for a particular atom. Thus we can say that there is a reduction in the binding energy as we move from

the K-shell to the L-shell to the M-shell, etc., within a particular atom.

The reason for the existence of the binding energy is the electrostatic attraction between the nucleus and the electrons in the shells. Thus we would expect to find an increase in the K-shell binding energy with an increase in the atomic number of the element. This is found to be the case in practice.

A knowledge of the binding energy of the various electron shells in different elements is important in radiation physics for the following reasons:

• A knowledge of the binding energies of the different shells allows us to predict the energies of the characteristic radiations which the atom might produce (see Ch. 28 for further details)
• A knowledge of the binding energies of different electron shells within an atom of an element will allow us to determine the likely position of absorption edges during photoelectric absorption (see Ch. 30 for further details)
• If we know the energy of the characteristic radiation from an element and we know the position of absorption edges when radiation is attenuated by this material, then this allows us to explain why elements are relatively transparent to their own characteristic radiation (see Ch. 30 for further details).

SUMMARY

In this chapter you should have learnt:

- The main subatomic particle which can be joined together to produce matter (see Sect. 26.2)
- A basic planetary model of the atom which consists of a nucleus containing protons and neutrons and has electrons in specific orbitals around this nucleus (see Sect. 26.2)
- The basic structure of the atomic nucleus and the reasons for its stability or otherwise (see Sects 26.3 and 26.3.1)
- The configuration of electron orbitals for differing atoms and the factors which determine the maximum number of electrons in an orbital (see Sects 26.4 and 26.5)
- The basic structure of the periodic table of elements and the electron configuration of elements (see Sect. 26.5)
- The meaning of the term *ground state* when applied to an atom and the consequences of raising the energy of the electrons above the ground state (see Sect. 26.6)
- An explanation of the term *binding energy* and a brief outline of areas where a knowledge of the binding energy of electron shells is of importance in radiation physics (see Sect. 26.7).

SELF-TEST

a. With the aid of a diagram, describe the $^{14}_{7}N$ atom.

b. Explain the meaning of the following:

  (i)   a nuclide

  (ii) a radionuclide

  (iii) an isotope

  (iv) an isobar

  (v)   atomic number

  (vi) atomic mass number.

c. What is meant by the following terms:

  (i)   discrete electron orbital

  (ii) electron shell

  (iii) electron-binding energy?

d. List the Bury–Bohr rules for electron configuration and hence describe the electron configuration of potassium, which has an atomic number of 19.

e. Explain what the electron configurations are in the following situations:

  (i)   ionic bonds

  (ii) covalent bonds.

f. What is meant by the terms excitation and ionisation when used to describe changes in electron energy within an atom?

FURTHER READING

Ball J L, Moore A D 1997 Essential physics for radiographers, 3rd edn. Blackwell Scientific Publications, London, ch 4

Bushong S C 2004 Radiologic science for technologists: physics, biology and protection. Mosby, New York, ch 4

Curry T S III, Dowdey J E, Murry R C Jr 1990 Christensen's physics of diagnostic radiography, 4th edn. Lee & Febiger, London, ch 2

Dowsett D J, Kenny P A, Johnston R E 1998 The physics of diagnostic imaging. Chapman & Hall Medical, London, ch 2

CHAPTER CONTENTS

27.1   Aim   246

27.2   Introduction   246

27.3   Nuclide Chart   247

27.4   Alpha Decay or Alpha-Particle
         Emission   248

27.5   Beta Decay or Beta-Particle Emission   249
         27.5.1 Negatron (β⁻) Emission   249
         27.5.2 Positron (β⁺) Emission   250
         27.5.3 The Fate of the Positron   251
         27.5.4 The Neutrino   252

27.6   Gamma Decay or Gamma-ray
         Emission   253
         27.6.1 Metastable States and Isomeric
                  Transitions   253
         27.6.2 Internal Conversion   254
         27.6.3 X-rays and Auger Electrons   254

27.7   Electron Capture   255

27.8   Branching Decay Programmes   256

27.9   Fission   256
         27.9.1 The Nuclear Reactor   258

27.10   Summary of Radioactive Nuclear
         Transformations   259

27.11   Artificially Produced Radionuclides   259
         27.11.1 The Technetium Generator   259
         27.11.2 Growth of Activity   261
         27.11.3 Production of Radionuclides
                  Using a Cyclotron   262

27.12   Clinically Useful Radionuclides   263

Self-Test   265

Further Reading   265

27.1 AIM

The aim of this chapter is to discuss the various types of radioactive decay which can occur. Within the chapter the relevance of these processes to nuclear medicine will be considered along with a list of clinically useful radionuclides.

27.2 INTRODUCTION

Radioactive decay has already been considered as an example of exponential decay in Chapter 4 where we also looked at concepts like half-life and decay constant (if the memory of these concepts is getting dim, please refer to the appropriate section(s) of Ch. 4).

In Chapter 26 we also referred to various terms which may be used to define nuclear structure. This chapter will now look at the changes which may take place in the nucleus during radioactive decay and we will also look at the production of artificial radionuclides.

The term *radioactive* is applied to nuclei that are unstable. In these nuclei the forces disrupting the nucleus are stronger than the forces holding the nucleus together. The instability of the nucleus is demonstrated by the fact that it changes its internal structure to a more stable form, often (but not always) ejecting a charged particle from the nucleus in the process. Each time a nucleus changes its structure it is called a

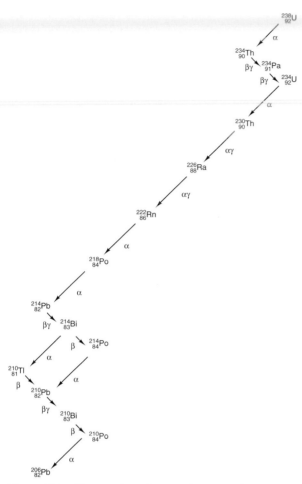

Figure 27.1 The uranium decay series. *Note* that arrows to the right indicate an increase in the atomic number while arrows to the left indicate a decrease. The downward direction of the arrows indicates that the nucleus loses energy with each transformation (downward direction not drawn to scale).

radioactive disintegration or a *nuclear transformation* and may result in a change in the atomic number (and therefore element) or a change in the mass number or a change of both the atomic number and the mass number.

A pictorial representation of the decay process (Figure 27.1) is called a *decay scheme*. In addition to this, it is possible for a nucleus to undergo more than one type of transformation (see Figure 27.12, later in this chapter) and this type of decay is called a *branching scheme*.

It is impossible to determine the exact time when a particular nucleus will transform, but the laws of probability may be used to determine the behaviour of a large number of nuclei (see Sect. 4.3 for a discussion of radioactive decay and the exponential law).

The unit of radioactivity is the becquerel (Bq) where 1 becquerel is 1 nuclear disintegration per second.

INSIGHT

Before the introduction of International System of Units (SI) units, radioactivity was measured in curie (Ci). 1 curie was equal to 3.7×10^{10} nuclear disintegrations per second. Thus, an activity of 1 Ci is the same as an activity of 3.7×10^{10} Bq or 37 GBq. From this it can be seen that the curie was a much larger unit than the becquerel.

It is often useful to know the specific activity of a sample. This is the activity of radionuclide per unit mass of the sample and so is measured in $Bq.kg^{-1}$ or submultiples thereof.

27.3 NUCLIDE CHART

It is often useful to draw a graph, plotting the number of neutrons in a nucleus against the number of protons, as all nuclides may be included in this *nuclide chart*. Such a chart is shown in simplified form in Figure 27.2. Note that isotopes (lines of equal atomic number) are given by any vertical line on the figure. In such a graph, an angle of 45° to the *x*-axis represents a situation where the nucleus contains equal numbers of protons and neutrons ($Z = N$).

It is found on such a graph that there is a broad band of nuclides with low atomic numbers at about 45° to the *x*-axis and these are all stable or only weakly radioactive. Thus for the lighter elements, nuclear stability can be produced with equal numbers of protons and neutrons. From the graph it can be seen that, as the atomic number increases, a proportionately larger number of neutrons is necessary to produce nuclear stability. Thus we can say that, as the Coulomb repulsion (see Sect. 9.4) between the protons increases, then more neutrons are required to produce

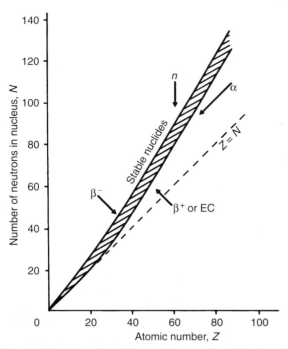

Figure 27.2 A graph of the neutron number (*N*) plotted against the atomic number (*Z*), showing the position of the stable nuclides as a shaded band. *Note* that, as the atomic number increases, a higher proportion of neutrons to protons is required to achieve stability. Also shown are the directions which a nucleus takes for various forms of radioactive decay (these movements are not to scale). EC, electron capture.

the short-range nuclear forces (see Sect. 26.3.1), thus producing the cohesive forces required for a stable nucleus. Nuclei which have atomic numbers greater than 83 (bismuth) are so large that it is impossible to produce a stable nuclear configuration.

Nuclides whose combination of neutrons and protons means that they land outside the band of stability shown in Figure 27.2 have nuclei possessing higher energies than those within the band. As a consequence, such a nucleus is unstable and tends, on decay, to produce a new nucleus of lower energy which is closer to or within the stable band. The energy difference between the nucleus before and after decay is emitted either as a charged particle or as a quantum (or quanta) of electromagnetic radiation. The decay scheme towards stability may be in the form of a single step (e.g. $^{14}_{6}C$ decays to stable $^{14}_{7}N$ by the emission of a beta-particle – see

Figure 27.4) or it may be in the form of a very circuitous route involving many nuclear transformations (e.g. the decay of $^{238}_{92}U$ to $^{206}_{82}Pb$ involves at least 14 steps – see Figure 27.1). As a general rule, the greater the mass number of the nuclide, the more complicated the decay path to eventual stability.

The effect of different decay modes is illustrated using arrows on Figure 27.2. The direction of the arrow shows the direction of change of position on the chart before and after the decay process. You may find it helpful to refer back to this chart while studying the decay processes in more detail in the following sections of this chapter.

27.4 ALPHA DECAY OR ALPHA-PARTICLE EMISSION

For the spontaneous emission of an alpha-particle from a nucleus, the nuclide must have an atomic mass number greater than 150. The nucleus must also have *too few neutrons for the number of protons* – a higher neutron-to-proton ratio would be required to produce nuclear stability. The alpha-particle consists of two protons and two neutrons tightly bound together (a helium nucleus). It may be considered as a free particle having high kinetic energy, which is trapped in the nucleus. Thus the daughter nucleus has two protons and two neutrons fewer than the parent nucleus (see Equation 27.1).

The mechanism of production of the alpha-particle is quite complex. As we have already identified (see Sect. 26.3.1), the nucleus depends on a balance of disruptive electrostatic (Coulomb) forces and attractive forces between the nucleons caused by the short-range nuclear forces. In very large nuclei there is a large amount of electrostatic repulsion between the protons which extends across the whole nucleus. This is balanced by the short-range nuclear force which exists between adjacent nucleons. Thus, if the nucleus becomes elongated, the electrostatic forces dominate and the nucleus becomes even more elongated. This process continues until the nucleus divides into two fragments, the daughter nuclide and the alpha-particle.

An example of alpha-decay is the decay of bismuth-212 to thallium-208 with the emission of alpha-particles. This process is shown in the equation below:

$$^{212}_{83}\text{Bi} \rightarrow {}^{208}_{81}\text{Tl} + {}^{4}_{2}\alpha \qquad \textit{Equation 27.1}$$

Note that there is a reduction of four in the atomic mass number and two in the atomic number between parent and daughter product.

This reaction can also be written as shown in Figure 27.3 (the decay of $^{212}_{83}$Bi also includes the emission of a beta-particle and is discussed later as an example of a branching programme; for simplicity, only the alpha-particle reaction is shown in Figure 27.3 and the percentages shown refer only to the alpha-particles). Because the daughter product is to the left of the parent nuclide this shows that there is a reduction in the atomic number. The reaction also shows that the difference in energy between the parent nuclide and the daughter nuclide is 6.08 MeV. If we consider only the alpha-particles emitted we find that approximately 71% of these have an energy of 6.04 MeV and 29% have an energy of 6.08 MeV. In the case of the first group of alpha-particles, the nucleus is left in an excited state with excess energy of 0.04 MeV which it emits as a gamma-ray.

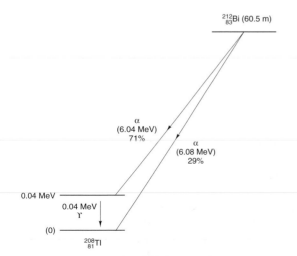

Figure 27.3   An example of alpha-particle emission. The nucleus decreases its atomic number and energy as shown.

The ejection of an alpha-particle means that, to preserve momentum, the nucleus must also recoil with an equal and opposite momentum to that of the alpha-particle. The energy of the recoiling nucleus is typically about 2% of that of the emitted alpha-particle. (Recoil also exists for beta-decay but is much smaller due to the tiny mass of the beta-particle.)

Alpha-particles are intensely ionising but have a very short range in tissue so have little practical application in radiology.

27.5 BETA DECAY OR BETA-PARTICLE EMISSION

In the process of beta decay a particle, having a mass equal to that of an electron, is ejected from the nucleus. The ejected particles, however, may have either a positive or negative charge and so, although they are known collectively as beta-particles, negative beta-particles (β^-) or *negatrons* and positive beta-particles (β^+) or *positrons* both exist. Although the negatron is exactly the same as an electron, in this and subsequent chapters the term *negatron* will be used to describe the particle which exits from the nucleus of an atom while the term *electron* will be used to describe particles which orbit the nucleus of the atom. Because the processes are different for the production of the negatron and the positron they will be dealt with under separate headings.

27.5.1 Negatron (β^-) Emission

As we can see from Figure 27.2, β^--particles are emitted from nuclei which have too many neutrons for nuclear stability. As we saw in Chapter 26, nucleons are constantly being changed from proton to neutron and back within the atomic nucleus. A neutron may be thought of as consisting of a proton and a negatron:

$$n \rightarrow p^+ + \beta^- \qquad \textit{Equation 27.2}$$

It appears that, in nuclei which have too many neutrons, there is a finite possibility that a neutron becomes isolated within the nucleus and then decays to form a proton and a negatron. The proton rejoins the nucleus and the negatron is ejected. This transformation results in the atomic mass number remaining unchanged (the combined number of protons and neutrons is still the same) but the atomic number will increase by one as one extra proton has been added to the nucleus (this results in the formation of a different element with the consequent rearrangement of electron orbitals to suit the new element).

An example of β⁻-particle decay is shown below, where carbon-14 decays to form nitrogen with the emission of a β⁻-particle.

$$^{14}_{6}C \rightarrow ^{14}_{7}N + \beta^{-} \qquad \textit{Equation 27.3}$$

This can also be illustrated using the methods discussed for alpha-particle emission to show the transformation from parent to daughter product. Such a diagram is shown in Figure 27.4.

Note that this time there is an increase in the atomic number so the line is down and to the right. This simple decay process is an example of *pure beta emission* since no other transformations are involved.

Figure 27.5 shows a more complex emission pattern where the parent and daughter nuclei are separated by an energy difference of 2.81 MeV. The β⁻-particle has an energy of 0.31 MeV and so the nucleus is left in an excited state – 2.50 MeV above its ground state. The nucleus emits this energy in the form of two gamma-rays, one of energy 1.17 MeV and the other of energy 1.33 MeV. (This will be discussed further when we consider gamma-ray emission in Sect. 27.6.)

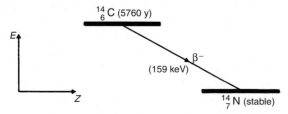

Figure 27.4 An example of pure beta-particle (negatron) emission. The nucleus increases in atomic number and loses energy as shown.

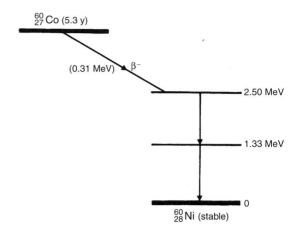

Figure 27.5 The decay of cobalt-60 as an example of beta decay followed by a gamma decay of the daughter nucleus.

27.5.2 Positron (β⁺) Emission

As mentioned earlier, protons are continuously changing into neutrons and back. In these reactions we can consider a proton as consisting of a neutron and a positron.

$$p^{+} \rightarrow n + \beta^{+} \qquad \textit{Equation 27.4}$$

If we consider Figure 27.2, we see that positron emission takes place from nuclei that have too many protons to achieve stability. In such cases protons appear to become isolated within the nucleus and then decay to form a neutron which rejoins the nucleus and a positron which is ejected from the nucleus. In this reaction the atomic mass number will remain the same but the atomic number will decrease by one (the total number of protons and neutrons is unchanged but one proton has been converted into a neutron).

An example of such a reaction is the decay of carbon-11 to boron, as shown below:

$$^{11}_{6}C \rightarrow ^{11}_{5}B + \beta^{+} \qquad \textit{Equation 27.5}$$

If we consider the energy changes that take place within the nucleus, as shown in Figure 27.6, we see that the situation regarding energy of the β⁺-particle is not as simple as it is for the β⁻-particle.

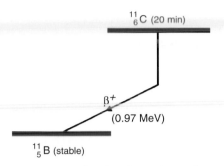

Figure 27.6 An example of positron decay. The nucleus experiences a decrease in the atomic number and loses energy, as shown.

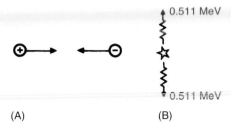

(A)   (B)

Figure 27.7 (A) A collision between a positron and an electron where both have a minimal kinetic energy. (B) The annihilation radiation where two photons, each of 0.511 MeV, are produced at 180° to each other.

The energy difference between the parent and daughter nucleus in this case is 1.99 MeV. An energy loss of $2mc^2$ is required to create the positron and allow it to escape from the nucleus, where m is the mass of the positron and c is the velocity of electromagnetic radiation. As the mass of the positron is the same as the mass of the electron, then 1.02 MeV is required to create the positron and eject it from the nucleus and any remaining energy (in this case 0.97 MeV) is given to the positron as kinetic energy.

INSIGHT

A negatron or a positron is influenced by the electrostatic forces which exist between it and the nucleus until it is able to escape from the atom. As a result the kinetic energy of the β⁻-particle is reduced by the force of attraction which exists between it and the nucleus, while the kinetic energy of the β⁺-particle is increased by electrostatic repulsion. Energy and momentum are conserved in this process.

27.5.3 The Fate of the Positron

An energetic positron emitted by a nucleus will move through the surrounding atoms and will lose kinetic energy because of collisions with them. As its momentum decreases, it is more likely to interact with a free electron in the material. The positron is the *antiparticle* of the electron and

when they meet they completely annihilate each other to form two gamma-rays of annihilation radiation. This process is shown diagrammatically in Figure 27.7 where the annihilation radiation consists of two photons, each of energy 0.511 MeV, ejected at 180° to each other. In this way both energy and momentum are conserved. The mutual annihilation of the electron and the positron is an example of the principle of mass–energy equivalence (see Sect. 24.4.1) as given by Einstein's equation $E = mc^2$, and shows that each particle has a mass–energy of 0.511 MeV, in agreement with Table 26.1.

The annihilation radiation produced by the reaction may now interact with neighbouring atoms by the processes of Compton scattering and photoelectric absorption (see Ch. 30) and may produce characteristic radiation and Auger electrons (see Sect. 27.6.3) by processes that will be discussed later in this chapter.

INSIGHT

The positron and the electron may annihilate each other when the positron still has considerable kinetic energy. In this case the two quanta are not emitted at 180° to each other and each has an energy higher than 0.511 MeV. The excess of energy of the positron is divided equally between each quantum. In each case energy and momentum are conserved. A diagrammatic representation of the process is shown in the figure.

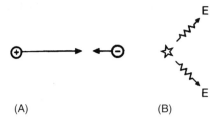

(A) A collision between a positron and an electron where the positron has significant kinetic energy; (B) the direction of propagation of the annihilation radiation where the photons have energy in excess of 0.511 MeV each.

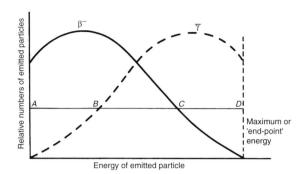

Figure 27.8 The sharing of energy between the beta-particle and the neutrino in beta decay – the case shown is for negatron emission.

27.5.4 The Neutrino

Consider the carbon-14 reaction which we discussed earlier. Here the carbon-14 decayed to nitrogen, where the difference in energy between the parent and the daughter nucleus was 159 keV. As only beta decay takes place we could confidently expect that all the β^--particles should have an energy of 159 keV. If we plot a graph of the energy of the beta-particles against the numbers emitted we get a graph similar to the β^- graph shown in Figure 27.8. The maximum or end-point energy of the β^--particles in this case is 159 keV. The graph means that, although only beta decay takes place and although the difference between the parent and the daughter nucleus is 159 keV, some of the β^--particles have energies less than 159 keV. Such a situation would appear to suggest that this does not obey the law of conservation of energy (see Sect. 24.4). This difficulty was overcome by Wolfgang Pauli in 1933, when he postulated that another particle – the *neutrino* – is always ejected with a beta-particle. Pauli suggested that a neutrino (symbol ν) is ejected at the same time as a positron and that an antineutrino (symbol ν̄) is ejected at the same time as a negatron. The *total energy* of the emitted negatron and antineutrino corresponds to the energy difference between the parent and daughter nucleus. How this energy is shared between the two particles will differ for each decay of the nucleus. In this way a continuous distribution of energies is obtained both for the β^--particle and the antineu-

trino, as shown in Figure 27.8. Because of the presence of the neutrino and antineutrino we now need to modify some of the equations we considered earlier:

$$^{14}_{6}C \rightarrow {}^{14}_{7}N + \beta^- + \bar{\nu}$$

$$^{11}_{6}C \rightarrow {}^{11}_{5}B + \beta^+ + \nu \qquad \textit{Equation 27.6}$$

INSIGHT

Although Pauli postulated the existence of neutrinos and antineutrinos in 1933, the presence of these particles proved difficult to detect until much later. There is now conclusive proof of their existence because of experiments performed using nuclear reactors and particle accelerators. The neutrino and the antineutrino differ in their direction of spin relative to their direction of motion – the neutrino spins anticlockwise and the antineutrino spins clockwise. They are antiparticles and if they are made to collide they will produce electromagnetic radiation in the form of annihilation radiation. The reason the particles are so difficult to detect can be seen by considering their three major properties:

1. zero rest mass
2. zero charge
3. extremely small interaction with matter.

Because of these properties it is extremely difficult to detect the presence of neutrinos (or antineutrinos) – they have a half-value thickness (see Sect. 4.8) of many miles in lead!

27.6 GAMMA DECAY OR GAMMA-RAY EMISSION

Gamma-rays are part of the electromagnetic spectrum and are similar in many ways to X-rays. Gamma-rays are emitted from a nucleus which has excess energy whereas X-rays are from electrons as they lose energy (this will be further discussed in Ch. 28). It is possible for gamma-rays to have lower energies than X-rays and vice versa. However, the maximum energy possible from gamma-rays exceeds that of X-rays.

We discussed in this chapter (see Sect. 27.5.1) the fact that cobalt-60 decayed with the emission of a β-particle but the daughter nucleus was left in an excited state. The situation for this daughter nucleus is depicted in Figure 27.9A. The figure illustrates the energy states of the daughter nucleus by means of horizontal lines above the thick line representing the ground state of the nucleus. In this case, the $^{60}_{28}$Ni nucleus is left at an energy 2.5 MeV above its ground state. It immediately decays to its ground state in two jumps:

1. It decays to 1.33 MeV above its ground state by the emission of a 1.17 MeV gamma-ray
2. It then drops to its ground state by the emission of a second gamma-ray of energy 1.33 MeV.

Figure 27.9B shows the line spectra of the gamma radiation emitted by the nucleus where each gamma-ray has a precise energy corresponding to the discrete energy transformations within the nucleus.

27.6.1 Metastable States and Isomeric Transitions

In the case of $^{60}_{27}$Co decaying to $^{60}_{28}$Ni the nucleus remains in an excited state before the emission of the gamma-rays for a time so short that it is incapable of accurate measurement. However, this is not always the case, and those excited states that last sufficiently long for their durations to be measured are known as *metastable states*. The transition from a metastable state to a more stable state is known as an *isomeric transition*. Such metastable radionuclides prove to be useful in nuclear medicine because of the low dose which they deliver to the patient – the patient gets no dose from β⁻-particles emitted before metastability. Technetium-99m (usually written $^{99}_{43}$Tc^{m} or, less commonly, $^{99m}_{43}$Tc) is a radionuclide which is widely used in nuclear medicine. A simplified decay scheme for it is shown in Figure 27.10 and it will be discussed in more detail later in this chapter (see Sect. 27.11.1). The half-life of $^{99}_{43}$Tc^{m} is 6 hours and it emits a gamma-ray of energy 140 keV when it decays to $^{99}_{43}$Tc. The half-life of $^{99}_{43}$Tc is so long (2.1 × 10^5 years) that it can be considered stable for all practical purposes.

The reaction can be written as:

$$^{99}_{43}\text{Tc}^{m} \rightarrow \,^{99}_{43}\text{Tc} + \gamma \qquad \textit{Equation 27.7}$$

The next section of this chapter considers the possible effects of gamma emission from the nucleus on the whole atom rather than on the nucleus only.

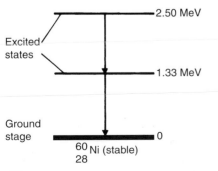

(A)

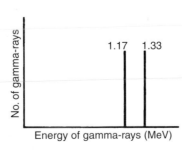

(B)

Figure 27.9   (A) The excited states of a nickel-60 nucleus which is left in an excited state as the result of the previous decay of a cobalt-60 nucleus. This decays to its ground state by the emission of two gamma photons, each representing the difference in energy between the excited states. (B) The line spectrum produced by the gamma radiation.

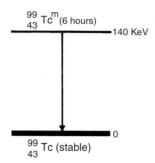

Figure 27.10 An example of the decay of technetium from a metastable to a stable state with the emission of a 140 keV gamma photon.

27.6.2 Internal Conversion

When a nuclide is decaying by gamma emission there is a competing process within the atom called *internal conversion*. This process results in electrons with discrete energies (unlike the continuous spectrum of energies of negatrons) being emitted from the atom. The process is a result of a direct interaction between the nucleus and an orbiting electron such that the nucleus is able to drop to its ground state by giving all of its excess energy to the electron.

The innermost electrons of the atom have orbitals which pass close to or even through the nucleus. Thus it is a matter of statistical probability whether the excess energy of the nucleus will result in a gamma-ray emission from the nucleus or electron emission from the inner shells. The K-shell is situated closest to the nucleus so is most likely to participate in such a reaction, followed by the L-, M-shells, etc. The *converted electron* escapes from the atom with an energy equal to the energy donated by the nucleus minus the binding energy of that particular electron. This can be stated:

> KE of converted electron = nuclear energy
> transition – BE   *Equation 27.8*

where KE = kinetic energy and BE = binding energy of the electron.

The *internal conversion coefficient*, α, is defined as the ratio of the number of nuclear transformations which result in internal conversion to the number which result in gamma-ray emission.

Thus, α may take a value between 0, resulting in no internal conversions, and infinity, corresponding to complete internal conversion. This can be illustrated by considering the figures for the decay of $^{99}_{43}\text{Tc}^{m}$ to $^{99}_{43}\text{Tc}$. Approximately 9% of the nuclear transitions result in internal conversions of electrons from the K-shell, 1.1% from the L-shell and 0.3% from the M-shell. This means that 10.4% of the nuclear transitions result in internal conversions and 89.6% result in gamma-ray emission. This gives an internal conversion coefficient (α) for $^{99}_{43}\text{Tc}^{m}$ of 0.116.

27.6.3 X-rays and Auger Electrons

If a radioactive decay results in a vacancy occurring within one of the inner electron shells of the atom, then electrons from orbitals further away from the nucleus will perform quantum jumps inwards until there are no inner shell vacancies. Each such quantum jump will result in the emission of electromagnetic radiation from the atom equal to the energy difference between the two shells. For inner-shell transitions the energy of this electromagnetic radiation may be in the X-ray part of the spectrum. Such radiation is known as *fluorescent radiation* and its energy is characteristic of the atom concerned.

If we consider the internal conversion process which we have just described and take a situation where a K-shell electron is removed from the atom, the vacancy thus created in the K-shell may be filled from the L-shell (a K_{α} transition) or from the M-shell (a K_{β} transition). Such a quantum jump would be accompanied by the emission of a photon of electromagnetic radiation equivalent to the energy difference between the two shells. If it was a K_{α} transition, there would now be a vacancy in the L-shell and this might be filled from the M-shell, etc. This would again be accompanied by the emission of a photon of electromagnetic radiation equal to the energy difference between the L- and M-shells. This process continues until the atom is able to capture a free electron to fill the vacancy – usually in one of its outermost shells. Until this occurs the atom contains more protons than electrons and so is regarded as a *positive ion*.

This already rather complex situation is further complicated by the fact that some of the photons emitted by such transitions may have sufficient energy to interact with other electrons in the atom and to remove them from their orbitals and eject them from the atom. This process is called the *photoelectric effect* and may occur if the photon energy is greater than the binding energy of the electron (see Ch. 30 for a more detailed description). The electrons thus ejected are called *Auger electrons* and have discrete energies equal to the photon energy minus the binding energy of the electron. The ejection of an Auger electron from a shell leaves a vacancy in that shell which will be filled by electrons jumping down from orbitals even further away from the nucleus, with the release of more fluorescent radiation and perhaps the release of even more Auger electrons.

From the above we can see that the ejection of an electron from one of the orbitals by internal conversion may result in a complicated sequence of orbital quantum jumps accompanied by the release of photons of electromagnetic radiation and the ejection of Auger electrons from the atom. The term *fluorescent yield* is used to describe the fraction of the electron transitions which result in the production of fluorescent radiation.

If we consider $^{99}_{43}\text{Tc}^m$ from the previous discussion, you may remember that 11.6% of the energy from the nucleus results in internal conversion ($\alpha = 0.116$). Of the resulting electron quantum jumps, 80% of the transitions result in fluorescent radiation and 20% result in the production of Auger electrons. Thus the fluorescent yield for technetium is 0.8. Some typical fluorescent radiation energies for $^{99}_{43}\text{Tc}^m$ are:

$$K_\alpha = 18.4 \text{ keV}, L_\alpha = 2.4 \text{ keV}, M_\alpha = 0.2 \text{ keV}$$

Note: The fact that the electrons emitted by this process carry discrete amounts of energy makes it easy to distinguish them from negatron emission where there is a continuous spectrum of energies.

INSIGHT

For each decay, the total energies for all the fluorescent radiation and of all the electrons emitted from the shells of the atom equal the energy lost by the nucleus in the nuclear transition. This is because the binding energy of each ejected electron is recovered in the fluorescent radiation emitted in the subsequent cascade of orbital jumps. Thus the whole process obeys the law of conservation of energy (see Sect. 5.3).

27.7 ELECTRON CAPTURE

If a nucleus of low mass number has too few neutrons for stability but has insufficient excess energy (<1.02 MeV) to eject a positron, then an alternative way by which the nucleus may undergo an isobaric transformation and lose energy is *electron capture*. In this process the nucleus captures one of the orbiting electrons, the most likely being a capture of a *K*-shell electron. Sometimes the terms '*K* capture' and '*L* capture' are used to denote the shell from which the electron was captured. A situation where electron capture is the only process involved is shown in Figure 27.11A where $^{131}_{55}\text{Cs}$ decays to $^{131}_{54}\text{Xe}$.

In the diagram, the atomic number is reduced by one because the capture of an electron by the nucleus results in one of the protons in the nucleus changing into a neutron. Also note that, during the process of electron capture, a neutrino is emitted by the nucleus. The processes involved in electron capture may be shown by Equation 27.9.

$$p^+ + e^- \rightarrow n + \nu \qquad \text{\textit{Equation 27.9}}$$

In situations where a low-mass nucleus has too few neutrons and an excess energy greater than 1.02 MeV, then the process of electron capture may compete with the process of positron emission. An example of such a competing process is shown in the decay of $^{58}_{27}\text{Co}$ into stable $^{58}_{26}\text{Fe}$ in Figure 27.11B.

Note that both the process of electron capture and the process of positron emission involve the conversion of a proton to a neutron. Thus the atomic mass number remains unaltered but the atomic number is reduced by one.

As we mentioned earlier in this chapter (Sect. 27.6.2), creating a vacancy in an inner electron

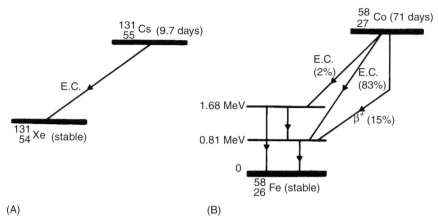

(A)   (B)

Figure 27.11 (A) Pure electron capture decay. (B) Electron capture (EC) and positron decay occurring in the same nuclide (85% EC and 15% positron decay). Also emitted are the X-rays from the iron-58 atoms and the 0.511 MeV annihilation radiations from the positron–electron annihilations.

shell will result in the emission of characteristic fluorescent radiation from the atom. It is interesting to note that, in the case of electron capture this is characteristic of the *daughter* product. This means that the electron orbitals of the daughter product are established before the consequent electron transitions occur.

27.8 BRANCHING DECAY PROGRAMMES

If the nucleus is very large, it is possible that it may disintegrate in more than one way. We have already encountered this – although it was not described in detail – in the uranium series in Figure 27.1. In this case $^{214}_{83}$Bi can either decay to $^{214}_{84}$Po by β⁻-particle emission or it can decay to $^{210}_{81}$Tl by alpha-particle emission.

Another isotope of bismuth, $^{212}_{83}$Bi, decays in a similar branching programme. The decay process for this isotope involves the emission of alpha-particles of energies 6.04 and 6.08 MeV, gamma-rays of energy 0.04 MeV and β⁻-particles of maximum energy 2.25 MeV. The initial decay scheme for the $^{212}_{83}$Bi nuclide is shown in Figure 27.12. *Note* that for simplicity only the first disintegrations are shown. As can be seen from the diagram, both $^{208}_{81}$Tl and $^{212}_{84}$Po have short half-lives and so are also radioactive.

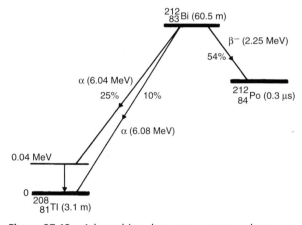

Figure 27.12 A branching decay programme where alpha and beta decay processes compete in the decay of bismuth-212.

27.9 FISSION

As we mentioned in our discussion of alpha-decay (see Sect. 27.4), the short-range forces holding the nucleus together exist between adjacent nucleons, whereas the Coulomb forces act across the whole of the nucleus. This fact becomes increasingly important as the size of the nucleus increases. A very large nucleus may be pictured as being rather like a liquid drop in which the nucleons are moving about with very high energy and continuously deforming the shape of the nucleus.

During this process, it is possible for the nucleus to become very elongated and then to break into two fragments, usually of fairly similar sizes. Such a phenomenon is known as *spontaneous fission* and can occur for very large nuclei, e.g. thorium-232 is capable of spontaneous fission. As well as the *fission fragments* from such a reaction, one or more neutrons are usually liberated and the whole fission process is accompanied by the release of large amounts of energy.

Neutron-activated fission is a more controllable process than spontaneous fission. This occurs as a result of a heavy nucleus capturing an incoming neutron and then breaking into large fragments in a similar way to spontaneous fission. An example of such a reaction is the disintegration of $^{238}_{92}U$ into two fission fragments of $^{145}_{56}Ba$ and $^{94}_{36}Kr$ if the uranium-238 nucleus is made to absorb a neutron. The fission of the nucleus is normally accompanied by the release of gamma-rays and neutrons. Both of the fissile fragments are extremely rich in neutrons and so each will usually release a neutron. The neutrons from both of the above processes can now react with two $^{238}_{92}U$ nuclei, resulting in the release of four fissile fragments and four neutrons, and so a chain reaction can be set up. Such a process is accompanied by the release of large amounts of energy (see Insight).

INSIGHT

On average, a uranium-238 nucleus will release an energy of 200 MeV on fission. If we consider the complete fission of a 1-kg mass of uranium (this is about the size of a golf ball), we need to consider the energy released by all the uranium atoms in a 1-kg mass. By applying Avogadro's equation (see Sect. 5.6) to this we can calculate that 1 kg of uranium-238 contains 2.5×10^{24} atoms. If each of these atoms releases 200 MeV of energy, the total energy released will be 5.1×10^{26} MeV. This is the same as 8.1×10^{13} joules of energy.

A pictorial representation of the neutron-activated fission process is shown in Figure 27.13. The incoming neutron is captured in Figure 27.13A and delivers sufficient energy to the nucleus (Figure 27.13B) to elongate its shape into an ellipsoid. As mentioned earlier, the Coulomb forces

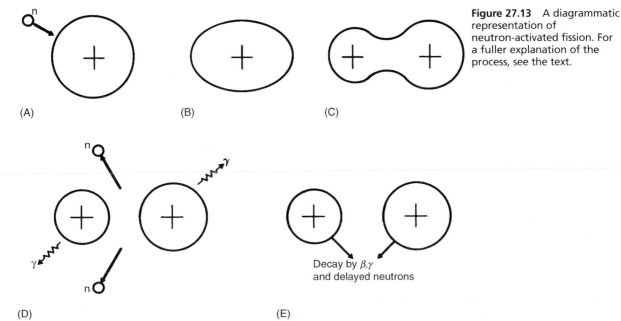

(A)   (B)   (C)

Figure 27.13   A diagrammatic representation of neutron-activated fission. For a fuller explanation of the process, see the text.

Decay by β,γ and delayed neutrons

(D)   (E)

across the nucleus are now at an advantage over the short-range nuclear forces and the nucleus further distorts to form a 'peanut' shape (Figure 27.13C) and eventually breaks to form two fragments because of the electrostatic repulsion between the two main nuclear masses. The two fragments fly apart (their kinetic energy accounts for about 80% of the total disintegration energy) and several neutrons and gamma-ray photons are usually emitted (Figure 27.13D). The neutrons emitted by this reaction may now interact with other atoms to cause fission and the release of further neutrons and so a chain reaction is set up, with the consequent liberation of large amounts of energy. The fissile fragments (Figure 27.13E) are themselves rich in neutrons for their atomic numbers and so will undergo further disintegration to move towards more stable nuclei. This initial process results in the production of β⁻-particles (with associated gamma-rays), which produces a more stable proton/neutron configuration or, if the nucleus is very excited, the ejection of a neutron from the nucleus. These neutrons are known as *delayed neutrons* to distinguish them from the *prompt neutrons* which are emitted at the moment of fission.

Fission products from any type of nucleus are not always the same and may have different relative sizes on each disintegration. Thus a great range of other decay chains is possible from other fissile fragments.

INSIGHT

It is also possible to initiate fission in the nucleus by bombarding it with proton (or with alpha-particles) or by striking it with high-energy photons. Examples of these are:

- Copper ($^{63}_{29}$Cu), if bombarded with protons, can be made to undergo fission to produce sodium ($^{24}_{11}$Na) and potassium ($^{39}_{19}$K). This process is accompanied by neutron emission
- Uranium-238 ($^{238}_{32}$U), if it is bombarded by photons of energy equal to or greater than 5.1 MeV, will undergo fission. This latter process is known as *photofission*.

27.9.1 The Nuclear Reactor

The nuclear reactor (or pile) produces heat energy by controlled fission. The heat generated within the reactor raises the temperature of a coolant which in turn is used to heat water to produce steam. The steam then drives very powerful electric generators.

A simplified diagram of such a reactor is shown in Figure 27.14. The controlled fission is produced by using the neutrons of fissile decay to produce further fission in other atoms. Thus, a sustained reaction can be set up where one neutron released during the fission of a nucleus will interact with another nucleus to produce fission of that nucleus with the release of further neutrons.

Nuclear reactors are important in radiation medicine in that they allow us to insert samples

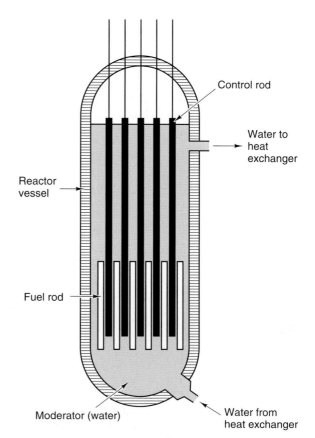

Figure 27.14 Simplified diagram of a pressurised water nuclear reactor.

into the neutron flux within the reactor. This results in neutrons being inserted into nuclei to allow the manufacture of *artificial radionuclides*.

INSIGHT

In 1986 the operators of the nuclear reactor at Chernobyl, near Kiev, lost control of the reactor by a somewhat bizarre set of operator errors. As a result, the reactor went hypercritical and power surged to about 100 times its normal value. This caused serious overheating of the core which caused it to explode and start a fire in the graphite moderator. The debris from this explosion contained many byproducts of fission and was carried over a large area of northern and western Europe, causing serious radioactive contamination. An area of 30-km radius around the reactor is so seriously contaminated that it has had to be permanently evacuated.

27.10 SUMMARY OF RADIOACTIVE NUCLEAR TRANSFORMATIONS

Table 27.1 is a summary of the types of radioactive decay discussed so far in this chapter. You may find it useful to refer back to this table when considering the production of artificial radionuclides and also in considering the use of radionuclides in medicine.

27.11 ARTIFICIALLY PRODUCED RADIONUCLIDES

Radionuclides may be artificially produced by bombarding the nuclei of elements with particles, e.g. neutrons from either a nuclear reactor or a particle accelerator such as a cyclotron. These particles are captured by the nucleus, making it unstable and causing it to decay by one or more of the methods described above.

Many of the artificially produced radionuclides that are relevant to nuclear medicine are produced in this way. The capture of a neutron is immediately accompanied by the ejection of a gamma-ray or particle. The daughter nucleus produced by neutron capture is obviously rich in neutrons and so is likely to decay by β^--emission. This may be accompanied by gamma emission. It is not feasible to produce nuclei with very short half-lives at a remote site and then transport these to the hospital. Such radionuclides are produced at the hospital's radiopharmacy by the use of either a technetium generator or a medical cyclotron. The increasing use of medical cyclotrons to produce radionuclides for positron emission tomography (PET) scanning merits a brief description of the physics of such a device. Such a discussion is included in this chapter (see Sect. 27.11.3) but first, the more common technetium generator will be considered.

27.11.1 The Technetium Generator

The *technetium generator* used in nuclear medicine is an important example of the production of artificial radionuclides. If molybdenum-98 is placed in a neutron stream, the nuclei of the molybdenum atoms can be made to absorb the neutrons to produce molybdenum-99. The capture of a neutron raises the energy of the resulting molybdenum-99 nuclei and each loses this energy by the prompt emission of a gamma-ray. The reaction may be shown using the equation below:

$$^{98}_{42}\text{Mo} + n \rightarrow {}^{99}_{42}\text{Mo} + \gamma \qquad \textit{Equation 27.10}$$

The molybdenum-99/alumina column is in the centre of the generator, as shown in Figure 27.15. The molybdenum-99 has a half-life of 67 hours and decays to form technetium-99m by β^--particle emission, as shown below:

$$^{99}_{42}\text{Mo} \rightarrow {}^{99}_{43}\text{Tc}^m + \beta^- + \bar{\nu} \qquad \textit{Equation 27.11}$$

The $^{99}_{43}\text{Tc}^m$ is eluted (or flushed) from the generator at regular intervals as sodium pertechnetate. This isotope, which is in liquid form, may be used for a number of radionuclide imaging situations. The $^{99}_{43}\text{Tc}^m$ decays to $^{99}_{43}\text{Tc}$ by the emission of a gamma-ray of energy 140 keV. The metastable isotope, as we saw earlier in this chapter, has a half-life of 6 hours.

Table 27.1 Summary of the effects of radioactive decay

Type of decay	Symbol	Effect on nucleus			Effect on atom	Comments
		Z	N	A		
Alpha	α	$Z-2$	$N-2$	$A-4$	Electron orbits change to that of daughter nucleus	Occurs in elements with a mass number greater than 150. Daughter products may undergo further decay by a variety of processes mentioned below
Negatron emission	β^-	$Z+1$	$N-1$	–	Electron orbits change to that of daughter nucleus	Proton changes to neutron in nucleus. Negatron emitted from the nucleus with a spread of energies but the energy of the negatron plus the energy of the antineutrino is constant for a given nuclide. Daughter nucleus may further decay by prompt or delayed gamma-ray emission competing with internal conversion (IC)
Positron emission	β^+	$Z-1$	$N+1$	–	Electron orbits change to that of daughter nucleus	Neutron changes to proton in nucleus. The positron is emitted with a neutrino and the sum of their energies is constant for a given nuclide. The process only occurs if the energy loss by the parent nucleus can be greater than 1.02 MeV. Positron is annihilated by collision with electron and two photons of annihilation radiation, each of energy 0.511 MeV, are produced. Daughter nucleus may decay by gamma radiation and/or IC
Gamma radiation	γ	–	–	–	No effect on the number of nucleons in the nucleus but the process may compete with IC	Produced by the quantum jump from excited state of the nucleus to a lower energy. Excited states of measurable half-life are defined as *metastable* and the transition is *isomeric*
Internal conversion	IC	–	–	–	Characteristic radiation and Auger electrons emitted	An inner orbital electron of the atom interacts with the nucleus and is ejected from the atom. The electron is given the excess nuclear energy. This creates a vacancy in the shell and results in the emission of characteristic radiation and Auger electrons
Electron capture	EC	$Z-1$	$N+1$	–	Characteristic radiation and Auger electrons of the daughter nucleus are emitted	An inner orbital electron is captured by the nucleus and changes a proton to a neutron. A neutrino is emitted, carrying energy changes of the nucleus. The nucleus may decay spontaneously by gamma-ray emission. The vacancy left in the electron orbit results in the emission of characteristic radiation and Auger electrons
Fission	f	Size and structure of the fragments may vary			Bonds may be broken or ionisation caused by fragment	Fission may be spontaneous or neutron-activated. The nucleus splits, producing two or more fragments, gamma-rays and neutrons. Controlled fission is used in nuclear reactors (see text) and the neutrons can be used to produce artificial radionuclides

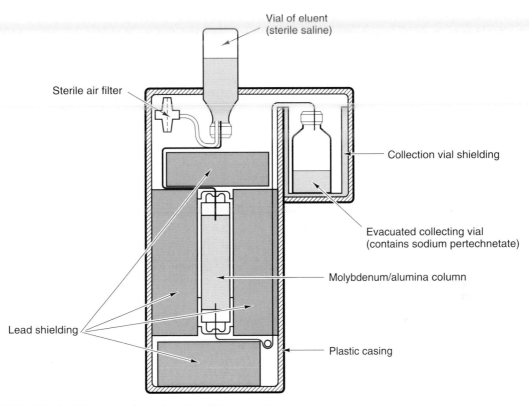

Figure 27.15   Principal features of a technetium-99m generator.

A number of other isotopes used in nuclear medicine can be produced from stable materials when they are bombarded with particles but further discussion about their production is beyond the scope of this book.

27.11.2 Growth of Activity

If we consider the molybdenum-98 which has been placed within a neutron stream in a nuclear reactor, then the number of daughter nuclei formed by the capture process increases over a period of time. However, the number of daughter nuclei formed does not increase indefinitely for the following reasons:

- As more of the original nuclei have captured neutrons, there are fewer left to do the same
- Daughter nuclei themselves may capture further neutrons and form a different isotope of that element. (In practice, the probability of this happening for most of the isotopes used in nuclear medicine is very low)
- Daughter nuclei undergo radioactive decay during the irradiation time.

The relative importance of the above processes depends on factors such as the sample material, the half-lives involved, the neutron flux and the neutron energy spectrum. The growth of the activity of the daughter product is in exponential form and is described by the equation:

$$A_t = kF(1 - e^{-\lambda t}) \qquad \textit{Equation 27.12}$$

where A_t is the radioactivity (measured in becquerels) after a time t, k is a constant for a given sample and a given reactor, F is a measure of the neutron flux (number of neutrons per unit area per second), and λ is the decay constant of the daughter radionuclide formed.

The growth curve of the activity of the daughter nuclide is shown in Figure 27.16 for

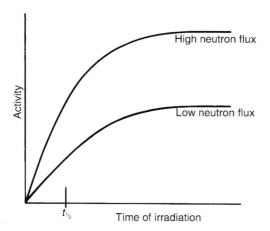

Figure 27.16 A graphical representation of the growth of activity induced by irradiating a suitable sample with neutrons.

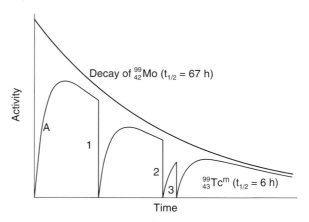

Figure 27.17 An example of radioactive equilibrium. Molybdenum-99 decays with a half-life of 67 hours to technetium-99m (half-life = 6 hours). At time 0, the Tc-99m grows in activity (A in the figure) – this is removed by elution from a technetium generator (1, 2, 3), after which the activity grows again.

two levels of neutron flux (note the similarity between these growth curves and the exponential curves obtained when a capacitor is charged through a resistor – Figure 16.5). In both cases, the activity produced in the sample reaches a maximum value after about four half-lives. It is usual in most cases, however, to irradiate the sample for only two or three half-lives as this time produces the maximum gain for the time of irradiation.

As can be seen from the graphs, when the activity reaches its maximum value there is a constant value of activity produced even if the sample is further irradiated. This is because equal numbers of daughter nuclei are being produced and decaying each second. This situation is known as *radioactive equilibrium*. Radioactive equilibrium may also occur in decay chains where the daughter nuclide is also decaying into another nuclide (see Insight below).

INSIGHT

Another example of radioactive equilibrium is the decay of $^{99}_{42}$Mo into $^{99}_{43}$Tc^m that takes place in the technetium generator. The half-life for the $^{99}_{42}$Mo is 67 hours and for the $^{99}_{43}$Tc is 6 hours. If we start the process at a time when there is no $^{99}_{43}$Tc^m present, the activity of the $^{99}_{43}$Tc^m will rise until it reaches 90% of the activity of the molybdenum.

This is shown in section A of the graph in Figure 27.17. The curves for both the isotopes now run in parallel – they are in radioactive equilibrium. Elution of the generator removes all the activity due to the technetium (see 1, 2 and 3 in Figure 27.17) but it will again return to 90% of the activity of the molybdenum unless two elutions follow each other too rapidly, as in 2 and 3. The generator may thus be used as a source of the daughter nuclide for a much longer time than the half-life of the daughter would otherwise permit.

27.11.3 Production of Radionuclides Using a Cyclotron

The type of cyclotron used in nuclear medicine to produce artificial radionuclides by the bombardment of stable substances will briefly be described. A simple diagram of such a device is shown in Figure 27.18.

The cyclotron consists of an evacuated cylinder which has an ion source placed at its centre. Ions from this source are influenced by strong axial and radial magnetic fields. This causes acceleration of the ions in circular paths of increasing radius. This ion beam achieves significant velocity and can be made to interact with materials placed at the exit port of the cyclotron. This interaction causes

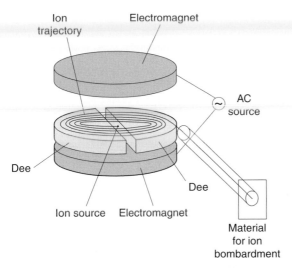

Figure 27.18 The main components of a medical cyclotron.

nuclear changes in these materials and we can produce neutron-deficient nuclei (see Sect. 27.5.1) which are capable of positron emission. Such materials form the basis of the radiopharmaceuticals used in PET scanning.

27.12 CLINICALLY USEFUL RADIONUCLIDES

Radionuclides are used to diagnose and to treat certain conditions. When they are used for diagnosis, they may be *labelled* (chemically linked) to a certain *radiopharmaceutical*, thus encouraging their uptake by specific body parts. The labelled radionuclide may then be injected into, or ingested by, the patient. Such diagnostic techniques in nuclear medicine have three main uses:

1. to provide numerical or graphical information on organ physiology, e.g. technetium-labelled diethylene triamine pentaacetic acid (DTPA) will give information on the rate of excretion of this radionuclide by the kidneys, thus giving information on renal function
2. to produce an image of organ physiology on a gamma camera, e.g. $^{99}_{43}Tc^m$ as pertechnetate may be injected into the patient to produce images of the skeletal physiology; this is very

useful for early detection of metastatic spread into bone
3. to produce information on organ physiology using PET scanning, e.g. brain scans using fluorodeoxyglucose can produce images of cerebral physiology indicating the levels of cerebral activity for specific tasks.

A list of the radioisotopes which are commonly used is given in Table 27.2.

For the diagnostic purposes of imaging or charting organ physiology, only gamma-ray emission or positron emission is useful. This is because particles (α or β) emitted are absorbed very efficiently by the patient's tissues. If the particles are absorbed by the patient and do not reach the imaging or counting device, they contribute a radiation dose to the patient but give no diagnostic information. In the case of positron emission, the positron itself is rapidly annihilated by collision with an electron (see Sect. 27.5.3) but the annihilation radiation is detected by suitable detectors in a PET scanner (see Appendix B).

The ideal radionuclide for imaging should:

- have a short half-life – approximately twice the length of time from injection into the patient to completion of the scan
- emit gamma-rays of relatively low energy, so that these are easily detected and do not pose a major hazard to others because of their penetrating power
- emit no particles as part of its decay pattern as these add significantly to the patient dose
- be readily labelled to allow its uptake by specific organs
- be readily excreted by the patient
- be easily generated in the radiopharmacy.

In many ways $^{99}_{43}Tc^m$ is the almost ideal radionuclide for scanning purposes.

As can be seen from Table 27.2, other radionuclides can be used for a variety of purposes in medicine. Detailed discussion of their use is the subject of a specialised text and beyond the scope of this book. A number of specialist texts on this topic may be found in the list of further reading at the end of this chapter.

Table 27.2 Radionuclides commonly used in medicine

Application	Radionuclide	$t^{1}/_{2}$	Decay mode	Gamma energy (MeV)	Maximum beta energy (MeV)	Comments
Diagnostic						
Organ physiology	$^{131}_{53}$I	8.04 days	β^-, γ	0.364	0.61	Thyroid uptakes (NaI)
	$^{132}_{53}$I	2.3 h	β^-, γ	0.67 0.78	2.12	Renal function (iodohippurate)
	$^{99}_{43}$Tc^m	6 h	IT	0.140	–	Renal function (DTPA)
Organ imaging	$^{99}_{43}$Tc^m	6 h	IT	0.140	–	Imaging of brain, kidney, liver, lung, skeleton, spleen
	$^{113}_{49}$In^m	90 min	IT	0.390	–	Imaging of brain, kidney, liver
	$^{75}_{34}$Se	121 days	EC	0.14 0.27	–	Imaging of pancreas
	$^{68}_{31}$Ga	68 min	β^+, EC	0.51	1.89	Imaging of tumours and inflammatory lesions
	$^{81}_{36}$Kr^m	13 s	IT	0.19	–	Pulmonary function (ventilation) studies
	$^{133}_{54}$Xe	5.3 days	β^-, γ	0.081	0.34	Cerebral blood flow, pulmonary function (ventilation) studies
Tracers	$^{3}_{1}$H	12.3 years	β^-	–	0.018	Used for a large variety of studies
	$^{14}_{6}$C	5760 years	β^-	–	0.115	
	$^{35}_{16}$S	87.2 days	β^-	–	0.167	Used in the estimation of cellular volumes
	$^{43}_{19}$K	22 h	β^-, γ	0.37 0.61	0.83	
	$^{51}_{24}$Cr	27.8 days	EC	0.32	–	Used for a variety of blood studies
	$^{59}_{27}$Fe	445 days	β^-, γ	1.10 1.29	0.46	
	$^{57}_{27}$Co	270 days	EC	0.112	–	Used for the investigation of pernicious anaemia
	$^{58}_{27}$Co	71 days	β^+, EC	0.51 0.81	0.485	
Therapy						
By injection	$^{32}_{15}$P	14.3 days	β^-	–	1.71	Phosphate used for the treatment of polycythaemia vera
	$^{90}_{39}$Y	62.2 h	β^-	–	2.27	Used as a colloid in the treatment of some lymphatic cancers
By ingestion	$^{131}_{53}$I	8.04 days	β^-, γ	0.364	0.61	Treatment of hyperthyroidism or thyroid cancer
Interstitial	$^{182}_{73}$Ta	115 days	βs, γs	Wide range	Wide range	Localised treatment of cancer by the insertion of needles, tubes or wires of the radionuclide
	$^{192}_{77}$Ir	74 days	βs, γs	Wide range	Wide range	
	$^{137}_{55}$Cs	30 years	β^-, γ	0.662	0.51	
Teletherapy	$^{137}_{55}$Cs	30 years	β^-, γ	0.662	0.51	External beams of gamma radiation from the radionuclides are used to treat cancers
	$^{60}_{27}$Co	5.3 years	β^-, γ	1.17 1.33	0.31	
Radioimmunoassay	$^{125}_{53}$I	60 days	EC	0.027 0.035	–	Used to detect small quantities of hormones

IT, isomeric transition; EC, electron capture; DTPA, diethylene triamine pentaacetic acid.

SUMMARY

In this chapter you should have learnt:

- The mechanism for alpha decay and alpha-particle emission (see Sect. 27.4)
- Beta decay leading to negatron emission (see Sect. 27.5.1)
- Beta decay leading to positron emission (see Sect. 27.5.2)
- The fate of the positron after emission (see Sect. 27.5.3)
- The fact that a neutrino or an antineutrino forms part of beta emission (see Sect. 27.5.4)
- The mechanism of gamma decay and gamma-ray emission (see Sect. 27.6)
- The meaning of metastable nuclei and isomeric transitions (see Sect. 27.6.1)
- The mechanism of the process of internal conversion (see Sect. 27.6.2)
- The mechanisms involved in the emission of X-rays and Auger electrons from the atoms of radionuclides (see Sect. 27.6.3)
- The mechanism of electron capture and the subsequent changes within the atom (see Sect. 27.7)
- Branching decay programmes (see Sect. 27.8)
- The processes involved in nuclear fission (see Sect. 27.9)
- The use of nuclear fission in the nuclear reactor (see Sect. 27.9.1)
- The mechanisms for the production of artificial radionuclides (see Sect. 27.11)
- The construction and operation of the technetium generator (see Sect. 27.11.1)
- The production of radionuclides using a cyclotron (see Sect. 27.11.3)
- The clinical uses of radionuclides and examples of radionuclides which can be used for each purpose (see Sect. 27.12).

SELF-TEST

a. Discuss the conditions necessary for alpha-particle emission and describe the mechanism of alpha decay. Give an example of alpha decay.

b. Discuss the conditions necessary for negatron and positron decay and give an example of each. For the purposes of this description, the emission of the neutrino and the antineutrino may be ignored.

c. Discuss gamma-ray emission and explain what is meant by *metastable atoms* and *isomeric transitions*.

d. Describe the process of electron capture.

e. Describe what is meant by nuclear fission, distinguishing between spontaneous fission and neutron-activated fission.

f. With the aid of a diagram, discuss the construction and operation of a technetium generator.

g. List the desirable properties of a radionuclide to be used in medical imaging and show how $^{99}_{43}\text{Tc}^{m}$ fulfils these properties.

FURTHER READING

Ball J L, Moore A D 1997 Essential physics for radiographers, 3rd edn. Blackwell Scientific Publications, London, ch 17

Carter P H 1994 Chesney's equipment for student radiographers, 4th edn. Blackwell Publishing, London, ch 5

Curry T S III, Dowdey J E, Murry R C Jr 1990 Christensen's physics of diagnostic radiography, 4th edn. Lee & Febiger, London, chs 5, 9, 10, 11, 14 and 15

Dowsett D J, Kenny P A, Johnston R E 1998 The physics of diagnostic imaging. Chapman & Hall Medical, London, chs 15 and 16

Webb S (ed) 2000 The physics of medical imaging, 2nd edn. Institute of Physics Publishing, Bristol, ch 2

Part 5

X-rays and Matter

PART CONTENTS

28. The Production of X-rays   269

29. Factors Affecting X-ray Beam Quality
    and Quantity   277

30. Interactions of X-rays with Matter
    284

31. Luminescence and
    Photostimulation   298

32. The Radiographic Image   306

Chapter 28

The Production of X-rays

CHAPTER CONTENTS

28.1 Aim   269

28.2 Interactions of Electrons with Matter   269

28.3 Interactions between Electrons from the Filament and the Outer Electrons of the Target Atoms in the X-ray Tube   270

28.4 Interactions between Electrons from the Filament and the Nuclei of the Target Atoms in the X- ray Tube   271
    28.4.1 Elastic Collisions with the Nuclei   271
    28.4.2 Inelastic Collisions with the Nuclei – Production of Bremsstrahlung Radiation   271

28.5 Inelastic Collisions with the Electrons of the Target Atoms – Production of Characteristic Radiation   272

28.6 The X-ray Spectrum   273

Self-Test   276

Further Reading   276

28.1 AIM

The aim of this chapter is to consider the mechanisms by which X-rays are produced at the target of the X-ray tube. The concept of the X-ray spectrum will be introduced and this chapter will act as a foundation for Chapter 29, where the factors affecting the X-ray spectrum will be considered.

28.2 INTERACTIONS OF ELECTRONS WITH MATTER

In Chapter 21 we discussed the construction of the X-ray tube and the functions of its various components. In that chapter we stated that electrons are produced at the filament by thermionic emission, they are accelerated towards the tungsten target and, on impact with the target, they suffer sudden deceleration to produce X-rays and heat. In this chapter we will look in more detail at the processes involved at subatomic level in the target of the X-ray tube.

There are a number of ways in which high-energy electrons from the filament of the X-ray tube may lose their energy when they collide with the atoms of the target. These are shown in Figure 28.1:

- The loss of energy by the electrons from the filament because of interactions between them and the outer electrons surrounding the atoms of the target material (see electron 1 in Figure 28.1)
- The loss of energy by electrons from the filament because of interactions between them

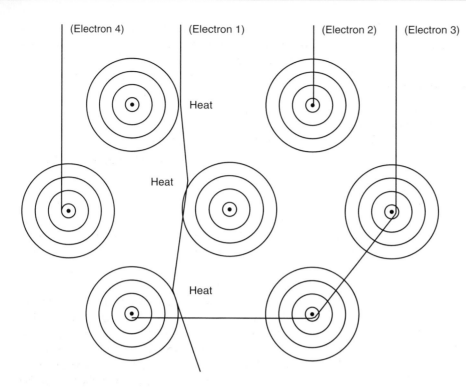

(Electron 4)   (Electron 1)   (Electron 2)   (Electron 3)

Heat

Heat

Heat

Figure 28.1 Diagrammatic representation of possible interactions between electrons from the filament and target atoms in an X-ray tube. An explanation of the interactions is given in the text.

and the nuclei of the atoms of the target material (see electrons 2 and 3 in Figure 28.1)

• The loss of energy by electrons from the filament because of interactions between them and individual inner electrons of the target atoms (see electron 4 in Figure 28.1).

The interactions between electrons and target atoms may be *elastic* where there is conservation of kinetic energy or *inelastic* collisions in which kinetic energy is lost (see Sect. 5.4). It is also important to realise that an electron from the filament may experience many interactions (typically about 1000) before it is brought to rest within 0.25–0.5 mm of the target surface.

28.3 INTERACTIONS BETWEEN ELECTRONS FROM THE FILAMENT AND THE OUTER ELECTRONS OF THE TARGET ATOMS IN THE X-RAY TUBE

As you may remember from Chapter 21, the main material of the X-ray tube target is tungsten, which has an atomic number of 74. Thus each target atom is surrounded by 74 electrons in various orbitals. These electrons have the effect of deflecting the approaching electron from the filament because of the electrostatic repulsion between them and the filament electron. Such deflections from the electron's original path are small and so the loss of kinetic energy is small. The kinetic energy lost by the electron is emitted as a photon of electromagnetic radiation. The energy of this photon is such that it falls into the infrared part of the spectrum and so heat is produced in the target material. If we consider the statistical probability of this process occurring rather than the other three processes identified in Section 28.2, we can see that it has a very high probability of occurring.

This is because the other three processes involve an interaction between either the incoming electron and the nucleus or the incoming electron and the inner orbital electrons. The area occupied by the nucleus and the inner electron orbitals is very small compared to the size of the whole tungsten atom and so an incoming electron has a much greater chance of interacting with the whole atom. For the above reasons, about 95–99% of the energy produced at the target of the X-ray tube is in the form of heat.

28.4 INTERACTIONS BETWEEN ELECTRONS FROM THE FILAMENT AND THE NUCLEI OF THE TARGET ATOMS IN THE X-RAY TUBE

As mentioned at the beginning of this chapter, the interactions of electrons from the filament with the nuclei of the target atoms can be elastic interactions or inelastic interactions. As each of these results in a different outcome they will now be considered separately.

28.4.1 Elastic Collisions with the Nuclei

The electron has a relatively low mass and a negative charge, while the tungsten nucleus has a larger mass (about 334 000 times that of the electron) and a positive charge (74 times that of the electron). Thus the electron is attracted to the more massive tungsten nucleus.

As shown in Figure 28.2, the closer the electron travels to the nucleus, the more it is deflected from its original path by the attraction of the positive nucleus. Because the mass of the electron is so tiny compared to that of the nucleus, the amount of energy it transfers to it is proportionately small.

These events therefore serve only to produce very tortuous paths for the electrons within the tungsten, without transferring much energy to

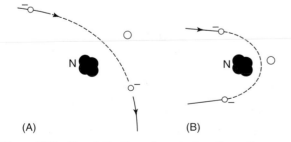

(A)   (B)

Figure 28.2   The deflection of an electron from the filament when it interacts with the nucleus of a target atom in the X-ray tube. (A) is a small deflection and (B) is a large deflection.

the tungsten. The number of such events compared to the number of inelastic collisions, discussed in the next section, increases with the atomic number of the target material and so they are very frequent in tungsten.

28.4.2 Inelastic Collisions with the Nuclei – Production of Bremsstrahlung Radiation

Classical physics concluded that when a charged particle changed its velocity this *always* resulted in the emission of electromagnetic radiation. However, we have already seen that this is not the case, as the electrons in the Bohr model of the atom are continuously changing their velocity (see Sect. 26.4). We have also seen in the previous section that electrons can undergo elastic collisions with the nucleus which result in no electromagnetic radiation being produced. As shown in Figure 28.2, the electron must accelerate towards the nucleus during its deflection but, despite this acceleration, a quantum of electromagnetic radiation is emitted in only a small percentage of cases. When such a quantum is emitted, the kinetic energy of the electron is suddenly reduced by an amount equal to the energy of the quantum, and so the electron is suddenly slowed down or *braked*.

This is an example of an inelastic interaction since the total kinetic energy of the electron and of the nucleus is not conserved because some energy is removed by the emission of the quantum of radiation. The energy of the quantum may be in the X-ray part of the electromagnetic spectrum and the radiation is known as *braking* or *Bremsstrahlung* radiation. The exact energy of this quantum will vary and may be very small if the electron does not lose much energy in its interaction with the nucleus or it may be up to the total kinetic energy of the electron if it is involved in a direct collision with the nucleus (see electron 2 in Figure 28.1).

Note that not every electron passing close to the nucleus will emit such a photon of radiation but only those which are able to undergo a sudden loss of energy by an inelastic interaction with the nucleus.

The Bremsstrahlung process is illustrated in Figure 28.3, where the X-ray photon is emitted at the point, and the electron continues with reduced energy on the pathway shown. The probability of Bremsstrahlung radiation being produced is very small (about 1–5% for diagnostic X-ray tubes). The intensity of the radiation produced is related to the atomic number of the target material (Z) and the energy of the electron beam (E) by the equation:

$$I \propto ZE^2 \qquad \qquad Equation\ 28.1$$

In diagnostic X-ray tubes, tungsten is used as the target material as its high atomic number (74) leads to a higher intensity of X-ray production.

The effect on the X-ray spectrum of changing the energy of the electron beam will be discussed in more detail in Chapter 29, but it is worth noting at this stage that the higher electron energies used in linear accelerators mean that there is more efficient X-ray production and that a smaller percentage of the energy is converted into heat.

If the law of Conservation of Momentum (see Sect. 5.4) is applied, then, in order to conserve momentum, the greater the energy of the incident electrons, the more likely the Bremsstrahlung radiation is to be emitted in the same direction as the electrons. Thus, for low-electron-energy beams the X-rays are directed almost isotropically, in diagnostic X-ray tubes (medium-energy range) the central ray of the X-ray beam is at right angles to the electron beam and in linear accelerators (high-energy range) the useful X-ray beam is transmitted forward through the anode in the same direction as the electrons.

28.5 INELASTIC COLLISIONS WITH THE ELECTRONS OF THE TARGET ATOMS – PRODUCTION OF CHARACTERISTIC RADIATION

As can be seen from Figure 28.1 (see route of electron 4), it is also possible for an electron from the filament to be involved in an inelastic collision with one of the orbital electrons of the target atoms. Such interactions are shown in more detail in Figure 28.4. Depending on the energy transferred to the orbital electron, such collisions may result in either excitation of the atom (Figure 28.4A) or ionisation of the atom (Figure 28.4B). For excitation to occur, the electron must be given sufficient energy to raise it to its new orbital, whereas for ionisation the

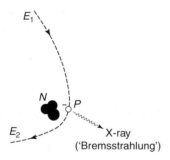

Figure 28.3 The production of Bremsstrahlung X-rays. An electron at point *P* suddenly loses energy by the emission of an X-ray photon. The electron continues with a reduced energy, E_2.

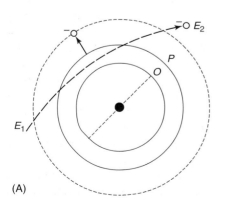

(A)

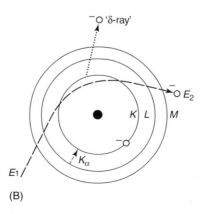

(B)

Figure 28.4 (A) Excitation and (B) ionisation caused by the passage of an energetic electron through a tungsten atom. Both processes result in the production of heat and ionisation produces characteristic radiation (K_α radiation is shown in the diagram). E_2 is less than E_1 in both diagrams. Note that, for clarity, only the electron orbitals that have a direct bearing on the interaction are shown.

electron must be given sufficient energy to overcome its binding energy and thus be liberated from the atom. In the case of ionisation of the target atom, the electron is ejected from its orbital with a given kinetic energy and is often referred to as a *delta-ray*. This electron may have sufficient energy to excite or ionise other atoms in its path.

The process of excitation or ionisation causes a vacancy in the electron shell involved – the K-shell in the atom shown in Figure 28.4B. This vacancy is quickly filled by one of the outer electrons undergoing a quantum jump downwards to fill the vacancy and emitting a quantum of electromagnetic radiation in the process. The energy of the quantum emitted is given by:

$$E = E_1 - E_2 \qquad \text{Equation 28.2}$$

where E_1 is the energy of the electron before the jump and E_2 is the energy of the electron after the jump. As this energy varies for the same transition in different materials it is known as *characteristic radiation* as it is characteristic of the material emitting the radiation.

If we consider Figure 28.5, where a vacancy has been created in the K-shell of the atom, then the most probable jump is from the L-shell with the next probability being a jump from the M-shell followed by the probability of a jump from the N-shell. These are known as K_α, K_β, K_γ transitions and the radiation known as K_α-characteristic radiation, etc. If we assume that the vacancy in the K-shell has been filled by a transition from the L-shell, there will now be a vacancy in this shell which can be filled from the M-shell or the N-shell, etc., with the emission of L_α- or L_β-characteristic radiation. In this way a cascade of electrons will occur, with each one emitting a photon of energy, given by Equation 28.2. In the diagnostic X-ray tube only the K- and L-characteristic radiations are of any significance as the others are absorbed by the target material or the insert envelope.

As well as the characteristic radiation produced, both excitation and ionisation result in the production of heat within the target. In *excitation* this is achieved by the absorption of energy by the target as the electron falls back to its original orbital, while in *ionisation* it is produced by the increased kinetic energy received by the tungsten atoms as they slow down the electrons ejected by the collision.

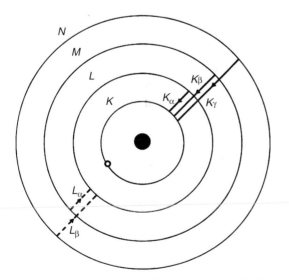

Figure 28.5 The production of characteristic radiation. The K-lines are formed by quantum jumps down to the K-shell. Also note that the energy of the K_α-line must be less than the binding energy of the K-shell. (The significance of this fact is discussed when photoelectric absorption edges are considered in Sect. 30.5.)

28.6 THE X-RAY SPECTRUM

So far in this chapter we have considered the production of X-ray quanta by two major mechanisms:

1. Energetic electrons from the filament interact with the nuclei of target atoms and are slowed down, thus giving off energy in the form of X-ray quanta – Bremsstrahlung radiation. As we mentioned earlier, the energy of the quantum may be very small if the interaction with the nucleus is small, or it may be up to the energy of the incoming electron if this electron is brought to rest by the nucleus. All energies between the two extremes are possible and so it can be seen that the Bremsstrahlung radiation will form a continuous spectrum (see Sect. 25.6)

2. Vacancies created in inner electron orbitals are filled by the electrons from orbitals further

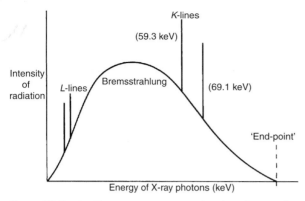

Figure 28.6 An X-ray spectrum as emitted at the anode of an X-ray tube with a tungsten target. (For an explanation of this spectrum, see the text.)

away from the nucleus making a quantum jump to fill the vacancy and giving off a photon of radiation in the process. This is the characteristic radiation from the atom. As the energy differences between specific orbitals is constant for an atom, this will take the form of a series of line spectra (see Sect. 25.6).

If the overall X-ray intensity is plotted against the energy of the radiation, a summation of the two effects, known as the *X-ray spectrum,* is produced. Such a spectrum produced at the tungsten target of an X-ray tube is shown in Figure 28.6.

Certain important features of this spectrum are worthy of further discussion:

- The energy of the Bremsstrahlung radiation is expressed in keV and lies somewhere between zero and a maximum value. This maximum photon energy is achieved if an electron which has the maximum kinetic energy gives up all its energy to form a single photon. The value of this photon for a specific beam may be deduced as follows. Suppose the potential difference across the X-ray tube is 100 kVp. An electron accelerated across the tube when the peak voltage is applied would have achieved a kinetic energy of 100 keV at its point of contact with the anode. If it now gives up all this energy as a single photon, the energy of the photon will be 100 keV and this will be the maximum photon energy for a tube operating at this kVp. Similarly, for an X-ray tube operating at 50 kVp the maximum photon energy will be

50 keV. Thus it can be seen that *the maximum photon energy is dependent on the potential difference across the tube (kVp) but is independent of the material of the target*

- The Bremsstrahlung radiation is a continuous spectrum. The intensity of the low-energy photons within this spectrum is decreased because of absorption of these photons by the target material; as will be seen in Chapter 29, the intensity is further decreased by the filtration of the X-ray beam before it leaves the tube

- The *average energy* of the X-ray beam is about one-third to one-half of its maximum energy – this is related to the *quality* of the X-ray beam (see Ch. 29)

- The total intensity of the beam – the *quantity* of the radiation – is given by the area under the curve

- The energies of the K, L, M, etc. lines are always in the same position, although the energy of lines from M onwards is so small that it is likely to be totally absorbed in the X-ray tube. These discrete energies form a line spectrum – the exact energy of the line is determined by Equation 28.2

- The line spectra will not be produced unless the energy of the electron beam from the filament exceeds the binding energy of the appropriate electron shell of the atom. To produce the K-characteristic lines at a tungsten target, electrons must have an energy >69 keV and to produce L-lines electrons must have an energy >11 keV. In practice this means that K-lines are not produced when the potential across the tube is less than 70 kVp.

In the spectrograph in Figure 28.6 we have considered the intensity of the radiation plotted against the photon energy. It is sometimes useful to calculate the wavelength of the radiation rather than know its photon energy. As you may remember from Section 25.3.2, the photon energy and its associated wavelength are related by Planck's equation (see Equation 25.6). From this we can see that the maximum photon energy corresponds to the minimum wavelength. Since the numerical value of the maximum photon energy is the same as the kVp, we can calculate the minimum wavelength from the equation:

$$\lambda_{min} = \frac{1.24}{kVp}$$ *Equation 28.3*

INSIGHT

Although we have explained the maximum and minimum energies in the continuous spectrum, we have not explained the shape – the distribution of energies – of the spectrum. This is quite a complicated process and involves consideration of the chances of photons of various energies being produced, the direction of the radiation emitted and the chances of this radiation being absorbed or scattered within the target.

Consider an ultra-thin target, which is constructed in such a way that there are only a few layers of target atoms and so incoming electrons from the filament are only likely to have one interaction and there is negligible attenuation by the target of the radiation produced. In such circumstances the number of photons of each energy produced will be related to the statistical chance of an electron losing that amount of energy in its Bremsstrahlung interaction with the nucleus. As the nucleus of the atom is relatively small compared with the whole atom, the chance of an electron from the filament colliding with it and so producing a maximum-energy photon, is equally small. The chance of a filament electron getting close to the nucleus is statistically larger and so there should be more photons produced which have less than the maximum energy compared with the number which have the maximum energy. Thus, as we increase the diameter of the circle around the nucleus within which we consider electrons interacting to produce X-ray photons, so we increase the statistical possibility of producing photons with that energy. As these electrons are further from the nucleus of the atom, the energy of the photon produced would be smaller.

The production of lower-energy photons is further increased in a target with a finite thickness if we still ignore any radiation attenuation by the target. A target of finite thickness – normally a few millimetres – can really be considered as a series of ultra-thin targets one on top of the other. Because of this, the energy of the electrons reaching the second ultra-thin layer is less due to

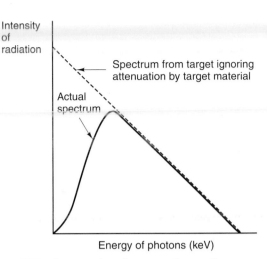

Figure 28.7 A comparison between the continuous spectrum produced if attenuation by the target material is ignored and the actual spectrum produced from a tube target.

their energy loss in the first layer – this again favours the production of lower-energy X-ray photons. Thus the deeper we go into the target, the lower the predicted energy of the photons produced.

Because of the two processes described, we would expect the number of photons produced to increase as the photon energy decreases. This is shown by the broken line in Figure 28.7.

In an X-ray tube the target is just a few millimetres thick so we must consider X-rays being produced below the surface of the target. As these photons leave the target they are attenuated by the target atoms. Both scattering and absorption (see Ch. 30) favour attenuation of the lower-energy photons. Thus lower-energy photons are heavily attenuated by the target atoms. The attenuation of the lower-energy photons is increased because they are more likely to be produced deeper in the target material and so have further to travel through the target. This attenuation of the photons produced by the target material produces a continuous spectrum similar to the solid line in Figure 28.7.

The effect of various parameters on the spectrum of radiation emitted from the X-ray tube will form the material of the next chapter.

SUMMARY

In this chapter you should have learnt:

- The three major mechanisms by which electrons from the filament of the X-ray tube may lose energy when they interact with the atoms of the target (see Sect. 28.2)
- The result of interactions between electrons from the filament of the X-ray tube and the outer electrons around atoms of the target material (see Sect. 28.3)
- The result of elastic interactions between electrons from the filament and the nuclei of atoms of the tube target (see Sect. 28.4.1)

- How inelastic collisions between electrons from the filament and the nuclei of atoms of the target of the X-ray tube result in the production of Bremsstrahlung radiation (see Sect. 28.4.2)
- How inelastic collisions between electrons from the filament and the orbital electrons of target atoms may result in the production of characteristic radiation (see Sect. 28.5)
- The graphical representation of the X-ray spectrum and the significant features of this graph (see Sect. 28.6).

SELF-TEST

a. With the aid of a diagram, identify the principal interactions which cause the electrons from the filament to lose energy when they interact with the target atoms of the X-ray tube.

b. Describe the mechanism by which Bremsstrahlung radiation is produced at the target of the X-ray tube.

c. Describe the production of characteristic radiation at the target of the X-ray tube and list the conditions necessary for characteristic radiation to be produced.

d. With the aid of a line graph, describe the X-ray spectrum produced at the target of an X-ray tube operating at 100 kVp. Give an equation to show the relationship between the minimum photon wavelength and the kVp across the X-ray tube.

FURTHER READING

You will find that Chapter 20 of this text deals in further detail with the factors that affect the spectrum of X-rays from the X-ray tube. In addition, you may find that the chapters from the following texts provide useful further reading:

Ball J L, Moore A D 1997 Essential physics for radiographers, 3rd edn. Blackwell Scientific Publications, London, ch 16

Bushong S C 2004 Radiologic science for technologists: physics, biology and protection. Mosby, New York, chs 11 and 12

Curry T S III, Dowdey J E, Murry R C Jr 1990 Christensen's physics of diagnostic radiography, 4th edn. Lee & Febiger, London, ch 2

Dendy P P, Heaton B 1999 Physics for diagnostic radiology, 2nd edn. Institute of Physics Publishing, ch 2

Dowsett D J, Kenny P A, Johnston R E 1998 The physics of diagnostic imaging, Chapman & Hall Medical, London, ch 3

Webb S (ed) 2000 The physics of medical imaging, 2nd edn. Institute of Physics Publishing, Bristol, ch 2

Chapter 29

Factors Affecting X-ray Beam Quality and Quantity

CHAPTER CONTENTS

29.1 Aim   277

29.2 Introduction   277

29.3 The Effect of mA on the X-ray Beam   278

29.4 The Effect of kVp on the X-ray Beam   278

29.5 The Effect of the Target Material on the X-ray Beam   279

29.6 The Effect of Rectification on the X-ray Beam   279

29.7 The Effect of Filtration on the X-ray Beam   280

29.8 Summary of the Factors Affecting the Quantity, Quality and Intensity of the X-ray Beam   282

Self-Test   283

Further Reading   283

29.1 AIM

The aim of this chapter is to consider the various factors that have an influence on the quantity and/or the quality of the beam of radiation from the X-ray tube.

29.2 INTRODUCTION

In Chapter 28 we considered the mechanisms by which X-rays were produced at the anode of the X-ray tube. In this chapter we will consider the various factors that influence the *quantity* and/or the *quality* of the X-ray beam and hence its *intensity* at a given point. Before we look at this in any more detail, it is first important to ensure that we understand the meaning of the terms *quantity, quality* and *intensity* as applied to a beam of X radiation.

DEFINITIONS

The *quantity* of radiation in an X-ray beam is a measure of the number of photons in the beam. The terms *quantity* and *exposure* are often interchanged in radiography as the higher the quantity or amount of radiation, the greater the exposure to a structure. In fact, probably the simplest method of comparing the quantity of two beams of radiation is to compare the exposure received by a structure. As we shall see in Chapter 33, the exposure is measured using the unit of *air kerma*. As the quantity of radiation increases, so does the *intensity* of the beam.

The *quality* of a beam of X-rays is a measure of its penetrating power. As we saw in Section 28.6, the quality of the beam is related to its average photon energy. In Sections 4.7 and 4.8 we saw that a monochromatic beam of radiation is exponentially absorbed by a uniform medium and so the penetrating power of two beams may be compared by comparing their half-value thickness – the higher the value of the half-value thickness, the more penetrating the beam. Although the beam of X-rays from the tube is not monochromatic, but has a continuous spectrum over a wide range of energies, the half-value layer is a useful way of comparing the penetrating power of X-ray beams.

However, changing the quality of the radiation beam also affects the *intensity* of the beam. For a given quantity of radiation, the higher the quality of the radiation, the greater the intensity of the radiation beam.

The *intensity* of a beam of X radiation is defined as the total amount of energy – measured at right angles to the direction of the beam – passing through unit area in unit time. Although measured in units of joules per metre squared per second, in radiography we tend to use one of its effects – the ionisation of air or of *air kerma* – as a measurement of radiation beam intensity.

As can be seen from the definitions of quantity and quality, any factors that change the quantity or the quality of the radiation beam will bring about a change in the beam's intensity.

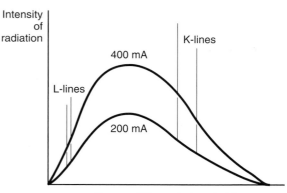

Figure 29.1   The effect of the mA on the X-ray spectrum. *Note* that the *quantity* of the radiation changes – as shown by the alteration of the area under each curve – but the *quality* of the radiation is unaltered – as shown by the maximum photon energy and the peak photon energy being at the same energy for each graph. Thus we can say that the mA selected for an exposure affects the quantity of the X-ray beam but does not affect the quality of the beam – an increase in the mA will produce an increase in the quantity of radiation from the target.

that the quantity of the X-ray beam per unit time (or the beam intensity) is directly proportional to the mA through the tube.

$$I \propto mA \qquad\qquad \textit{Equation 29.1}$$

The effect on the X-ray beam of altering the mA is shown in Figure 29.1. Note that the area under the graph for 200 mA is half the area under the graph for 400 mA. The maximum photon energy and the minimum photon energy are the same in each case and the average photon energy remains unaltered.

29.3 THE EFFECT OF MA ON THE X-RAY BEAM

If the current through the X-ray tube (mA) is, for example, doubled, the number of electrons flowing across the tube in unit time is doubled. If all the other factors remain unchanged, each electron will have the same chance of creating X-ray photons and so the number of photons of each energy produced per unit time will be doubled. If the mA is halved, the same argument can be used to show that the number of X-ray photons of each energy is also halved. Thus we can say

29.4 THE EFFECT OF KVP ON THE X-RAY BEAM

The kVp across the X-ray tube influences the force of attraction experienced by an electron released by the filament as it moves towards the anode. Thus, if the kVp is increased, then the kinetic energy of the electron at the point when it starts to interact with the target will be increased. As we saw in Section 28.4.2, the efficiency of X-ray production by Bremsstrahlung is proportional to E^2 and so this improved efficiency means that:

$$I \propto kVp^2 \qquad \textit{Equation 29.2}$$

As we already discussed in Section 28.4.2, increasing the kVp will also increase the energy of the maximum-energy photons in the beam – if the kVp is 50, then the maximum photon energy is 50 keV and if the kVp is 100, then the maximum photon energy is 100 keV. As the average photon energy is approximately 30–50% of the maximum photon energy, increasing the maximum photon energy will also increase the average photon energy.

As mentioned earlier, increasing the kVp will increase the kinetic energy of the electrons from the filament when they reach the target and so this may mean that characteristic radiation is seen on the higher kVp spectrum but not at the lower value – at 100 kVp the electrons reaching the target have energies up to 100 keV and so can displace K-shell electrons in tungsten, whereas at 50 kVp the 50-keV electrons have insufficient energy to displace a K-shell electron from the tungsten atom.

The spectrum produced at 100 kVp and at 50 kVp is shown in Figure 29.2, where the changes mentioned above can be identified.

Thus we can say that the kVp selected for an exposure affects both the quantity and the quality of the X-ray beam produced – an increase in kVp will produce an increase in the quantity and the quality of the radiation from the target.

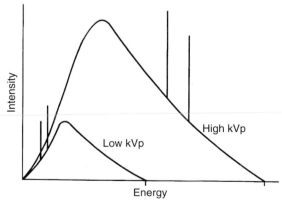

Figure 29.2   The effect of kVp on the X-ray spectrum. *Note* that the kVp affects both the *quantity* and the *quality* of the radiation beam. Also note that the lower of the two curves is unable to produce K-characteristic radiation, although both curves can produce L-lines.

29.5 THE EFFECT OF THE TARGET MATERIAL ON THE X-RAY BEAM

As mentioned in Section 28.4.2, the atomic number of the target material has an effect on the X-ray beam from the tube. The higher the atomic number of the target material, the more positive the nucleus of the target atom and so the more it attracts the electrons from the filament which pass close to it. Thus the production of X-rays by the Bremsstrahlung process is more efficient and the intensity of the beam is increased. The maximum and minimum photon energies in the beam are not affected by the target material.

The target material also affects the characteristic radiation produced. The energies of the characteristic radiations from a tungsten and a molybdenum target are shown in Table 29.1.

Thus, although the target material does not affect the quality of the Bremsstrahlung radiation, it does affect the energy of the characteristic radiation and this does have some effect on the overall quality of the X-ray beam – this effect may be enhanced by filtering the radiation with the same material as the target (this will be considered further in Ch. 30 when absorption mechanisms are discussed).

The radiation spectra from a tungsten and a molybdenum target are shown in Figure 29.3.

29.6 THE EFFECT OF RECTIFICATION ON THE X-RAY BEAM

The type of high-tension rectification of the X-ray generator affects the spectrum of radiation

Table 29.1   Comparison of characteristic radiation energies produced from a tungsten target and a molybdenum target

	Energy of K_α characteristic radiation (keV)	Energy of L_α characteristic radiation (keV)
Tungsten	59.32	8.39
Molybdenum	17.48	2.22

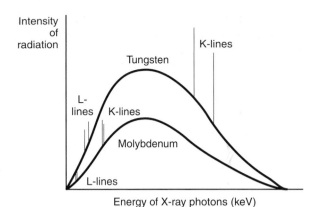

Figure 29.3 The effect of the target material on the X-ray spectrum. *Note* that the lower atomic number of molybdenum means that there is a reduction in the *quantity* of the radiation but the *quality* of the Bremsstrahlung radiation is not affected. The *characteristic radiation* is at a lower photon energy for the target with the lower atomic number.

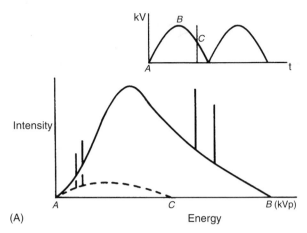

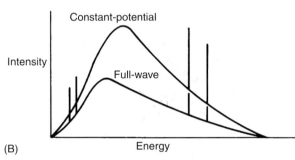

Figure 29.4 (A) The spectrum of radiation produced with a single-phase two-pulse rectified waveform as kVp values *B* and *C* are applied across the X-ray tube. (B) The effect of rectification on the X-ray spectrum where the constant potential generator produces radiation of higher *quantity* and higher *quality*.

produced at the target of the X-ray tube. This is because of the changing energy of the electron beam striking the target each half-cycle. If we consider full-wave rectification with no capacitor smoothing, as produced by the two-pulse generator (see Sect. 19.4), then the potential across the tube varies from zero to the kVp each half-cycle. Thus the energy of the electrons striking the target varies from zero to a keV with a numerical value equal to that of the kVp. The maximum photon energy at differing stages in the half-cycle will vary across the same range as the electron energies.

We can see how this affects the spectrum produced if we consider Figure 29.4A and consider the spectra produced at point *B* in the voltage waveform and at point *C*. The time-averaged spectrum for full-wave rectification is shown in Figure 29.4B. Now consider a constant potential being applied to the X-ray tube during the entire exposure. This would be the same as if voltage *B* is applied for the whole exposure, and so the spectrum for voltage *B* is labelled in Figure 29.4B as the spectrum from a constant-potential unit. Note that, for constant potential, the area under the graph is increased and the value of the photon energy of the average photon is also increased – the graph for a medium frequency

generator is almost identical to that for the constant potential generator.

Thus we can say that the rectification – or the type of X-ray generator – affects both the quantity and the quality of the X-ray beam produced. The nearer the voltage across the tube is to a constant potential, the higher the quantity and the quality of the radiation produced at the target.

29.7 THE EFFECT OF FILTRATION ON THE X-RAY BEAM

In all the discussion so far we have considered the beam of X radiation produced at the target of the X-ray tube. Before this radiation can be utilised in radiography or radiotherapy, it must first leave the tube. In leaving the tube the radiation beam must first pass through the glass of the tube insert, the oil in the housing and finally the window of the housing – plus any additional filtration – and it is filtered at each stage of this process. Thus, to consider the beam which will interact with the patient, we need to consider the effect of filtration on the spectrum of radiation produced at the tube target.

Spectrum A in Figure 29.5 shows the distribution of energies emitted from the tube target. This would be the spectrum of the radiation before it leaves the glass envelope of the tube. As we will discuss in Chapter 30, when a beam of radiation passes through any medium, the beam is attenuated by the processes of absorption and scattering. We will see that the lower the photon energy, the higher the chance of it being absorbed or scattered. So the passage of the X-ray beam through the glass envelope, the oil and the exit window of the shield results in selective attenuation of the lower-energy photons. Since this filtration is inherent to the tube construction, it is known as the *inherent filtration* of the X-ray tube. The spectrum emitted after the inherent filtration is shown as spectrum B in Figure 29.5.

This beam still contains a significant number of low-energy photons. If these were allowed to interact with the tissues of a patient, they would be absorbed by superficial tissues and so would contribute to the patient dose but would make no contribution to the radiograph – or to the tumour treatment in the case of radiotherapy. The amount of low-energy photons in the spectrum can be significantly reduced by incorporating additional filtration into the beam, near the exit port of the tube, before it interacts with the patient's tissues. Such a spectrum is shown as line C in Figure 29.5. The inherent filtration of diagnostic X-ray tubes is usually expressed in *millimetres of aluminium-equivalent*, i.e. the inherent filtration is equivalent to the filtration of the beam achieved by the stated number of millimetres of aluminium. The inherent filtration of most diagnostic X-ray tubes is between 0.5 and 1.0 mm of aluminium-equivalent. The total filtration in the beam is the sum of the inherent filtration and the additional filtration. This total filtration is between 1.5 and 2.5 mm depending upon the maximum kVp at which the tube is designed to operate.

As can be seen from Figure 29.5, filtration affects both the quantity and the quality of the X-ray beam – the greater the thickness of the filtration in the X-ray beam, the less the quantity but the greater the quality of the X-ray beam emerging from the X-ray tube.

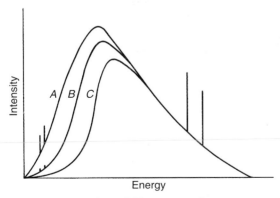

Figure 29.5 The effect of filtration on the X-ray spectrum. Line *A* represents the spectrum produced at the target of the X-ray tube; line *B* shows how this spectrum is modified because of the inherent filtration of the tube; and line *C* shows how the spectrum is modified because of the total filtration. Note that filtration causes a reduction in the *quantity* of the radiation but an increase in the *quality*.

INSIGHT

Aluminium has a low atomic number (13) and so is able to absorb many of the low-energy X-ray photons in a beam of diagnostic energy, by photoelectric absorption (see Ch. 30). High-energy X-ray photons have a low probability of being absorbed or scattered by the aluminium and so are relatively unaffected by the filtration. This makes aluminium the ideal material for filtration of diagnostic energy X-ray beams.

The radiation beam from the therapy X-ray tube has a much higher average energy than the diagnostic beam. This beam is often hardened – low-energy radiations are removed – by the use of a composite filter. An example of this is when the beam is first filtered through copper ($Z = 29$) and

Table 29.2 Factors affecting the quantity and quality of the X-ray beam

Factor	Effect on the quantity of the X-ray beam	Effect on the quality of the X-ray beam
Increase in the tube current (mA)	Produces an increase in the quantity of radiation directly proportional to the increase in mA	The quality of the radiation from the tube is unaffected by the tube current
Increase in the potential difference (kVp) across the X-ray tube	An increase in kVp produces an increase in the quantity of radiation produced at the target proportional to the kVp^2	An increase in the kVp produces an increase in the average energy of the photons in the X-ray beam and an increase in beam quality
Target material	An increase in the atomic number of the target material will produce an increase in the quantity of radiation produced which is directly proportional to the change in the atomic number	A change in the atomic number will produce no change in the quantity of the beam produced by the Bremsstrahlung process. A higher atomic number will produce characteristic radiation of higher energy and, if this is in significant amounts, it may increase the quantity of the overall spectrum
Rectification	The closer the voltage waveform across the X-ray tube is to a constant potential, the greater the quantity of radiation produced	The closer the voltage waveform across the X-ray tube is to a constant potential, the greater the quality of radiation produced
Filtration	Filtration reduces the quantity of radiation emerging from the X-ray tube. The reduction is related to the thickness and the atomic number of the filter	Filtration improves the quality of radiation from an X-ray tube by the selective removal of low-energy photons

then is further filtered through an aluminium filter. The copper is responsible for the initial filtration but transmits some low-energy radiation due to the photoelectric absorption edge of copper. The copper also produces low-energy characteristic radiation as a result of photoelectric absorption in the copper atoms. The function of the aluminium filter is to absorb the radiation transmitted through the copper because of the K-shell photoelectric absorption edge of copper and also to remove the characteristic radiation produced by the photoelectric absorption in the copper. These concepts will be further discussed in the next chapter.

29.8 SUMMARY OF THE FACTORS AFFECTING THE QUANTITY, QUALITY AND INTENSITY OF THE X-RAY BEAM

The factors which affect the quantity and/or quality of the beam of X-radiation emerging from an X-ray tube are summarised in Table 29.2.

SUMMARY

In this chapter you should have learnt:

- The meaning of the terms *quantity* and *quality* as applied to the X-ray beam (see Sect. 29.2)
- The effect of the current through the X-ray tube (mA) on the quantity of the X-ray beam produced (see Sect. 29.3)
- The effect of the potential difference across the X-ray tube (kVp) on the quantity and the quality of the X-ray beam produced (see Sect. 29.4)
- The effect of the atomic number of the target material on the quantity of the radiation produced and on the characteristic radiation from the target (see Sect. 29.5)
- The effect of the voltage waveform applied to the X-ray tube (rectification) on the quantity and the quality of the X-ray beam produced (see Sect. 29.6)
- The effect of filtration on the quantity and the quality of the radiation beam emerging from the X-ray tube (see Sect. 29.7).

SELF-TEST

a. What is meant by the terms *quantity* and *quality* when used to describe an X-ray beam?

b. With the aid of a graph, discuss the effect of the tube current (mA) on the spectrum of radiation from the X-ray tube.

c. With the aid of a graph, discuss the effect of the potential difference across the X-ray tube (kVp) on the spectrum of radiation from the tube.

d. With the aid of a graph, discuss the effect of the target material on the spectrum of radiation from the tube.

e. With the aid of a graph, discuss the effect of the high-tension rectification on the spectrum of radiation from the tube.

f. With the aid of a graph, discuss the effect of filtration on the spectrum of radiation from the tube.

FURTHER READING

Ball J L, Moore A D 1997 Essential physics for radiographers, 3rd edn. Blackwell Scientific Publications, London, ch 16

Carter P H 1994 Chesney's equipment for student radiographers, 4th edn. Blackwell Publishing, London, chs 2 and 3

Curry T S III, Dowdey J E, Murry R C Jr 1990 Christensen's physics of diagnostic radiography, 4th edn. Lee & Febiger, London, ch 2

Johns H E, Cunningham J R 1983 The physics of radiology, 4th edn. Charles C Thomas, Illinois, USA, ch 2

Webb S (ed) 2000 The physics of medical imaging, 2nd edn. Institute of Physics Publishing, Bristol, ch 2

Chapter 30

Interactions of X-rays with Matter

CHAPTER CONTENTS

30.1 Aim   284

30.2 Outline of Possible Interactions   284
   30.2.1 Probability and Cross-Sections   285
   30.2.2 The Total Linear Attenuation Coefficient (μ)   286
   30.2.3 The Total Mass Attenuation Coefficient (μ/ρ)   286

30.3 Attenuation and Absorption   287

30.4 Elastic (Coherent) Scattering   287

30.5 Photoelectric Absorption   289
   30.5.1 Photoelectric Absorption, Attenuation and Absorption Coefficients   290

30.6 Compton Scattering   291
   30.6.1 Compton Attenuation, Absorption and Scatter Coefficients   292

30.7 Pair Production   293
   30.7.1 Attenuation, Absorption and Scatter Coefficients for Pair Production   294

30.8 Relative Importance of the Attenuation Processes in Radiography   294

30.9 Conclusion   296

Self-Test   297

Further Reading   297

30.1 AIM

The aim of this chapter is to introduce the reader to the interaction processes that may occur when radiation photons interact with matter. The factors that influence such interaction processes will be discussed. An understanding of the processes is important for consideration of both the production of the radiograph and of the biological effects of radiation on tissue.

30.2 OUTLINE OF POSSIBLE INTERACTIONS

When a beam of X-rays interacts with a medium, e.g. an area of patient tissue, there are a number of possible interactions between the photons and the atoms of the medium. These are outlined in Figure 30.1. If we consider photon *A*, we can see that this interacts with an atom of the medium and is deflected from its path – this deflection may or may not be accompanied by a loss of photon energy. This process is known as *scattering*. Photon *B*, on the other hand, interacts with an atom of the medium and loses all of its energy to the atom. This process is known as *absorption*. The third photon, photon *C*, passes through the material without interacting with any of the atoms. If we measure the intensity of the radiation in a given area before it interacts with the medium and again in a similar area after the interactions, we find that there is a lower intensity of radiation after passing through the medium – *the beam of radiation has been attenuated* (see Sect. 4.7).

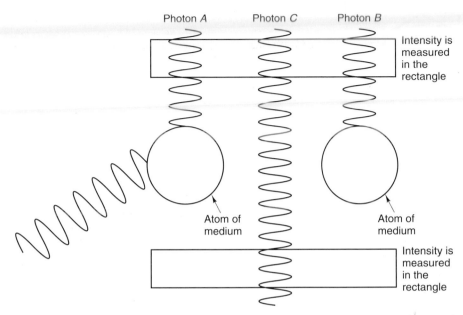

Figure 30.1 Mechanisms of interaction of X-ray photons with matter. Photon *A* is scattered, photon *B* is absorbed and photon *C* is transmitted. *Note* that the number of photons passing through the lower rectangle is less than the number passing through the upper rectangle and so attenuation has taken place.

Thus we can say:

When a beam of radiation passes through a medium it is attenuated by the processes of absorption and scattering.

The reactions considered above involve an interaction between a photon and an orbiting electron rather than between a photon and the nucleus of the atom (this will be discussed in more detail in the rest of this chapter) and so, for an interaction to occur, a photon must pass close to the electron orbiting the atom with which it is capable of interacting. Thus we can consider the atoms in a medium as targets which, if hit, will attenuate a photon from the primary radiation beam.

30.2.1 Probability and Cross-Sections

The probability of an X-ray photon interacting with a *particular atom* is low, but the very large number of atoms in even a small volume of a solid substance makes the probability of a photon interacting with *some atom* much greater. In Figure 30.2, a beam of X-rays of area *A* is incident upon a medium whose atoms appear to the beam

each to have an area of *a*. This area is called the cross-section of the atom to a particular type of radiation, a typical area being 1.5×10^{-28} m^2. If an X-ray photon hits one of the atoms, it is either absorbed or scattered from the primary beam.

Note that the area *a* is not the true size of the atom but is the apparent area of the atom likely to interact with the X-ray beam. The value of *a* depends on a number of things, including the atomic number of the material and the energy of the X-ray photon.

The probability of an interaction occurring can be predicted by dividing the total area of the atoms within the irradiated area by the size of this area. If we consider Figure 30.2 and take it that there are *N* atoms per unit volume of the material, then the number of atoms in the irradiated cylinder of cross-sectional area *A* is $N \times A \times x$. Thus the total area of the atoms in the irradiated area is $a(N \times Ax)$ or $aNAx$.

The probability of an interaction

$$= \frac{aNAx}{A}$$

$$= aNx \qquad \qquad Equation\ 30.1$$

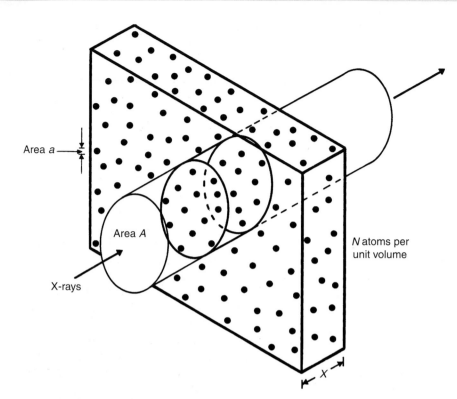

Figure 30.2   Consideration of the area of individual atoms as part of the total irradiated area. If any of the X-ray photons passing through area A hits an atom (area a) then the photon is removed from the beam. As fewer photons will exit from the medium than entered the same area, the beam is said to be attenuated. For further explanation, see the text.

Area a

Area A

X-rays

N atoms per unit volume

x

30.2.2 The Total Linear Attenuation Coefficient (μ)

As we discussed in Section 4.7, a parallel beam of monoenergetic radiation will undergo exponential attenuation as it passes through a uniform medium. The intensity of the incident beam (I_0) and the intensity after a thickness x are given by the equation:

$$I_x = I_0 e^{-\mu x}$$ *Equation 30.2*

where μ is the total linear attenuation coefficient. If we now consider Equations 30.1 and 30.2, it can be seen that, as the probability of an interaction increases (aNx), the linear attenuation coefficient (μ) will also increase. The total linear coefficient may be defined:

DEFINITION

The total *linear attenuation coefficient*, μ, is the fraction of the X-rays removed from a beam per unit thickness of the attenuating medium.

30.2.3 The Total Mass Attenuation Coefficient (μ/ρ)

As we have seen from Equation 30.1, the probability of an interaction between an X-ray photon and a medium containing N atoms is proportional to N. If we consider the medium shown in Figure 30.2 and take a situation where it is heated until it has expanded to a thickness of $2x$, then the number of atoms in the thickness x will be $N/2$ and the linear attenuation coefficient (μ) will also be halved. As the number of atoms per unit volume has halved, the density of the material (ρ) will also have halved. However, the ratio μ/ρ will be the same in both cases. This ratio μ/ρ is known as the *total mass attenuation coefficient* and is defined:

DEFINITION

The *total mass attenuation coefficient*, μ/ρ, is the fraction of the X-rays removed from a beam of unit cross-sectional area by unit mass of the medium.

INSIGHT

Note the use of the term *total* in both of the above coefficients. This is because there is a mass attenuation coefficient due to each of the attenuation processes and so the total linear attenuation coefficient is the sum of the individual linear attenuation coefficients and the total mass attenuation coefficient is the sum of the individual mass attenuation coefficients. Thus:

$$\mu = \tau + \sigma + \pi \qquad \textit{Equation 30.3}$$

where μ is the total linear attenuation coefficient, τ is the linear attenuation coefficient due to the photoelectric effect, σ is the linear attenuation coefficient due to Compton scattering and π is the linear atttenuation coefficient due to pair production. Similarly:

$$\frac{\mu}{\rho} = \frac{\tau}{\rho} + \frac{\sigma}{\rho} + \frac{\pi}{\rho} \qquad \textit{Equation 30.4}$$

where μ/ρ is the total mass attenuation coefficient, τ/ρ is the mass attenuation coefficient due to the photoelectric effect, σ/ρ is the mass attenuation coefficient due to Compton scattering and π/ρ is the mass attenuation coefficient due to pair production.

If we wish to calculate the amount of radiation which would pass through a given *length* of a material, then we would use the linear attenuation coefficient. In most other cases the mass attenuation coefficient would be used as this is unaffected by the state of the medium: it may be solid, liquid or gas as long as the changes in density are taken into account. Thus, if we wish to consider the effect of a change, for instance, of photon energy on the transmitted beam, this type of calculation would be undertaken using the mass attenuation coefficient.

The following sections of this chapter will consider the effect on the mass attenuation coefficient of the different types of X-ray inter-actions and of different attenuating materials. An understanding of these is fundamental to a consideration of the formation of the radiograph (see Ch. 32).

30.3 ATTENUATION AND ABSORPTION

The four interaction processes described in the rest of this chapter involve *attenuation* since the intensity of the primary X-ray beam is reduced as a result of each process. In some of the processes, energy is transferred from the photons in the X-ray beam to the atoms of the medium and so *absorption* is said to have taken place. Thus an absorption process must involve the transfer of energy from the photons to the atoms of the material.

In other processes, the photon is deflected from its original path and so is said to be *scattered*. This may involve no transfer of energy to the medium (see coherent or elastic scatter, Sect. 30.4) or it may involve deflection of the photon and a transfer of energy to the medium (see Compton scattering, Sect. 30.6).

As we have already noted, attenuation con-sists of both absorption and scattering and the contribution of each of the individual processes to the whole is shown in Table 30.1.

As can be seen from the table, the *total mass absorption coefficient* will be composed of the mass absorption coefficients from each of the attenua-tion processes. This may be defined as follows:

DEFINITION

The *total mass absorption coefficient* is the fraction of the energy contained in the X-ray beam which is absorbed per unit mass of the irradiated medium.

30.4 ELASTIC (COHERENT) SCATTERING

When the energy of a photon is considerably less than the binding energies of orbiting electrons of the atoms of the attenuator, the photon may be deflected from its path with no loss of energy after it has interacted with one of the electrons. This process is known as *elastic* scattering or *coherent* scattering (sometimes also known as *classical scattering* or *Rayleigh scattering*).

Table 30.1   Contribution of each of the attenuation processes to absorption and scatter

Process	Description of interactions	Effect of Z, E	Comments
Elastic scattering	Photon interacts with bound atomic electron. Photon energy is less than the electron-binding energy. Photon is re-radiated from the material with no energy loss	$\sigma_{coh}/\rho \propto Z^2E$	No energy absorption in the medium. Photon scattered in the forward direction. Effect is neglible in biological tissues because of low Z
Photoelectric absorption	Photon of energy ≥ the binding energy of an electron interacts with bound electron and ejects it from its orbital. Photon disappears as all its energy is absorbed by the electron. Kinetic energy of the electron = E-binding energy. Atom recoils, conserving momentum	$\tau/\rho \propto Z^3/E^3$	Ejected electron loses velocity to surrounding atoms, giving energy to them, i.e. absorption takes place. The electron vacancy created is filled by electrons making quantum jumps and so characteristic radiation is emitted
Compton scattering	Photon behaves like a particle and collides with a free electron. Energy of the incident photon is shared between the electron and the scattered photon	$\sigma/\rho \propto$ electron density/E	Energy of the displaced electron is absorbed by the medium, so Compton process produces attenuation and partial absorption. Electron densities of all materials except hydrogen are similar and so σ/ρ values are largely independent of the type of attenuator
Pair production	Photon of energy ≥1.02 MeV may spontaneously disappear in the vicinity of the nucleus of an attenuator atom, producing an electron and a positron. Atom recoils and preserves momentum. Positron eventually annihilated with an electron to form two photons of annihilation radiation, each with energy of 0.51 MeV	$\pi/\rho \propto (E - 1.02)Z$	Probability of pair production increases with E above 1.02 MeV. Contribution of πs is very small compared to π and is often ignored (see Sect. 30.7.1)

In this process the incoming photon interacts with an electron and raises its energy but does not give it sufficient energy to become excited or ionised. The electron then returns to its previous energy level by the emission of a photon which is equal in energy to the incoming photon but is in a different direction, hence scattering has occurred. The photon is scattered predominantly in the forward direction, because elastic scattering cannot occur if the recoil experienced by the atom as a whole during the scattering process is sufficient to produce excitation or ionisation. There is no absorption since no energy has been given permanently to the material and the attenuation, although present, is small since the majority of the photons are only scattered through a small angle. This is particularly so if the energy of the photon is higher than 100 eV and the atomic number of the attenuator is relatively low. The factors affecting the mass attenuation coefficient due to elastic scattering are shown in Equation 30.5.

$$\frac{\sigma_{coh}}{\rho} \propto \frac{Z^2}{E} \qquad \textit{Equation 30.5}$$

where σ_{coh}/ρ is the mass attenuation coefficient due to elastic scattering, Z is the atomic number of the attenuator and E is the photon energy.

In medical radiography, the effect of elastic scattering can be largely ignored since the average atomic number of tissue is low (approximately 7.4) and the photon energy is too high to allow significant elastic scatter.

Elastic scattering may occur as a result of a photon interacting with the nucleus of an atom of the attenuator but the effect is even less and so may safely be ignored in medical radiography.

INSIGHT

In X-ray diffraction studies of crystals it is the elastic scattering that is responsible for the coherent 'reflections' from the various atomic planes within the crystal lattice. Low-energy, monoenergetic X-rays are used for this purpose but only a small percentage are able to take part in the elastic scattering process.

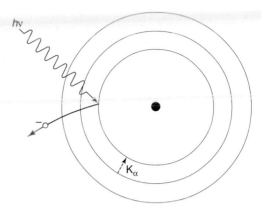

Figure 30.3 The process of photoelectric absorption and the subsequent emission of a quantum of characteristic radiation. The incoming photon (h_v) is absorbed by the K-shell electron, which is then displaced from that shell. The vacancy is filled from the L-shell with the emission of K_a-characteristic radiation.

30.5 PHOTOELECTRIC ABSORPTION

The previous section has shown that elastic scattering has little significance for radiography except at extremely low photon energies. The process of photoelectric absorption, which we will now discuss, is important even at very low energies and continues to be important at the photon energies found in the typical X-ray spectrum for diagnostic radiography.

In photoelectric absorption, the X-ray photon is involved in an *inelastic* collision with an orbiting electron of an atom of the absorber. The photon gives up all its energy to the electron (and thus disappears) and the electron is ejected from the atom. As ejection of the electron from the atom is a necessary part of the process, photoelectric absorption can only take place if the photon energy is equal to, or greater than, the binding energy of the electron.

The process of photoelectric absorption is shown schematically in Figure 30.3, where it is assumed that the X-ray photon of energy hv ejects an electron from the K-shell of the atom. Some of the energy of the photon is used in overcoming the binding energy of the electron and the rest is given to the electron as kinetic energy. If we assume that the electron has a binding energy of B, then the kinetic energy after ejection (it is then referred to as *a photoelectron*) is ($hv - B$). The vacancy thus created in the K-shell will be filled by electrons in orbitals further from the nucleus performing a series of quantum jumps downwards, producing characteristic radiation (see Sect. 28.5) and the possible emission of Auger electrons (see Sect. 27.6.3) from orbitals further out from the nucleus. As

you may remember from Section 28.5, the energy of the characteristic radiation is equal to the difference in energy of the electron before and after the quantum jump. In the case of X-ray photons interacting with atoms of body tissue, this energy difference is very small (normally between 1.2×10^{-2} and 1.8×10^{-2} eV) and so is in the infrared part of the electromagnetic spectrum.

The probability of a photoelectric interaction occurring at a particular shell depends on the binding energy of the electrons in the shell and the energy of the incoming photon. The probability is zero when the energy of the photon is less than the binding energy of the electron; it is greatest when the photon energy is equal to the binding energy and thereafter decreases rapidly with increasing photon energy. A graph of the mass absorption coefficient for photoelectric absorption in lead is shown in Figure 30.4 to illustrate these points.

The outer orbital shells of the atom are affected by the lower photon energies, only to have a reducing absorption as the photon energy increases. When the photon energy reaches the binding energy of the orbital then electrons in that orbital can take part in photoelectric absorption, thus producing a sudden increase in the amount of absorption. Such an increase is shown for the K-shell electrons of the lead atom in

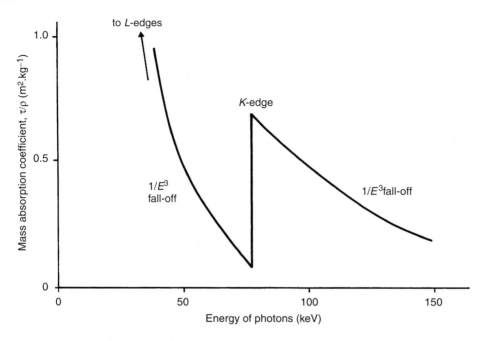

Figure 30.4 The mass absorption coefficient for the photoelectric effect in lead and its variation with photon energy.

Figure 30.4. This sudden increase is known as an *absorption edge* and so Figure 30.4 shows the K absorption edge for the lead atom. Between the absorption edges the mass attenuation coefficient due to the photoelectric effect (τ/ρ) is approximately proportional to $1/E^3$.

30.5.1 Photoelectric Absorption, Attenuation and Absorption Coefficients

The mass attenuation coefficient for the photoelectric effect (τ/ρ) is related to the atomic number (Z) of the absorber and the photon energy of the radiation (E). A very approximate guide to this relationship is given by the equation:

$$\frac{\tau}{\rho} \propto \frac{Z^3}{E^3} \qquad \text{Equation 30.6}$$

This equation applies to energies up to about 200 keV. At higher energies the E^3 term approximates to E^2 and eventually to E.

In photoelectric absorption, the X-ray beam is both attenuated and absorbed since individual photons are removed from the beam (attenuation) and energy is imparted to the absorbing medium (absorption). The absorbed energy is composed of the following parts:

- kinetic energy of the ejected photoelectron
- energy of recoil of the absorbing atom
- the energy of the photons of characteristic radiation and Auger electrons.

The ejected photoelectron is quickly brought to rest by the surrounding atoms and delivers its energy to them in the process. A similar thing happens with the Auger electrons. It is possible, however, for the characteristic radiation to escape from the absorber, especially if the energy of the characteristic radiation is high and it is produced near the surface of the absorber. In such cases, the *mass absorption coefficient* is slightly less than the *mass attenuation coefficient* since not all of the energy of the original photon has been absorbed by the medium. For this difference to be significant, the characteristic radiation must have high photon energy. The effect is thus only important in materials with high atomic numbers. As most of the atoms which make up body tissues have low atomic numbers, it may be considered that the mass absorption coefficient and the mass attenuation coefficient are equal for photoelectric absorption in practical radiography.

When we consider the absorption of X-ray photons to produce a radiographic image we need to look at the linear attenuation coefficient.

From Equation 30.6 we can see that, for the photoelectric effect at a given photon energy, this is proportional to the density of the absorber and its atomic number cubed. Bone is approximately twice as dense as soft tissue and its atomic number is also approximately twice that of soft tissue. For these reasons, the linear attenuation coefficient for photoelectric absorption for bone is approximately 16 times that of soft tissue (or, put another way, soft tissue will transmit 16 times as much radiation as bone). As the blackening (or optical density) on a radiograph is proportional to the radiation dose it receives, this explains why bones appear lighter than the same thickness of soft tissue.

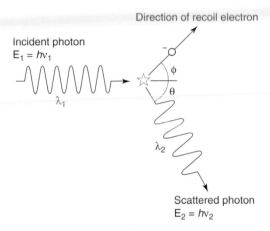

Figure 30.5 The process of Compton scattering. The scattered photon has less energy than the incident photon and may be scattered through any angle. The recoil electron is always scattered in a 'forward' direction.

30.6 COMPTON SCATTERING

In the case of the photoelectric effect, the X-ray photon has an energy close to or just above the binding energy of the electron. If the energy of the X-ray photon is very much higher than the binding energy of the electron, the electron may be regarded as a *free electron*. The reaction between an X-ray photon and a free electron is known as *Compton scattering* and results in the partial absorption of the energy of an X-ray photon which undergoes such scatter. Because the interaction is between a photon and a free electron, the electron density of the material is important in determining the probability of Compton scatter occurring.

The Compton scattering process is shown diagrammatically in Figure 30.5. The incident X-ray photon has an energy E_1 (= hv_1) and collides with the electron, which recoils, thus taking some of the photon energy. The energy remaining, E_2 (=hv_2), is the energy of the deflected (or scattered) photon. Since E_2 is less than E_1, then the wavelength of the scattered photon must be greater than the wavelength of the incident photon, as shown in Figure 30.5 (see Sect. 25.3.2 for the relationship between photon energy and wavelength). Compton scattering interactions are termed *inelastic* in that the photon energy is not conserved, although the total energy of the interaction is conserved.

After a Compton scattering process, the photon may travel in any direction but the electron can only travel in a forward direction relative to the incident photon. Thus, in Figure 30.5, θ may be any value, while Φ lies between 1° ± 90° relative to the direction of the incident photon. The division of the energy of the original photon between the electron and the scattered photon depends on the original photon energy (E_1) and the angle through which it has been scattered. It may be shown that in order to preserve both energy and momentum the following equation must be obeyed:

$$\lambda_2 - \lambda_1 = \frac{(h(1 - \cos \theta))}{mc} \qquad \textit{Equation 30.7}$$

where the quantity $\lambda_2 - \lambda_1$ is called the *Compton wavelength shift*, h is Planck's constant, m is the mass of the electron and c is the velocity of light.

Two important conclusions may be drawn from Equation 30.7:

1. $\lambda_2 - \lambda_1$ depends only on h, m, c and θ and so is not dependent on the wavelength of the incident photon or the composition of the attenuating material
2. For a given value of scattering angle, θ, the value of $\lambda_2 - \lambda_1$ is constant. Low-energy photons have longer wavelengths, so that the wavelength change represents a smaller *fractional* change in λ and hence only a slight reduction in the energy of the scattered

photons. By applying the same argument, high-energy photons scattered through the same angle will experience a much larger fractional change in their wavelength and energy.

Equation 30.7 shows what happens to the photon wavelengths when scattered through an angle of θ. It does not give any information on the relative probability of a photon actually being scattered through that angle. Mathematical predictions based on quantum mechanics, and practical measurements have shown that low-energy photons (up to about 100 keV) are scattered in all directions with almost equal probability. High-energy photons (greater than 1 MeV) are scattered predominantly in a forward direction, i.e. they have small scattering angles.

An alternative way of writing Equation 30.7 using the photon energy change instead of the wavelength change is given below:

$$\frac{1}{E_2} - \frac{1}{E_1} = \frac{(1 - \cos \theta)}{511} \qquad \textit{Equation 30.8}$$

where E_1 and E_2 are in keV.

30.6.1 Compton Attenuation, Absorption and Scatter Coefficients

The mass attenuation coefficient for Compton scattering (σ/ρ) is given by the equation:

$$\frac{\sigma}{\rho} \propto \frac{\text{electron density}}{E} \qquad \textit{Equation 30.9}$$

As shown in the above equation, the probability of Compton scattering occurring in unit mass is inversely proportional to the energy of the photon – the amount of Compton scattering occurring in unit mass decreases as the photon energy increases.

It can also be seen from the above equation that the probability is also directly proportional to the electron density. As we saw in Section 5.6, it is possible to use Avogadro's number to calculate the number of atoms per mole of an element ($N_a = 6 \times 10^{23}$ mol^{-1}). We can therefore calculate the number of atoms per unit mass by simply dividing this by the mass number (A) for the element:

number of atoms per unit mass

$$= \frac{N_a}{A} \qquad \textit{Equation 30.10}$$

The number of electrons in a normal atom is the same as the number of protons and is given by Z, the atomic number (see Sect. 26.3). The electron density is the number of electrons per unit mass and is given by the equation:

$$\text{electron density} = N_a \times \frac{Z}{A} \qquad \textit{Equation 30.11}$$

If we assume that most elements have approximately equal numbers of protons and neutrons in the atomic nucleus, then the value of Z/A is 0.5. The exception to this rule is hydrogen, which contains no neutron in its nucleus, and so $Z/A = 1$. Thus hydrogen contains 6×10^{23} electrons per gram (or 6×10^{26} electrons per kilogram), whereas all other substances contain approximately half this value (between 2.5 and 3.5×10^{23} electrons per gram). The lower values are for the heavier elements, which have a larger neutron-to-proton ratio.

Thus we can see from Equation 30.9 that, at a given photon energy, the mass attenuation coefficient due to Compton scattering is very similar for all elements except hydrogen, where it is twice as large.

The *mass absorption coefficient* for Compton scattering (σ_a/ρ) represents the average energy transferred to the electron (and hence the medium) as a fraction of the total energy in the beam. As shown in the previous section, the higher the energy of the photon, the higher the average energy lost by the photon as a result of Compton scattering. This means that the electron takes more energy in the recoil process as the photon energy increases. As a result of this, the values for the mass absorption coefficient (σ_a/ρ) and the mass attenuation coefficient (σ/ρ) are closer to the same value at higher photon energies than they are at lower photon energies. This situation is shown in Figure 30.6.

As we have already noted in Equation 30.9, the *mass attenuation coefficient* (σ/ρ) is *inversely* proportional to the photon energy and so we would expect σ/ρ to decrease as the photon energy increases. This is also shown in Figure 30.6.

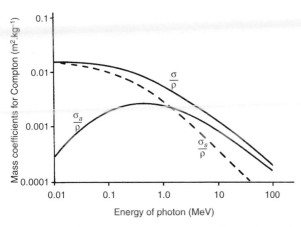

Figure 30.6 The mass attenuation, mass absorption and mass scattering coefficients for Compton scattering. As the energy increases, the absorbed energy (σ_a/ρ) becomes an increasing proportion of the total energy of the interaction (σ/ρ). See text for further details.

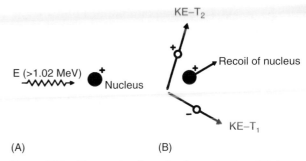

Figure 30.7 The mechanism of pair production. (A) A photon of energy (E) >1.02 MeV approaches the nucleus of an atom of the attenuating material. When the photon passes close to the nucleus it produces a positron and a negatron, as shown in (B). KE, kinetic energy.

Also shown in Figure 30.6 (represented by the broken line) is the *mass scattering coefficient* (σ_s/ρ). This represents the fraction of the total beam energy left to the photons after a Compton scattering event. At the point where the two curves cross (approximately 1.5 MeV), the electrons and the photons share equal amounts of energy. Below this energy the scattered photon carries more energy than the electron and above the energy the reverse is true.

When considering the coefficients it is important to remember that the mass attenuation coefficient is a measure of the *total* energy removed from the primary beam, whereas the absorption coefficient and the scattering coefficient are a measure of the proportion of energy removed from the beam by the electron and scattered photon respectively.

Since the sum of the energies of the electron and the scattered photon must equal the energy of the incident photon, then we can say:

$$\sigma = \sigma_a + \sigma_s$$

and $$\frac{\sigma}{\rho} = \frac{\sigma_a}{\rho} + \frac{\sigma_s}{\rho}$$ *Equation 30.12*

30.7 PAIR PRODUCTION

Pair production resulting in the formation of two charged particles from a single high-energy

photon can only occur at photon energies of 1.02 MeV or above. This is because this value represents the energy equivalent of the masses of two electrons. One of these, the negatron, has a negative charge, just like a normal electron, while the other particle, the positron, has an equal and opposite positive charge. The total charge present as a result of the interaction is therefore zero and equal to the uncharged photon creating the interaction. The process is illustrated in Figure 30.7.

The interaction, which occurs as the photon interacts with the electrical field of the nucleus, is an example of mass–energy equivalence (see Sect. 24.4.1) as the energy from the photon is converted into mass. Any photon energy remaining after the interaction is passed to the particles as kinetic energy. This can be stated using the following equation:

$$E = (m_0c^2 + T_1) + (m_0c^2 + T_2)$$

where E is the energy of the photon, m_0 is the rest mass of positron or electron, c is the velocity of electromagnetic radiation, T_1 is the kinetic energy of the electron and T_2 is the kinetic energy of the positron.

This equation can be further simplified to give:

$$E = 2m_0c^2 + T_1 + T_2$$

If we consider the rest mass of the electron and positron pair then we can calculate that $2m_0c^2$ is equal to 1.02 MeV. This explains why pair production will not take place if the photon energy is less than 1.02 MeV as this amount of energy is required to create the electron and positron pair. The equation may now be written in the form:

$$E \text{ (MeV)} = 1.02 + T_1 + T_2 \qquad \textit{Equation 30.13}$$

This shows that 1.02 MeV of the energy of the photon is used to create the electron and positron pair and the rest is given to the two particles in kinetic energy.

30.7.1 Attenuation, Absorption and Scatter Coefficients for Pair Production

The linear attenuation coefficient for pair production is usually given the symbol π so that the mass attenuation coefficient is π/ρ. This is related both to the photon energy and the atomic number, as shown by Equation 30.14:

$$\frac{\pi}{\rho} = (E - 1.02)Z \qquad \textit{Equation 30.14}$$

where E is the photon energy in MeV and Z is the atomic number of the attenuation material. (*Note* that this is the only process where the amount of attenuation increases with an increase in the photon energy.)

The kinetic energies of the electron and positron pair are absorbed by the medium as the particles slow down in it. Thus the energy absorbed by the medium is less than the energy of the original photon and is equal to $(E - 1.02)$ MeV from Equation 30.14. The electron will eventually lose all its kinetic energy and come to rest. However, the positron will eventually collide with an electron and both will disappear with the emission of two photons of annihilation radiation, where each photon has an energy of 0.51 MeV. This is the conversion of matter into energy, sometimes termed annihilation, and it is the reverse of pair production. If the two photons of annihilation radiation produced by this reaction are completely absorbed by the material, then the total energy absorbed is given by the relationship $(E - 1.02) + (2 \times 0.51) = E$, i.e. the whole of the energy of the original photon which caused the pair production.

There is, however, no certainty that this will happen. In such cases the absorption coefficient (π_a) is less than the attenuation coefficient (π) by a fraction: $(E - 1.02)/E$. This can be rewritten as $1 - (1.02/E)$ and so we have:

$$\pi_a = \frac{\pi(1 - 1.02)}{E} \qquad \textit{Equation 30.15}$$

By analogy with the absorption and scatter coefficient for Compton scatter (see Equation 30.12), in the case of pair production, we may write:

$$\pi = \pi_a + \pi_s$$

$$\frac{\pi}{\rho} = \frac{\pi_a}{\rho} + \frac{\pi_s}{\rho} \qquad \textit{Equation 30.16}$$

where π_s is the fraction of the energy carried by the two annihilation photons each of energy 0.51 MeV, so $\pi_s = 1.02/E$.

However, in all but the most accurate work, it is usual to ignore the scattering coefficient, π_s, since it is usually very small at the photon energies used in therapeutic radiography and so the more exact Equation 30.16 is replaced by more approximate relationships which assume that $\pi_s = 0$:

$$\pi = \pi_a$$

$$\frac{\pi}{\rho} = \frac{\pi_a}{\rho} \qquad \textit{Equation 30.17}$$

30.8 RELATIVE IMPORTANCE OF THE ATTENUATION PROCESSES IN RADIOGRAPHY

As we have already established in Equations 30.3 and 30.4, at a particular photon energy, some or all of the above processes may be competing to remove photons from the radiation beam. Thus the total linear attenuation coefficient, μ, is the sum of the linear attenuation coefficients due to photoelectric absorption, Compton scattering and pair production. Thus the relationship $I_x = I_0 e^{-\mu x}$ can be rewritten as:

$$I_x = I_0 e^{-(\tau + \sigma + \pi)x} \qquad \textit{Equation 30.18}$$

where τ is the linear attenuation coefficient due to photoelectric absorption, σ is the linear

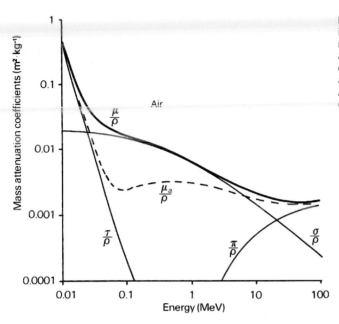

Figure 30.8   Mass attenuation coefficients for air – μ/ρ is the total mass attenuation coefficient, τ/ρ is the mass attenuation coefficient due to photoelectric absorption, σ/ρ is the mass attenuation coefficient due to Compton scattering and π/ρ is the mass attenuation coefficient due to pair production. Also shown (broken line) is the total mass absorption coefficient (μ_a/ρ).

attenuation coefficient due to Compton scattering and π is the linear attenuation coefficient due to pair production. From the above equation we can also deduce the relationships given in Equations 30.3 and 30.4:

$$\mu = \tau + \sigma + \pi$$

$$\frac{\mu}{\rho} = \frac{\tau}{\rho} + \frac{\sigma}{\rho} + \frac{\pi}{\rho} \qquad \textit{Equation 30.19}$$

By applying the same argument to absorption, we can arrive at very similar equations:

$$\mu_a = \tau_a + \sigma_a + \pi_a$$

$$\frac{\mu_a}{\rho} = \frac{\tau_a}{\rho} + \frac{\sigma_a}{\rho} + \frac{\pi_a}{\rho} \qquad \textit{Equation 30.20}$$

Similarly, for scatter, we can write equations:

$$\mu_s = \sigma_s$$

$$\frac{\mu_s}{\rho} = \frac{\sigma_s}{\rho} \qquad \textit{Equation 32.21}$$

where the contribution to the scattering from pair production is ignored. It should also be remembered that photoelectric absorption contributes to energy absorption but not to scatter.

These points are illustrated in Figures 30.8 and 30.9, where the mass attenuation coefficients for photoelectric absorption (τ/ρ), Compton scattering (σ/ρ) and pair production (π/ρ) are shown

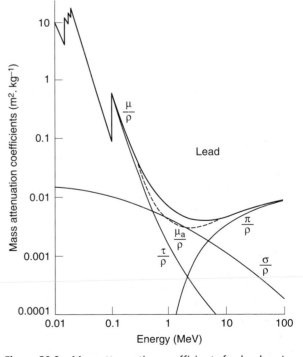

Figure 30.9   Mass attenuation coefficients for lead – μ/ρ is the total mass attenuation coefficient, τ/ρ is the mass attenuation coefficient due to photoelectric absorption, σ/ρ is the mass attenuation coefficient due to Compton scattering and π/ρ is the mass attenuation coefficient due to pair production. Also shown (broken line) is the total mass absorption coefficient (μ_a/ρ).

for air and for lead. The total mass attenuation coefficients (μ/ρ) are shown as thick lines and the total mass absorption coefficients (μ_a/ρ) are shown as broken lines.

The following important points about the attenuation processes should be noted from the graphs:

- Photoelectric absorption dominates at low energies (up to 50–500 keV, depending on the atomic number of the absorber)
- The absorption edges become more pronounced as the atomic number of the absorber increases
- Compton scattering dominates over a wide range of energies ($\simeq$50 keV to 5 MeV) in all materials
- The Compton region is almost identical in all attenuating materials (except hydrogen) because of the similarity of electron density of all materials. Thus the shape of the Compton curve is independent of the attenuator (the curve for σ/ρ is the same shape for both air and lead)
- Pair production is only significant for high energies (> 1.02 MeV) and for attenuating materials of high atomic number
- The significance of the contribution of pair production increases as the photon energy increases above 1.02 MeV. This is the opposite to the effect on the other processes of increasing the photon energy.

30.9 CONCLUSION

As can be seen from the above, the attenuation of an X-ray beam as it passes through a patient's tissues is a complicated affair depending on the energy of the photons, the tissue thickness and the atomic number of the tissue through which the beam passes. In both radiography and radiotherapy we are able to alter the photon energy and this has important consequences for the absorption pattern and the intensity pattern of the beam emerging from the patient. These will be discussed in more detail in Chapter 32

when the formation of the radiographic image is considered.

The significance of the high absorption of materials with high atomic numbers (as shown by the graph for lead in Figure 30.9) will also be considered in Chapter 34, which considers the topic of radiation protection.

A summary of the interaction processes, which may be useful in subsequent chapters of this text, is given in Table 30.2.

SUMMARY

In this chapter you should have learnt:

- The meaning of the terms *attenuation*, *absorption* and *scattering* as applied to a beam of radiation passing through matter (see Sect. 30.2)
- The factors which control the probability of an interaction taking place between the X-ray photon and an atom of the attenuator (see Sect. 30.2.1)
- The meaning of the terms *total linear attenuation coefficient* and *total mass attenuation coefficient* and where it is appropriate to use each (see Sects 30.2.2 and 30.2.3)
- The interrelationships between attenuation and absorption (see Sect. 30.3)
- The mechanism of elastic (coherent) scattering and the factors affecting it (see Sect. 30.4)
- The mechanism of photoelectric absorption and the factors affecting it (see Sect. 30.5)
- The mechanism of Compton scattering and the factors affecting it (see Sect. 30.6)
- The mechanism of pair production and the factors affecting it (see Sect. 30.7)
- The relative importance of each of the attenuation processes in radiography (see Sect. 30.8).

Table 30.2   Summary of interaction processes

Process	Description of interaction	Effect of Z, E	Comments
Elastic scattering	Photon interacts with bound atomic electron. Photon energy is less than the electron-binding energy. Photon is reradiated from the material with no energy loss	$\sigma_{coh}/\rho \propto Z^2/E$	No energy absorption in the medium. Photon scattered in the forward direction. Effect is negligible in biological tissues in radiology because of low Z
Photoelectric absorption	Photon of energy $\geq$ the binding energy of an electron interacts with a bound electron and ejects it from its orbital. Photon disappears as all its energy is absorbed by the electron. Kinetic energy of the electron = E-binding energy. Atom recoils, conserving momentum	$\tau/\rho \propto Z^3/E^3$	Ejected electron loses velocity to surrounding atoms, giving energy to them, i.e. absorption takes place. The electron vacancy created is filled by electrons making quantum jumps and so characteristic radiation is emitted
Compton scattering	Photon behaves like a particle and collides with a free electron. Energy of the incident photon is shared between the electron and the scattered photon	$\sigma/\rho \propto$ electron density/E	Energy of the displaced electron is absorbed by the medium, so Compton process produces attenuation and partial absorption. Electron densities of all materials except hydrogen are similar and so σ/ρ values are largely independent of the type of attenuator
Pair production	Photon of energy greater than 1.02 MeV may spontaneously disappear in the vicinity of the nucleus of an attenuator atom, producing an electron and positron pair. Atom recoils and conserves momentum. Positron eventually annihilated with an electron to form two photons of annihilation radiation, each of energy 0.51 MeV	$\pi\rho \propto (E - 1.02)Z$	Probability of pair production increases with E above 1.02 MeV. Contribution of π_s is very small compared to π and is often ignored

SELF-TEST

a. 'When a beam of radiation passes through matter it is attenuated by absorption and scattering.' What is meant by the terms:

   (i)   attenuation

   (ii) absorption

   (iii) scattering?

b. What is meant by the terms *total linear attenuation coefficient* and *total mass attenuation coefficient*? Give a different situation where each might be used as a measure of attenuation.

c. Describe the process of photoelectric absorption and give an equation which shows the factors which influence the mass attenuation coefficient due to this effect.

d. Describe the process of Compton scattering and give an equation which shows the factors which influence the mass attenuation coefficient due to this process.

e. Describe the process of pair production and give an equation which shows the factors which influence the mass attenuation coefficient due to this process.

FURTHER READING

Ball J L, Moore A D 1997 Essential physics for radiographers, 3rd edn. Blackwell Scientific Publications, London, ch 16

Bushong S C 2004 Radiologic science for technologists: physics, biology and protection. Mosby, New York, ch 13

Curry T S III, Dowdey J E, Murry R C Jr 1990 Christensen's physics of diagnostic radiography, 4th edn. Lee & Febiger, London, ch 2

Dendy P P, Heaton B 1999 Physics for diagnostic radiology, 2nd edn. Institute of Physics Publishing, ch 3

Dowsett D J, Kenny P A, Johnston R E 1998 The physics of diagnostic imaging. Chapman & Hall Medical, London, ch 6

Webb S (ed) 2000 The physics of medical imaging, 2nd edn. Institute of Physics Publishing, Bristol, ch 2

Chapter 31

Luminescence and Photostimulation

CHAPTER CONTENTS

31.1 Aim 298

31.2 Introduction 298

31.3 Luminescence, Fluorescence and
       Phosphorescence 298
       31.3.1 Mechanism of Fluorescence 299
       31.3.2 Mechanism of
                Phosphorescence 300

31.4 Mechanism of Thermoluminescence 301

31.5 Fluorescent Screens in Radiography 301
       31.5.1 Construction of an X-ray
                Intensifying Screen 302
       31.5.2 Phosphor Materials Used in
                Intensifying Screens 303
       31.5.3 Comparison of Intensifying
                Screens 303

31.6 Further Examples of Fluorescence 304

31.7 Photostimulation 304

Self-Test 305

Further Reading 305

31.1 AIM

The aim of this chapter is to introduce the reader to the topics of luminescence, fluorescence, phosphorescence, thermoluminescence and photostimulation. In the case of each of the processes the relevance to radiographic imaging will be briefly discussed.

31.2 INTRODUCTION

If we irradiate a material with high-energy photons and this causes the material to emit photons of lower energy, then the material is exhibiting the property of luminescence. Within the strict laws of physics, provided that the energy is lower than that of the original radiation beam, the emitted radiation can be in any part of the electromagnetic spectrum, but in radiography we are generally more interested in luminescence when the radiation emitted falls in the visible part of the spectrum. Before we can discuss the process in detail there are some basic terms that we need to define.

31.3 LUMINESCENCE, FLUORESCENCE AND PHOSPHORESCENCE

As mentioned above, if we irradiate a material and it emits visible light, then that material is said to exhibit *luminescence*.

Fluorescence occurs when the light emission ceases almost immediately after the irradiation has stopped (the time interval is about 10^{-8} s). If we consider the use of luminescent materials in radiography (see Sect. 31.5), then it can be seen that we require materials that exhibit fluorescence as this allows us to remove the film from the cassette and process the film immediately after the X-ray exposure has taken place.

Phosphorescence occurs if the material continues to emit light for a significant time after the initial period of radiation. For this reason, phosphorescence is often referred to as *afterglow*. Such a phenomenon is generally not desirable in radiography – if we got significant afterglow then we would have to wait before cassettes could be emptied and refilled with film.

From the above we can say that luminescence occurs when we irradiate a material and the substance produces light. If the production of light ceases within 10^{-8} s of the end of the irradiation, then the process is one of fluorescence; if it continues beyond this point, then we have phosphorescence.

INSIGHT

Fluorescence was first demonstrated in salts of phosphorus and so fluorescent materials in radiography are often referred to as phosphors, even though they contain no traces of phosphorus! Some of the phosphors used in intensifying screens (see Sect. 31.5.2) exhibit both fluorescence and phosphorescence. We can

encourage fluorescence (and hence discourage phosphorescence) by the addition of activators to the phosphor material. This will also be discussed in the rest of this chapter.

31.3.1 Mechanism of Fluorescence

The mechanism of fluorescence can be explained by reference to the electron band theory (see Sects 10.3 and 18.3). Fluorescence is caused by an electron in a high-energy state dropping to a lower-energy state and thereby emitting a quantum of radiation (Figure 31.1). If the wavelength of this quantum is in the range 400–700 nm, this will form part of the visible spectrum. If we consider a phosphor used in radiography being irradiated with X-ray photons, then the first process necessary is that some of the electrons of the phosphor atoms are involved in photoelectric interactions with the X-ray photons raising the energy of the electrons. As already mentioned, the overall efficiency of a phosphor may be improved by the addition of activators. These impurities encourage the formation of luminescent centres within the phosphor – the efficiency of lanthanum oxybromide will be increased by the addition of terbium as an activator. The activators possess discrete electron energy levels which are different from that of the phosphor crystal and these are used to form the luminescent centre. This is shown diagrammatically in Figure 31.1, where part A shows the electron

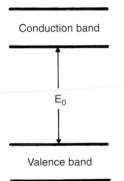

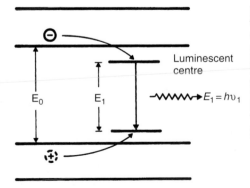

Figure 31.1 Mechanism of fluorescence in a crystal. (A) The outer electron structure of a pure crystal; (B) the effect of an impurity atom on the electron levels. Such impurities enhance fluorescence by forming luminescent centres. These impurities are known as activators. The explanation of the fluorescent process will be found in the text.

(A)

(B)

energy level arrangement in a pure crystal and part B the arrangement in a crystal with a luminescent centre. These centres will produce fluorescence more efficiently than the pure crystal.

The sequence of events occurring within the crystal is as follows:

- An X-ray photon undergoes a photoelectric interaction with an electron of one of the crystal atoms
- The photoelectric interaction liberates the electron and gives it some kinetic energy so that it is free to move within the conduction band, leaving a 'hole' in the valence band
- The energetic electron, on passing close to other atoms, excites and ionises these atoms and so more electrons are raised into the conduction band (leaving more holes in the valence band)
- Some of the electrons so liberated will lose small amounts of energy which will allow them to adjust their energy to the energy level of the luminescent centres
- At the same time, some of the holes in the valence band will have their energy raised to allow them to reach the lower energy level of the luminescent centre
- Some of the electrons at the upper level of the luminescent centre will perform a quantum jump to neutralise the holes at the lower level of the centre. This is shown diagrammatically in Figure 31.1B where the energy of the emitted photon is $E_1 = h v_1$, where v_1 is the frequency of the emitted photon and h is Planck's constant
- The difference in energy between the upper and lower levels in the luminescent centre controls the photon energy E_1 and hence the colour of the emitted (fluorescent) light
- As more electrons enter the luminescent centres than are involved in the initial photoelectric interactions, the number of fluorescent photons is greater than the number of absorbed photons.

As can be seen from the above, the process of fluorescence occurs as a number of stages and inefficiency at any one stage can affect the efficiency of the whole process. This allows us to compare the operation of different phosphors by comparing efficiency at each of the stages.

The *quantum detection efficiency* (QDE) is a measure of the percentage of the quanta (e.g. X rays) incident on the phosphor which are stopped by the phosphor.

The *quantum conversion efficiency* (QCE) is a measure of the percentage of the quantal energy stopped by the phosphor which is converted into light photons.

The *scintillation efficiency* (ScE) is a measure of the percentage of the quantal energy incident on the phosphor which is converted into useful light photons.

As the ScE is a measure of the overall process, it is affected by changes in the QDE or QCE: if the QDE is 50% and the QCE is 20%, then the ScE will be 10% (ScE = QDE × QCE). These measures of efficiency are shown in Table 31.1 for two phosphors used in radiography.

31.3.2 Mechanism of Phosphorescence

Phosphorescence is caused by the presence of electron traps within the crystal structure of the phosphor. The mechanism is as follows:

- An X-ray photon undergoes a photoelectric interaction with an electron of one of the crystal atoms
- The photoelectric interaction liberates the electron and gives it some kinetic energy so that it is free to move within the conduction band, leaving a 'hole' in the valence band
- The energetic electron, on passing close to other atoms, excites and ionises these atoms and so more electrons are raised into the conduction band (leaving more holes in the valence band)

Table 31.1 Measures of the efficiency of two phosphors used in radiography (the photon energy of the incident radiation was 60 keV)

Phosphor	Quantum detection efficiency (%)	Quantum conversion efficiency (%)	Scintillation efficiency (%)
Calcium tungstate	13	5	0.65
Gadolinium oxysulphide	51	20	10.2

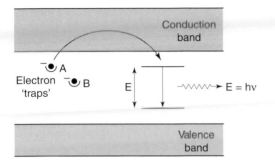

Figure 31.2 The production of phosphorescence or afterglow. An electron enters trap A as a result of energy absorbed from the radiation beam striking the material. This electron can subsequently enter the conduction band as a result of thermal agitation and hence produce fluorescent photons, as shown. (The electron in trap B will only be released if the material is heated and this will be discussed in Sect. 31.4.)

- Some of the electrons so liberated will lose small amounts of energy which will cause them to fall into the electron traps
- The electrons remain in the traps until they are released as a result of interatomic vibrations. If the traps are sufficiently near the conduction band this may happen without the application of additional energy (see trap A in Figure 31.2)
- Some of these released electrons will find luminescent centres and light will be produced by the process described for fluorescence.

Because there is a measurable length of time when the electron is 'stuck' in the electron trap, the luminescence will occur after the irradiation of the material has ceased. This is phosphorescence or afterglow. The phenomenon diminishes exponentially from the time of cessation of the irradiation. Such a process is generally regarded as a nuisance in radiography, especially for image intensifier and television phosphors, since the phosphor may still 'remember' the previous image when a new one is being produced.

31.4 MECHANISM OF THERMOLUMINESCENCE

If we refer to Figure 31.2 we can see that trap B is too 'deep' below the conduction band for the electrons in it to leave and enter the conduction

band. This is a typical arrangement for a thermoluminescent material, e.g. lithium fluoride. This material contains deep traps in the forbidden energy gap between the valence and conduction bands. The mechanism of thermoluminescence is as follows:

- An X-ray photon undergoes a photoelectric interaction with an electron of one of the crystal atoms
- The photoelectric interaction liberates the electron and gives it some kinetic energy so that it is free to move within the conduction band, leaving a 'hole' in the valence band
- The energetic electron, on passing close to other atoms, excites and ionises these atoms and so more electrons are raised into the conduction band (leaving more holes in the valence band)
- Some of the electrons so liberated will lose small amounts of energy which will cause them to fall into the electron traps
- These electrons get stuck in the traps (see trap B in Figure 31.2), but these traps are too deep in the forbidden energy gap for normal interatomic vibration to release them. If more energy is applied to the substance by heating it, the electrons will gain energy as a result of the increased interatomic vibrations and can move up to the conduction band
- Some of these electrons will find luminescent centres and light will be produced by the process described for fluorescence
- Thus the intensity of the light emitted from the thermoluminescent material is directly proportional to the amount of radiation incident on the material. This is the basis of thermoluminescent dosimetry, which will be discussed in Chs 33 and 34.

31.5 FLUORESCENT SCREENS IN RADIOGRAPHY

Fluorescent screens are used in a number of situations in radiography but probably the most common use is as intensifying screens in the X-ray cassette. Figure 31.3 shows an open cassette; note the position of the back and the front

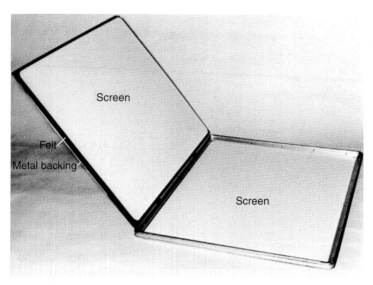

Figure 31.3 The structure of a radiographic cassette. The film is placed between the two screens prior to the X-ray exposure being made.

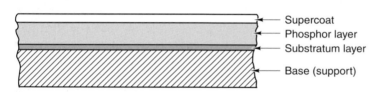

Figure 31.4 A cross-section through a typical X-ray intensifying screen (not drawn to scale).

intensifying screen. It helps to understand the function of such screens if we know their basic construction.

31.5.1 Construction of an X-ray Intensifying Screen

Figure 31.4 shows a cross-section through a typical intensifying screen.

The base material of the screen is usually a flexible white plastic. Its function is to give support to the rest of the screen.

The film side of the base is coated in the *substratum layer*. The function of this layer varies depending on the type of intensifying screen. In a fast intensifying screen it has the function of reflecting the light from the phosphor layer forward on to the film and so increasing the speed screen. In a high-resolution (or detail) intensifying screen the substratum layer has an absorptive function – it absorbs the light from the back of the phosphor layer, thus preventing it being reflected

forward to the film. This increases the resolving power of the screen but diminishes its speed.

The phosphor layer is responsible for converting the X-ray photon energy to light photons. It usually consists of phosphor material crystals (e.g. gadolinium oxybromide activated with terbium) suspended in a clear binder. A colour tint may be added to this binder or it may have carbon microgranules added to it. Both will cause selective absorption of the more oblique light rays from the phosphor crystals and therefore increase the resolution of the screen (but, once again, this improvement is produced at the expense of a loss of speed).

Finally, the *supercoat is* a clear layer of varnish which protects the phosphor layer from abrasion and contamination. This layer is usually smooth so that there is close contact between the film and the intensifying screen. Some screen manufacturers add clear microspheres to this layer. This improves the resolution of the screen and also ensures that the film and screen separate easily in daylight-film-handling devices.

31.5.2 Phosphor Materials Used in Intensifying Screens

The traditional material for the phosphor of X-ray intensifying screens was calcium tungstate ($CaWO_4$). This produced light mainly in the blue part of the visible spectrum which allowed a good match with monochromatic film emulsions. However, as can be seen from Table 31.1, the scintillation efficiency for calcium tungstate is fairly low (0.65%) and so it has been replaced over the last 20 years by more efficient phosphors in the form of 'rare earths'.

The first generation of rare-earth phosphors were terbium-activated gadolinium oxysulphide (Gd_2O_2S:Tb) or lanthanum oxysulphide (La_2O_2S:Tb). These emitted a line spectrum with the peak emission in the green part of the visible spectrum. This necessitated a switch from monochromatic (blue-sensitive) film emulsions to orthochromatic (green-sensitive) film emulsions. The spectral characteristics of the two phosphors and the corresponding film emulsions are shown in Figure 31.5.

The second-generation rare-earth phosphors are now more common. These are again activated with terbium and are the oxybromide salts of lanthanum (LaOBr:Tb) or gadolinium (GdOBr:Tb). These have the advantage of fluorescence in predominantly the blue part of the visible spectrum and so they may be used with monochromatic film emulsions.

31.5.3 Comparison of Intensifying Screens

A detailed comparison of different intensifying screens is beyond the scope of this text and is covered by one of the radiographic photography texts listed at the end of this chapter. However, some of the basic terminology is useful in understanding the formation of the radiographic image, which we will cover in Chapter 32.

X-ray photons incident on the intensifying screens cause the screens to fluoresce and the light from this fluorescence will create an image on the film emulsion. At first this may seem a rather inefficient process as the scintillation efficiency of most phosphors is less than 10%. However, it should be remembered that one captured X-ray photon can cause the emission of thousands of light photons. Because the light photons have lower energy, they are much more likely to undergo photoelectric interactions with the crystals of the photographic emulsion. In a typical situation, about 99% of the image on the film is created by the action of the light from the screens and about 1% by the direct action of the X-ray photons on the photographic emulsion.

As a general rule, provided we use the same phosphor material, an increase in the screen speed will cause a reduction in the resolution of the system. In a modern diagnostic imaging department it is therefore necessary to have intensifying screens of differing speeds for differing imaging

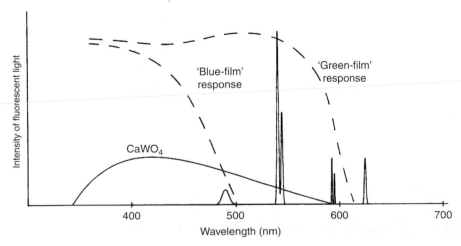

Figure 31.5 The fluorescent spectrum of a rare-earth screen (line spectra) compared to the spectrum from a calcium tungstate screen (continuous spectrum). Also shown as broken lines are the photographic sensitivities of conventional (monochromatic or blue-sensitive) and extended (orthochromatic or green-sensitive) film.

situations. The speed of different screens may be compared by comparing their intensification factors thus:

$$\text{Intensification factor (IF)} = \frac{E}{E_s} \quad \textit{Equation 31.1}$$

where E is the exposure without screens and E_s is the exposure required to produce the same image using screens. Thus if 100 mAs is required to produce a certain image density without screens and the same density is produced by 2 mAs when using screens, the intensification factor of these screens is 50. Intensification factors of up to 50 were available for calcium tungstate screens, while intensification factors of up to 500 are available for rare-earth screens.

INSIGHT

In many cases in a modern imaging department the speed of the imaging system is stated by quoting the speed class. This takes account of the speed of the intensifying screens and film – the class speed of the system can be altered by altering the speed of either the intensifying screens or the film.

31.6 FURTHER EXAMPLES OF FLUORESCENCE

Four further examples of fluorescence applicable to radiographic imaging will now be briefly considered (more detailed descriptions may be found in specialist textbooks on X-ray equipment):

1. If we use an image intensifier in fluoroscopy, then this contains an input phosphor and an output phosphor. The input phosphor is usually made of caesium iodide and absorbs X-ray photons and re-emits the energy as light photons. The light photons fall on a photocathode which will emit electrons when bombarded by light. The electrons are accelerated and focused on to an output phosphor where their energy is used to create light photons by the fluorescent effect. The net result of this is that the image is intensified by about 5000 times between the input phosphor and the output phosphor

2. In the television monitor the phosphor on the face of the monitor is bombarded by electrons. Such high-energy electrons are capable of causing the phosphor to fluoresce, thus producing the image on the television monitor

3. Scintillation counters made of sodium iodide crystals coupled with photomultiplier tubes can be used to detect small amounts of X-rays and gamma-rays. The intensity of the fluorescence from the crystal is measured by the photomultiplier tube and this is proportional to the intensity of the radiation hitting the crystal. Such devices are used in nuclear medicine, computed tomographic scanners and osteoporosis scanners

4. Radiographic viewing boxes contain fluorescent tubes. An electrical discharge in the gas in the tube causes the emission of ultraviolet radiation. This is absorbed by a suitable phosphor coated on to the inside of the tubes which then emits light.

31.7 PHOTOSTIMULATION

The process of photostimulation is very similar to the process of thermoluminescence. A suitable material (normally a barium fluorohalide) is irradiated and the following process takes place:

- An X-ray photon undergoes a photoelectric interaction with an electron of one of the crystal atoms
- The photoelectric interaction liberates the electron, giving it some kinetic energy so that it is free to move within the conduction band, leaving a 'hole' in the valence band
- The energetic electron, on passing close to other atoms, excites and ionises these atoms, liberating more electrons and raising them into the conduction band and leaving more holes in the valence band
- Some of the liberated electrons lose small amounts of energy, causing them to fall into the electron traps in the forbidden gap between the valence and conduction bands. This stage is

analogous to the production of the latent image of the photographic image production process

- The trapped electrons do not have sufficient energy to 'escape' from the traps and remain there. At a later time the material is then scanned with a laser beam at a particular frequency; the trapped electrons gain energy from this process and can leave the traps and move up to the conduction band
- Some of these electrons will find luminescent centres and light will be produced by the process described for fluorescence
- Thus the intensity of the light emitted from each area of the material is proportional to the amount of radiation each area received
- Finally, the material is exposed to an intense white light. This imparts more energy to the material, releasing all 'trapped' electrons and preparing the material for another exposure to X radiation.

This process is the basis of photostimulable plates which are used in computed radiography imaging systems (see Appendix E).

SUMMARY

In this chapter you should have learnt:

- The meaning of the terms *luminescence, fluorescence,* and *phosphorescence* (see Sect. 31.3)
- The mechanism of fluorescence (see Sect. 31.3.1)
- The meaning of the terms *quantum detection efficiency, quantum conversion efficiency* and *scintillation efficiency* (see Sect. 31.3.1)
- The mechanism of phosphorescence (see Sect. 31.3.2)
- The mechanism of thermoluminescence (see Sect. 31.4)
- The construction and practical application of intensifying screens (see Sect. 31.5)
- Other uses of fluorescence in radiography (see Sect. 31.6)
- The mechanism of photostimulation radiography (see Sect. 31.7).

SELF-TEST

a. Distinguish between the terms *luminescence, fluorescence* and *phosphorescence*.

b. Describe the mechanism of fluorescence.

c. Describe the mechanism of thermoluminescence.

d. Briefly describe the construction of a typical X-ray intensifying screen.

e. Outline the basic physics of photostimulation.

FURTHER READING

Carter P H 1994 Chesney's equipment for student radiographers, 4th edn. Blackwell Publishing, London, chs 2 and 3
Curry T S III, Dowdey J E, Murry R C Jr 1990 Christensen's physics of diagnostic radiography, 4th edn. Lee & Febiger, London, ch 2

Roberts D P, Smith N L, Gunn C 1994 Radiographic imaging: a practical approach. Churchill Livingstone, Edinburgh, chs 2 and 5
Webb S (ed) 2000 The physics of medical imaging, 2nd edn. Institute of Physics Publishing, Bristol, ch 2

Chapter 32

The Radiographic Image

CHAPTER CONTENTS

32.1 Aim 306

32.2 Introduction 306

32.3 The X-ray Image Pattern 307
    32.3.1 Attenuation of the X-ray Beam by the Body 307
    32.3.2 Scatter and the Radiographic Image 309
    32.3.3 Limiting Scattered Radiation Formation 309
    32.3.4 Stopping Scatter from Reaching the Image Receptor 309
    32.3.5 Effect of kVp on the X-ray Image 310

32.4 The Radiographic Image Pattern 311

32.5 The Characteristic Curve for an Emulsion 311
    32.5.1 Uses of Characteristic Curves 312

32.6 Practical Considerations in Exposure Selection 313

Self-Test 314

Further Reading 315

32.1 AIM

The aim of this chapter is to consider the major factors involved in the production of a radiographic image. The chapter will first consider the attenuation patterns in a patient that will produce an X-ray image and will then consider how this reacts with a recording medium to produce a radiograph. The chapter also summarises how the selection of exposure factors affects the quality of the radiographic image produced.

32.2 INTRODUCTION

The geometrical factors that contribute to the quality of the radiographic image have already been discussed in some detail in Chapter 2 of this text. These factors determine the magnification of the image and the amount of geometric unsharpness produced. The radiographic image depends on more than geometrical considerations. The purpose of this chapter is to consider the other factors which contribute to the image quality. To understand this it is necessary to understand the contribution of photoelectric absorption (Sect. 30.5) and Compton scattering (Sect. 30.6) to the final radiographic image.

It is easier to understand the final image quality if we consider image formation as a two-stage process:

- the production of an X-ray image pattern as the beam of radiation is attenuated by the patient

• the production of a radiographic image as this radiation pattern interacts with a recording medium.

This chapter will therefore consist of two halves, each looking at one of these stages.

32.3 THE X-RAY IMAGE PATTERN

32.3.1 Attenuation of the X-ray Beam by the Body

We will assume, for simplicity, that the radiation beam from the X-ray tube striking the body is of uniform intensity across the beam. When this beam interacts with the body substance, different structures will cause different amounts of attenuation and thus 'a pattern of radiation intensities' is transmitted to the imaging device. If all structures in the beam attenuated the radiation by the same amount, there will be no such pattern and consequently no image of any structures will be seen on the radiograph. A simple example of such differential absorption is shown in Figure 32.1, where two separate rectangular blocks of bone and soft tissue are shown interacting with the X-ray beam. The profiles of the incident (I_0) and the transmitted (I_T) radiation

intensifies are also shown. If again we assume, for simplicity, that the attenuation of the radiation beam is exponential, then we get:

$$I_B = I_0 e^{-\mu(B)d}$$
$$I_T = I_0 e^{-\mu(T)d}$$

Equation 32.1

where I_0 is the intensity of the X-ray beam before it enters the patient, $\mu(B)$ is the total linear attenuation coefficient for bone and $\mu(T)$ is the total linear attenuation coefficient for soft tissue. I_B is the intensity of the radiation transmitted through a thickness d of bone and I_T is the intensity transmitted through a similar thickness of soft tissue. As can be seen from Figure 32.1, I_B is less than I_T. This is because $\mu(B)$ is greater than $\mu(T)$. There are two physical reasons for this:

1. the density of bone is approximately twice that of soft tissue ($\rho_B = 1.8$; $\rho_T = 1.0$)
2. the average atomic number of bone is approximately twice that of soft tissue ($Z_B = 14$; $Z_T = 7.5$).

As we saw in Section 30.2.2, the total linear attenuation coefficient is proportional to the number of atoms present in unit volume and hence the density of the medium. As the density of bone is twice that of soft tissue, then there must be twice as many atoms in unit volume and

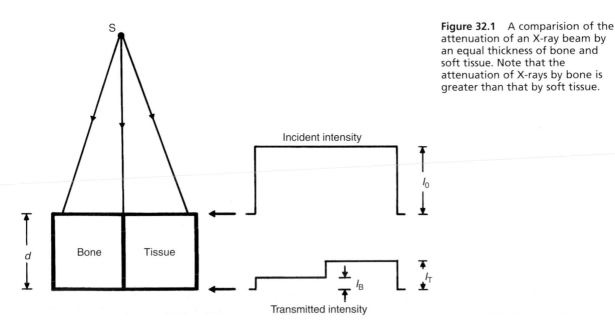

Figure 32.1 A comparision of the attenuation of an X-ray beam by an equal thickness of bone and soft tissue. Note that the attenuation of X-rays by bone is greater than that by soft tissue.

so, all other things being equal, the linear atten-uation coefficient for bone would be twice that for soft tissue.

To appreciate the importance of the difference in atomic number we must consider the attenuation process occurring (see Sect. 30.5 and 30.6). The equations for each process are summarised below:

$$\tau \propto \rho \times \frac{Z^3}{E^3}$$

$$\sigma \propto \rho \, \frac{(\text{electron density})}{E} \qquad \textit{Equation 32.2}$$

where τ is the linear attenuation coefficient for the photoelectric effect, σ is the linear attenuation coefficient for Compton scattering, ρ is the density of the attenuator, Z is its atomic number and E is the photon energy. The higher atomic number of bone means that it will greatly attenuate suitable radiation by the photoelectric effect.

As the total attenuation is a combination of both the photoelectric effect and Compton scattering, in the diagnostic energy ranges a given thickness of bone will attenuate radiation approximately 12 times the level of an equal thickness of soft tissue.

The findings are summarised in Table 32.1. The essential points to be taken from the table are that in the diagnostic range of photon energies the higher atomic number of bone results in pho-toelectric absorption being the main attenuation process, whereas the lower atomic number of soft tissue means that Compton scattering is the main attenuation process. (In the therapy range of photon energies the dominant attenuation processes are Compton scattering and pair production, both of which are less dependent on the atomic number of the attenuator.)

A more realistic example of attenuation is given in Figure 32.2. This simulates the presence of a piece of bone surrounded by soft tissue. A profile of the transmitted radiation intensity is also shown and it can be seen that its minimum corresponds to the maximum thickness of the bone (point A in the figure).

The *fraction* of the incident radiation trans-mitted through the thickness, d, of bone is $e^{-\mu(B)d}$. Similarly, the fraction transmitted through the thickness $D-d$ of soft tissue is $e^{-\mu(T)(D-d)}$. Thus, the total fraction can be found by *adding* the two fractions so that:

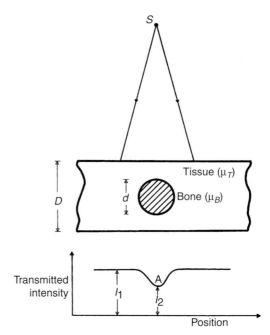

Figure 32.2   A profile of transmitted X-ray intensity obtained from a bone embedded in soft tissue.

Table 32.1	Comparison of linear attenuation in bone and soft tissue		
Attenuator	Photoelectric $\tau \propto \rho \times Z^3/E^3$	Compton scattering $\sigma \propto \rho$ (electron density)/E	Total attenuation $\mu = \tau + \sigma$
Bone $Z = 14$ $\rho = 1.8$	Photoelectric absorption is high when photon energy is low: 12–16 times greater than soft tissue	Predominates at high photon energies 500 keV to 5 MeV	Mainly photoelectric absorption at diagnostic energies
Soft tissue $Z = 7.5$ $\rho = 1.0$	Significant at low energies < 25 keV	Predominates at photon energies > 30 keV	Compton scattering is the dominant process if the average photon energy is greater than about 30 keV

$$\frac{I_2}{I_0} = e^{-\mu(B)d} + e^{-\mu(T)(D-d)}$$

so $I_2 = I_0\, e^{-\mu(B)d} + e^{-\mu(T)(D-d)}$
or $I_2 = I_0 e^{-\mu(T)D - [-\mu(B) - \mu(T)]d}$
and $I_1 = I_0 e^{-\mu(T)D}$ *Equation 32.3*

The difference between I_2 and I is responsible for the contrast on the radiograph.

32.3.2 Scatter and the Radiographic Image

So far, the sections of this chapter have been oversimplified in that the emerging radiation beam is assumed to be composed only of transmitted primary beam. If only photoelectric absorption took place this would be true, but it is not true in the case of Compton scatter where only partial absorption of the photon energy occurs. This scattered radiation may escape from the patient and reach the image-recording medium. Unfortunately, such scatter will form an image on the medium, *but the image formed by the scatter forms an overall fog and so is not a useful image.* Unless this scatter can be limited, serious image degradation can occur.

Scatter to the radiograph may be limited in two ways:

1. limiting the amount of scatter formed
2. stopping any scatter formed from reaching the image-recording medium.

Each of these will now be considered in turn

32.3.3 Limiting Scattered Radiation Formation

The amount of scatter formed in the patient depends on the number of atoms involved in scattering interactions. Thus, scatter formation is volume-dependent, i.e. *the greater the volume of patient irradiated, the greater the quantity of scatter formed.* One of the major ways a radiographer may limit scatter formation is to reduce the volume of tissue irradiated. This can be done by collimation using a light-beam diaphragm or cones (see Figure 21.1) or, in some cases, by tissue displacement. Both these methods will not only produce an improvement in image quality but also reduce the radiation dose to the patient and others by limiting the scatter formation.

INSIGHT

Most radiographers know from experience that the scattered radiation to the radiograph is increased as kVp is increased. This process is a somewhat complicated one. If the kVp is increased then photon energy is increased and from Equations 30.9 and 32.2 we see that σ/ρ is proportional to $1/E$. Thus, with higher-energy photons there are fewer scattering events within a given volume of tissue. However, with higher photon energy, the angle of scatter is smaller and consequently the scatter has a higher energy and is more likely to leave the body. We thus have more scatter leaving the patient and the scatter is in a more forward direction and so is more likely to hit the image receptor.

32.3.4 Stopping Scatter from Reaching the Image Receptor

The most common way of stopping scatter, once formed, from reaching the image receptor is to use a secondary radiation grid. The use of such a grid can remove about 90% of the scatter from the beam. A secondary radiation grid consists of strips of high-atomic-number material (e.g. lead) interspaced with strips of low-atomic-number material (e.g. carbon fibre). A section through such a grid is shown in Figure 32.3, where the lead strips are shaded. Primary radiation should

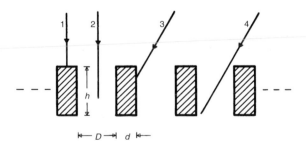

Figure 32.3 The principle of action of a secondary radiation grid. Scattered rays (3 and 4 in the diagram) are more likely to strike the lead and be absorbed by the lead than the primary rays (1 and 2 in the diagram).

hit the grid at right angles to its surface (or nearly right angles to it) and so will easily pass between the lead strips (see ray 2 in Figure 32.3). Some of the primary radiation will however strike a lead strip and be absorbed. The fraction of the primary beam stopped is given by the ratio $d/(D + d)$, since this is the fraction of the grid covered by lead; in practice this means we must increase the exposure when using a grid. Because scattered radiation is at an oblique angle to the primary beam it has an increased probability of striking a lead strip and being absorbed. If the angle is very small, such scatter may be able to pass between the strips and reach the image receptor, but such rays do not contribute as much to image degradation as the more oblique rays.

Various factors of grid design may be chosen to optimise the performance of a secondary radiation grid for a particular application:

- The *grid ratio* (r) is the height of the strips (h) to the width (D):

$$r = \frac{h}{D} \qquad \text{Equation 32.4}$$

It can be appreciated from Figure 32.3 that increasing the height of the lead strips or reducing the space between (i.e. increasing the grid ratio) them will increase the efficiency of the grid in absorbing scattered radiation with a relatively small scatter angle

- The *grid lattice* or *lattice density* is a measure of the number of lines of lead per centimetre. If we consider that space between each strip is controlled by the grid ratio, then the number of lines per centimetre will affect the thickness of the individual lines. Grids with a high lattice density (i.e. 30–40 lines per centimetre) will have very fine lines and so do not degrade the image. If grid lattice density is low it is possible to see the grid lines and this detracts from image quality. A solution to this problem is to move the grid during the exposure so that the grid lines are blurred out. Such a device is known as a *Potter–Bucky diaphragm* or, more commonly, a *Bucky*

- As mentioned earlier, the grid will absorb some of the primary radiation and so it is necessary to increase the exposure when using a grid to compensate for this. The amount by

which the exposure must be increased is known as the grid factor.

$$\text{Grid factor} = \frac{\text{exposure with grid}}{\text{exposure without grid}}$$

Equation 32.5

Note. This equation is only accurate if the kVp used for the exposure remains constant. A change of kVp will result in a change in the amount and type of scatter produced (see Insight, Sect. 32.3.3). It will also change the contrast range of the image (see Sect. 32.3.5). For most grids encountered in a diagnostic department, the grid factor will be between 2 and 6.

32.3.5 Effect of kVp on the X-ray Image

The effect of a change of kVp on the spectrum of radiation produced by the X-ray tube has already been discussed in Section 29.4 and, as can be seen from Figure 29.2, the average energy for a single-phase two-pulse generator is about one-third to one-half of the maximum photon energy. This means that if 90 kVp was applied across the X-ray tube, the maximum photon energy would be 90 keV, but the *average* photon energy would be approximately 40 keV. We can therefore apply the various scattering and attenuation coefficients to a beam of radiation generated at 90 kVp that we would apply to a monoenergetic beam of photon energy of 40 keV.

The effect of increasing kVp is to increase the average photon energy and reduce the linear attenuation coefficients of both bone and soft tissue. The radiation beam is more penetrating. From Equation 32.2 it can be seen that increasing photon energy will reduce the amount of photo-electric absorption (τ) more than it will reduce Compton scattering (σ) because the photoelectric effect is proportional to $1/E^3$. Because of less photoelectric absorption there is less differentiation in absorption between bone and soft tissue – there is less contrast between the densities in the radiographic image. As already mentioned (see Insight, Sect. 32.3.3) an increase in kVp will also result in more scatter reaching the image receptor, further reducing contrast. Increasing kVp degrades image contrast in the ways mentioned above. However, there are practical advantages in using a high kVp. These are:

- It increases the intensity of the radiation beam, allowing a reduction in exposure time
- It results in a higher percentage of the radiation beam being transmitted through the patient, again allowing a reduction in the exposure time
- Because a higher percentage of the incident beam is transmitted through the patient, the absorbed radiation dose received by the patient is reduced.

INSIGHT

The 'best' image is the one that most clearly demonstrates the structures we wish to see! There are some situations in which a low kVp is used to produce a high contrast between tissues of almost the same density (e.g. mammography) and others where we may wish to use a high kVp to demonstrate structures of very different radiopacity in the same image (e.g. high kV chest radiography).

32.4 THE RADIOIGRAPHIC IMAGE PATTERN

The X-ray image pattern discussed so far in this chapter may be used to form an image on a number of different image receptors, for instance on a visual display unit (VDU), an imaging plate or even a conventional film–intensifying screen combination. Where the image is displayed on a VDU the light intensity is directly proportional to the radiation intensity. This is not so when the radiation image is transferred to a photographic emulsion. If we consider the film–intensifying screen combination, the intensifying screen produces light in proportion to the intensity of the X-ray image pattern. This light produces a latent image in the film emulsion. Processing then converts the invisible latent image into a visible permanent image. A similar process occurs in the laser imager. The intensity of the laser beam is directly related to the intensity of the radiation

pattern and the laser beam produces a latent image on the film's emulsion. Processing converts the invisible latent image into a permanent one. In both instances the higher radiation intensity results in a greater exposure being received by the emulsion and a blacker image being produced. However, this blackening effect is not linear. An instrument called a *densitometer*, which is calibrated to measure optical density, is used to measure the amount of blackening or density produced. Density is defined as $\log_{10}(I_0/I_t)$, where I_0 is the intensity of the light on the processed emulsion and I_t is the intensity of the light transmitted through it. Examination of a processed image will show that the darker the image, the less light transmitted through it and hence the higher the optical density. A graph of optical densities produced by various exposures given to a film is known as the *characteristic curve* for that emulsion.

INSIGHT

Optical density, like the response of the eye to differing light intensities, is a logarithmic function. If we consider two points, where the light intensity is I_1 and I_2, the difference between these two levels is the amount of contrast present. Because of the logarithmic function of our eyes our perception of this contrast is given by $(\log_{10} I_1 - \log_{10} I_2)$. However if we measure the two densities D_1 and D_2, then our perception of this contrast is simply the difference between them $(D_1 - D_2)$. *Note* that density does not have any units.

32.5 THE CHARACTERISTIC CURVE FOR AN EMULSION

The characteristic curve for an emulsion can be shown graphically by plotting the densities that result from a known series of relative photographic exposures. The use of relative rather than absolute simplifies the scaling of the x-axis. It is usual to plot density against the logarithm of

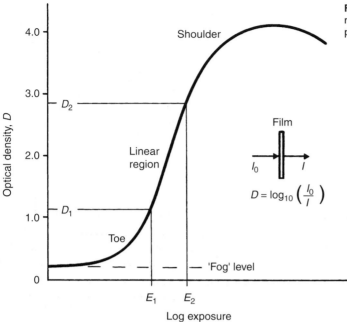

Figure 32.4 A characteristic curve for a radiographic emulsion showing optical density plotted against the log of the relative exposure.

$$D = \log_{10}\left(\frac{I_0}{I}\right)$$

the relative exposure to accommodate the wide range of exposures to which the emulsion can respond. A graph of a typical emulsion is shown in Figure 32.4.

Features of this graph will now be discussed:

- Even when the relative exposure is zero, the emulsion will show some density. This is referred to as *base plus fog*. It results from the small amount of fog produced by the chemical activity of the developing process and any tint that may be present in the base material of the film. The density of this region is normally less than 0.2
- There follows an initial horizontal portion where an increase in exposure produces no increase in density. This is often referred to as the *threshold* of the curve
- The *toe* of the curve is the point at which the emulsion is becoming increasingly responsive to differences in exposure
- There follows a region where an increase in exposure produces a linear increase in density. We aim to set X-ray exposure factors so that the exposure to the film falls in this part of the characteristic curve
- The linear increase 'flattens' off at the *shoulder*. This usually occurs at densities between 3 and

4. We can only see contrasts between densities of just over 2 with the unaided eye; densities above this are seen as black. Industrial radiography makes use of this region.

32.5.1 Uses of Characteristic Curves

Characteristic curves have many uses. We will only discuss a few in this chapter. Further information on uses of the characteristic curve can be found in the further reading listed at the end of the chapter. Referral to Figure 32.4 shows that exposure E_1 produces density D_1 and exposure E_2 produces density D_2. The contrast is the difference in density between the two areas. Not all emulsions respond at the same rate. Emulsion A in Figure 32.5 is an example of the type of curve produced by a high-contrast emulsion whereas emulsion B is that of a low-contrast emulsion. Notice that the same increase in exposure produces a bigger density difference with emulsion A. This example shows one of the fundamental rules of sensitometry:

Contrast and film latitude are reciprocal relationships. Emulsions with high contrast have a narrow exposure range and latitude,

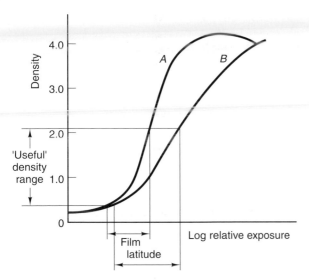

Figure 32.5   Characteristic curves for two film emulsions showing different film latitudes. Film *B* has shallower gradient and wider latitude than film *A*.

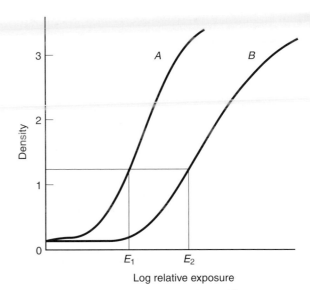

Figure 32.6   Characteristic curves for two film emulsions showing films of different speeds. Film *B* requires more exposure to reach the same density as film *A* and so is slower.

while low-contrast emulsions have wide exposure latitude and range.

Finally, comparison of the amount of exposure required to produce a given density (usually taken at density 1 above base plus fog) permits the relative sensitivity (or speed) of an emulsion or imaging system to be assessed. In Fig. 32.6 we can see that film *B* requires a larger exposure (E_2) than film *A*. Thus we can say that film *A* is faster. We can say how much faster from the formula:

$$\text{Relative speed of } A = \text{antilog } (E_2 - E_1)$$

With digital image manipulation these differences are less obvious but they are still important in minimising the radiation dose delivered to the patient.

32.6 PRACTICAL CONSIDERATIONS IN EXPOSURE SELECTION

The interrelationships between the various factors that affect image quality are complex and require considerable skill to master. There is a strong subjective element in selecting the 'best' image but no absolute rules can be laid down for exposure

factors. The wide degree of variability in shape and size of the patients themselves, together with other practical difficulties (e.g. patients who are unable to keep still during the exposure) would provide so many exceptions that it is impossible to adhere to a strict set of rules. The radiographer's experience is therefore critical in producing images of consistently high quality under all conditions. The following paragraphs should be considered with these general comments in mind.

The value of the kVp selected is critical in determining the contrast and average density in the image. This is because the linear attenuation coefficients of various body structures vary with the photon energy of the beam. Thus the selection of too high a kVp will result in loss of contrast, but an increase in the contrast range and structures will be demonstrated due to the decrease in photoelectric absorption. The increased amount of scatter to the image receptor will result in further loss of image contrast, although this can be counteracted by using a secondary radiation grid and by limiting the radiation beam to the smallest possible field size. On the other hand, if a lower kVp is selected, the image contrast is increased, but the range of contrast present and structures demonstrated are lowered. If the kVp is too low, denser body structures (e.g. the bony skeleton) will not be penetrated by the radiation beam, resulting in excessive contrast and an increase in the absorbed radiation dose to the patient.

As we saw in Section 29.4, the kVp also affects the amount of radiation from the X-ray tube. Too low a kVp results in an image with insufficient density, while too high a kVp results in an image with excessive density, unless this effect is compensated for by changing the current (mA) across the X-ray tube.

The tube current (mA) and duration of the exposure time affect the quantity of radiation produced by an X-ray tube for a given kVp selection (see Sect. 30.3). If the mA is too low, the radiograph will lack optical density and an underexposed image will be produced. Conversely, if the mA is too high, this will result in excessive density producing an overexposed radiograph. It is also important to remember that our ability to perceive contrast is inhibited if the density on the radiograph is much above 2.

Digital image manipulation (which is designed to produce a suitable range of contrasts automatically) masks these effects to an extent but can produce a pixellated image if insufficient density is present. This will again result in increased radiation dose to the patient. If too high a kVp is used, this effect is not present in the image. However, the patient will still have received more radiation than is necessary to produce a suitable image.

SUMMARY

In this chapter, you should have learnt:

- How the X-ray beam is attenuated by bone and soft tissue (see Sect. 32.3.1)
- The effect of scattered radiation on the X-ray image and subsequently on the radiograph (Sect. 32.3.2)
- Methods of limiting the amount of scattered radiation formed (see Sect. 32.3.3)
- Methods of reducing the amount of scatter reaching the image receptor, including factors that affect the efficiency of a secondary radiation grid (see Sect. 32.3.4)
- The effect of a change of kVp on the X-ray image pattern (see Sect. 32.3.5)
- How the X-ray image pattern is changed into the radiographic image (see Sect. 32.4)
- What is meant by the characteristic curve of an emulsion (see Sect. 32.5)
- How the characteristic curve can be used to compare the latitude of two emulsions and the relationship between latitude and contrast (see Sect. 32.5.3)
- Practical considerations in the choice of exposure factors (see Sect. 32.6).

SELF-TEST

a. Explain why, when a uniform beam of radiation is directed at a given thickness of bone and the same thickness of soft tissue, less radiation is transmitted through the bone than the tissue.

b. Discuss the effects of kVp selection on the quality of the subsequent image.

c. Explain how the amount of scattered radiation reaching the image receptor can be limited.

d. List three items of information that may gained from the characteristic curves of the emulsions shown in Figure 32.6.

FURTHER READING

Ball J L, Moore A D 1997 Essential physics for radiographers, 3rd edn. Blackwell Scientific Publications, London, ch 16

Carter P H 1994 Chesney's equipment for student radiographers, 4th edn. Blackwell Publishing, London, chs 2 and 3

Curry T S III, Dowdey J E, Murry R C Jr 1990 Christensen's physics of diagnostic radiography, 4th edn. Lee & Febiger, London, ch 2

Fauber T 2005 Radiographic imaging and exposure, 2nd edn. Mosby, New York, chs 3 and 4

Gunn C 2002 Radiographic imaging – a practical approach, 3rd edn. Churchill Livingstone, Edinburgh, chs 4, 5 and 8

Johns H E, Cunningham J R 1983 The physics of radiology, 4th edn. Charles C Thomas, Illinois, USA, ch 2

Webb S (ed) 2000 The physics of medical imaging, 2nd edn. Institute of Physics Publishing, Bristol, ch 2

Part 6

Dosimetry and Radiation Protection

PART CONTENTS

33. Radiation Dosimetry **319**

34. Radiation Protection **333**

Chapter 33

Radiation Dosimetry

CHAPTER CONTENTS

33.1 Aim 319

33.2 Introduction 319

33.3 Units of Exposure and Dose 320
    33.3.1 Exposure and Air Kerma 320
    33.3.2 Absorbed Dose and Kerma 320
    33.3.3 Effects of Different Media 322

33.4 Quality Factor and Dose-Equivalent 323

33.5 Absolute Measurement of Absorbed
    Dose 325
    33.5.1 Calorimetry 325
    33.5.2 The Free-Air Ionisation
        Chamber 325
    33.5.3 Chemical Methods of Dose
        Measurement 327

33.6 Types of Detectors and Dosimeters 328
    33.6.1 The Thimble Ionisation
        Chamber 328
    33.6.2 The Geiger–Müller Counter 329
    33.6.3 Scintillation Detectors 330
    33.6.4 Thermoluminescent Dosimetry
        (TLD) 330
    33.6.5 Photographic Film 331
    33.6.6 Semiconductor Detectors 331

Self-Test 332

Further Reading 332

33.1 AIM

The aim of this chapter is to introduce the reader to the concepts of exposure, absorbed dose and dose-equivalent. The chapter then goes on to consider methods of absolute measurement of radiation dose and different relative methods of dose measurement.

33.2 INTRODUCTION

As we saw in Chapter 1 of this book, we live in an environment where we are continuously subjected to ionising radiation from natural causes such as cosmic rays and naturally occurring radionuclides. In fact, about 90% of the average UK radiation dose comes from natural sources. In addition to this, there are artificial contributions to the radiation dose because of fallout from weapons testing, leakage from nuclear power plants, manufacture of radionuclides and medical exposure to radiation. All ionising radiations, whether natural or artificial, constitute a hazard. It is assumed that the greater the radiation dose to which the population is exposed, the greater the hazard. The accurate measurement of radiation dose received by the population is therefore important in trying to quantify the hazard. As can be seen from Figure 1.3 in Chapter 1, medical radiation constitutes the largest single contribution of the artificial radiation exposure to the population in the UK and so it is important to minimise this radiation dose and hence the total population dose. However, the hazards associated with medical irradiation must be considered against the benefits the patients receive from diagnosis and treatment. This risk–benefit will be discussed in detail in Chapter 34.

33.3 UNITS OF EXPOSURE AND DOSE

When an X-ray beam passes through air, it produces excitation and ionisation of the air molecules. The electrons ejected in this first inter-action (e.g. during photoelectric absorption) can have sufficient energy to ionise other atoms and so produce more electrons – the delta-rays. Such delta-rays are responsible for the great majority of ionizations, often referred to as secondary ionisations. The net effect on the air is:

- the formation of electrical charges in the air by ionisation
- the absorption of energy by the air as the electrical charges are slowed down by collision with the air molecules (thus producing further ionisation)
- the consequent production of heat energy because of the transfer of energy to the air molecules.

The traditional measure of exposure concerns the first of these effects only and is a measure of the amount of ionisation that occurs in air. The unit of exposure is defined thus:

DEFINITION

The exposure at a particular point in a beam of X- or gamma radiation is the ratio Q/m, where Q is the total electrical charge of one sign produced in a small volume of air of mass m.

Thus the units of exposure are coulombs per kilogram ($C.kg^{-1}$) of air. It is important to remember that exposure can only be defined for air and only for X- or gamma radiation.

Exposure rate ($C.kg^{-1}.s^{-1}$) is a measure of the intensity of a beam of given quality since the greater the number of photons at a given energy passing through unit area, the greater the amount of ionisation of air in unit time.

In air, the proportions of ionisation and heat produced by the absorption of radiation are approximately constant and therefore do not depend on the energy of the radiation. The total amount of ionisation produced in air is thus proportional to the energy absorbed from the beam, e.g. the average energy required to produce ionisation in air is about 33 eV, so an X-ray photon of energy 33 keV which is fully absorbed in air produces about 1000 primary ionisations.

The atomic number of air is 7.64, which is close to that of muscle, at 7.42. For this reason the mass absorption coefficients of air and muscle are very similar. This means that the energy absorbed from an X-ray beam by a given *mass* of air is very similar to the energy absorbed from the beam by the same *mass* of muscle. The energy absorbed by both air and muscle is thus proportional to the exposure measured in air. This is the main reason for the importance of air as a medium in radiation dosimetry as it allows the dose in tissue to be calculated from knowledge of the air exposure.

33.3.1 Exposure and Air Kerma

In recent years the term 'exposure' has gradually fallen out of common usage and has been replaced by *absorbed dose in air* or *air kerma* (the initials of kerma stand for *k*inetic *e*nergy *r*eleased per unit *m*ass of *a*bsorber); for instance, the maximum permissible radiation leakage rate from the X-ray tube is now quoted in air kerma. The main reason for this is that it is much easier to calculate the absorbed dose in a structure from the air kerma.

33.3.2 Absorbed Dose and Kerma

The measurement of the quantity of electrical *charge* produced in air by ionisation is not the same as the measurement of the *energy* actually absorbed, although the two quantities are proportional to each other. The energy absorbed by unit mass of the medium is stated as the *absorbed dose* and is defined thus:

DEFINITION

The *absorbed dose* in a medium is in the ratio E/m, where E is the energy absorbed by the medium due to a beam of ionising radiation being directed at a small mass m.

The unit of absorbed dose is the *gray* (Gy) and so we can say that 1 gray = 1 joule per kilogram (1 Gy = 1 J.kg^{-1}).

Note that *exposure* is defined in terms of X- or gamma radiation only, while *absorbed dose* is defined in terms of any ionising radiation. Thus, the absorbed dose from alpha-particles, beta-particles and neutrons are all measured in grays. However, ultraviolet radiation is only capable of excitation rather than ionisation of the atoms of the medium and so is outside the scope of the definition of absorbed dose.

If all the electrons produced by the primary and secondary ionisations within a medium are stopped within it, then it can be seen that the energy *removed* from the beam of ionising radiation is the same as the energy *absorbed* by the medium (this makes the assumption that all the fluorescent or characteristic radiation is absorbed, as is the case in body tissues). However, this does not necessarily apply to a very small volume within the medium – such a volume may be removing energy from the beam but the absorbed energy may be deposited *outside* the volume (but still within the body) due to the distance travelled by the electrons before coming to rest. Electrons with an energy of 1 MeV travel for about 5 mm in tissue before coming to rest. This effect is illustrated in Figure 33.1, where an incoming X-ray beam of high energy interacts with a volume element V within the medium. Because of the high energy of the beam the electrons produced by Compton scatter are scattered in a forward direction, so much of their energy is absorbed outside the volume V. There will also be secondary ionisations resulting in the production of delta-rays but for simplicity these are not shown in the figure. In general, if the secondary electrons produced within the volume deposit a total energy E within the medium, and E_{IN} and E_{OUT} are the total energies of the electrons entering and escaping

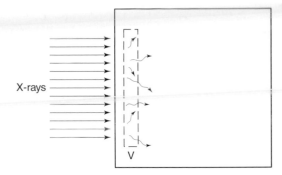

Figure 33.1 X-rays interacting with atoms in volume V produce electrons that may travel outside V.

from the volume, then the absorbed dose in grays is given by:

$$\text{absorbed dose} = (E + E_{IN} - E_{OUT})/m$$

Equation 33.1

where m is the mass of the particular small volume considered. If a larger volume is considered, then this formula can be used to calculate the average absorbed dose in that volume.

Electronic equilibrium is said to occur if $E_{IN} = E_{OUT}$, since there is no net loss or gain of the electrons over the small volume being considered. If $E_{IN} - E_{OUT}$ is a constant value not equal to zero, there is said to be *quasielectronic equilibrium*. If the intensity of the radiation is varied, the net loss or gain of electrons will vary in proportion. An example of electronic equilibrium occurs in the free-air ionisation chamber, which will be discussed later in Section 33.5.2.

The absorbed dose expresses the quantity of energy absorbed in the medium due to a beam of ionising radiation passing through it. However, as stated at the beginning of this section, the site of the attenuating events (e.g. photoelectric absorption) may be at some distance from the absorption process because of the distance travelled by the ejected electrons before coming to rest. The quantity which measures the amount of attenuation in a small volume is called the kerma (see Sect. 33.3.1). Kerma is also measured in grays and may differ significantly from the absorbed dose at any particular position within the medium.

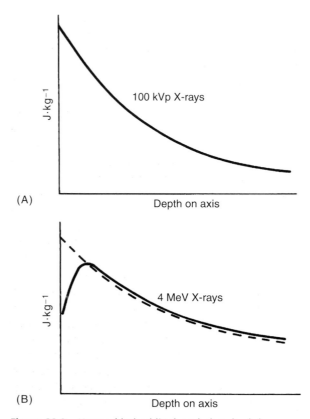

(A)

(B)

Figure 33.2 Kerma (dashed line) and absorbed dose for (A) 100 kVp diagnostic beam and (B) 4 MeV therapy beam. In (A) the two curves are coincident, but they are different in (B) because of the increased energy – and hence range – of the secondary electrons produced.

The absorbed dose and kerma along the axis of a beam of X radiation are shown in Figure 33.2. Figure 33.2A shows the case where an X-ray beam generated at 100 kVp is incident upon soft tissue: this type of situation might occur in diagnostic radiography. The electrons released in the primary and secondary ionisations are of relatively low energy and so are absorbed close to the site of the initial attenuating interactions. Hence, the kerma and absorbed dose at any particular point along the beam axis are essentially the same and the curves are coincident in the figure. This is not the case if the X-ray beam has high photon energy, since electrons produced by the initial ionisation have considerable energy and so deposit their energy some distance from the point of the original attenuation process. As can be seen in Figure 33.2B, the kerma and the

absorbed dose due to 4 MeV X-rays interacting with tissue are not the same. It may be easier to understand these curves if it is remembered that:

- the *kerma* is a measure of the *attenuation* – the number of photoelectric and Compton events
- the *absorbed dose* is a measure of the *energy deposited* in the medium by the primary and secondary electrons being brought to rest.

33.3.3 Effects of Different Media

Instruments that are used to measure absorbed dose or absorbed dose rate are called *dosemeters* and *dose-rate meters* respectively. Some of these instruments are described in more detail in later sections of this chapter (see Sect. 33.5 onwards). It is common practice to calibrate these meters to read the absorbed dose or dose rate in air through which the X- or gamma-rays are passing. Such a dosemeter may read 0.5 mGy as the total absorbed dose in air at a point within an X-ray beam. *It must not be inferred, however, that this is the absorbed dose that would be received by any other medium if placed in the same position.* For two media to receive the same absorbed dose, each must absorb the same energy from the beam per unit mass (remember, 1 Gy = 1 J.kg⁻¹). This is the same as saying that the mass absorption coefficient (μ_a/ρ) of the two media must be equal. Thus if D_{air} is the absorbed dose in air and D_m the absorbed dose in a medium when both are irradiated with the same beam of X-rays, it follows that if the mass absorption coefficients are not equal, this equation may by drawn up:

$$\frac{D_m}{D_{air}} = \frac{(\mu_a/\rho)_m}{(\mu_a/\rho)_{air}}$$

or $D_m = D_{air} \times \dfrac{(\mu_a/\rho)_m}{(\mu_a/\rho)_{air}}$ *Equation 33.2*

Thus, if the mass absorption coefficient of air and the given medium are known at the energy of the X-ray quanta, the absorbed dose in the medium may be calculated using Equation 33.2. In practice, this allows us to measure the absorbed dose in air at a certain point and then calculate the absorbed dose in the patient at the same point without subjecting the patient to a great degree of discomfort.

The mass absorption coefficients of both air and bone vary with photon energy. These variations of the two coefficients are shown in Figure 33.3A and the variations in the ratio of the two coefficients are shown in Figure 32.3B. As can be seen from the graphs, at low photon energies (50 keV is shown with the broken line in Figure 33.3A), the mass absorption coefficient of bone is considerably higher than that of air. This is because, at low energies, the photoelectric effect predominates ($\tau/\rho \propto Z^3/E^3$) and the atomic number of bone ($Z = 14$) is approximately double

that of air ($Z = 7.64$). For this reason and because of the large difference in density, we get a high level of contrast between bone and air on a radiograph (this can be seen on the chest radiograph or on radiographs of the paranasal sinuses). At an energy of about 1 MeV, however, the two graphs are very close and the ratio of the two coefficients approaches 1. This is because of the dominance of Compton scatter in this region ($\sigma/\rho \propto$ electron density and the electron density for bone and air is approximately the same). This means that there would be a low level of contrast between the two if they were radiographed using 1-MeV photons. At above about 10 MeV the curves again diverge owing to the greater amount of pair production in bone compared to air ($\pi/\rho \propto Z$). Thus it is clear that an instrument calibrated to read absorbed dose in air must be used with caution when calculating the absorbed dose in another medium as the relationships between the absorption coefficients vary with the photon energies. This is particularly the case in the diagnostic range of energies where absorption is principally by the photoelectric effect, which is very sensitive to both atomic number and photon energy.

33.4 QUALITY FACTOR AND DOSE-EQUIVALENT

As described in the previous section, the *absorbed dose* measures the energy absorbed per unit mass of the medium when it is subjected to any type of ionising radiation. However, the *biological effects* of the radiation on tissue, for instance, do not depend solely on the absorbed dose, but also on the *type of radiation* and on the *absorbed dose rate*. It is found that alpha-particles will cause considerably more damage (about 20 times as much) in a biological specimen compared to the same absorbed dose of X-rays. It is also found that radiation delivered as a single large dose will generally cause more biological damage than the same dose fractionated into multiple small doses and delivered over a period of time.

The differences in biological effects of different types of ionising radiations are due to the different densities of ionisations they produce in

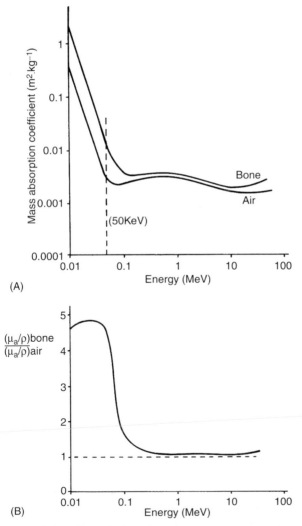

(A)

(B)

Figure 33.3 The variation of energy of (A) the mass attenuation coefficients of air and bone and (B) the ratio of the two coefficients.

a sample. Radiation, which causes large numbers of ionisation per unit length of tract through a material, will cause large amounts of biological damage. As you may remember, when an atom is ionised (e.g. by a photoelectric interaction) an electron (negative ion) is released and the atom now becomes a positive ion – an ion pair has been formed. X-rays and beta-particles do not produce ion pairs as close together as do the more massive protons or alpha particles of the same energy. Thus, protons or alpha-particles are brought to rest quickly within the medium by losing their kinetic energy in the production of many ions over a short distance – an alpha particle of energy 1 MeV will only travel 5×10^{-3} mm in tissue, protons will travel 3×10^{-2} mm and beta-particles will travel 5 mm before being brought to rest. Because of this, the larger particles break chemical bonds, which are very close together, and so the chance of repair is reduced. This means that they have a greater biological effect on the specimen. It is also found that neutrons will produce dense ionisation by the ejection of protons from the nuclei or by nuclear recoil. The absorbed dose in grays is thus not an accurate measure of the biological effects of different types of radiation owing to the very different patterns of ionisation produced. The unit used to measure the overall biological effects of different types of radiation is called the *unit of dose-equivalent* and is measured in sieverts (Sv). The absorbed dose in grays and the dose-equivalent in sieverts are related to each other, as shown in Equation 33.3:

dose equivalent (Sv) = $Q \times$ absorbed dose (Gy) $\times N$ *Equation 33.3*

where Q is known as the *quality factor* for the radiation and is related to the number of ion pairs produced per unit length by the radiation. N includes other factors that may affect the biological process, such as the *dose rate*. In many cases, the value of N is 1 and so the equation is frequently quoted without the factor N appearing.

Table 33.1 shows the value of the quality factor for different types of radiation.

Note that Q is unity for X-rays and gamma-rays so the absorbed dose is the same as the dose

Table 33.1 Quality factors for different ionising radiations

Type of ionising radiation	Quality factor(Q)
X-rays or gamma-rays	1
Electrons or beta-particles	1
Thermal neutrons	2.3
Fast neutrons (or neutrons of high energy)	10
Protons	10
Alpha-particles	20
Recoil nuclei (e.g. in alpha decay)	20
Fission fragments	20

equivalent for these radiations. The biological effect of particulate radiations is therefore compared to that of X-rays or gamma rays by means of the value of Q. As can be seen from Table 33.1, electrons also have a quality factor of unity. This is because an external beam of electrons will produce secondary electrons with the same ionisation density as X-rays and gamma-rays. However, alpha-particles have a Q of 20, indicating that the same absorbed dose will produce 20 times as much biological damage as the same absorbed dose of X-rays.

Since Q is a comparative number, the sievert has the same units as the Gray (J.kg^{-1}). The quality factor may therefore be considered a scaling factor relating the biological effect of absorbed dose to the same dose of X-rays or gamma rays.

Dose-equivalent in sieverts has a vital role to play in radiation protection, where it is required to consider the sum of the effects of exposure to different types of radiation.

INSIGHT

The dose-equivalent is too crude a unit for use in radiobiology as it considers the *average effect(s)* on a group of cells. In radiobiology, we wish to look more precisely at individual effects on cells, e.g. impairment of cell reproduction. For this, we use a more precise scaling factor – the *relative biological effectiveness* (RBE). The RBE compares the absorbed doses of different ionising radiations required to produce the same biological effect. As with the quality factor (Q), these are usually compared to the same dose of X- or gamma radiation.

The remainder of this chapter is concerned with a brief overview of some of the methods used to measure exposure and absorbed doses.

33.5 ABSOLUTE MEASUREMENT OF ABSORBED DOSE

The absolute measurement of absorbed dose in air due to a beam of X-rays requires very careful techniques and very specialised equipment. It is therefore more suited to a specialised laboratory than to a hospital or university department environment. In the UK, the National Physics Laboratory and in the USA, the National Bureau of Standards calibrate and check specialised dosemeters under carefully controlled conditions. Such dosemeters are termed *absolute standards*. Dosemeters used in hospitals and universities are sent to such centres on a regular basis to be calibrated against the absolute standards: such dosemeters are then known as *secondary standards*. Further dosemeters are calibrated against these secondary standards. Such dosemeters are known as *substandards*. This initial section considers the manner in which an *absolute measurement* of absorbed dose may be made and the following section (Sect. 33.6) is an overview of the most common of the *relative methods* of assessing absorbed dose.

33.5.1 Calorimetry

A beam of X-rays or gamma-rays will be attenuated as it passes through a medium and the attenuation processes (see Ch. 30) will produce many ionisations within the medium. The atoms of the medium eventually absorb the kinetic energy of the electron ejected from their atoms. This results in these atoms having an increase in their kinetic energy – heat will be produced in the medium. The medium thus experiences a temperature rise that is proportional to the heat energy absorbed by the medium and therefore

the absorbed dose. In Section 8.3.2 we have shown that:

$$Q = mc(T_2 - T_1)$$

where Q is the heat energy, m is the mass of the body, c is its specific heat capacity and $(T_2 - T_1)$ is the temperature rise experienced by the body.

We also know from the earlier sections of this chapter (see Sect. 33.3.2) that absorbed dose is energy per unit mass of the medium and so:

$$D = \frac{Q}{m}$$

Thus, we can produce the equation

$$D = c(T_2 - T_1) \qquad \text{Equation 33.4}$$

Using the above equation, if we know the specific heat capacity of the medium, the absorbed dose may be calculated from the temperature rise produced in an irradiated medium. This is known as the calorimetric method of absorbed dose measurement. However, the temperature rise produced is very small: 1 Gy will produce a temperature rise of about $2 \times 10^{-4}\,\mathrm{C}^\circ$ and so the process needs very controlled conditions and is most appropriate when measuring very large absorbed doses of radiation. A more sensitive method is to collect the charge produced in an ionisation chamber: this is described below.

33.5.2 The Free-Air Ionisation Chamber

The ions produced by the absorption of an X-ray beam in air may be collected by oppositely charged plates situated in the air. The liberated electrons are attracted towards the positive plate and the positive ions are attracted towards the negative plate. Thus charge, whose magnitude is proportional to the exposure in coulombs per kilogram and the absorbed dose in grays, flows through the chamber. Certain precautions are necessary, however, to achieve accurate results:

• As shown in Figure 33.4, the central lower disc is surrounded by an annulus which is at earth potential. (*Note* that, as Figure 33.4 is a vertical section through such a chamber, the annulus

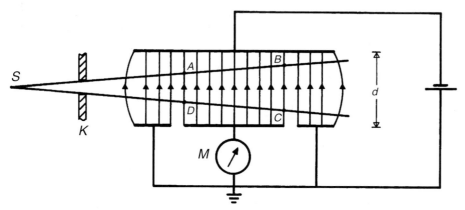

Figure 33.4 A diagrammatic vertical section through a free-air ionisation chamber. *S* is the radiation source and *K* is a collimator. The electrons resulting from the ionisation that takes place in the area *ABCD* are collected on the collecting plate *CD* which is connected to the meter *M*. This measures the negative charge produced as a result of the radiation.

appears as if it were two separate plates.) This construction enables an accurate estimation of the volume of air from which the ion pairs are collected, as it ensures that the lines of electrical force are at right angles to both the collecting plates. *Note* that this is not the case at the outer edge of the annulus, where the lines of electrical force are bowed outwards, thus including an unknown quantity of air beyond the edge of the plates. The volume of air from which the ion pairs are collected may be calculated by knowing the geometry of *ABCD*. Ion pairs produced outside this volume are still collected by the annulus but do not pass through the meter *M* and its associated electronic amplifier and thus do not contribute to the current indicated by the meter

- Some electrons produced by ionisation in the region *ABCD* will escape and produce further ionisations over the annulus rather than the central disc. This suggests that the current measured by the meter, *M*, is too low, but this is not the case because on average the same number of electrons are gained by the volume under consideration. This is a case of electronic equilibrium, described earlier (Sect. 33.3.2)
- The potential difference across the plates must be sufficiently high to collect all the ion pairs produced in the air. If we irradiate a free-air ionisation chamber with a steady beam of radiation, the current flowing through the chamber will vary with the potential difference across the plates, as shown in Figure 33.5
- Below the saturation voltage, some of the positive and negative ions recombine by mutual

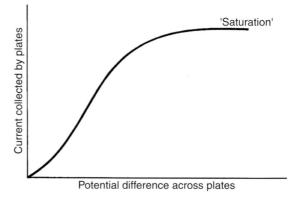

Figure 33.5 The variation of current flowing through meter *M* in Figure 33.4 with the applied potential across the plates.

attraction (or germinal recombination) and so not all ions are collected. Above saturation voltage the electrical field strength between the plates is large enough to ensure that all the ions move to the appropriately charged plate for collection. The actual voltage depends on the separation on the plates, but typically this in the region of a few hundred volts

- The separation of the plates, *d*, shown in Figure 33.4, must be sufficiently large to enable the production of all the secondary ionisations in air. No electron produced during the ionisation process must reach the plates before it produces all the ion pairs of which it is capable. If *d* is too small, then the current measured by the meter, *M*, will be too low since there are too few ion pairs produced in the air volume and hence the estimate of the exposure or absorbed dose will be too low. The required plate separation depends on the energy of the X- or gamma-ray beam, since photons with high energies will produce electrons with correspondingly high energies that will travel further in air. Typical values vary from about 20 cm for photon energies up to 250 keV to several metres for photons of energy above 1 MeV. From this it can be seen that the greater the energy of the beam, the more cumbersome the measurement, due to the necessity for greater separation of the plates.

- The total charge in coulombs measured by the free-air ionisation chamber is a direct measure of the exposure in $C.kg^{-1}$ and is proportional to the absorbed dose in grays ($J.kg^{-1}$). The mass of the air irradiated depends on the temperature and the pressure of air and must therefore be corrected for the effects of these variations. If ρ_0 is the density of air at a known temperature and pressure, then the mass of the air m_0 in the irradiated volume, v, can be calculated as $m_0 = \rho_0 v$. At a new temperature and pressure (T_1 and P_1), the density changes to $\rho_0 T_0 P_1 / T_1 P_0$ so the mass of the air, m', being irradiated is given by:

$$m' = m_0 \times \left(\frac{T_0}{T_1}\right) \times \left(\frac{P_1}{P_0}\right) \qquad \text{Equation 33.5}$$

The exposure (in $C.kg^{-1}$) is therefore the ratio of the total charge collected to the mass of air irradiated (m'). The absorbed dose (in grays) is calculated from the energy absorbed divided by m' – the energy absorbed can be calculated from the charge collected since it takes about 33 eV to produce one ion pair in air.

The ionisation method is not suitable for use with liquids owing to the very rapid germinal recombination of the ions and the relatively high current, which flows through many liquids, even when they are not being irradiated. A semiconductor (see Sect. 33.6.6) may, however, be used to collect the ion pairs produced by irradiation.

From the above it can be seen that the free-air ionisation chamber is suitable for the absolute measurement of exposure and absorbed dose in air. The absorbed dose, which would have occurred in another medium, placed in the same beam of radiation may be calculated from the mass absorption coefficients, as explained earlier in Section 33.3.3.

33.5.3 Chemical Methods of Dose Measurement

We have already established that radiation affects the chemical bonds between atoms of a material through which it passes by both ionisation and excitation of electrons. Research by Fricke has shown that ionising radiation is able to transform a dilute solution of ferrous sulphate, $FeSO_4$, to ferric sulphate, $Fe_2(SO_4)_3$, by rearrangement of the chemical bonds. The number of ferric ions so produced is proportional to the absorbed dose – 100 eV of absorbed dose will produce about 15 ferric ions. Thus, a chemical measurement of the concentration of the ferric ions produced at a given energy of a given radiation beam may used as a measure of the absorbed dose in water.

Such a chemical dosimeter may be calibrated against either of the two preceding methods of absorbed dose measure. It is included in this section *on absolute methods of dose measurement* because, once the conversion factor between the absorbed dose and the quantity of ferric ions is known, no further calibration is necessary. The process of calibration is therefore similar to the calculation of absorbed dose in the free-air ionisation chamber from the knowledge of the energy required to produce an ion pair in air.

The above method of dose measurement is known as the *Fricke dosemeter*, but it is only suitable for the estimation of very large doses, in excess of 20 Gy. This is because of chemical impurities present in the solution, the rapid rate of germinal recombination of the ions produced and relatively insensitive methods of chemical estimation of the quantity of ferric ions produced. It is, however, particularly suitable for use with high-energy radiation beams and for irregular shapes of irradiated volumes The advent of conformational radiotherapy treatment and the requirement under the Ionising Radiations (Medical Exposure) Regulations (IR(ME)R: see Ch. 34) to optimise radiation dose to the patient have resulted in the development of a number of polymer gels. These are tissue-equivalent with a density of 0.99 g.cm⁻¹ and show a linear response to high-energy photons from 300 keV to in excess of 8 MeV. Ionising radiation also has a polymerisation effect on the gel supporting the ferrous sulphate atoms; this reduces germinal recombination and prevents migration of the ferric sulphate atoms formed outside the beam area. Magnetic resonance spectrometry is used to estimate the number of ferric sulphate atoms present. If placed (in a suitable container) in an amorphic phantom, such dosemeters may be used to confirm the steep dose gradients that are an essential feature of conformational therapy treatments.

33.6 TYPES OF DETECTORS AND DOSEMETERS

So far in this chapter we have considered the measurement of absorbed dose by *absolute* methods. These form a standard against which other types of dosemeter can be compared or calibrated. There are many such *relative methods* by which absorbed dose may be estimated, each with some advantages and disadvantages. The most common of these methods are briefly outlined below.

33.6.1 The Thimble Ionisation Chamber

The size and configuration of the free-air ionisation chamber discussed so far make it a suitable instrument for the standardisation of radiation dose measurement but totally unsuitable for routine dose measurement in a hospital environment – a plate separation of 5 metres would be required if we needed to measure the dose rate at a patient's skin from a cobalt-60 source! The thimble ionisation chamber shown in Figure 33.6 circumvents some of these difficulties by, as it were, 'condensing' the air into a solid medium surrounding the central electrode. The cap of the thimble chamber is said to be *air-equivalent*, i.e. it is made of a material that has the same atomic number as air (e.g. graphite, bakelite, plastic) and so its absorption properties

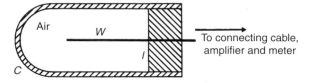

Figure 33.6 Construction of a thimble ionisation chamber. C, cap; W, central wire; I, insulator.

are the same as the *same mass of air*. The central aluminium electrode has a fixed amount of positive charge put on it from an external source. When the chamber is irradiated, some of the more energetic electrons liberated in the cap will penetrate into the air of the chamber and be attracted to the central electrode. Thus, the central electrode will lose some of its positive charge. By the choice of suitable materials, the thimble chamber can be made to have the same absorbing properties as the same mass of air. Such a device is calibrated for several photon energies against a standard chamber, such as the free-air chamber, described earlier in this chapter, and a correction factor is used to convert the indicated loss of charge from the central electrode to true absorbed dose. The choice of wall thickness of the cap is one of the factors that influence the applied correction, since a thin cap may not produce sufficient electrons entering the chamber, while too thick a cap will absorb more radiation than it needs to. *Note* that the vast majority of the electrons used to measure the change in charge or the current through the chamber are produced in the wall of the chamber and not in the air cavity of the chamber, but it is the passage of such electrons into the air cavity that enables the change in charge or the current to be measured. Corrections for variations in the temperature and pressure of the air must be made, as is the case for the free-air chamber.

Thimble-type chambers are still extensively used in radiation measurements in hospitals. For example, the calibration of the radiation output from a teletherapy machine is usually accomplished by the use of a thimble chamber connected to an electronic amplification system, which measures and displays the charge produced in the chamber during irradiation. However, in order to relate the reading obtained because of a

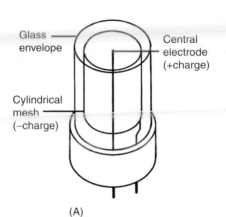

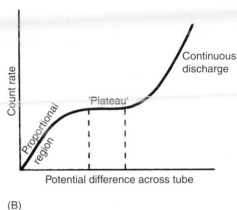

given exposure to the radiation output of the machine (usually expressed in cGy.min⁻¹), certain correction factors need to be applied. These include the following:

- the reading must be corrected for temperature and pressure
- the reading must be corrected by a factor which relates the reading of this *substandard unit* to a *secondary standard unit* calibrated by a national body (e.g. the Radiation Section of the Health Protection Agency) – this correction factor depends on the energy of the radiation
- the correction which requires to be applied to the secondary standard to compare it with the absolute standard – this is again related to the energy of the radiation and a factor to convert exposure to absorbed dose at the appropriate radiation energy.

In addition, there may be some machine-dependent correction factors, such as correction for 'switch-on' and 'switch-off' errors.

33.6.2 The Geiger–Müller Counter

The thimble chamber described in the previous section is an example of an ionisation chamber where the charge collected on the electrodes is proportional to the energy absorbed from the X-ray beam. The Geiger–Müller counter works on the principle of gas multiplication and gives the same magnitude of electrical pulse per absorption event whatever the energy of the absorbed radiation. The structure of a typical Geiger–Müller tube is shown in Figure 33.7A.

A glass envelope contains an inert gas (argon) at low pressure and two electrodes – a positively charged central electrode and a negatively charged mesh cylinder. Ionisation is caused in the gas by the entry of a photon or by the entry of particulate radiation if the window is sufficiently thin to allow particles to enter the envelope. The ions are attracted to the appropriate electrode and, as they pass through the gas, they will gain sufficient energy to eject electrons from the gas atoms if the potential difference between the electrodes is sufficiently great. The electrons so produced continue this process and rapid gas multiplication takes place, especially near the central electrode, since the field strength is great in this region. The effect of gas multiplication is such that well in excess of 1 million electrons are collected by the central electrode for every single ion produced in the primary absorption process. These 'electron avalanches' form the pulses, which allow the system to count the number of initial ionisation events. The presence of a small quantity of alcohol vapour in the gas helps to quench the gas multiplication process so that it does not become continuous. It does this by absorbing the kinetic energy of the positive ions in the gas so that they are prevented from striking the mesh with sufficient energy to release further electrons and so keep the process going indefinitely. Alternatively, the potential difference between the electrodes may be momentarily reduced after an electron avalanche, thus terminating the gas multiplication. In either case, there is a *dead time* after each pulse, where another absorption event, if present, is not recorded. A typical dead time is 5 μs and so the differences between the observed count rates and the real count rates are negligible except at high count rates – at an observed count rate of 1000 per second, the true count rate is 1005, whereas at an observed count rate of 100 000 per second the true count rate is 200 000! The correct potential difference to be applied to a Geiger–Müller tube is determined in practice by plotting a graph of the count rate obtained when a small radioactive source is placed near the tube, against the applied voltage. Such a graph is shown in Figure 33.7B. Three distinct regions of such a graph exist:

1. the *proportional region*, where some gas multiplication takes place and the sizes of the electrical pulses are proportional to the energy deposited in the gas by the radiation
2. the *plateau region*, where maximum gas amplification takes place and all electrical pulses have the same size, irrespective of the energy of the radiation
3. the *continuous-discharge region*, where the electrical field strength is sufficient to ionise the gas atoms and so produce continuous unwanted gas multiplication. The plateau is usually between 100 and 1500 V, depending on the size of the Geiger–Müller tube.

As can be seen, the Geiger Müller tube is suitable for detecting the presence of radiation rather than for an accurate estimation of absorbed doses, since the pulses bear no relationship to the energy of the radiation causing them. It is therefore often used as a contamination monitor for radioactive spillage or as a method of determining whether radiation is present in a specific area.

33.6.3 Scintillation Detectors

The operation of a scintillation detector employing a sodium iodide crystal and a photomulti-

plier tube is described in Appendix B, which considers radionuclide imaging and nuclear medicine in more detail.

Any suitable scintillating material can be used, whether solid or liquid, and the principle of operation is that the size of the electrical pulse produced by the photomultiplier is proportional to the energy deposited in the scintillator. Scintillation plastics have been produced which have an atomic number close to that of air and tissue. These can therefore be termed as being *air-equivalent* and so have similar variations of absorption to air, with variations in photon energy. They are therefore useful in estimating absorbed dose in air. Sodium iodide has a much higher atomic number than air and will therefore show a marked variation in absorption with photon energy, especially near its absorption edges (see Sect. 30.5). This requires correction factors to be applied for different photon energies if an accurate estimation of the absorbed dose in air is to be made. This is particularly so for thin crystals, which show a more marked variation in absorption with photon energy, compared with thick crystals.

Scintillation counters are very sensitive devices and are used in many applications in radiography and radionuclide imaging, e.g. for the detection of radioactive contamination, for estimation of in vitro radioactivity, as radiation detectors on computed tomography and osteoporosis scanners and as the detection mechanism in gamma cameras.

33.6.4 Thermoluminescent Dosimetry (TLD)

The basic physics of thermoluminesce has already been described (see Sect. 31.4). Thermoluminescence may be used to estimate radiation doses by the use of lithium fluoride in the form of powder, extruded chips or impregnated Teflon discs or rods. The impurities in the lithium fluoride generate electron traps and the number of electrons which are 'stuck' in these traps is proportional to the absorbed dose in the lithium fluoride. The average atomic number of lithium fluoride is 8.2 so it is close to soft tissue ($Z = 7.5$)

and both have similar absorption variations with photon energy. The small discs do not show up on radiographs and so may be strapped to the part of the body where we wish to measure the absorbed dose. After irradiation, the discs are heated and the amount of light emitted is compared to a standard dosimeter to which a known dose has been given. The dose to the disc can then be calculated by direct proportion. The discs are then annealed and may be reused.

The fact that the discs have radiolucency similar to tissue allows us to use them to estimate radiation dose without interfering with the radiograph or radiotherapy treatment. The discs are small, measuring only a few millimetres across, and so may be used to estimate the dose to different structures in the body during a diagnostic or therapeutic procedure.

The role of TLD in personnel monitoring will be considered in Chapter 34.

33.6.5 Photographic Film

Photographic film will produce an increase in optical density when it is irradiated. The response, however, is not in linear proportion to the absorbed dose of the emulsion. A calibration graph for the particular film at known radiation doses and specific processing conditions must therefore be produced. This is a major disadvantage if it is to be used as a method of dose estimation. It is also true that the film emulsion has a higher atomic number than tissue (AgBr has an average atomic number of 41) and so has significantly higher photoelectric absorption at low energies. Therefore, the relationship between photographic density and dose must be corrected for the energy of the radiation to allow us to estimate the absorbed dose in tissue. Photographic film forms the basis of the film-badge method of personnel monitoring and its role in this area will be described in more detail in Chapter 34. Photographic film is also useful, for instance, in checking the accuracy of the light-beam diaphragm on a diagnostic X-ray machine, or the accuracy of the jaws on a therapy machine.

33.6.6 Semiconductor Detectors

As we saw in Section 18.3, electrons in a semiconductor can readily have their energy raised to that of the conduction band and so can take part in electrical conduction. The absorption of energy from an X-ray photon (by either photoelectric absorption or Compton scattering) can raise an electron to the conduction band energies. This electron causes secondary electrons from the atoms of the material to be raised to the conduction band, by imparting some of its energy to them. If a potential difference is placed across the semiconductor, then these electrons are collected before they have time to recombine. Thus there is a current pulse whose magnitude is proportional to the number of electrons and hence the absorbed dose within the semiconductor. This is similar to the current through an irradiated ionisation chamber and the semiconductor detector can be thought of as a solid-state ionisation chamber. It has the great advantage over the air ionisation chamber that it produces 10 times as many ion pairs for a given dose of radiation and so is much more sensitive to small doses. This is because only 3 eV is required to produce an ion pair in a semiconductor, compared to 33 eV to produce an ion pair in air. The electrical signal obtained from the semiconductor device is thus more accurate – it has a smaller statistical uncertainty – and may, for example, be used to produce very accurate gamma-ray spectra.

Semiconductor detectors may be calibrated against a thimble chamber, for example, for a given energy of radiation.

Semiconductor detectors tend to be used for more specialised forms of radiation detection, e.g. a small semiconductor detector may be inserted into the rectum to measure rectal dose.

SUMMARY

In this chapter, you should have learnt:

- The definition of exposure and the relationship between exposure and absorbed dose (see Sect. 33.3)
- The definition of and the relationship between absorbed dose and kerma (see Sect. 33.2)
- The effects of different media on the absorbed dose (see Sect. 33.3.3)
- The meaning of the terms *quality factor* and *dose-equivalent* and how their values vary for different types of radiation (see Sect. 33.4)
- Measurement of radiation exposure and absorbed dose by the free air ionisation chamber (see Sect. 33.5.2)
- Measurement of radiation exposure and absorbed dose by chemical dosemeters (see Sect. 33.5.3)
- Measurement of radiation exposure and absorbed dose by the thimble ionisation chamber (see Sect. 33.6.1)
- Detection of the presence of radiation by the Geiger–Müller counter (see Sect. 33.6.2)
- Measurement of radiation exposure and absorbed dose by scintillation detectors (see Sect. 33.6.3)
- Measurement of radiation exposure and absorbed dose by thermoluminescent dosimetry (see Sect. 33.6.4)
- Measurement of radiation exposure and absorbed dose by photographic film (see Sect. 33.6.5)
- Measurement of radiation exposure and absorbed dose by semiconductor detectors (see Sect. 33.6.6).

SELF-TEST

a. Outline the differences between exposure, absorbed dose and dose-equivalent in the measurement of radiation. Explain why the three units are necessary.

b. List the methods that can be used for the absolute measurement of exposure or absorbed dose of radiation. Describe one of those in detail.

c. Describe the use of a thimble ionisation chamber in the measurement of exposure or absorbed radiation dose.

d. List six methods that may be used to detect radiation. Describe one of those methods.

FURTHER READING

Ball J L, Moore A D 1997 Essential physics for radiographers, 3rd edn. Blackwell Scientific Publications, London, ch 16

Ball J, Price T 1995 Chesney's radiographic imaging, 6th edn. Blackwell Scientific Publications, London, ch 5

Curry T S III, Dowdey J E, Murry R C Jr 1990 Christensen's physics of diagnostic radiography, 4th edn. Lee & Febiger, London, ch 2

Dowsett D J, Kenny P A, Johnston R E 1998 The physics of diagnostic imaging, Chapman & Hall Medical, London, chs 21 and 22

Johns H E, Cunningham J R 1983 The physics of radiology, 4th edn. Charles C Thomas, Illinois, USA, ch 2

Keall P, Baldock C 1999 A theoretical study of the radiological properties and water equivalence of Fricke and polymer gels used for radiation dosimetry. Australasian Journal of Physics and Engineering Sciences in Medicine 22(3):85–91

Chapter 34

Radiation Protection

CHAPTER CONTENTS

34.1   Aim 333

34.2   Purpose and Scope of Radiation Protection 333

34.3   Ionising Radiation Regulations 334

34.4   Biological Effects of Ionising Radiation 335
        34.4.1 Stochastic Effects 335
        34.4.2 Deterministic (Non-Stochastic) Effects 337

34.5   Risk–benefit, ALARA (ALARP) and Detriment 337

34.6   Radiological Examinations of Women of
        Reproductive Capacity 338

34.7   Dose-Equivalent Limits 339

34.8   Effective Dose 341

34.9   Committed Dose 342

34.10   Designation of Radiation Workers 343
        34.10.1 Dose Limitations for Employees
                Who have been Overexposed to
                Radiation 345

34.11   Practical Radiation Protection 345
        34.11.1 Radiation Protection Advisers and
                Radiation Protection Supervisors 346
        34.11.2 Local Rules 346
        34.11.3 Personnel Monitoring 347
        34.11.4 Designation of Work Areas 349
        34.11.5 Duties of Designated Individuals as
                Defined by IR(ME)R 2000 349
        34.11.6 Good Radiographic Practice 350
        34.11.7 Room Design 350

Self-Test 352

Further Reading 353

34.1 AIM

The aim of this chapter is to introduce the reader to the basic legal requirements for the safe use of ionising radiation. This will cover the main documents involved and will then look at practical ways in which these are implemented in radiology or radiotherapy departments. Note that only limited reference is made to nuclear medicine and any reader who requires further information in this area is recommended to consult one of the nuclear medicine texts listed at the end of this chapter.

34.2 PURPOSE AND SCOPE OF RADIATION PROTECTION

The purpose of radiation protection is to produce and maintain an environment, both at work and in the outside world, where the levels of ionising radiation pose a minimal acceptable risk for human beings. *Natural ionising radiations* (Table 34.1) have always existed and our bodies are subject to these radiations at all times. Those natural sources of radiation thus constitute a radiation dose received by the whole population and radiation protection procedures can do little or nothing to reduce this limit.

At the beginning of any discussion on radiation protection it is important to realise that our environment can only be described as *relatively safe* from the effects of such radiations. It follows from this that one of the basic tasks of radiation

Table 34.1 Average radiation doses to the population in the UK from various sources

Natural/artificial	Source	Percentage of total UK dose	Average annual whole-body dose equivalent (μSv)
Natural radiation	Radon gas from rocks	47	1200
	Gamma-/X-rays from rocks	14	350
	Ingested radiation from food and drink	12	300
	Cosmic radiation	10	250
	Radiation from thoron (byproduct of radon)	4	100
Artificial radiation	Medical irradiation	12	300
	Nuclear discharges	0.1	2.5
	Occupational exposure (radiation workers)	0.2	5
	Fallout from weapons testing	0.4	10
	Miscellaneous other sources	0.4	10

protection is to establish *levels of risk* to the population due to natural and artificial radiation sources and then to take steps to keep these levels of risk as low as possible. The average doses received by the UK population from the various sources of radiation are shown in Table 34.1.

Once the levels of risk from such radiation have been ascertained, appropriate dose-equivalent limits (see Sect. 34.7) may be set so that the risk associated with such radiations is no greater (and frequently is much less) than other aspects of life, e.g. the risk of injury as a result of mechanical accident. Establishing such dose-equivalent limits, and ensuring that staff work within these limits, helps to prevent the suffering and early deaths that were experienced by the pioneering radiation workers who were exposed to very large doses of radiation.

A full study of radiation protection would need to cover the following topics:

- radiobiology
- genetics
- statistical analysis of risk
- methods of reducing radiation doses to workers
- the fate and decay patterns of radioactivity released into the environment
- the absorbing power of different materials to different radiations.

Such a vast scope of study cannot be covered in one chapter, or even in one book. Only a simplified – but sufficient to allow safe working – treatment of these topics is considered in the remainder of the chapter. For coverage at greater depth the reader is referred to some of the more specialist texts on this topic listed at the end of the chapter.

34.3 IONISING RADIATION REGULATIONS

The above comments indicate the wide scope of radiation protection and the need for multidisciplinary collaboration in tackling some of the problems. Radiation protection is a developing subject where the acquisition of new knowledge is used to formulate safer procedures and lower radiation doses or risks.

In the UK protection policy is subject to centralised policy decisions from Brussels. The *Euratom Directives* are an attempt to standardise and modernise radiation protection practice in all member states of the European Community (EC). The International Commission for Radiation Protection (ICRP) has produced a number of recommendations on radiation protection. These have been incorporated in these Directives, and have had a significant impact on British law. The Euratom Directives 90/641, 96/29 and 97/7 resulted in the publication of the Ionising Radiation Regulations 1999 (IRR 1999). Similarly, Euratom Directive 97/43 has resulted in the publication of the Ionising Radiation (Medical Exposure) Regulations 2000 (IR(ME)R 2000). The inspectorate of the *Health and Safety Executive*

(HSE) is responsible for ensuring that employers and employees comply with the above regulations. IRR 1999 applies to all radiation work and radiation workers in both the private and public sectors of the nuclear industry and those who may be affected by such work activities. In contrast, IR(ME)R 2000 applies whenever humans are irradiated for diagnostic, therapeutic, research or other medical or dental purposes, and where in vitro medical tests are conducted. These regulations apply to staff, students, patients and their friends and relatives who are acting as comforters or carers, volunteers in research projects and members of the public. Details of acceptable methods of meeting the requirements of these laws have been published as the *Approved Code of Practice* (for IRR 1999) and *Medical and Dental Guidance Notes – A Good Practice Guide on All Aspects of Ionising Radiation Protection in the Clinical Environment* (for IR(ME)R 2000). The main points of these documents will be discussed within the context of this chapter but the reader is strongly recommended to study both documents as space permits the consideration of only a few essential regulations in this chapter.

34.4 BIOLOGICAL EFFECTS OF IONISING RADIATION

As we saw in Chapter 30, X- and gamma-rays are capable of ionising matter through which they pass – hence the term *ionising radiation*. The ejection of an electron from an atom or molecule of the material means that *atomic bonds are broken*. This is true even if the electron ejected is from an inner shell, as the resulting cascade of electrons falling into the inner orbitals results in an electron vacancy in the outer, valence shell, and so disrupts the valency bonding between the atoms (see Sect. 26.6).

Such an ejection of an electron from an atom or molecule results in the formation of a negative ion (the electron) and a positive ion (the remaining part of the atom or molecule). If the ions so formed in tissue by the primary or secondary ionisation processes (see Sect. 33.3) are capable of recombining exactly as they were before, then no radiation damage will occur in the tissue. Some such recombinations take place (in about 10^{-11} s) but the breaking of chemical bonds produces free radicals which are chemically highly reactive ions capable of forming new bonds to other ions. Thus new chemicals have been formed within the cells of the tissue. If the original chemical was important to the normal function of the cell then the cell can behave abnormally and so *the radiation has caused biological damage*. A typical sequence of events may run as follows:

1. Photon of ionising radiation absorbed by atom of the cell, causing *ionisation*
2. The ejected electron has sufficient energy to cause ionisation of other atoms in the material – *secondary ionisation* has occurred
3. Some of the free radicals so produced combine with others to form new chemicals within the cell, producing a *chemical change*
4. This chemical change causes abnormal behaviour of the cell, resulting in a *biological change*.

The effects of the biological changes so caused may be categorised under two headings:

1. stochastic effects
2. deterministic (non-stochastic) effects.

34.4.1 Stochastic Effects

A stochastic effect is one where *the probability* of the effect occurring is governed by the laws of chance. In the case of radiation-induced stochastic effects we can say that the greater the radiation dose received, the greater the probability of the effect occurring. This has two important consequences in terms of stochastic effects:

1. *There is no 'safe dose limit'. All doses of radiation carry some risk.* The greater the dose, the greater the risk – this allows us to define an acceptable level of risk and hence calculate *dose-equivalent limits*
2. Since the probability of the effect occurring is chance-related, *the severity of the effect is unrelated to the radiation dose received*. This can be seen more easily if we look at radiation-induced cancers as an example of a stochastic

effect. If we increase the dose to a population sample, we will see a corresponding increase in the *number* of radiation-induced cancers, but no increase in the *severity* of the cancers produced.

Two important stochastic effects due to exposure to ionising radiation are:

1. radiation-induced cancers
2. genetic effects.

These will now be discussed in more detail.

34.4.1.1 Radiation-Induced Cancers

Most radiation-induced cancers develop some years after the radiation was received. This is known as the *latent period* and may extend up to 30 years.

The risk of inducing a particular type of cancer is measured by comparing the number of cancers produced in the irradiated population sample in excess of those expected in the same size of unirradiated population sample. This is known as the *risk factor* for the particular cancer.

DEFINITION

The *risk factor* is the estimated likelihood of the occurrence of a particular radiation-induced effect per unit dose-equivalent received by each member of the population considered.

If the risk factor for a particular effect is r, then we may express r mathematically as:

$$r = \frac{\left(\dfrac{\text{no. of cases}}{\text{size of population}}\right)}{\text{dose-equivalent received by population}}$$

Equation 34.1

The units of r are fraction per sievert, i.e. Sv^{-1}.

INSIGHT

The risk factor for radiation-induced leukaemia is estimated at about 2×10^{-3} Sv^{-1}. This means that if members of a population each receive 1 Sv then the fraction of the population developing leukaemia is 2×10^{-3}. Hence, if a population of 1 million individuals were to receive 1 Sv of radiation, then $10^6 \times 2 \times 10^{-3} = 2000$ leukaemias will be likely to occur within that sample. While this may look an alarming number, it should be remembered that 1 Sv is a large amount of radiation – about equivalent to the dose received if each member of the sample had 50 000 chest radiographs – so the risk factor, although not zero, is very small.

The risk factors for most other radiation-induced cancers are of a similar or smaller value than that for leukemia. Some tissues are, however, more radiosensitive than others. This is particularly true of tissues where the cells are rapidly dividing. The positive side of this is that cancer cells, because of their rapid division, are more susceptible to radiation damage than healthy cells. On the negative side, the fetus is sensitive to radiation damage, especially at the early stages of its development. Hence pregnant women, or women who suspect they might be pregnant, should only be X-rayed under very specific conditions (see Sect. 34.6).

As radiation-induced cancers are stochastic effects, the incidence of such cancers in a population sample may be reduced by minimising the radiation dose received. Thus in medical exposure to radiation we aim to keep the radiation dose received by individuals as low as reasonably practicable.

34.4.1.2 Genetic Effects

Genetic effects are caused by radiation-induced damage to the genes or chromosomes in the ova or spermatozoa. Biological damage to the chromosomes occurs due to ionisation and subsequent faulty recombination of the molecules which make up the chromosomes. The biological code contained by the genes on the chromosomes has been altered and this constitutes an abnormality in the structure of the chromosomes which will be passed on to future generations if reproduction is possible. Thus *the genetically significant radiation* dose is the radiation dose to the gonads of persons of reproductive capacity. Severe genetic effects tend to be eliminated from the population because of the short life span of those affected or their inability to reproduce. However, less severe effects are more likely to become part of the human gene pool as a result of human reproduction. Thus, future generations may be protected from an unacceptably high proportion of defective genes by the reduction of the radiation dose to members of the population who are (or, in the case of children, will be in the future) of reproductive capacity. In practice this means reducing the contribution of artificial radiations to a minimum, by the use of appropriate radiation protection procedures. The gonad dose in radiographic investigations must therefore be reduced as far as possible by the use of good technique and appropriate equipment (see Sect. 34.11.5).

34.4.2 Deterministic (Non-Stochastic) Effects

A deterministic effect of radiation is one:

- whose severity increases with radiation dose (death being the exception to the rule – although the time between the radiation incident and death decreases with an increase in dose)
- for which there is usually a threshold below which the effect will not occur.

Thus we can say that a stochastic effect *may* occur, whereas for a deterministic effect, above a certain dose value, the effect *always* occurs. Examples of deterministic effects include erythema (skin reddening) or epilation (hair dropping out). The radiation doses required to produce such effects are very large and are likely to occur only as the result of radiation accidents, although some of the deterministic effects may occur as a result of radiotherapy treatment. Some such effects with the associated doses are given in Table 34.2.

INSIGHT

The classification of radiation-induced damage into stochastic and deterministic effects is relatively recent. The previous classification was

Table 34.2 Deterministic effects and radiation doses required to produce them

Radiation dose (as a single whole-body exposure: Sv)	Deterministic effect
20	Death within a matter of hours, due to severe damage to central nervous system
10	Death is likely to occur within days due to damage to lining of gastrointestinal tract. Infection is likely to enter blood stream; patient will die of either septicaemia or haemorrhage as a result of breakdown of the gut lining
5	Death likely to occur within weeks due to bone marrow damage (may be prevented by radical medical intervention)
1	Temporary depression of blood count. (Patient may develop stochastic effects)

into *somatic* effects and *genetic* effects. Somatic effects referred to damage caused to the individual and genetic effects to damage passed on to future generations. Thus somatic damage includes stochastic and deterministic effects, as can be seen from the above discussion.

34.5 RISK–BENEFIT, ALARA (ALARP) AND DETRIMENT

In view of the possible adverse effects of radiation on individuals and on future generations, it is logical to suggest that no unnecessary radiation dose should be received by any person. Thus no radiological investigation should be undertaken unless there is sound clinical evidence to suggest that the patient is likely to benefit from the investigation – all radiological investigations need to be *justified*. Even when it is decided that the patient is likely to benefit from a radiological procedure, the radiation dose received by staff and patients should be kept as low as possible. Examples of how this can be done have already been covered – patient dose may be reduced by the use of filtration (see Sect. 29.7), collimation of the X-ray beam (see Sect. 32.3.3) and by the use of fast film/screen combinations (see Sect. 31.5), while dose to patients and staff may be reduced by good radiographic technique (see Sect. 34.11.5). As we have already discussed when we considered stochastic effects, all exposure to ionising radiation carries a risk: the smaller the dose, the smaller the risk. Thus all radiographic procedures carry a risk – albeit a small one – that irreversible damage *may* be done to the patient as a result of the radiation exposure. However, it is necessary to quantify this risk against the potential benefit to the patient as a result of radiography. If we consider a patient with a suspected fracture of the femur, the patient is likely to get a greater benefit out of having this fracture diagnosed and treated than the extremely small chance that he or she may develop leukaemia in later life as a result of the radiation exposure – in this case the decision to expose the patient to ionising radiation can clearly be justified. As we have already considered, the risk of radiation-induced injury is decreased when the radiation dose received is reduced. However, it is not practical in a modern society to reduce the radiation dose (and consequently the risk) to zero. A balance must be achieved between the desirability of low radiation doses and the difficulty and cost of achieving these low doses. This leads to the so-called ALARA principle, introduced in ICRP 26, which states that doses to patients and staff should be kept *as low as reasonably achievable*. The IRR 1999 has a very similar concept – the ALARP principle – which states that radiation doses should be kept *as low as reasonably practicable*.

Radiation exposure reduction due to a particular investigation or technique must therefore be analysed in terms of the benefits likely to be achieved and the difficulty or cost of reducing the detrimental effects of the radiation received to lower levels. An appropriate practical compromise must then be reached between the cost or difficulty and the likely improvement produced. For instance, the use of robotic arms in a hospital radiopharmacy would undoubtedly reduce the radiation dose received by staff by a small amount but at a very high cost in terms of financial outlay and would also cause considerable inconvenience to the staff involved. On the other hand, the use of lead covering on the benches is a much cheaper solution and is likely to produce a greater reduction in radiation doses. Thus it should be remembered that the high-cost, high-technology solution is not always the most appropriate.

It would often be difficult to choose between various practical solutions to working safely with radiation unless a *quantitative* assessment of the detrimental effects of radiation were possible. The *detriment* due to radiation has a precise mathematical meaning and is defined in ICRP 26 thus:

DEFINITION

The *detriment* is the expectation of harm incurred from an exposure to radiation, taking into account not only the probability of each type of deleterious effect, but also the severity of the effect.

The risk factors discussed above are of value in assessing such detriment.

34.6 RADIOLOGICAL EXAMINATIONS OF WOMEN OF REPRODUCTIVE CAPACITY

The relative sensitivity of the fetus to ionising radiation (see Sect. 34.4) means that it is good radiographic practice to avoid radiological investigations of the lower abdomen and pelvis of women who are or may be pregnant unless there are overriding clinical reasons why such investigations must be performed. (In many cases, in the modern diagnostic imaging department, we can get the required information using ultrasound, which is a non-ionising type of radiation.) The ovum also is particularly sensitive to ionising radiation in the 7 weeks prior to ovulation. The risk to the fetus from radiation diminishes as the pregnancy progresses but at no stage is this risk zero. It is therefore important to attempt to ensure that the benefits of a radiological investigation of *a woman who is pregnant or may be pregnant* outweigh the risks involved, as outlined in the previous section of this chapter – remember that both the mother and the fetus are being irradiated and so both are at risk. An earlier recommendation of the ICRP was that *women of reproductive capacity should only be X-rayed within 10 days of the commencement of their last menstrual period* since pregnancy at that time was highly unlikely. This was known as the *10-day rule*.

In 1984, as a result of a more accurate estimate of the risks and benefits associated with radiography of the lower abdomen of such women before and after conception, the ICRP issued new recommendations. The relevant paragraph reads as follows:

> **During the first ten days following the onset of a menstrual period, there can be no risk to any conceptus, since no conception will have occurred. The risk to a child who had previously been irradiated in utero during the remainder of a four-week period following the onset of menstruation is likely to be so small that there need be no special limitation on exposures required within these four weeks.**

Following the publication of the ICRP Recommendations, the National Radiological Protection Board (NRPB) added its own recommendations, which are applicable in the UK. These are summarised below:

- Any woman who has an overdue or missed period should be treated as though she were pregnant
- If the woman cannot answer 'no' to the question 'are you, or might you be pregnant?' then she should be regarded as if she were pregnant
- If the clinical indications are that an exposure should be made where the primary beam irradiates the fetus, then great care must be taken to minimise the number of views and the absorbed dose per view, but without jeopardising the diagnostic value of the investigation
- Provided good collimation is used, and properly shielded equipment, radiographs of areas remote from the fetus (e.g. chest, skull, hand)

may be done safely at any time during the pregnancy.

The demise of the 10-day rule in favour of the new recommendations does not reduce the care that should be taken in limiting the potential radiation dose to the fetus. The change in emphasis of the recommendations is that special precautions need only be taken if the woman is, or may be, pregnant – where 'pregnant' is defined as beginning when a menstrual period is overdue. Other than this, there is no need for special limitations of exposures during a menstrual cycle except for the normal requirements to keep all absorbed radiation doses as low as reasonably practicable. Good radiographic techniques should thus be used at all times to minimise radiation doses for all exposures.

A flow chart showing the progress of a woman of reproductive capacity presenting for a radiographic examination is given in Figure 34.1.

34.7 DOSE-EQUIVALENT LIMITS

IRR 1999 has followed the recommendations of ICRP 26 in using the term *dose-equivalent limits* or dose limits in preference to the term *maximum permissible dose*, which was used in the previous Code of Practice. The new terminology will be used throughout this chapter.

The setting of dose limits for individuals and groups of individuals is an extension of the risk–benefit principle outlined above (see Sect. 34.4.1). In the estimation of such limits, the effects of natural background radiation and radiation to the individual from medical exposure are excluded. This is because the former is largely beyond our control and so no practical purpose is served by its inclusion, and the latter is because individuals irradiated during a medical investigation are assumed to benefit directly from such irradiation.

The limits discussed should not be considered as constituting boundary lines between safety and danger. Rather, they should reflect levels of risk, either to the individual or to groups within the population, which are comparable to the risks from other activities within society that are

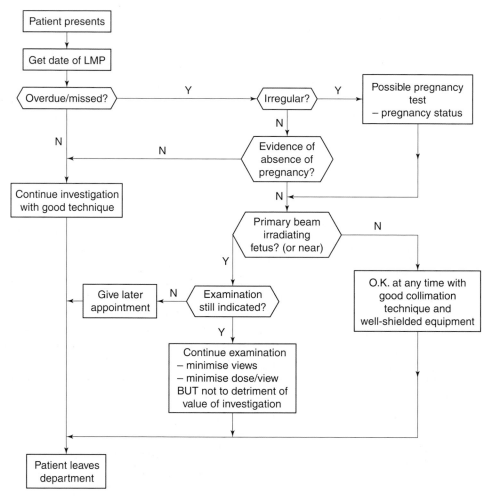

Figure 34.1 A flow chart which can be used to ensure that the radiation protection requirements are met during radiography of women who are of reproductive capacity. LMP, last menstrual period.

already considered to possess an adequate degree of safety and represent what is considered to be an acceptable risk. There is therefore no abrupt increase in hazard if the radiation dose limit is exceeded, only an increasing probability of a stochastic effect occurring after some suitable latent period. If the limit is grossly exceeded, various prompt deterministic effects will occur.

INSIGHT

The assessment of socially acceptable risk in various occupations and to the general public produces figures in the range 10^{-5} to 10^{-6} per year.

It is regarded as an acceptable risk that between 1 in 100 000 and 1 in a million of the population sample may die each year as a result of the hazard involved. The average risk in the UK of death due to an accident at work is approximately 10^{-5}. If we take the figure of 10^{-5} and apply it to Equation 34.1, then the annual dose-equivalent limit (see Sect. 34.7) is 1 mSv if it is assumed that the total risk factor from all stochastic effects is 10^{-2} Sv^{-1}. The use of stochastic effects to derive the dose-equivalent limits is chosen because such effects show no threshold and are therefore more significant than deterministic effects for the lower radiation doses. The dose-equivalent limits are thus chosen to *prevent* deterministic effects and to *limit* the occurrence of stochastic effects to a socially acceptable level.

34.8 EFFECTIVE DOSE

When ICRP 26 was published in 1977, it introduced the concept of *effective dose equivalent* in order to take account of the fact that different organs in the body show different sensitivities to radiation. This concept has been continued in future ICRP publications (notably ICRP 60, published in 1990 and ICRP 75, published in 1997), although the weighting factors (Table 34.3) given to the various organs are slightly different from ICRP 26 and the term was changed to *effective dose*. Using the concept of effective dose we can state that a specific dose given to an organ of high radiosensitivity carries a higher risk than if the same dose is given to an organ of lower sensitivity. In the former case a *higher effective dose* is received. Each organ is therefore given a *weighting factor* which represents its sensitivity to radiation in relation to that of the whole body when the whole body receives the same dose. Thus the weighting factor can be defined:

Table 34.3 Weighting factors for different tissues irradiated singly

Tissue	Weighting factor (w_t)
Testes and ovaries	0.20
Red bone marrow	0.12
Colon	0.12
Lung	0.12
Stomach	0.12
Breast	0.05
Urinary bladder	0.05
Thyroid	0.05
Liver	0.05
Oesophagus	0.05
Bone surfaces	0.02
Other tissues not listed above	0.05

DEFINITION

The *weighting factor* (W_t) of a particular tissue or organ is the risk of stochastic effects being induced in the organ when singly irradiated, compared to the total risk of inducing stochastic effects if the same radiation dose is received by the whole body.

The various weighting factors for different tissues are shown in Table 34.3. As can be seen, the testes and ovaries are the most radiosensitive tissues as they have the highest value of weighting factor. The weighting factors quoted are those from ICRP 60. Notice also that the sum of the weighting factors is unity.

The unit of effective dose is just the same as the unit of dose equivalent (Sv or mSv) since the weighting factors are constants.

The following example shows how the weighting factors given in Table 34.3 are used to calculate the effective dose-equivalent received from radiography of the chest.

EXAMPLE

Radiography of the chest produced the following doses: gonads 0.01 mSv, breast 0.05 mSv, red bone marrow 0.005 mSv, lung 0.15 mSv, thyroid 0.02 mSv, bone 0.005 mSv, stomach 0.05 mSv, liver 0.002 mSv, colon 0.002 mSv and bladder 0.001mSv. What is the effective dose equivalent received by the patient?

We can calculate the effective dose-equivalent by taking the dose equivalent for each structure and multiplying it by the appropriate weighting factor. Thus we have:

$$
\begin{aligned}
\text{Dose equivalent} = {} & (0.01 \times 0.2) + (0.05 \times 0.05) + \\
& (0.005 \times 0.12) + (0.15 \times 0.12) + \\
& (0.02 \times 0.05) + (0.005 \times 0.05) + \\
& (0.05 \times 0.12) + (0.002 \times 0.05) + \\
& (0.002 \times 0.12) + (0.001 \times 0.05)
\end{aligned}
$$

$$
\begin{aligned}
= {} & 0.002 + 0.0025 + 0.0006 + \\
& 0.0027 + 0.001 + 0.00025 + \\
& 0.006 + 0.0001 + 0.00024 + \\
& 0.00005
\end{aligned}
$$

$$
= 0.01544 \text{ mSv}
$$

Thus a chest radiograph produced using the above technique is equivalent to 0.01544 mSv to the whole body for radiation protection purposes.

34.9 COMMITTED DOSE

When we consider committed dose, we are considering the absorbed dose which a person receives as a result of the intake of radioactive material. In such a case the person will continue to receive a dose of radiation as long as any traces of radioactivity remain within the body. The factors which affect the activity remaining in the body are the effective half-life, which is related to the physical half-life, and the biological half-life, as shown in the equation below (this has been discussed in more detail in Sect. 4.6):

$$\frac{1}{t_{1/2(\text{eff})}} = \frac{1}{t_{1/2(\text{phys})}} + \frac{1}{t_{1/2(\text{biol})}} \qquad \textit{Equation 34.2}$$

where $t_{1/2(\text{eff})}$ is the effective half-life, $t_{1/2(\text{phys})}$ is the physical half-life and $t_{1/2(\text{biol})}$ is the biological half-life. It is not possible to alter the physical half-life of a radionuclide as this depends on the structure of the nucleus, but it may be possible to reduce the biological half-life, e.g. by increasing the rate of excretion of the nuclide from the body (in nuclear imaging, patients are encouraged to drink fluid, after the scan is completed, to help eliminate technetium from the body). This results in a reduction of the effective half-life, as shown by Equation 34.2.

The effective half-life is, however, only one of a number of factors that determine the magnitude of the radiation dose-equivalent delivered to the body. Other factors include:

- the concentration of the activity in the organ (measured in MBq.kg^{-1})
- whether the concentration is uniform or localised within 'hot spots' within the organ
- the decay system (see Sect. 27.3) of the radionuclide
- the quality factors (see Sect. 33.4) of the radiations emitted
- the size and shape of the organ
- the proximity of other organs which might be irradiated
- the weighting factor for the organ.

The decay system is particularly relevant if alpha- or beta-particles are emitted as they have a very short range in tissue and alpha-particles have a high quality factor (20). Gamma-rays, however, are exponentially absorbed by the organ and so will contribute a smaller dose to that organ but may contribute a significant dose to other surrounding organs. The higher the energy of the gamma-rays, the lower the attenuation within the organ.

The *committed dose-equivalent* is a quantitative assessment of the effect of a particular intake of radioactivity over the whole of a person's working life. It may be defined as follows:

DEFINITION

The *committed dose-equivalent* is the dose-equivalent accruing over a period of 50 years following the intake of radioactive material.

The *committed effective dose* is obtained using the weighting factors in Table 34.3, and, once this figure is obtained for a given intake over a given period of time, it is compared with equivalent limits laid down by the IRR 1999 for the same period (e.g. annual or quarterly dose limit) for the appropriate category of person (radiation worker, member of the public, etc.). The dose limits stipulated by the IRR 1999 are shown in Table 34.4.

Table 34.4A shows the dose limits for two categories of radiation workers and also for other persons who are not radiation workers. Note that in all cases the dose limits for radiation workers under 18 years of age are three-tenths of the adult radiation worker doses, and the dose limits for members of the public are one-twentieth of the adult radiation worker doses. The whole-body dose limits are expressed in *effective dose* units (including the contributions of the committed dose), whereas the dose limits to individual organs are in *dose-equivalent* units. The use of weighting factors in the determination of effective dose is described above. These are required to calculate the effective whole-body dose.

Table 34.4A   Dose limits (mSv) per calendar year specified by Ionising Radiation Regulations 1999

Category of person	Dose to whole body	Dose to lens of the eye	Dose to skin averaged over an area of 1 cm²	Dose to hands, forearms, feet and ankles
Employee aged 18 or over	20	150	500	500
Trainees aged under 18	6	50	150	150
Comforter or carer: no specific dose limit stated in IRR 1999[a]	1	15	50	50
Other persons	1	15	50	50

[a]National Radiological Board (now Radiological Protection Section of Health Protection Agency) recommends that the dose should not exceed 5 mSv over a five year period.

Table 34.4B   Dose-equivalent limits (in mSv) for women of reproductive capacity and pregnant radiation workers set by the Ionising Radiation Regulations 1999

Category of person	Dose-equivalent to the abdomen	Time interval
Women of reproductive capacity who are radiation workers	13	Any consecutive 3-month period[a]
Pregnant women who are radiation workers	10	During the declared term of pregnancy

[a]Note: the whole-body dose must still not exceed the annual restrictions for employees over 18 years of age or for trainees under 18 years of age (whichever is relevant).

Table 34.4B shows the dose limits specified by the IRR 1999 in order to protect the fetus. The dose-equivalents shown refer to the maximum value which may be received from *external radiation*, i.e. the committed dose from the intake of radioactive materials is not included. Hence there is a need to restrict the possible intake of radioactivity, especially in working environments where radioactive material is more easily dispersed into the air. *Note* that a woman who is not a radiation worker is already subject to the limit of 1 mSv per calendar year, as shown in Table 34.4A.

INSIGHT

It is worth recalling at this point that the unit of dose-equivalent, the sievert, is the product of the absorbed dose and the quality factor for the radiation. Now the absorbed dose (measured in grays) is measured in $J.kg^{-1}$ and so relates to *unit mass.* Thus the total energy absorbed in a man weighing 70 kg who has received a whole-body dose of 3 Gy is $3 \times 70 = 210$ J. For the same person, the lungs might weigh approximately 0.5 kg and so the energy absorbed by the lungs for an absorbed dose of 3 Gy is $3 \times 0.5 = 1.5$ J. Thus the lungs would absorb 0.007 of the energy absorbed by the whole body, while they have a weighting factor of 0.12.

From this it can be seen that the same value of absorbed dose or dose-equivalent in different organs does not imply the same total absorption of energy but the same energy per unit mass. The biological effects of the absorbed energy depend on the radiosensitivity of the organ, as described above.

34.10 DESIGNATION OF RADIATION WORKERS

If an employee is likely to receive a whole-body dose-equivalent of ionising radiation which exceeds 6 mSv per annum then that person must be designated as a classified radiation worker, provided that:

- the employee is aged 18 years or more
- the employee has been certified as fit on medical grounds to be designated a classified person

- the employee is informed of being so designated.

Some of the practical ways of implementing the designation of employees as required by IRR 1999 regulation 20 are summarised below:

- It is not sufficient to rely on an individual's history of doses received if they are less than the three-tenths limit. The *potential doses* which may be received in a set of circumstances must be assessed
- The reason for designation may be that the individual works in *controlled areas* (see Sect. 34.11.4) but this is not, on its own, sufficient reason for designation
- Even if the *local rules* (see Sect. 34.11.2), when strictly obeyed, indicate that doses in excess of the three-tenths limit will not occur, persons who work with radiation sources which are capable of producing an overdose in a few minutes will need to be classified. (This has limited applications in the medical field for diagnostic imaging since it was intended to apply to personnel working with industrial rather than medical sources)
- When considering the classification of persons in relation to the intake of radionuclides from unsealed sources, the following factors should be taken into account:
  the potential for any intake to occur
  the likely magnitude of any intake
  the radiotoxicity of any intake.

A person who is a *classified radiation worker* must be subject to *medical surveillance*, with periodic reviews of health at least every 12 months. The health records for such an individual must be kept on a suitable form until the person has attained the age of 75 years or at least 50 years from the date of the last entry (IRR 1999 regulation 24). The employer must also arrange for the radiation dose which the classified person receives to be measured using a suitable *personal dosemeter* (see Sect. 34.11.3). Such doses must be measured by an approved *dosimetry service* on the basis of accepted national standards. Again, the employer must keep records of all doses recorded for such individuals until the person has attained the age of 75 years or at least 50 years after the last entry.

It should be noted that the above discussion does not mean that radiation workers who are not classified should not have dose records and/or medical records kept, but that there is no legal requirement to do so. However, the *radiation protection adviser* (RPA: see Sect. 34.11.1) may use personnel and site dose records to justify their designation (or lack of it) for both personnel and for working areas.

Any employee whose annual whole-body dose exceeds 15 mSv shall be subject to an investigation to see if the working practices involved are in keeping with the ALARA principle (see Sect. 34.5) or whether improvements may be made which would lead to a reduction in the dose. Records of such investigations must be kept for at least 50 years (IRR 1999 regulation 23).

In a medical environment, employees such as radiographers, medical laboratory scientific officers and medical physics technicians are involved in working with ionising radiation in the fields of diagnostic radiography, therapeutic radiography, nuclear medicine and pathology investigations using radionuclides. Each of these procedures contributes to the radiation doses received by appropriate personnel and these must be analysed to see if a particular individual needs to become a classified person to conform to the requirements of the IRR 1999. For example, a diagnostic radiographer is subject to ionising radiation from scatter from the patient and the walls of the X-ray room, while a therapy radiographer may receive some radiation through the walls of the treatment room and may receive an unexpected dose if the therapy source sticks in the exposed position after a treatment.

Staff in the nuclear medicine department will receive doses to the hands due to the preparation of radiopharmaceuticals and the handling of 'flood sources' for gamma cameras. They will also receive a whole-body dose due to being in close proximity to patients who have received diagnostic or therapeutic quantities of radiopharmaceuticals. Laboratory technicians who perform tests using radioactivity will also receive a dose to their hands and may receive doses from spills or airborne contamination.

However, it is unlikely that any of those workers will need to be classified, although the radiological monitoring of their received doses and that of their environment is a precaution, and one which may be used to justify their non-classified status.

34.10.1 Dose Limitations for Employees who have been Overexposed to Radiation

IRR 1999 lays down the procedures to adopt if it is known, or suspected, that an employee has been subject to overexposure to radiation. This overexposure may be the result of a single incident or because the total radiation dose received by the person during the period in question exceeds the relevant dose limit for that period. Again, it must be remembered that this is considered *occupational exposure* and any radiation exposure received by the person due to medical investigation or treatment does not count. After an overexposure has been reported to the employer, he or she must notify the HSE and the appropriate medical doctor. The employer must then carry out a detailed investigation into the circumstances of the overexposure. The HSE, the appointed doctor and the employee must receive a copy of the report and it must be kept by the employer until the person has attained the age of 75 years or at least 50 years after the last entry.

The overexposed person may be allowed to continue to work with ionising radiation provided the above notifications and investigations have been carried out, and under any condition(s) which the appointed doctor may specify. The dose limit for the individual for the remainder of the dose-limiting period (usually 1 year or 5 years) must be calculated and necessary steps taken to ensure that it is not exceeded.

34.11 PRACTICAL RADIATION PROTECTION

As described in the preceding sections of this chapter, radiation protection is based on three general principles:

1. Every practice resulting in an exposure to ionising radiation should be *justified* by the advantages it produces

2. All exposures should be kept *as low as reasonably achievable* (ALARA)

3. The sum of the doses and committed doses *should not exceed specified limits* (Table 34.4).

The first two principles show that it is not merely sufficient to observe the current dose limits for staff and diagnostic reference levels for investigations, since the possible health detriment from a given exposure must be compared to the overall benefit of that exposure. This may result in certain procedures involving ionising radiation being replaced by others that do not, e.g. ultrasound or magnetic resonance scans.

IRR 1999 indicates the legal and procedural framework in which these principles may be achieved in practice. Additionally, IR(ME)R 2000 considers ways in which the patient must be protected while undergoing an examination which involves exposure to ionising radiations. The main requirements of both documents are listed below:

- the provision of *suitable environments* for all employees, such that those areas where they are likely to receive a significant radiation dose, are suitably restricted and controlled (see Sect. 34.11.4)
- the *designation of employees* into classified and non-classified groups on the basis of the doses that they are likely to receive
- the establishing of a suitable personnel-monitoring service to ensure that radiation doses received are measured and recorded on a regular basis (whether or not non-classified radiation workers are monitored depends on local circumstances)
- the keeping of health records and radiation dose records for all classified radiation workers for the statutory period required by IRR 1999 (50 years)
- notification to the HSE of all radiation incidents and overexposures, and the writing of reports subsequent to the investigation of these incidents
- the establishment of *environmental monitoring* to establish that the working conditions of the employees and the doses received by the general public are in accordance with IRR 1999
- the appointment of a *suitably qualified and experienced* person as *RPA* to act in an advisory

capacity to the employer to ensure that IRR 1999 and IR(ME)R 2000 are being suitably implemented

- the appointment of one or more suitably qualified persons as *radiation protection supervisors* (RPSs) in each area of the department where work with ionising radiation takes place; such individuals are usually line managers and have sufficient understanding and authority to enforce the *local rules* for the area for which they are responsible
- the writing of suitable *local rules* for the establishment of safe working practices for employees
- the drawing-up of reasonable contingency plans, e.g. the procedure in the event of fire in a radiation area
- the duties of the employer with regard to radiation protection
- the duties of the referrer with regard to radiation protection
- the duties of the practitioner with regard to radiation protection
- the duties of the operator with regard to radiation protection.

The designation of workers, personnel record-keeping and the notification of incidents and overexposure have been discussed in previous sections of this chapter. The appointment of RPAs and RPSs, the formulation of local rules, personnel-monitoring methods and the designation of working areas will now be considered in the following sections. When this framework has been established, the duties of the employer, the referrer, the practitioner and the operator as defined by IR(ME)R 2000 will be identified.

34.11.1 Radiation Protection Advisers and Radiation Protection Supervisors

Regulation 13 of IRR 1999 states that every employer shall consult such suitable RPAs as are necessary for the purpose of advising the employer. Any RPA must be a *suitably qualified and experienced person* and is appointed for the purpose of advising the employer as to the observance of IRR 1999 and on all other aspects of the safe use of ionising radiation. The HSE must have been notified of the person's details, including qualifications and experience, at least 28 days before the appointment, or at shorter notice if this is unavoidable.

In order that RPAs may perform the advisory role, the employer must provide them with an adequate job description, preferably written, detailing the extent of their responsibilities and adequate information regarding the activities of the employees and adequate facilities with which to perform their duties.

The RPA must be consulted on the following matters, which are listed in Schedule 5 of the regulations:

- the implementation of requirements as to controlled and supervised areas
- the prior examination of plans for installation and the acceptance into service of new or modified sources of ionising radiation in relation to any engineering controls, design features, safety features and warning devices provided to restrict exposure to ionising radiation
- the regular calibration of equipment provided for monitoring levels of ionising radiation and the regular checking that such equipment is serviceable and correctly used
- the periodic examination and testing of engineering controls, design features, safety features and warning devices and the regular checking of systems of work provided to restrict exposure to ionising radiation.

The RPA is also involved in the selection of RPSs, who are persons directly involved in working with ionising radiation on a day-to-day basis. It is normal to have an RPS in each department to ensure safe working practice within that department. RPSs must have sufficient knowledge, experience and authority to allow them to carry out their duties in their department. Details of the RPAs and RPSs will normally be contained in the local rules.

34.11.2 Local Rules

Under IRR 1999, the employer has a legal responsibility to ensure that written local rules are produced for departments where employees are

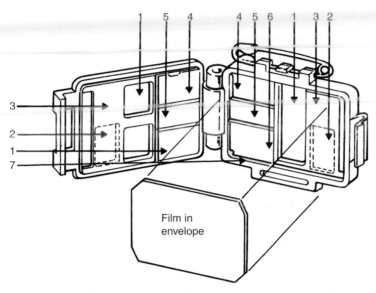

Figure 34.2 The film-badge-holder and film, as used in personnel monitoring. The optically sealed film has a fast emulsion on the side facing the front of the badge and a slow emulsion on the other side. If a high exposure to radiation has occurred, the fast emulsion may be removed, thus allowing a dose estimation to be made using the slow emulsion. Various filters are used to separate the effects of different types and energies of radiations. Key to structure of the holder: 1, open window; 2, thin plastic filter (0.5 mm); 3, thick plastic filter (2.8 mm); 4, dural (alloy of aluminium) filter (1.0 mm); 5, tin filter (0.7 mm) + lead filter (0.3 mm); 6, cadmium filter (0.7 mm) + lead filter (0.3 mm); 7, strip of lead (0.3 mm) which shields filters 5 and 6 to prevent radiation entering the holder through the side of the badge and thus affecting the film under these filters. Beta-particles are absorbed by filters 3 onwards. Only high-energy X-rays and gamma-rays are able to penetrate the tin + lead filter (5) significantly, so that an estimate may be made of the relative amounts of low- and high-energy X- and gamma-rays by comparing the photographic densities between filters 4 and 5. The cadmium + lead filter (6) is used to estimate exposure to thermal neutrons (for workers in the nuclear industry) because neutron capture by the cadmium nuclei results in gamma photon emission which creates an exposure to the film. Courtesy of the Radiological Protection Section, of the Health Protection Agency.

involved in work with ionising radiation. These rules must be brought to the attention of all employees working in these departments. In practice, the RPAs have the necessary knowledge and experience to formulate these rules and it is the task of the RPSs to ensure that the rules are known and put into practice by colleagues in their own departments.

The local rules for a department should be displayed in a prominent position, or positions, within the department concerned, and should contain the following information:

- the name of the RPA and RPS for the department
- a description of each restricted area (see Sect. 34.11.4)
- details of restrictions of access to such areas
- written systems of work detailing the working procedures and protocols for the department
- details of any contingency plans.

34.11.3 Personnel Monitoring

It is necessary to measure the radiation doses received by radiation workers in the course of their work to verify that these doses are within the recommended limits. This is known as *personnel monitoring* and acts not only as a check of the actual doses received but also as a scrutiny of the various radiation protection policies formulated by the RPA. It also allows the RPA and the RPSs to identify individuals who habitually have higher doses and counsel such individuals before their neglectfulness reaches serious proportions.

There are three main methods of personnel monitoring currently used in the UK. These are:

1. the film-badge method
2. thermoluminescent dosimetry (TLD)
3. pocket dosimeters.

34.11.3.1 The Film-Badge Method

This method is based on the principle that the optical density produced by processing on photographic film increases with the amount of radiation received by the film. This principle has already been discussed in Section 33.6.5. The use of plastic, tin and aluminium filters in the badge-holder enables the distinction to be made whether the dose was the result of beta-particle or low- or high-energy X- or gamma-rays. The films must be processed and read by an approved dosimetry service. Details of the construction of the film-badge-holder and film are given in Figure 34.2.

The main advantage of the film-badge method of monitoring is that the film may be kept as a permanent record of the dose received. It does, however, have the disadvantage that the dose reading takes place some time after the exposure to radiation. Film is expensive, not reusable and can deteriorate if not stored in proper conditions prior to processing. In addition to this, film is less sensitive than other methods and makes it difficult to estimate if some of the new lower dose limit restrictions have been met.

34.11.3.2 Thermoluminescent Dosimetry

Some of the disadvantages of the film-badge method of monitoring are overcome by the use of TLD. The basic principles of this process have already been discussed in Section 33.6.4. An example of a TLD badge used for monitoring purposes is shown in Figure 34.3. This badge contains an identified holder which contains two discs of thermoluminescent material. One disc is positioned behind the open window of the badge and estimates the skin dose while the other disc is behind the plastic dome and is used to estimate the whole-body dose.

Thermoluminescent materials may also be used to measure doses to specific organs, e.g. they can be wrapped round a finger to measure the dose to that finger.

34.11.3.3 Pocket Dosimeters

There are a number of specialised electronic devices available which will measure the radia-

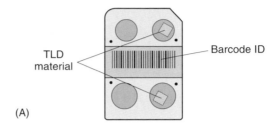

(A)

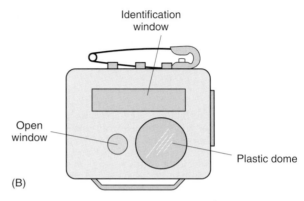

(B)

Figure 34.3   The thermoluminescent dosimeter badge as supplied by the Health Protection Agency (HPA: formerly the National Radiological Protection Board). (A) The plastic Harshaw card, without its Melinex wrapping. This wrapping protects the lithium fluoride/polytetrafluoroethylene (PTFE) thermoluminescent dosimetry (TLD) inserts on the card from light and alpha radiations, as well as providing chemical protection and a measure of physical protection. *Note*: the card is designed so that it can only be inserted into the holder in the correct way. Each card is identified by a unique barcode, used in the automated dose-reading process. (B) The card holder has two windows – a long rectangular window along the top edge to display the wearer's identity and an open window that lies directly over one of the TLDs on the card. The other TLD lies under the dome, which is made of thick (90 mg.cm^{-2}) plastic. This TLD is used to record the more penetrating and gamma radiations producing the Hp10 dose or depth received by the wearer. The TLD under the open window records all weakly and strongly penetrating radiations, including beta radiation. This dose reading produces the Hp0.07 or skin dose.

tion dose *at the time of exposure* and warn the wearer of any unusually high dose. These may be worn in the pockets of laboratory coats and so are known as *pocket dosimeters*. The dose is usually displayed on a digital readout on the dosemeter or can be linked to a suitable PC to give a printout

Table 34.5 Description of designation of areas

Type of designation	Requirements for designation	Permitted access
Controlled area	An area where any person is likely to receive an effective dose greater than 6 mSv per year or three-tenths of any <u>relevant</u> dose limit	A. Classified radiation workers B. Radiation workers who follow a written system of work, designed to restrict significant radiation exposure in that area C. Patients undergoing medical diagnostic or therapeutic exposures
Supervised area	A. Note that an area within a controlled area cannot also be designated as a supervised area B. An area where any person is likely to receive an effective dose greater than 1 mSv per year or one-tenth of any <u>relevant</u> dose limit An area where it is necessary to determine whether the area should be designated a controlled area	Persons whose presence is necessary during a radiation exposure

of doses. Such devices can not only show the total dose but can also give a breakdown of the rate at which the dose was received, e.g. dose rate per hour for a specific day.

The final choice of the most appropriate method of personnel monitoring is usually made by the RPA, who will assess the risk of receiving an unexpectedly high dose of radiation.

34.11.4 Designation of Work Areas

In order to protect employees and members of the public from unnecessary amounts of radiation when on an employer's property, the IRR 1999 (part 4, regulation 16) makes a distinction between two types of areas:

1. supervised areas
2. controlled areas.

The differences between the two areas are summarised in Table 34.5.

Once the employer has designated an area as a controlled area, access must be restricted to it, and the area should be demarcated or otherwise delineated by some suitable means. The area may be described with respect to existing walls if this is convenient but this may not always be possible, e.g. in the case of a mobile X-ray unit used in a ward. Access is best restricted using physical barriers; where the work is of short duration access may be restricted by continuous

supervision, e.g. mobile radiography in a ward. The limitations of access to a controlled area are listed in Table 34.5. Many X-ray departments have dispensed with the supervised area and simply regard the whole of the X-ray room and its protected cubicle as a controlled area.

34.11.5 Duties of Designated Individuals as Defined by IR(ME)R 2000

34.11.5.1 Duties of the Employer

To permit adherence to the regulations the employer is responsible for ensuring that written systems are in place for every type of standard radiological practice for each equipment. The employer shall establish recommendations concerning referral criteria for medical exposures, quality assurance programmes, diagnostic reference levels and dose constraints for biomedical and medical research programmes where no direct benefit to the individual is expected from the exposure. In addition, the employer has a responsibility to ensure that every practitioner and operator engaged by the employer complies with the regulations and undertakes continuing education and training after qualification. The employer must also investigate and report appropriately any overexposure to radiation and must also undertake appropriate reviews if diagnostic reference levels are consistently exceeded.

34.11.5.2 Duties of the Referrer

The referrer must supply the practitioner with sufficient medical data relevant to the medical exposure requested to enable the practitioner to decide whether there is sufficient net benefit to the patient to allow justification of the exposure.

34.11.5.3 Duties of the Practitioner

The practitioner is responsible for the justification of a medical exposure to radiation. The practitioner and the operator shall cooperate to ensure all exposures are optimised, i.e. radiation doses are kept as low as reasonably practicable for any medical exposure.

34.11.5.4 Duties of the Operator

The operator is responsible for checking that the exposure to radiation has been justified and for the practical aspects of making the exposure. In this process the operator should keep the radiation dose to the patient as low as reasonably practicable but consistent with the clinical requirements for the exposure and should ensure that the exposure is within the diagnostic reference level produced by the employer for the examination.

34.11.6 Good Radiographic Practice

As has already been discussed, it is always important to minimise the radiation doses received by patients and staff. Methods of achieving this are given in Table 34.6 (for patients) and Table 34.7 (for staff). It may be noted that some of the items listed are within the control of the operator and some are not. By careful attention to such detail the radiographer should be able to produce radiographs of high diagnostic quality with the lowest practicable radiation dose to the patient.

Fluoroscopy results in higher radiation doses than conventional radiography and therefore good technique is even more essential to keep radiation doses to a minimum. The use of a mod-ern fluoroscopic unit with pulsed fluoroscopy, image storage, automatic collimation and digitisation of the image all result in a reduction of the radiation doses to patients and staff.

34.11.7 Room Design

For radiation protection purposes the function of the X-ray room is to provide an enclosure for the X-ray unit and so limit the access to the radiation area. The room should also provide adequate

Table 34.6   Methods of minimising radiation dose to patients

Factors outside the radiographer's control
Filtration of the X-ray beam (see Sect. 29.7)
Rectification (see Sect. 29.6)
Tube shielding (see Ch. 21)

Factors within the radiographer's control
Limitation of field size by use of collimation
Use of the fastest image receptor system, consistent with the requirements of the examination
Use of the highest practicable kVp
Use of automatic exposure control systems
Selection of an appropriate secondary radiation grid
Tissue displacement with obese patients

In fluoroscopy
Use of a correctly set-up image intensifier
Use of automatic collimation
Use of pulsed fluorography and image storage systems
Use of digital fluorography

Table 34.7   Methods of dose reduction to staff

In radiography
Only those whose presence is required should be in the room during exposures
All staff should stand behind the protective barrier during the exposure
The X-ray tube must have adequate shielding
Restless patients should be supported by immobilisation devices. Radiographers *should not* support such patients

In fluorography
Staff must wear adequate protective clothing, as specified in the written systems of work
Use of automatic collimation
Staff should stand as far as possible from the primary beam
Protective shielding should be incorporated in the image intensifier to reduce dose from scattered radiation

shielding to the rest of the environment from the radiation produced. In addition, provision is made for a barrier inside the room behind which staff may be protected from the radiation while they operate the units – in therapy treatment rooms, the equipment is operated from outside the treatment room. If there is more than one X-ray tube operating from the generator in a diagnostic room, there must be a visual indication (usually a warning light) to indicate which tube is in circuit and so is capable of producing radiation if energised.

The level of radiation protection given by barriers and walls is usually stated in terms of their *lead-equivalent*.

DEFINITION

The lead-equivalent of an absorbing material is the thickness of lead which would absorb the same amount of radiation as the given material when exposed to radiation of the same type and quality.

The lead-equivalent thus gives a basis for comparing one barrier with another at a given beam energy.

In the diagnostic range of beam energies (up to 150 keV) the photoelectric absorption within lead is significant owing to its high atomic number (see Sect. 30.5). For this reason, many barriers (e.g. doors) in the diagnostic X-ray room incorporate a few millimetres of lead laminated with wood to give adequate radiation protection. Lead-glass windows are often fitted to such barriers to enable a visual contact to be maintained. The protection afforded by such a window must be at least the same amount as the protective barrier itself and there must be no gaps where the radiation is able to penetrate. The siting of such a barrier to protect the staff must be such that the radiation must be scattered at least twice (thus greatly reducing its intensity) before reaching the opening in the barrier.

Wall thicknesses between X-ray rooms and adjacent areas must be such that any transmitted radiation will not produce a dose in excess of 1 mSv per year, which is the maximum dose for the general public. This figure must be calculated for all walls, floors, ceilings and windows of the X-ray rooms and is calculated by applying a *use factor*. The use factor is an estimation of the time when the radiation beam will be pointing towards that area. As a result of this calculation, the maximum dose received by a person sited on the far side of the barrier may be estimated and it must not exceed 1 mSv per year. In previous legislation there was also an *occupancy factor* which looked at the fraction of time a person was likely to spend in this area, but this factor has now been discontinued.

The materials used in the construction of the walls and floor of the X-ray room may contain lead sheeting or there may be sufficient thickness of other materials, such as concrete, to provide adequate absorption of the primary and scatter radiation produced in the room. The lead-equivalent of a concrete wall 15 cm thick is approximately 1.5 mm within the diagnostic energy range – this reflects the superior absorption of lead compared with concrete in this energy range. The lead-equivalent of such walls may be increased by the use of *barium sulphate plaster* as a thin coating on the walls. This is because of the high atomic number of barium (56).

As the beam energy increases, the advantage of lead over concrete diminishes as there is a gradual shift from the predominance of photoelectric absorption to the predominance of Compton scattering. Thus the lead-equivalent of a barrier will increase with an increase in the photon energy – a greater thickness of lead will be required to give the same level of protection as the barrier. In the region of 1 MeV the Compton scattering process predominates and lead has no real advantage over concrete since all materials have similar mass attenuation coefficients due to the Compton process. Thus many of the barriers used in radiotherapy departments are made of large thicknesses of concrete.

In conclusion, the design of a room, its wall thickness and the barriers must be such that the radiation dose received by patients, staff and members of the public is kept to a minimum in accordance with the ALARA principle. Further details of the design of diagnostic and therapy rooms will be found in specialised publications on this topic.

SUMMARY

In this chapter you should have learnt:

- The purpose and scope of radiation protection (see Sect. 34.2)
- An outline of ionising radiation regulations (see Sect. 34.3)
- The biological effects of ionising radiation (see Sect. 34.4)
- The stochastic effects of ionising radiation, including radiation-induced cancers and genetic effects (see Sect. 34.4.1)
- The deterministic (non-stochastic) effects of ionising radiation (see Sect. 34.4.2)
- Risk–benefit, ALARA (ALARP) and detriment as applied to ionising radiation (see Sect. 34.5)
- Special precautions in the radiological examination of women of reproductive capacity (see Sect. 34.6)
- Dose-equivalent limits in radiation protection (see Sect. 34.7)
- The definition of effective dose and how this is used in radiation protection (see Sect. 34.8)

- The definition of committed dose and how this is used in radiation protection (see Sect. 34.9)
- The requirements for the designation of radiation workers (see Sect. 34.10)
- Dose limitations for employees who have been overexposed to radiation (see Sect. 34.10.1)
- Practical radiation protection measures (see Sect. 34.11)
- The appointment and work of RPAs and RPSs (see Sect. 34.11.1)
- Local rules and their uses in radiation protection (see Sect. 34.11.2)
- Methods of personnel monitoring (see Sect. 34.11.3)
- Designation of work areas in radiation protection (see Sect. 34.11.4)
- Duties of designated individuals as defined by IR(ME)R 2000 (see Sect. 34.11.5)
- Good radiographic practice and its role in radiation protection (see Sect. 34.11.6)
- The requirements for room design in radiography and radiotherapy (see Sect. 34.11.7).

SELF-TEST

a. Outline the sequence of events that can lead to ionising radiation having a biological effect on tissue.

b. Compare and contrast *stochastic* and *deterministic* effects of radiation.

c. If all the organs of the body receive an effective dose of 2 mSv, what is the effective whole-body dose?

d. List the factors to be considered when estimating the committed dose from an ingested radioactive material.

e. What are the annual whole-body radiation dose limits for the following categories of personnel:

(i) a radiation worker over 18 years of age

(ii) a trainee radiation worker under 18 years of age

(iii) a member of the public who is not a radiation worker

(iv) a female radiation worker of reproductive capacity

(v) a pregnant radiation worker?

f. Define a *classified radiation worker* and list the restrictions on the appointment of such a person.

g. List the three general principles of radiation protection.

h. Compare and contrast the role of the radiation protection adviser and the radiation protection supervisor.

i. List three methods of personnel monitoring and give the advantages and disadvantages of one of these methods.

j. List the requirements for the designation of a controlled area and list the persons who have access to such an area.

k. List the factors that a radiographer may use to limit the radiation dose to the patient during a diagnostic radiography procedure.

REFERENCES AND FURTHER READING

Allisy-Roberts P 2002 Medical and dental guidance notes – a good practice guide on all aspects of ionising radiation protection in the clinical environment. Institute of Physics and Engineering in Medicine, York, UK

Ball J L, Moore A D 1997 Essential physics for radiographers, 3rd edn. Blackwell Scientific Publications, London, ch 16

Ball J, Price T 1995 Chesney's radiographic imaging, 6th edn. Blackwell Scientific Publications, London, ch 5

Bushong S C 2004 Radiologic science for technologists: physics, biology and protection. Mosby, New York, chs 33–40

Curry T S III, Dowdey J E, Murry R C Jr 1990 Christensen's physics of diagnostic radiography, 4th edn. Lee & Febiger, London, chs 21 and 22

Dowd S B, Tilson E R 1999 Practical radiation protection and applied radiobiology, 2nd edn. W B Saunders, Philadelphia, PA

Dowsett D J, Kenny P A, Johnston R E 1998 The physics of diagnostic imaging. Chapman & Hall Medical, London, ch 19

Hay C A, Hughes D 1984 First year physics for radiographers. W B Saunders, London, ch 10

HMSO 1999 1999/3232 The ionising radiation regulations. HMSO, London

HMSO 2000 Statutory instrument 2000/1059. The ionising radiations (medical exposure) regulations. HMSO, London

HSE 2000 Working with ionising radiation – Ionising Radiation Regulations 1999. Approved code of practice and guidance. HSE Books, Sudbury

ICRP 1997 ICRP26 Annals of ICRP. Pergamon Press

IPEM 2002 Medical and dental guidance notes. A good practice guidance on all aspects of ionising radiation protection in the clinical environment. Institute of Physics and Engineering in Medicine, York

Johns H E, Cunningham J R 1983 The physics of radiology, 4th edn. Charles C Thomas, Illinois, USA, ch 2

Ohanian H C 1994 Principles of physics. W W Norton, London, ch 31

Sumner D, Wheldon T, Watson W 1991 Radiation risks: an evaluation. Tarragon Press, Glasgow

Thompson M A, Hattaway R T, Hall J D, Dowd S B 1994 Principles of imaging science and protection. W B Saunders, London, chs 18–21

Webb S (ed) 2000 The physics of medical imaging, 2nd edn. Institute of Physics Publishing, Bristol, ch 2

Appendices, Tables and Answers to Self-Tests

PART CONTENTS

Appendix A Mathematics for
    Radiography **357**

Appendix B Scintillation Counters **372**

Appendix C CT Scanning **377**

Appendix D Magnetic Resonance
    Imaging **383**

Appendix E Digital Imaging **387**

Appendix F Ultrasound Imaging **391**

Appendix G Positron Emission Tomography
    (PET Scanning) **394**

Appendix H Modulation Transfer Function
    (MTF) **397**

Appendix I SI Base Units **401**

Tables **403**

Answers to Self-Tests **409**

Appendix A

Mathematics for Radiography

This appendix on the revision of mathematics is directed primarily at those whose mathematics is a little weak. However, many of the worked examples shown are chosen from topics in radiography.

For those studying for examinations, the following remarks may be of help. Examiners frequently complain of cramped, untidy mathematics which is difficult to follow. What they are hoping to see in the answer is a clear statement of the problem and an easy-to-follow development of the mathematics used to obtain the solution. This may be more important (and hence gain more marks) than simply reaching the correct numerical answer. In fact, the correct answer simply recorded on its own with little or no supporting mathematical reasoning will not achieve many marks – remember that the examiner cannot know how you achieved the final answer unless you tell him/her. In practice, you should use phrases and sentences to tell the examiner how you have progressed from one step of the problem to the next as you move towards the eventual solution. This should also help you to think more clearly about what you are doing and also to check the integrity of your final answer – this is probably even more important with the widespread use of pocket calculators. A study of the worked examples in this appendix should clarify these points.

A.1 ALGEBRAIC SYMBOLS

The letters of the English and Greek alphabet (see Table D following the Appendices) are often used to represent the magnitude of an unknown quantity. For example, an electrical potential difference may be represented by V volts, an angle by θ (theta) degrees or radians and an energy by E joules. Such a practice enables the symbols to be used in place of the actual numerical values of the quantities, and is of great practical use in solving equations (see Appendix A.4).

A.1.1 Suffixes

Suffixes are used to denote a specific value of a particular quantity. If we use the symbol I to denote the intensity of radiation from a particular source, then I will depend upon the distance from the source at which the intensity is measured (see Ch. 3). We may call a particular distance x, say, and denote the intensity of this distance by I_x – meaning *the intensity at x*. For another distance y, the corresponding value of intensity is I_y.

Similarly, if a quantity N changes with time, t, the value of N at any given time may be denoted by N_t.

Suffixes are used, then, to avoid ambiguity and are used as such in many chapters of this book.

A.2 FRACTIONS AND PERCENTAGES

Although fractions are not commonly used in radiographic calculations since they have been largely replaced with decimals, nevertheless a knowledge of how to manipulate fractions mathematically is useful in calculations involving Ohm's law (see Ch. 10) and capacitors (see Ch. 16). For this reason a section on fractions and percentages is still included in this appendix.

A.2.1 Percentages

If a quantity increases in value by 50%, then this means that it has become greater by one-half of its previous value. Thus, if the electric current passing through an X-ray tube was 200 mA, then an increase of 50% would bring this to 300 mA. Alternatively, it may be said that the new value is 150% of the original value.

In general terms, if a is the original value of a quantity and b is its new value, then:

- the *percentage change* $= 100 \times \dfrac{b - a}{a}$

- $\dfrac{100b}{a}$ is the 'percentage of b compared to a'

- $y\%$ of a is just $\dfrac{y}{100} \times a$.

EXAMPLES

a. Original value = 60; new value = 80

The percentage change is then $100 \times \dfrac{20}{60} = 33\frac{1}{3}\%$

and the new value is $100 \times \dfrac{80}{60} = 133\frac{1}{3}\%$ of the original.

b. A quantity has reduced by 25%. What is the new value if it was 600 originally?

25% of 600 is just $\dfrac{25}{100} \times 600 = 150$, so that the new value is $600 - 150 = 450$.

A percentage is a special case of a fraction, where one number is divided by another. The following sections describe how fractions may be added together and multiplied.

A.2.2 Addition of Fractions

Suppose we have the fraction a/b, where a and b represent general numbers. Now the addition or subtraction of a/b to another fraction c/d rests on the fact that we can take any fraction and multiply top and bottom by the same factor (k, say) *without* altering its value,

i.e. $\dfrac{a}{b} = \dfrac{ka}{kb}$ (because the ks cancel)

It is the appropriate selection of k for each fraction which makes for the easy addition of fractions. For example, suppose we have:

$$\frac{2}{3} + \frac{5}{6}$$

If we multiply 2/3 by 2 (top and bottom), we will have a fraction expressed in sixths, just like the second fraction.

i.e. $\dfrac{2}{3} + \dfrac{5}{6} = \dfrac{2 \times 2}{2 \times 3} + \dfrac{5}{6} = \dfrac{4}{6} + \dfrac{5}{6} = \dfrac{9}{6} = 1\frac{1}{2}$

Notice that we multiplied only the first fraction – we need not do the same thing to the second. This method is often very quick, particularly when only two or three simple fractions are involved, and is in fact entirely equivalent to the more general method of using the lowest common denominator (LCD), as illustrated in the following example:

$$\frac{2}{3} + \frac{3}{4} - \frac{5}{6} = \frac{(4 \times 2 + 3 \times 3 - 2 \times 5)}{12}$$

$$= \frac{(8 + 9 - 10)}{12} = \frac{7}{12}$$

Here, the LCD of the denominators 3, 4 and 6 is 12 and is therefore used as the overall denominator on the right-hand side (RHS). The individual denominators are then divided into 12, the result being multiplied by the respective numerator and summed (observing the correct signs) as shown in the example.

EXERCISE A.1 (ANSWERS AT THE END OF THIS APPENDIX)

a. $\dfrac{11}{12} - \dfrac{5}{6}$

b. $\dfrac{7}{9} + \dfrac{2}{3}$

c. What is 20% of 50?

d. $\dfrac{2}{3} - \dfrac{1}{4} + \dfrac{3}{5}$

e. $\dfrac{7}{11} + \dfrac{2}{9} - \dfrac{2}{3}$

f. What is the percentage change if a quantity increases from 80 to 90?

A.3 MULTIPLYING AND DIVIDING

A.3.1 Positive and Negative Numbers

It is obvious that $1 \times 8 = 8$, but what are -1×8, -1×-8 and 8×-1?

To avoid having to work out such problems from first principles every time, a simple rule has been developed which we may call Rule 1.

> **Rule 1**
> When multiplying or dividing two numbers together:
> Two (+)s make a (+)
> Two (−)s make a (+)
> A (+) and a (−) make a (−)

i.e. only when the signs are dissimilar is the result negative.

EXAMPLES

a. $-3 \times 4 = -12$

b. $14 \div -7 = -2$

c. $\dfrac{-40}{-4} = 10$

d. $-2 \times -4 \times -3 = 8 \times -3 = -24$

EXERCISE A.2

a. $28 \div 7$

b. $\dfrac{-36}{6}$

c. $\dfrac{144}{-4}$

d. -13×-3

e. $-7 \times \dfrac{-8}{-2}$

A.3.2 Fractions

The *multiplication* of two or more fractions is just a matter of simplification by cancellation (where possible) and then multiplying all the numerators together to form the new numerator, and all the denominators together to form the new denominator.

EXAMPLES

a. $\dfrac{2}{3} \times \dfrac{7}{5} = \dfrac{14}{15}$ (no cancellation possible)

b. $\dfrac{2}{3} \times \dfrac{9}{4} = \dfrac{\cancel{2}^1}{\cancel{3}_1} \times \dfrac{\cancel{9}^3}{\cancel{4}_2} = \dfrac{3}{2}$

The *division* of two fractions is straightforward provided that the following rule is obeyed.

> **Rule 2**
> When dividing by one or more fractions, turn those in the denominator upside down and multiply.

Let us say, by way of illustration, that we wish to divide 4 by $\frac{1}{2}$,

i.e. $\dfrac{4}{\frac{1}{2}}$

Applying Rule 2, we turn $\frac{1}{2}$ upside down and multiply:

$$\dfrac{4}{\frac{1}{2}} = 4 \times \dfrac{2}{1} = 8$$

Is this the answer we would expect intuitively? Well, the problem may be expressed as 'how many halves are there in 4?', and then it is obvious that the answer is 8. Some more examples to clarify the method:

a. $7 \div \dfrac{14}{9} = 7 \times \dfrac{9}{14} = \dfrac{9}{2}$

b. $\dfrac{\frac{3}{8}}{\frac{7}{11}} = \dfrac{3}{8} \times \dfrac{11}{7} = \dfrac{33}{56}$

c. $\dfrac{\frac{4}{9}}{\frac{-8}{27}} = \dfrac{4}{9} \times \dfrac{-27}{8} = \dfrac{-3}{2}$

d. $\dfrac{\frac{2}{3}}{\frac{4}{7} \times \frac{3}{5}} = \dfrac{2}{3} \times \dfrac{7}{4} \times \dfrac{5}{3} = \dfrac{35}{18}$

EXERCISE A.3

a. $\dfrac{\dfrac{-4}{11}}{\dfrac{7}{22}}$

b. $\dfrac{\dfrac{2}{9}}{\dfrac{7}{3} \times \dfrac{-2}{11}}$

c. $\dfrac{\dfrac{1}{3} \times \dfrac{2}{9}}{\dfrac{9}{1} \times \dfrac{1}{2}}$

A.3.3 Brackets

A bracket links two or more quantities together such that the bracket and its contents may be treated mathematically as a single quantity. If we wish to *remove* the brackets, then care over the plus and minus signs must be taken (Rule 1).

EXAMPLES

a. $2 \times (a - b) = 2 \times a - 2 \times b = 2a - 2b$
   Thus, each term in the bracket is multiplied by the term outside the bracket, with due regard for the sign convention.

b. $-4(c - 2d) = -4c + 8d$
   Note that the multiplication sign, present in Example a, has been omitted, as is usually the case.

c. $-3\left(\dfrac{-2a}{3} + b - \dfrac{1c}{7}\right) = 2a - 3b + \dfrac{3c}{7}$

Multiplying two or more brackets together can become quite involved. However, it is rare for problems in radiography to require even the multiplication of two brackets, but the method is outlined below for the sake of completeness.
   Assume we wish to calculate:

$(a + b)(c + d)$
i.e. $(a + b)$ multiplied by $(c + d)$.

To perform this calculation, we take the first term of the first bracket, a, and multiply it by $(c + d)$. Then we add the result to the multiplication of the second term, b, by $(c + d)$:

i.e. $(a + b)(c + d) = a(c + d) + b(c + d)$
$$= ac + ad + bc + bd$$

Again, we must be careful of the sign convention (Rule 1), as the following two worked examples show.

EXAMPLES

a. $(7 + c)(d - 8) = 7(d - 8) + c(d - 8)$
   $$= 7d - 56 + cd - 8c$$
b. $(4 - a)(3 - b + 2c) = 4(3 - b + 2c) - a(3 - b + 2c)$
   $$= 12 - 4b + 8c - 3a + ab - 2ac$$

EXERCISE A.4

a. $7a - 4(a - 2)$
b. $-6(-x + y - 3)$
c. $2(3a - 4) - 3(-a + 6)$

A.4 SOLVING EQUATIONS

Many of the types of equations encountered in problems associated with radiography are those in which a single 'unknown' (whose numerical value we wish to calculate) is 'mixed up' with several other numbers which may occur on both sides of the equation. (The solution of several equations involving several unknowns, i.e. simultaneous equations, is not normally required, and so will not be discussed here.) Our task, then, in the equations encountered, is to 'unscramble' the unknown so as to leave it on one side of the equation and all the numbers on the other side – the equation is then said to be 'solved'. This process is straightforward, provided that the following simple rule is obeyed:

Rule 3
Always perform the same operation to both sides of an equation.

This rule is intuitively obvious if it is imagined that the equals sign of the equation is the pivot of a pair of scales which is in exact balance. Whatever weight we now add to or subtract from one scale-pan must be added to or subtracted from the other or the scales will no longer be in balance. Similarly, if we double (say) the weight on one side we must do the same to the other – thus, provided we multiply by the same factor, balance is preserved and one side is equal to the other side. For example, consider the simple equation:

$$x - 2 = 3$$

If we add 2 to the left-hand side (LHS) of this equation the –2 will be cancelled, leaving x only. However, in accordance with Rule 3 above, we must add 2 to the RHS in order to preserve equality.

i.e. $x - 2 + 2 = 3 + 2$ thus $x = 5$

Putting $x = 5$ in the original equation, we have $5 - 2 = 3$, which is correct.

As another example, consider: $15 - y = 7$. Subtracting 15 from both sides so as to eliminate it from the LHS:

$$15 - y - 15 = 7 - 15 \text{ i.e. } -y = -8$$

Multiplying both sides by –1 in order to make both terms positive (Rule 1), we have:

$$-1 \cdot -y = -1 \cdot -8 \text{ i.e. } y = 8$$

(*Note*: The symbol '·' is often used, as above, to denote multiplication.)

Substituting our solution into the original equation to serve as a check, as in the previous example, we have:

$$15 - 8 = 7, \text{ thus verifying our answer.}$$

It is apparent from these examples that a convenient way of picturing this type of mathematical operation is that of 'transferring a quantity from one side to the other and *changing its sign*'.

Obviously, this only applies to the elimination of variables by addition or subtraction, *not* multiplication, which will be discussed in the next example.

EXAMPLE

$$2 = 7 - \frac{5x}{2}$$

Proceeding as before, $\frac{5x}{2} = 7 - 2 = 5$

i.e. $\frac{5x}{2} = 5$

We cannot now add or subtract anything to leave x on its own – we have to multiply by 2/5:

i.e. $\frac{2}{5} \cdot \frac{5x}{2} = \frac{2}{5} \cdot 5$

i.e. $x = 2$

This last step is known as *cross-multiplication* and may be pictured in the following manner:

$$\text{(cross-multiplication)}$$

The double-ended arrows indicate that movement may be in either direction. Note that there is no change of sign.

One *incorrect* use of cross-multiplication occurs so frequently that it is worth a special mention here. Suppose we have the equation:

$$\frac{7x}{2} = \frac{3}{8} + \frac{x}{3}$$

If we cross-multiply in the following manner:

$$\frac{7x}{2} = \frac{3}{8} + \frac{x}{3} \text{ (incorrect)}$$

we obtain:

$$x = \frac{2 \cdot 3}{7 \cdot 8} + \frac{x}{3} \text{ (incorrect)}$$

The fault lies, of course, in the fact that Rule 3 has been disobeyed, i.e. the term $x/3$ remains unaltered although we were intending, by our cross-multiplication, to multiply both sides by 2/7. Hence, if we wished to cross-multiply at this stage, we should have obtained:

$$x = \frac{2 \cdot 3}{7 \cdot 8} + \frac{2 \cdot x}{7 \cdot 3} \text{ (correct)}$$

which may be further simplified to solve for x.

EXERCISE A.5

a. $\frac{2}{3}x = 4$

b. $\frac{7}{9}y - 1 = 13$

c. $q + \frac{3}{10} = \frac{5}{12}q$

d. $3\frac{3}{5}z - 12\frac{4}{5} = 1\frac{2}{5}z - \frac{7}{10}$

A.5 POWERS (INDICES)

An *index* is written at the top right of a quantity (the *base*) and refers to the number of times the quantity is multiplied by *itself*. For example, 5^3 means $5 \times 5 \times 5$ (i.e. 125). It is a convenient mathematical 'shorthand' to write powers of a number in this way. In this example, the index is a positive integer (i.e. 3), but this need not be the case for it may be positive, negative, fractional or decimal, as described below.

A.5.1 Combining Indices

Let us assume that we have two numbers, 2^3 and 2^2, which we wish to combine by addition, multiplication and division in order to elicit general rules for the handling of indices.

A.5.1.1 Addition

Using the definition of an index as described above:

$$2^3 + 2^2 = 2 \cdot 2 \cdot 2 + 2 \cdot 2 = 8 + 4 = 12$$

Thus, when adding such numbers, each term is calculated separately prior to addition (or subtraction).

A.5.1.2 Multiplication

Again, from first principles, we have:

$$2^3 \cdot 2^2 = (2^3) \cdot (2^2) = 2^5 = 2^{(3+2)}$$

Hence, when multiplying two or more such numbers together, the rule is to *add* the indices.

A.5.1.3 Division

$$\frac{2^3}{2^2} = \frac{2 \cdot 2 \cdot 2}{2 \cdot 2} = 2 = 2^{(3-2)}$$

Thus, when dividing such numbers, the rule is to *subtract* the indices.

A.5.2 Negative Indices

Suppose that we wish to divide 4^2 by 4^4. From first principles (Sect. A.5), we have

$$\frac{4^2}{4^4} = \frac{(4 \cdot 4)}{(4 \cdot 4 \cdot 4 \cdot 4)} = \frac{1}{4^2} \qquad \text{Equation A.1}$$

Also, by the rule on division as described above, we may subtract indices:

$$\frac{4^2}{4^4} = 4^{(2-4)} = 4^{-2} \qquad \text{Equation A.2}$$

Since Equations A.1 and A.2 are equal:

$$4^{-2} = \frac{1}{4^2}$$

In general, therefore:

$$x^{-n} = \frac{1}{x^n} \qquad \text{Equation A.3}$$

i.e. to change a negative index to a positive index, just take the reciprocal, as shown in Equation A.3.

EXAMPLES

a. $10^{-2} = \frac{1}{10^2} = \frac{1}{100}$

b. $\frac{1}{10^{-6}} = \frac{1}{\frac{1}{10^6}} = 1 \times \frac{10^6}{1} = 10^6$

c. $\frac{420 \times 10^2}{2 \times 10^4} = 210 \times 10^{-2} = \frac{210}{10^2} = \frac{210}{100} = 2.1$

A.5.3 Fractional Indices

What is meant by, say, $x^{1/2}$?

Now, $x^{1/2} \cdot x^{1/2} = x^{1/2 + 1/2} = x^1 = x$

Also, $\sqrt{x} \cdot \sqrt{x} = x$ from the definition of a square root.

Thus, from inspection of these two equations:

$$x^{1/2} = \sqrt{x}$$

i.e. $x^{1/2}$ is just the square root of x.

Similarly, $y^{1/3}$ is the cube root of y, $q^{5/8}$ is the eighth root of q raised to the fifth power, etc.

EXAMPLES

a. $9^{1/2} = \sqrt{9} = \pm 3$
b. $9^{3/2} = (9^{1/2})^3 = (\pm 3)^3 = \pm 27$
c. $64^{1/3} = \sqrt[3]{64} = 4$

A.5.4 The Zero Index – x^0

A general number x raised to a power m is x^m. If we divide x^m by itself, the answer will obviously be 1. But $x^m \div x^m$ is x^{m-m} by the rules discussed above. Thus $1 = x^{m-m} = x^0$. Since we took any general number, this result is also general (except for 0^0, which is indeterminate).

Thus any number raised to the power zero is *unity*.

A.5.5 Indices to Different Bases

A problem on the inverse-square law (see Ch. 3) frequently involves calculation of the form:

$$\frac{a \cdot b^2}{c^2}$$

Here a, b and c represent numbers whose values are known, having been specified by the problem. We wish to determine the best way of obtaining the final result, since b and c are frequently large numbers, whose squares are therefore even larger. This means that the probability of making an arithmetical error can be quite high if a laborious method of simplification is undertaken. However, a great simplification is possible if we remember that:

$$\frac{b^2}{c^2} = \left(\frac{b}{c}\right)^2 \qquad \textit{Equation A.4}$$

EXAMPLE

If $b = 90$ cm and $c = 60$ cm then b^2/c^2 the 'hard' way is:

$$\frac{b^2}{c^2} = \frac{90^2}{60^2} = \frac{8100}{3600} = \frac{81}{36}$$

which may be cancelled to give 2.25 – this exercise being left to the reader. The 'easy' way is to use Equation A.4:

i.e. $\dfrac{b^2}{c^2} = \left(\dfrac{b}{c}\right)^2 = \left(\dfrac{90}{60}\right)^2 = \left(\dfrac{3}{2}\right)^2 = 1.5^2 = 2.25$

Note that the answers are the same, as we should expect, but that the second method involves cancelling of smaller numbers so that there is less likelihood of an arithmetical error.

A.6 POWERS OF 10

When 10 is used as a base for indices, all the findings of the previous section apply. In addition, powers of 10 are very useful when measuring very large or very small quantities of a given unit, as shown in Table A.1.

Other names not shown in the table exist (see Table A after the Appendices), but these are all that we need. It is advisable for the student to memorise these terms as they are in very common usage in radiography. The following exercise is included for this purpose.

EXERCISE A.6

a. An X-ray tube has a current of 0.05 amperes passing through it. How many milliamperes (mA) does this correspond to?

Table A.1	Names for powers of 10		
Prefix	Symbol	Power of 10	Example
mega	M	10^6	1 MW = 10^6 watt
kilo	k	10^3	1 kV = 10^3 volt
milli	m	10^{-3}	1 mA = 10^{-3} ampere
micro	μ	10^{-6}	1 μF = 10^{-6} farad
nano	n	10^{-9}	1 nm = 10^{-9} metre
pico	p	10^{-12}	1 pF = 10^{-12} farad

b. If the X-ray tube has a peak potential difference of 125 000 volts across it, what is the value in kilovolts (kVp)?

c. Express a capacitance of 0.000065 farads in microfarads (μF).

d. A photon of light has a wavelength of 550 nanometres (nm). What is this in metres?

A.7 PROPORTIONALITY

A.7.1 Direct Proportion

If a car is travelling at constant speed such that the petrol consumption is a steady 60 km.l^{-1}, then:

0.5 litres have been used after 30 km
1.0 litres have been used after 60 km
1.5 litres have been used after 75 km, etc.

Thus, the amount of petrol consumed is in *direct proportion* to the number of miles travelled, and we may write:

litres $\propto$ mileage

where the sign '$\propto$' means 'is proportional to'. Alternatively, we may write:

litres $= \left(\dfrac{1}{60}\right) \times$ mileage

In general, therefore, if two quantities y and x are directly proportional to each other, then:

$y \propto x$ or $y = kx$

where k is called the 'constant of proportionality'. Some examples of direct proportionality which are discussed in the main text include:

• The electric current (I) through a metallic conductor is proportional to the potential difference (V) across it, i.e. $I \propto V$ (Ohm's law; Ch. 10).
• Intensity of an X-ray beam $\propto$ tube current (mA) (Ch. 29).
• Intensity of an X-ray beam $\propto$ kilovoltage squared, i.e. intensity $\propto$ kV^2 (Ch. 29).

A.7.2 Inverse Proportion

Suppose that we have many rectangles of equal area, k, but of differing heights (h) and widths (w). However, in each case the area is the same, so that:

$h \times w =$ constant (k)

Then, since k is constant, we may write:

$h \propto \dfrac{1}{w}$

In this case, therefore, h and w are in *inverse* proportion, since w is halved if h is doubled, and vice versa. This is opposite to *direct* proportion, of course, where doubling (say) one quantity also doubles the other.

Examples of inverse proportion discussed in the main text include:

• The capacity (C) of a parallel-plate capacitor is inversely proportional to the separation (d) between its plates, i.e. $C \propto 1/d$ (Ch. 16).
• The intensity (I) from a point source of electromagnetic radiation is inversely proportional to the square of the distance (x) from the course, i.e. $I \propto 1/x^2$ (Ch. 3).
• The electrical resistance (R) of a given length of wire varies inversely as the area of cross-section (A), i.e. $R \propto 1/A$ (Ch. 10).

A.8 GRAPHS

A.8.1 Drawing and Interpretation

A good understanding of the construction and interpretation of graphs is of great value in radiography, radiotherapy and nuclear medicine. The following simple but effective rules are offered in the drawing of good graphs:

• Each graph should take at least one-third of a page – use as large a scale as practicable so that you can make accurate readings
• Each graph should have a clear, appropriate title
• The axes, which should be drawn with a ruler, should be of approximately equal length
• Both axes must be clearly labelled to show what is being measured and should contain units (cm, s, kg, etc.) where appropriate.

- The *independent* variable is normally on the x-axis, and the *dependent* variable on the y-axis, i.e. the variable which is being measured is plotted on the y-axis while the variable causing the change in y is plotted on the x-axis. If we consider plotting the radioactivity from a sample over a period of time, then the independent variable is time (plotted on the x-axis) while the dependent variable is the radioactivity (plotted on the y-axis).

The following examples have been chosen to illustrate both the drawing and the interpretation of graphs.

EXAMPLE 1 – DIRECT PROPORTION

As described in the last section, two quantities, x and y, are directly proportional to each other if $y = kx$, where k is a constant. Figure A.1 shows $y = kx$ in graphical form.
   The following points should be noted:
- The graph passes through the origin, since when $x = 0$, y is also equal to zero
- The slope (or gradient) of the straight line produced is a measure of how steep it is and is defined as *the change in y divided by the corresponding change in x*. Since the graph passes through the origin, this is a convenient place from which to measure the changes. From this it can be seen that the slope is y/x. But from the equation $y = kx$ it can be seen that $y/x = k$. Thus the slope increases as k increases

- The general equation for a straight line will be in the form $y = mx + c$ where m is the gradient of the line and c is the intersection of the line with the y-axis – the value of x when $y = 0$.

EXAMPLE 2 – INVERSE PROPORTION

Figure A.2 shows a graph of the inverse relationship between the capacitance, C, of a parallel-plate capacitor and the distance of separation of its plates, d, where $C \propto 1/d$ or $C = k/d$ for a specific capacitor.
   From the graph it can be seen that, as the distance between the plates increases, so the capacitance of the capacitor decreases.

EXAMPLE 3 – RATING GRAPHS

Rating charts are supplied by the manufacturers of X-ray tubes, and contain a lot of information in graphical form which is an essential guide to the radiographer in the selection of 'safe' exposure factors, i.e. the combination of focal-spot size, kVp, mA and exposure time which will not cause damage to the X-ray tube. An example of a rating chart is given by Figure A.3, where a family of curves represent the maximum permissible exposure factors for different settings of kVp. The use of rating graphs is discussed in detail in Chapter 22 and we only

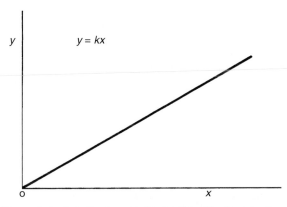

Figure A.1   Graph of $y = kx$, illustrating direct proportion.

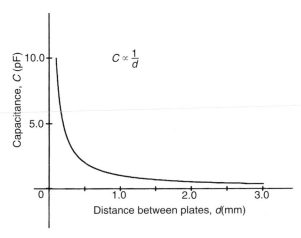

Figure A.2   Graph of $C \propto 1/d$, illustrating inverse proportion.

need to make the point here that points below a particular curve for one kVp setting are 'safe', while points above it lead to tube damage by overheating the anode.

Note the non-linear (logarithmic) scale on the x-axis. Logarithmic scales are discussed in Chapter 4.

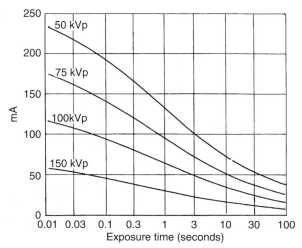

Figure A.3 Rating graph for an X-ray tube. Note the non-linear (logarithmic) scale on the x-axis.

A.8.2 Interpolation and Extrapolation

It is often the case that a graph is drawn using a relatively small number of points, and that these points are joined together with a curve or straight line passing through them. The smooth curve or line makes it possible to read off values from the graph, even when such values lie between the original points used to construct the graph. This procedure is known as *interpolation* and is one of the advantages of the graphical method.

If it is desired to determine the value of one of the plotted variables when it lies outside the range of the points used to plot the graph, the curve may be extended, or *extrapolated*, to reach this region. However, such an extrapolation can lead to large inaccuracies, since several different curves may seem equally suitable and there may be no way of knowing which one is correct!

EXERCISE A.7

a. Draw a graph of $y = 0.2x$, choosing values of x from 1 to 10 in steps of 1. Hence read from the graph the value of y when x is (i) 1.5, (ii) 9.5, (iii) 12, (iv) 0.5. Verify your answers by substitution into the original equation.

b. Repeat the same procedure for the equation $y = 0.2x^2$. (*Note* the increased uncertainty in obtaining the extrapolated value of y when x = 12.)

A.9 THE GEOMETRY OF TRIANGLES

A.9.1 The Right-Angled Triangle

Consider the right-angled triangle shown in Figure A.4. The trigonometric functions of sine, cosine and tangent are defined as:

$$\sin A = \frac{\text{opposite}}{\text{hypotenuse}} = \frac{a}{b}$$

$$\cos A = \frac{\text{adjacent}}{\text{hypotenuse}} = \frac{c}{b}$$

$$\tan A = \frac{\text{opposite}}{\text{adjacent}} = \frac{a}{c}$$

Note that:

$$\frac{\sin A}{\cos A} = \frac{\frac{a}{b}}{\frac{c}{b}} = \frac{a}{b} \times \frac{b}{c} \text{ (by Rule 2)}$$

i.e. $\dfrac{\sin A}{\cos A} = \dfrac{a}{c} = \tan A$

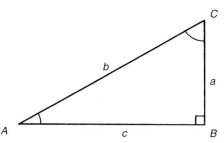

Figure A.4 A right-angled triangle. See text for definition of sine, cosine and tangent of an angle.

EXERCISE A.8

a. Write down expressions for sin C, cos C, tan C from Figure A.4.
b. What is the value of $\sin^2 A + \cos^2 A$?

The sine function occurs frequently throughout this book, e.g. in the geometry of triangles and in alternating current theory (Ch. 14). Its graphical form is shown in Figure A.5.

This graph is known as a sine wave, and always lies between +1 and –1. Also, the shape of the curve is *cyclical*, repeating itself every 360°.

A.9.2 Similarity of Triangles

The two triangles shown in Figure A.6 are said to be similar because one is just a bigger version of the other, while retaining the same *shape*. Thus, the corresponding angles of the two triangles are equal, but the lengths of the corresponding sides need not necessarily be so. However, if one side has a length which is double (say) that of the corresponding side of the other triangle, than *all* the sides will be doubled compared to the other triangle. Generally, then, we may write:

$$\frac{A}{a} = \frac{B}{b} = \frac{C}{c}$$

Equation A.5

In many practical examples in radiography, however, the similar triangles look more like those shown in Figure A.7.

These two types of similar triangles are discussed further in Chapter 2 (Sects 2.4–2.7). In each case, the ratios of the corresponding sides are equal, in agreement with Equation A.5.

A.10 POCKET CALCULATORS AND CALCULATIONS IN EXAMINATIONS

Because the price of pocket calculators now puts them within the range of even the most impoverished student, the purchase of such a calculator is strongly recommended. Scientific pocket calculators have the advantage that they can perform calculations which involve trigonometrical and logarithmic functions and so will be found especially useful. Many such calculators are also programmable, which means that formulae may be inserted into the calculator memory to allow it to perform certain calculations by simply inserting the appropriate data – a formula for Ohm's law could be inserted so that when the program

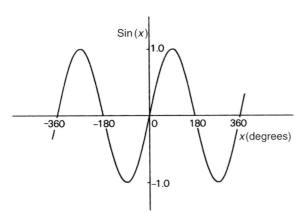

Figure A.5 A sine wave. The curve repeats itself every 360°.

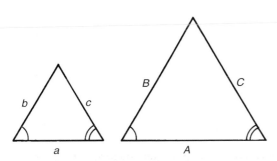

Figure A.6 Two similar triangles.

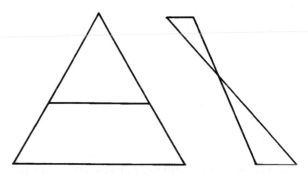

Figure A.7 Further examples of similar triangles.

is invoked the calculator will automatically calculate the resistance from the value of the potential and the current.

If you are to use a pocket calculator in examinations or if you are about to buy one, here are some suggestions that you might find helpful:

- Consider the types of calculations which you require from the calculator and do not buy one with lots of unnecessary functions – these simply increase your chance of error
- Try out a calculator before you buy it (if possible) and, if you are about to use one in an examination, make sure you are familiar with its layout and functions
- Find out the policy regarding the use of calculators in examinations at your university. Some universities will issue calculators for the purpose of examinations while others have specific regulations regarding programmable calculators
- Remember that the calculator will only give the correct answer if the correct information is keyed into it. It is important to remember indices and also try to get some 'feel' for the magnitude of the correct answer.

A.11 LOGARITHMS

Although few students would now undertake calculations using logarithms as the chosen method – thanks to the ease of use of the pocket calculator – it is nevertheless helpful to have a basic grasp of the theory of logarithms to explain certain functions in radiography, e.g. it may be easier to understand the exponential equations (see Ch. 4) in their logarithmic form.

DEFINITION

The *logarithm* of a number to a given *base* is the *power* by which the base must be raised to give the number.

Thus, the logarithm of 100 to the base 10 is 2 as $10^2 = 100$. This would normally be written as $\log_{10} 100 = 2$.

The base can be any number but, in practice, logarithms are usually to the base 10 or to the base e where e is the exponential number and is approximately equal to 2.7183.

Consider a situation where we wish to multiply two numbers a and b. If $a = 10^x$ and $b = 10^y$ then:

$$a \times b = 10^x \times 10^y$$
$$= 10^{(x+y)}$$

Thus from our initial definition of logarithms we can say:

$$\log_{10}(a \times b) = \log_{10}a + \log_{10}b$$

By a similar argument it can be shown that:

$$\log_{10}(a/b) = \log_{10}a - \log_{10}b$$

The main use of logarithms in radiography is to allow the simplification of complex formulae – if we consider the intensity of a beam of radiation which has travelled a distance x through a medium, this is given by the equation:

$$I_x = I_0 e^{-\mu x}$$

where I_x is the intensity of the radiation after a thickness x, I_0 is the initial intensity of the radiation, e is the exponential number and μ is the linear attenuation coefficient – these are all explained in Chapter 4. This equation is quite complicated to use in the above form but is much easier to use in its logarithmic form:

$$\log_e I_x = \log_e I_0 - \mu x$$

A.12 VECTOR QUANTITIES

In vector quantities the quantity concerned has direction as well as dimension. Thus in vector addition we need to take both these factors into account. This is probably best illustrated by two simple examples:

1. A man walks 30 metres in an easterly direction and then walks 20 metres in a northerly direction. How far must he walk in a straight line to get back to where he started? The situation may be visualised using Figure A.8.

By applying Pythagoras' theorem to this we can calculate that the distance from C to A is 36 metres.

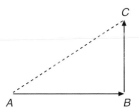

Figure A.8 Distances walked for calculation.

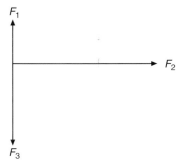

Figure A.9 Forces acting on a point.

2. Forces $F_1 = 1$ newton, $F_2 = 4$ newtons and $F_3 = 2$ newtons are applied to a point source, as shown in Figure A.9. What is the resultant force and what is its direction? As F_1 and F_3 are in opposite directions, the resultant force is the difference between F_1 and F_3 and is in the direction of F_3, as this is the larger of the two forces. We can now do vector addition (Figure A.10) where AB represents force F_2 and BD represents $(F_3 - F_1)$. The resultant force is represented by AD. By application of Pythagoras' theorem the length of this line is 4.12 newtons. Tan A is BD/AB and thus A can be calculated as approximately 14°. Thus we can say that the resultant force measures 4.12 newtons and is in a direction 14° below the horizontal.

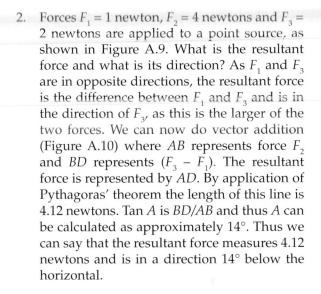

Figure A.10 Vector addition of forces.

APPENDIX SUMMARY

- If we multiply or divide two +s or two –s we get a +
- If we multiply or divide a + and a – sign we get a –
- When dividing by a fraction we can get the same result if we multiply by the fraction inverted (the fraction turned upside down)
- The following mathematical relationships have been established:
  $x^a \times x^b = x^{(a+b)}$
  $x^a/x^b = x^{(a-b)}$
  $x^{-a} = 1/x^a$
  $x^{1/2} = \sqrt{x}$
  $x^a/y^a = (x/y)^a$
- In direct proportion $y \propto x$ or $y = kx$ while in inverse proportion $y \propto 1/x$ or $y = c/x$, where k and c are constants of proportionality
- Sin θ = opposite/hypotenuse; cos θ = adjacent/hypotenuse and tan θ = opposite/adjacent

- Sine and cosine functions are cyclical, repeating themselves every 360°
- When drawing graphs, use a manageable scale, use a ruler, label both axes and use a title
- Similar triangles have the ratio of their corresponding sides equal
- There are certain factors to consider when purchasing or using a pocket calculator
- The basic theory of logarithms tells us that if $y = x^n$ then $\log_x y = n$
- $\log_{10}(x \times y) = \log_{10}x + \log_{10}y$
- $\log_{10}(x/y) = \log_{10}x - \log_{10}y$
- In vector addition we can get the resultant vector by joining the vectors end to end. The resultant vector is from the origin to the tip of the last vector.

ANSWERS TO EXERCISES

Exercises A.1

a. $\frac{11}{12} - \frac{5}{6} = \frac{11-10}{12} = \frac{1}{12}$

b. $\frac{7}{9} + \frac{2}{3} = \frac{7+6}{9} = \frac{13}{9} = 1\frac{4}{9}$

c. 20% of 50 $= \frac{20}{100} \times 50 = 10$

d. $\frac{2}{3} - \frac{1}{4} + \frac{3}{5} = \frac{40-15+36}{60} = \frac{61}{60} = 1\frac{1}{60}$

e. $\frac{7}{11} + \frac{2}{9} - \frac{2}{3} = \frac{63+22-66}{99} = \frac{19}{99}$

f. Percentage change $= 100 \times \frac{(90-80)}{80}$

$$= 100 \times \frac{10}{80} = 12.5\%$$

Exercises A.2

a. $28 \div 7 = 4$

b. $\frac{-36}{6} = -6$

c. $\frac{144}{-4} = -36$

d. $-13 \times -3 = 39$

e. $-7 \times \frac{-8}{-2} = -7 \times 4 = -28$

Exercises A.3

a. $\dfrac{\frac{-4}{11}}{\frac{7}{22}} = \frac{-4}{11} \times \frac{22}{7} = \frac{-8}{7} = -1\frac{1}{7}$

b. $\dfrac{\frac{2}{9}}{\frac{7}{3} \times \frac{-2}{11}} = \frac{2}{9} \times \frac{3}{7} \times \frac{11}{-2} = \frac{-11}{21}$

c. $\dfrac{\frac{1}{3} \times \frac{2}{9}}{\frac{9}{1} \times \frac{1}{2}} = \dfrac{\frac{2}{27}}{\frac{9}{2}} = \frac{2}{27} \times \frac{2}{9} = \frac{4}{243}$

Exercise A.4

a. $7a - 4(a - 2) = 7a - 4a + 8 = 3a + 8$

b. $-6(-x + y - 3) = 6x - 6y + 18$

c. $2(3a - 4) -3(-a + 6) = 6a - 8 + 3a - 18$
$$= 9a - 26$$

Exercise A.5

a. $\frac{2}{3}x = 4$

$2x = 12$

$x = 6$

b. $\frac{7}{9}y - 1 = 13$

$7y - 9 = 117$

$7y = 126$

$y = 18$

c. $q + \frac{3}{10} = \frac{5}{12}q$

$12q + \frac{36}{10} = 5q$

$12q - 5q = \frac{-36}{10}$

$7q = \frac{-36}{10}$

$q = \frac{-36}{70}$

$= \frac{-18}{35}$

d. $3\frac{3}{5}z - 12\frac{4}{5} = 1\frac{2}{5}z - \frac{7}{10}$

$3\frac{3}{5}z - 1\frac{2}{5}z = 12\frac{4}{5} - \frac{7}{10}$

$2\frac{1}{5}z = 12\frac{1}{10}$

$\frac{11}{5}z = \frac{121}{10}$

$110z = 605$

$z = \frac{605}{110}$

$= 5\frac{1}{2}$

Exercise A.6

a. 50 mA

b. 125 kVp

c. 65 μF

d. 0.00000055 m

Exercise A.7

a. From the graph you should obtain the following readings:

(i)   When $x = 1.5$, $y = 0.3$

(ii) When $x = 9.5$, $y = 1.9$

(iii) When $x = 12$, $y = 2.4$

(iv) When $x = 0.5$, $y = 0.1$.

b. From the graph you should obtain the following readings:

(i)   When $x = 1.5$, $y = 0.45$
(ii) When $x = 9.5$, $y = 18.05$
(iii) When $x = 12$, $y = 28.8$
(iv) When $x = 0.5$, $y = 0.05$.

Exercise A.8

A. From Figure A.4:

$\sin C = c/b$

$\cos C = a/b$
$\tan C = c/a$

b. From Figure A.4:

$$\sin^2 A + \cos^2 A = (a/b)^2 + (c/b)^2$$

$$= \frac{a^2 + c^2}{b^2}$$

But $a^2 + c^2 = b^2$ – by Pythagoras' theorem.
Thus, $\sin^2 A + \cos^2 A = 1$.

Appendix B

Scintillation Counters

A scintillation counter may be used to detect minute amounts of X- or gamma radiation. There are two main types of scintillation counter:

- a counter where the detector is in crystalline form, usually NaI(Tl)
- a counter where the detector is a liquid scintillation material.

B.1 NAI(TL) CRYSTALS AND PHOTOMULTIPLIERS

A crystal of sodium iodide with a thallium activator is one of the most efficient scintillators developed. The thallium impurities act as luminescent centres (see Sect. 31.3.1) and about 10–15% of the energy deposited in the crystal is converted to light energy. The maximum light emission is in the blue part of the spectrum, with a wavelength of 420 nm. The sodium iodide crystals are mounted in containers called cans to prevent them absorbing moisture from the atmosphere and becoming cloudy. One face of the crystal is attached to a transparent glass window and all other surfaces are in contact with a white reflective powder (magnesium oxide) so that as much light as possible is directed at the back of the crystal.

The back of the crystal is in optical contact with a photomultiplier tube, as shown in Figure B.1. If a gamma-ray is absorbed by the crystal (at point P on the diagram), this results in the emission of light in all directions. A fairly high percentage of this light reaches the photocathode of the *photomultiplier tube*. The photocathode consists of a thin coating of a mixture of alkaline salts deposited on

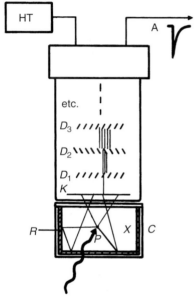

Figure B.1 A scintillation detector using sodium iodide. X, NaI(Tl) crystal; R, powdered reflector; C, crystal can; K, photocathode; D_1, D_2, etc., dynodes.

the inner wall of the face of the photomultiplier tube. About 10–25% of the light photons reaching the photocathode cause it to emit electrons by the photoelectric effect (see Sect. 30.5) and these electrons are accelerated through the tube to a series of positively charged plates called dynodes. The surface of these dynodes is coated with a layer of a secondary electron emitter so that each dynode produces approximately six times as many electrons as fall on it. As a result of this process, one electron released at the photocathode may result in one million electrons being collected by the anode of the photomultiplier. The collection of this charge occurs at a very short time interval after the initial electron is released by the photocathode (normally $<10^{-6}$s) and so a pulse of electricity is produced, the magnitude of the pulse being proportional to the energy of the absorbed gamma-ray photon.

INSIGHT

If the photomultiplier tube contains n dynodes, each of which releases six electrons for one incident electron, then the electron gain in the photomultiplier tube is 6^n. Thus, for a 10-dynode tube the gain would be 6^{10}, which is just over 60 000 000 electrons and represents a charge at the anode of about 10 picocoulombs.

A spectrum of these pulses will not produce the discrete gamma energies emitted by the radioactive source because of the statistical nature of the light production in the crystal and the electron multiplication in the photomultiplier. This is shown in Figure B.2, where the numbers of pulses of a given height are plotted. The true spectrum would be a line at the centre of the photopeak, as this corresponds to the energy of the gamma-rays absorbed by photoelectric absorption. In addition to the gamma-rays absorbed by photoelectric absorption, some of the gamma-rays undergo Compton scattering (see Sect. 30.6) within the crystal and then escape from the crystal with no further interactions. Gamma rays also undergo Compton scattering within the patient's tissues. Such scattering interactions result in energy being deposited in the crystal which is less than the energy of the gamma-rays and so smaller pulses are produced in the photomultiplier. These pulses produce a Compton peak, as shown in Figure B.2.

Some very-low-energy pulses are produced by the release of electrons from the photocathode by thermionic emission. There are also some positively charged ions produced at the dynodes which may strike the photocathode and cause it to release electrons. The electrons produced by both of the above mechanisms produce no useful signal and are referred to as 'noise pulses' (see Figure B.2).

B.2 THE USE OF SOLID SCINTILLATION COUNTERS IN MEDICINE

It is usual practice to count only the pulses that occur in the photopeak of the spectrum, particularly when investigating the activity and distribution of a radionuclide within a patient's body. This is achieved by the use of a *pulse height analyser* (PHA) which will only produce an electrical output signal if the input pulse lies within a certain range – this range is adjusted to cover the photopeak for the particular radionuclide. Pulses from the PHA are counted on a scalar for a time determined by the timer (Figure B.3). The number of counts obtained is directly related to the activity being measured and may be compared to a normal range of values for that structure.

An example of such a study will now be considered. The patient is given iodine-131 in the form of sodium iodide. The iodine component of this is taken up by the thyroid gland. The thyroid uptake may then be counted using equipment similar to that illustrated in Figure B.3. The gamma-rays emitted from the thyroid are detected by the lead-shielded sodium iodide crystal and those which lie within the photopeak are counted as described above.

The possibility of gamma-rays emitted outside the thyroid (see rays 3 and 4) being counted is reduced by the lead collimator – this is the shaded area in Figure B.3. The selection of a specific photopeak by the PHA allows the counter to

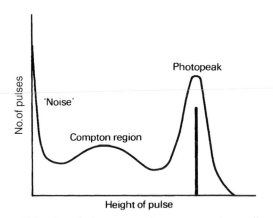

Figure B.2   A typical gamma-ray spectrum using sodium iodide.

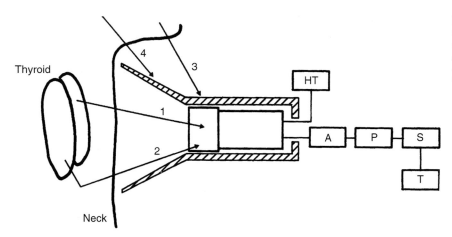

Figure B.3 A scintillation detector used to measure activity within a thyroid gland. A, amplifier; P, pulse height analyser (PHA); S, scalar; T, timer.

reject radiations which impinge on the crystals as a result of Compton scattering of the gamma-rays (see ray 2). The uptake count is obtained by expressing the thyroid uptake as a percentage of the total radiation ingested by the patient. Typical figures for a 24-hour uptake lie between 10 and 25%. An overactive thyroid will give a higher figure and an underactive thyroid has a lower figure.

B.3 THE GAMMA CAMERA

The gamma camera was first developed by H. O. Anger in 1958 and the camera and its associated technology have shown considerable progress since then. The gamma camera is a specialised type of scintillation counter where the position as well as the count of the scintillations within a thin NaI(Tl) crystal are obtained using a number of photomultipliers. Such a gamma camera and its associated circuitry are shown in Figure B.4. A multichannel parallel collimator similar to that shown in Figure B.4 ensures that only gamma-rays which are at right angles to the crystal face can enter the camera. A geometrical arrangement of photomultiplier tubes – of which there are typically between 61 and 75 – allows the position and the intensity of the scintillation produced in the crystal to be measured. This allows us to display a picture of certain physiological processes within the body. This ability to image a dynamic physiological process makes the gamma camera

a very powerful tool in the detection of pathologies where the physiology of the structure is disrupted.

B.4 LIQUID SCINTILLATION COUNTING

Radionuclides which decay solely by beta decay are not suitable for detection by NaI(Tl) crystals because of the low efficiency of detection. This is because many of the beta-particles are absorbed by the can around the crystal and others are scattered out of the crystal by interaction with the atoms of the crystal. If we wish to count the activity from samples containing such radionuclides, the most efficient way to do this is using liquid scintillation counting. A liquid scintillation solution is composed of:

- a solvent (e.g. benzene or toluene)
- a scintillation solute (the *primary* solute)
- a *secondary* solute.

A sample containing the beta-emitting radionuclide is dissolved in a liquid scintillation solution. The beta-particles from the radionuclide travel through the liquid and produce ionisation and excitation (see Sect. 26.6) within the molecules of the solvent. This excitation energy is transferred quickly (in less than 10^{-9}s) to the primary solute which fluoresces (see Sect. 31.3.1) when the electrons drop to their original lower-energy state. The secondary solute is introduced

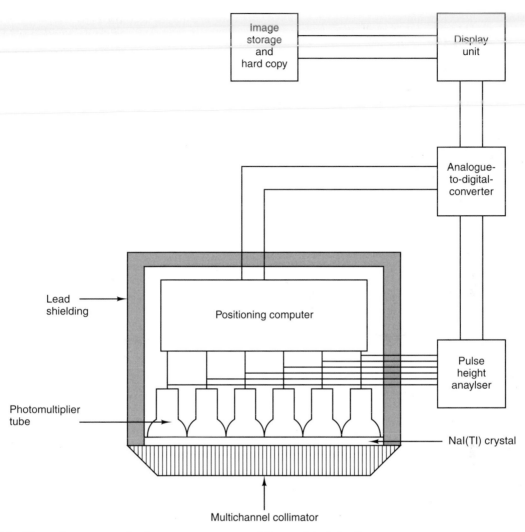

Figure B.4   The main components of a gamma camera and its associated circuitry.

into the solution as a *wavelength shifter* and so its function is to absorb photons emitted by the primary solute and reemit them as photons of a longer wavelength – this increases the efficiency of detection by the photomultiplier tubes. A typical efficiency for a liquid scintillation process is about 3%, i.e. 3% of the energy of the beta-particles is converted into photons which can be measured by the photomultiplier tubes.

A typical arrangement for counting the activity in a sample by liquid scintillation is shown in Figure B.5. Two photomultipliers, *A* and *B*, 'view' a plastic or glass bottle into which has been

introduced a small quantity (about 10 ml) of the liquid scintillation solution into which has been dissolved the radioactive sample. A scintillation event (for instance, at *P* in the liquid) produces light photons which are detected by both photo-multiplier tubes. The output from both photo-multiplier tubes is fed to a summing amplifier which is only switched on if the pulses from *A* and *B* are received at the same time – the pulses are in coincidence. In this way the random noise pulses from each photomultiplier tube are almost entirely eliminated. The output pulses from the summing amplifier are then a measure of the

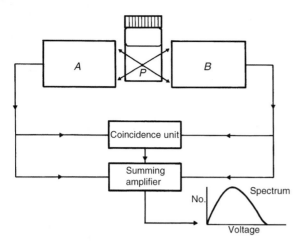

Figure B.5 A basic liquid scintillation counter.

continuous beta spectrum (see Figure 27.8) of the radioactive sample and may be counted using a scalar and timer, as described in Section B.3.

Liquid scintillation counting is an extremely sensitive method of measuring the activity of a beta-emitting sample because of the intimate contact between the sample and the scintillator. This means that very small quantities of beta-emitting radionuclide (as low as 1 part of nuclide in 10^{12} parts of solution) can be detected. Such techniques are used in biochemistry to detect small quantities of substances (e.g. hormones) which would be difficult to detect by other forms of chemical analysis.

Appendix C

CT Scanning

Since computed tomography (CT) was first demonstrated in 1973 by its inventor, Godfrey Hounsfield, CT has revolutionised the imaging of many body parts, especially soft-tissue and overlying structures, which are difficult to demonstrate using conventional techniques. The physics of CT is a complex topic. This appendix attempts to provide readers with an overview that will enable them to understand the basics of the process.

C.1 CT AND RADIATION DOSE

Although CT offers the ability to demonstrate structures that are difficult to visualise with conventional radiography, a survey by the UK National Radiological Protection Board (now the Health Protection Agency) showed that CT was used for only about 7% of all radiographic examinations in the UK, but that this modality accounted for more than 47% of the total radiation dose from the medical use of ionising radiation. Figure C.1 indicates reasons for this.

C.1.1 The CT Scanner

CT scanners can be broadly divided into conventional, spiral (or volumetric scanners) and multi-slice scanners. However all CT scanners have the same general appearance and operate on the principle of calculating the attenuation of the radiation beam as it passes through structures in its path.

A typical scanner consists of several subunits, in the following sections.

C.1.1.1 Patient Support Couch

This is about 1.5 metres long: the end nearest the gantry is narrowed to pass through the aperture of the gantry. Prior to the scan, couch position height and longitudinal movement can be adjusted by the user; during the scan couch movement is computer controlled.

C.1.1.2 Gantry

The gantry consists of a large box-like structure with a central aperture through which the patient is passed during the scan. On most machines the gantry may be tilted 20° each side of the vertical. Within the gantry are the X-ray tube, collimators, detectors, and the motor drive and control system to move the X-ray tube and detectors during the scan. Figure C.2 shows the geometry of the detectors and X-ray tube within the gantry.

C.1.1.3 X-ray Generator

This uses a three-phase mains supply and has a medium-frequency or constant-potential output. Radiation output is often pulsed, with each pulse lasting for about 3 milliseconds; this aids cooling and is necessary for the refreshment of the detectors. Generator output is monitored and controlled by an on-board microprocessor.

C.1.1.4 Computer and External Data Storage

The computer is possibly the most important part of the scanner and has many different functions (Figure C.3). It controls the operation of the

377

Effect on relative radiation dose

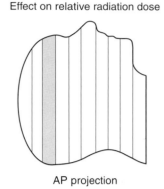

AP projection

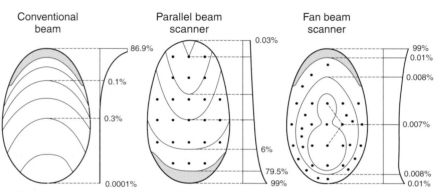

Figure C.1 Comparison of relative radiation dose delivered by conventional radiography and computed tomography for a single slice. AP, anteroposterior.

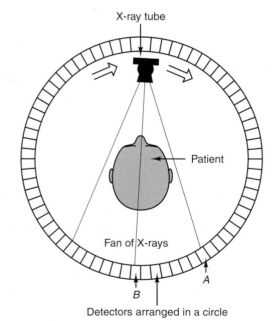

Figure C.2 Computed tomography gantry showing geometry of detectors, beam and X-ray tube.

scanner during the scan, collects the incoming data and processes it before passing the processed data to storage, and also displays the data as an image on the visual display unit (VDU) or other recording media. With fast processing times, this can be achieved within a few seconds of completion of the scanned slice. External or mass storage is usually to CD. The computer also has digital imaging and communications in medicine (DICOM) links to a laser imager for hard-copy production.

C.1.1.5 Diagnostic and Operator Consoles

These are used to input patient data and select operations to be carried out by the scanner and computer; in addition to facilities for the input of patient data, the operator's console offers a means of selecting the parameters to be used for the scan. Both types of console have some means of changing the window height and width of the displayed image. (*Note* that changing these parameters does not change the data sent for

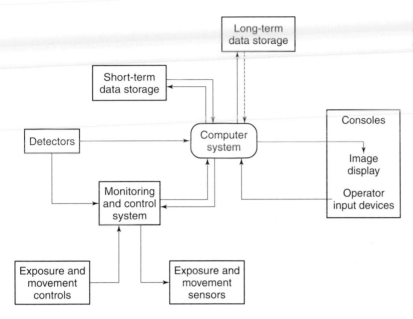

Figure C.3 Block diagram showing functions of the computer system in a computed tomography scanner.

processing, only the manner in which it is displayed.)

C.2 THE SCANNING PROCESS

The scanning process differs between conventional and spiral (or volumetric scanners). With a conventional scanner the tube rotates through an arc of approximately 350°. A number of pulsed exposures or views are made during this phase and the attenuation of the radiation beam is calculated for each pixel in the view. This process requires the simultaneous solution of several thousand simultaneous equations. On completion of the view the couch top is then advanced in a horizontal direction determined by the slice width and slice interval selected by the operator. Couch movement is computer controlled to ensure the selected slice increment is correct. When the movement has stopped the tube rotates in the opposite direction and the exposure process is repeated, producing another view. This process continues until the total of number of selected slices have been scanned. Scanning of the selected volume is then completed. As can be seen, each slice consists of several individual views. For each exposure:

- X-ray beam is attenuated as it passes through the patient
- Attenuated beam is detected by the detectors, which translate the incident X-ray intensity into an analogue electrical signal, which is directly proportional to the beam intensity on the detector
- The attenuated signal is subtracted from the incident-beam intensity signal
- The resultant number is converted into a digital number by the analogue-to-digital converter and passes to the computer.

Each view is processed as it is exposed, and the amount of radiation absorbed at each voxel in the slice is calculated. From the sum of the views a three-dimensional 'picture' of the absorption at different positions within the slice is constructed. Different algorithms may be used to manipulate the data, e.g. a bone algorithm will increase the differences between bone and soft-tissue absorption. The final stage of the processing is the allocation of a CT number (or Hounsfield number) to the value calculated for each voxel. This number represents the sum of all radiation absorbed by a voxel. Once this process is complete these values are stored prior to being mapped to the pixel display matrix of the VDU.

Lastly the values are changed to the display levels selected by the window selection set by the operator and passed to the VDU through the digital-to-analogue converter. These temporary values may also be sent to other image-recording devices attached to the scanner. Data for storage or plotting are taken from the stored values, not from the display values.

CT numbers range from −1000 (air) to +2000 (metallic implants). Water has a CT number of 0 (Figure C.4).

The display range of the VDU and the perception of the observer are limited so the full range of CT numbers cannot be used in any one display. To overcome this problem a method called windowing is used. We can select two factors: (1) the window level which selects the midpoint of our window; and (2) the window width which effectively limits the contrast range displayed. A wide window will give a wide contrast range with little density difference between adjacent pixels while a narrow one will result in higher density differences between adjacent pixels, but a much more restricted range of density contrasts (Figure C.5). To put it another way, window width governs the range of structures which may be viewed while window level governs the position of the window within the CT number scale.

Unlike ultrasound and radionuclide imaging, CT images show a clearly defined cross-sectional view of the structure of the body. The beam attenuation processes are exactly the same as those that occur in conventional radiographic examinations or radiotherapy treatments. Bony structures are well demonstrated and, because the detectors are more sensitive than the film screen combinations used in radiography, the small differences in absorption between soft-tissue structures can also be shown. If necessary, radiographic contrast agents can be used to enhance the contrast of selected soft-tissue structures.

C.3 SPIRAL CT

Spiral CT does not have the expose–move cycle of conventional CT; movement and exposure are simultaneous and continuous until the couch has moved through a pre-set distance.

Spiral CT produces a continuous output of raw data to the computer, representing a helical ribbon of information, probably best visualised as the spiral cord on a phone handset. Software in the computer processes this information as it is received, reconstructing it as a series of axial slices.

The scanning process differs from conventional scanning in that the X-ray tube rotates around the patient while couch movement and exposure occur simultaneously. This means, as

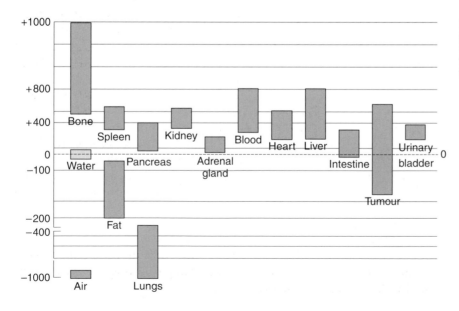

Figure C.4   Simplified diagram showing the relationship between computed tomography numbers and body tissues.

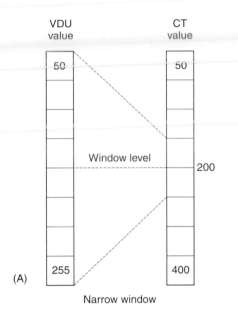

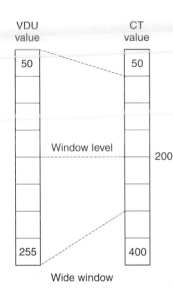

Figure C.5 Diagram showing how image contrast is affected by selection of window width. VDU, visual display unit; CT, computed tomography.

already mentioned, that the data are produced as a continuous stream of information, whereas in a conventional scan data are produced in distinct packages, separated by couch movement or slice. This places additional requirements on spiral scanners. These are:

- The X-ray tube must be able to rotate around the gantry continually during the exposure
- The X-ray tube should have a high heat capacity
- The computer must have sufficient power to be able to deal with the volume and rate of data generated.

Recent developments in X-ray tube and computer design have reduced the production costs of this type of scanner and they are becoming far more common.

The radiographer selects additional parameters (Table C.1) for volumetric scanning. There is very little difference in quality between a single CT slice and one produced by spiral CT. The most noticeable difference is that the actual slice width is slightly larger than the nominal slice width.

Pitch is defined as the amount of table feed per 360° rotation and, together with *collimation*, produces a nominal slice width. Most units offer a range of pitch values. The value is linked to table movement: the higher the value, the faster the

Table C.1 Comparison of parameters used in conventional and spiral (volumetric) computed tomographic (CT) scanning

Conventional CT	Spiral CT
Slice width	Collimation Pitch
Slice spacing	Index

movement. As pitch increases the degradation of the selection density profile becomes worse. This in turn affects spatial resolution along the Z-axis and also partial volume averaging. This also adversely affects contrast in the image. High pitch values have advantages: they reduce patient dose and permit a greater patient coverage in a given time, reducing the risk of movement artefacts.

As in conventional CT, once the scan has been carried out, the pitch and collimation, which effectively control slice width, cannot be changed.

Index determines where the computer commences a slice reconstruction.

As long as the raw data are available, the interpolation and reconstruction algorithms and the position of the *index* of the reconstructed slices may be altered, permitting changes in slice spacing.

C.3 IMAGE RECONSTRUCTION

As the information passes from the analogue-to-digital converter to the computer it is manipulated by a process termed *convoluted back-projection* and each pixel in the image is allocated a CT number. The higher the amount of radiation absorbed, the brighter the pixel and the higher the CT number. As with all digital images, the greater the number of pixels forming the image, the higher the resolution of the image and the higher the demands placed on the system's computer. With a 1 K image (1024 × 1024 pixel matrix), the image would contain 1 048 576 pixels.

C.4 MULTISLICE CT

Multislice CT offers further improvements on spiral CT and may be found on many modern CT scanners. This also places additional requirements on the scanner and involves changes to detector array. Additional bands of detectors are added to detector array, increasing its width.

Currently the most common number is four bands, although some scanners have as many as 16 bands of detectors. Multislice machines are capable of operating in a volumetric or conventional mode. In order that that radiation beam covers all the detector bands, the collimated slice width has to be increased. This in turn requires improved shielding (secondary collimation) of detectors, as well as an increased memory for image storage and faster processing time from the computer. The image-processing algorithms require modification to make allowance for distortion of image.

Multislice scanning offers the clinical advantages of a reduced risk of movement misregistration, a reduction in scanning times and a higher patient throughput.

Appendix D

Magnetic Resonance Imaging

D.1 NUCLEAR MAGNETIC RESONANCE (ALSO SEE CH. 11)

The phenomenon of nuclear magnetic spectrometry resonance has been used in chemistry since the early 1940s. However, the use of nuclear magnetic resonance (NMR) techniques for clinical imaging had to await the advances in computer technology that occurred in the 1970s, following the example of computed tomography (CT). Raymond Damadian from the USA had proposed in 1971 that the magnetic relaxation properties of tissues could be characteristic of tumour and normal tissue – this created a surge of interest in the potential of clinical magnetic resonance imaging (MRI). In the UK early research into the clinical use of MRI was carried out simultaneously in Aberdeen and Nottingham. The Nottingham group, headed by Peter Mansfield, produced the first images of a biological specimen (a grapefruit), while the Aberdeen group, headed by John Mallard, produced the first images of human anatomy. As a result of this MRI developed into a clinical technique used widely in radiology.

D.2 PULSE SEQUENCES

In Section 11.8.3 we mentioned that MRI uses sequences of radiofrequency (RF) pulses to generate signal information. The angle through which the net or overall magnetisation is 'flipped' depends upon the size and duration of the RF pulse. A flip angle, often of 90° but possibly of another value, puts the magnetisation into the transverse plane, facing the receiver coil. This is achieved by an *excitation pulse*. The spins relax (see Sect. 11.8.2) after the excitation pulse is turned off and are now refocused to produce a signal, either by a 180° pulse or by magnetic field gradients (magnetic fields which vary in strength in a linear way, like a slope). An example of a very basic pulse sequence is shown in Figure D.1.

If a 180° refocusing pulse is used, the relaxing spins are flipped completely over. They come back into phase to produce a signal or echo, as shown in Figure D.1. This is a spin-echo pulse sequence. If gradients are used, this is a gradient-echo pulse sequence. Again the spins are refocused to produce an echo. Gradient-echo sequences have the advantage of being fast, but do not correct local variations in field strength (and thus variations in signal) within the magnet.

The *time to repetition* (TR) is the time interval in milliseconds between the successive excitation pulses. The *time to echo* (TE) is the time interval in milliseconds between the excitation pulse and the echo. It is also double the time interval between the excitation pulse and the refocusing pulse or gradient. By varying the TR and TE we can alter the image weighting, making it T1, T2 or proton density. A short TR and TE gives a T1 sequence, while a long TR and TE gives a T2 sequence.

Many more complex pulse sequences exist. Fast spin-echo sequences consist of a chain of 180° refocusing pulses after the initial excitation pulse. This gives more pieces of signal in a short time, as each refocusing pulse produces an echo. Echo planar imaging is a very fast technique which uses a chain of gradient echoes.

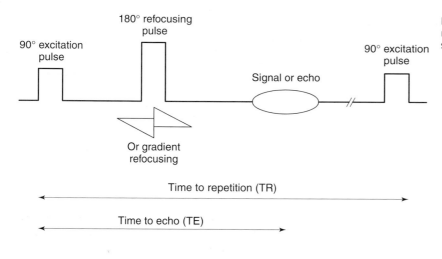

Figure D.1 A diagram of a simple magnetic resonance imaging pulse sequence.

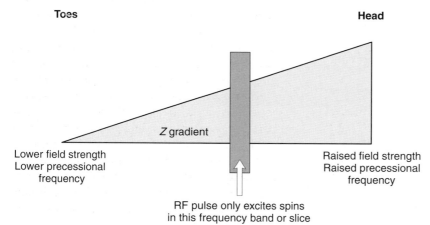

Figure D.2 Selection of an axial slice in magnetic resonance imaging. RF, radiofrequency.

D.3 IMAGE PRODUCTION

One of the most powerful features of MRI is its ability to image the body directly in any plane – axial, coronal, sagittal or even oblique. In order for it to achieve this, every volume element or *voxel* within the patient must return unique signal information. The spatial localisation or encoding is obtained by the application of three magnetic field gradients, in the x, y and z planes. The x gradient encodes for the horizontal axis of the magnet (i.e. patient's left to right), the y gradient for the vertical axis of the magnet (i.e. patient's anterior to posterior) and the z gradient for the longitudinal axis of the magnet

(i.e. patient's toes to head), with the patient lying supine in the magnet. Figure D.2 shows how the slice position is achieved.

The diagram assumes that we are choosing an axial slice in the patient, with a Z-gradient field superimposed on the main magnetic field. We can see that spins towards the feet will experience a lower field strength and thus precess at a slower rate. Spins towards the head will experience a greater field strength and precess at a faster rate. This is a consequence of the Larmor equation (see Sect. 11.8.2). If we apply an RF pulse with a narrow range of frequencies, termed the *transmit bandwidth*, we will only excite spins in a certain slice. The width of the slice is varied

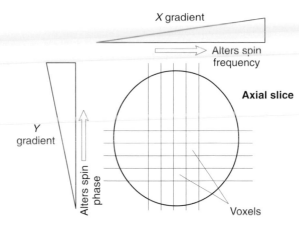

Figure D.3 Voxel localisation within the axial slice shown in Figure D.2.

a matrix of 256 pixels in the phase-encoding direction we have 256 lines of K space. Fast MRI techniques fill several, or even all, lines of K space in a single TR (see Sect. D.1). The slowest MRI technique, traditional spin echo, fills only one line of K space per TR.

D.4 MAGNET AND COIL DESIGN

There are three major types of MRI magnet:

1. *Superconducting magnets*. These are electro-magnets, using magnetic fields produced around coils of current-carrying wire. However they use wire materials such as niobium-tin or niobium-titanium alloy, which are superconducting at about 4 kelvin ($-269°C$) when cooled by liquid helium. This means that they have no electrical resistance and hence very large currents can flow without any losses. (The physics of superconductivity is discussed in Ch. 10.) This results in strong magnetic fields of several tesla. High-field-strength magnets obtain a good signal, which can be used to reduce scan times and improve scan resolution. Superconducting magnets normally also supply good field homogeneity, which is important for reduction of image noise and also for magnetic resonance spectroscopy (MRS).

2. *Resistive magnets*. These are again electro-magnets, but operating at room temperatures. Maximum field strength is only about 0.5 tesla, but they have the advantage that they can be turned off if needed. They may also have more open architecture, permitting easier access and interventional procedures and reduced patient claustrophobia. Their *fringe field* in the areas surrounding the magnet is low, reducing safety concerns. They may suffer from relatively poor field homogeneity.

3. *Permanent magnets*. These are based around large ferromagnetic iron or alloy cores and weigh several tons. Their maximum field strength is usually low. They may permit easy open access and are cheap to run once installed as they need minimal electrical

by adjusting the range of transmitted RF frequencies. The position of the slice is varied by altering the centre frequency in the z direction. If we were taking a sagittal or coronal slice we would use the X gradient or Y gradient respectively as the slice select gradient.

How about localising a point within the axial slice itself? This is illustrated by Figure D.3. We can use the X gradient to vary the precessional frequencies across the image, from left to right. This is now called the *frequency-encoding gradient*. But how can we use the Y gradient to encode uniquely from the anterior to the posterior of the patient? We cannot use frequency variations again this time, as we will obtain duplicate values. But we have a solution: when we vary the spin frequency using a gradient we are also varying the phase. Spins in a stronger part of the gradient field will be precessing faster. If we think of a clock face they might, for example, be in the 6 o'clock position, ahead of slower spins in the 3 o'clock position. Thus we measure the phase of the spins in the Y direction and the Y gradient is termed the *phase-encoding gradient*.

Information from within the imaging slice is stored in the MRI system's computer within something called K space. This consists of various lines of image information. The lines do not correspond directly to the rows of pixels on our final image. In fact, the centre of K space contains signal data and the outer margins of K space contain edge or resolution data. However, if we have power. They also have minimal fringe fields. However their field homogeneity may be poor.

Gradient coils in all of the above systems vary the field strength linearly either side of the magnetic isocentre in the x, y and z directions. They switch on and off rapidly and their uses include spatial localisation and gradient-echo imaging.

RF coils are simply loops of wire that transmit and/or receive RF energy to and from the patient. They may be of a volume design, completely enclosing the patient's anatomy, or of a surface coil design – a small coil placed on the surface of the patient. Volume coils are often transmit–receive coils, while surface coils are usually receive-only. Volume coils such as the body coil or the head coil provide a good image uniformity and coverage but a relatively weak signal. Surface coils tend to provide strong signal but weak uniformity and narrow anatomical coverage. Phased-array coils consist of a network of linked surface coils, providing the dual advantages of good signal and anatomical coverage. It should be noted that signal collection is maximised if a coil is placed as close as possible to the patient.

D.5 SAFETY

Although MRI does not employ ionising radiation, there are a host of biological effects associated with the procedure. There is no known risk of cancer induction and most effects are transient and reversible. However it should be noted that death could result in the case of a patient with a pacemaker or a ferromagnetic artery clip. Also death has been reported following the projectile effect of ferromagnetic objects pulled into the magnet.

A patient undergoing MRI is subjected to various fields: (1) the static magnetic field; (2) changing gradient magnetic fields; and (3) pulsed RF fields. The most important consequences of these three are: (1) the previously mentioned motion (torque) effect; (2) electrical current induction and acoustic noise; and (3) tissue heating.

There are no human studies that support the idea that pregnant staff or patients are at risk in MRI. However certain animal experiments have suggested a risk of reduced birth weight and length if fetuses are exposed long-term to magnetic fields. Thus MRI is not normally undertaken during the first trimester of a patient's pregnancy.

Appendix E

Digital Imaging

E.1 THE DIGITAL IMAGE

A conventional radiograph produced using film and intensifying screens is an example of an *analogue image*. The information (or data) it contains is represented by a range of continuously varying densities or shades of grey. If such an image is scanned as a series of horizontal lines and the densities plotted on a graph, we would see an appearance similar to that shown in Figure E.1A.

A digital image is divided into a series of small boxes called *pixels*, arranged in a series of rows and columns called a *matrix* (Figure E.2). The density of each pixel has a numerical integer value. If we consider our initial radiograph we could allocate the value 0 to the most dense value and 255 to the least dense value, giving a digital scale of 256. Thus, any single pixel would have a discrete value between 0 and 255 and our line would appear as a series of steps, as shown in Figure E.1B.

DEFINITION

An analogue image is one where the information it contains is presented as a range of continuously varying densities, whereas a *digital* image is any image in which the information is represented in discrete units, with integer values.

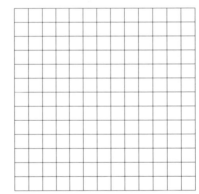

Figure E.2 An example of the matrix used for a digitised image. Each box of this matrix is a pixel.

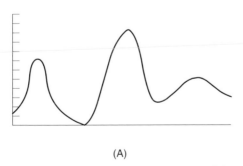

(A)

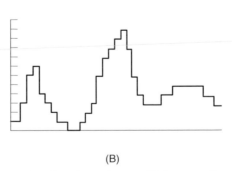

(B)

Figure E.1 A horizontal line drawn across an image. (A) A conventional analogue image; (B) the same line as a digital image.

The smaller the image size and the larger the value of the image matrix, the better the spatial resolution of the image. Most modern digital imaging systems have a matrix of 1024×1024 pixels; the resultant image has 1 048 576 individual pixels. If such an image is displayed on a visual display unit (VDU) in a 20-cm^2 section of the monitor image, each pixel will be a square of side just under 0.2 mm and so will be below the resolving power of the eye; thus we are aware of the overall image and do not see the individual pixels.

Digital imaging is used in the following imaging modalities and is also available for intraoral dental radiography:

- computed radiography
- digital fluorography
- digital mammography
- magnetic resonance imaging
- nuclear medicine
- direct array radiography
- digital subtraction angiography
- computed tomography
- ultrasound
- image transmission systems.

The process of converting the analogue radiation image from the patient into a digital image differs with each modality and application. However, the principle of changing this analogue signal into a digital one is common to all modalities and applications.

Digital imaging allows the construction of an image with a high spatial resolution, large dynamic range and good contrast resolution. In addition the imaged data may also be processed by a computer to enhance the diagnostic value of the raw unprocessed image. The data for these images, as already mentioned, can come from a variety of sources and will be received by some form of image receptor (imaging plate, digital array or transducer, for example). The signal then passes through several basic stages before a visible image is produced.

E.2 DIGITAL IMAGE PRODUCTION

If the image is not already in the form of an electrical signal, the first stage of the conversion process is to convert the image to an electrical signal. (This may not be necessary with all imaging modalities.) The analogue electrical signal passes into a digital one using a device known as an *analogue-to-digital converter* (ADC). Within the ADC the signal undergoes three stages: scanning, quantisation and coding.

E.2.1 Scanning

The incoming signal is scanned as a series of equally spaced horizontal lines. Each line is divided into a number of equally spaced points, producing a series of small 'boxes'. Each 'box' forms a single picture cell element or pixel. To eliminate display errors the scanning frequency must be at least twice the highest frequency present in the analogue image signal. This produces the *image matrix*. As already mentioned, the number of pixels per line is important as this controls the horizontal resolution of the image. A high rate of sampling produces a high-resolution image but is more demanding on the computing facilities.

The effect of pixel size on resolution can be seen by viewing Figure E.3. If viewed at close range the individual pixels are quite noticeable. However when viewed from a distance of about 1 meter, the eye cannot resolve the individual pixels.

E2.2 Quantisation

This process allocates a numerical integer to each pixel. On a scale of 1024, for example, each pixel can have an integer value between 0 and 1023. A typical TV camera video signal has a range from 0 to 700 mV at peak white intensity. This scale permits the ADC to detect changes in the video signal as low as 0.7 mV.

E2.3 Coding

The final stage, coding, converts the numerical value produced by quantisation into a binary number that can be understood by the computer, which cannot understand conventional numbers. The data then pass from the ADC to the computer.

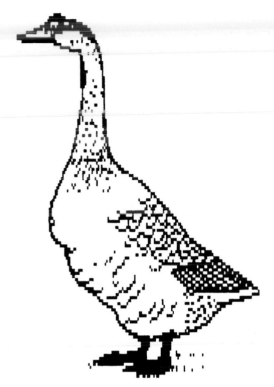

Figure E.3   An example of a digitised image where the pixels are so large that they can be seen at close range.

Where the signal is part of a moving image such as is produced during fluoroscopy it is also important that the ADC can sample and process each individual frame of the image before it is replaced by the next frame in the sequence, and therefore it is desirable that the ADC has a high sampling rate.

E.3 STORAGE AND MANIPULATION AND DISPLAY

The second stage of the conversion is carried out by the computer. The binary number passes to the central processing unit (CPU) of the computer which directs the data to an area of computer memory termed a *frame store*. When the data for the image is complete it is recalled by the CPU and, if required, manipulated. This facility allows us, for instance, to alter the contrast and brightness of the image, to window on specific values within the image so that only structures of interest are displayed, to enhance the edges of structures or to subtract one image from another. These facilities are especially useful in studies using a contrast agent.

Having manipulated the image as required, the binary values are recalled from the frame store and if necessary matched to the display capabilities of the VDU or monitor and passed to an output buffer (a storage area in the computer memory). Finally, once all data is modified and stored, the CPU monitors the transfer of the data to the appropriate output device. This process is shown diagrammatically in Figure E.4.

The final stage is the conversion of the digital signals from the computer back into an analogue signal. This process is carried out by a device known as a *digital-to-analogue converter* (DAC), which operates in a reverse manner to the ADC. As each binary number is received by the DAC it is allocated a discrete absolute numerical value; this current then passes through an output resistor, resulting in an analogue voltage output.

This is necessary as the monitor requires an analogue signal to control the electron 'gun' in the monitor tube. Finally, the electron beam from the cathode of the monitor tube is converted into a visible image by the phosphors of the monitor screen. Alternatively the signal may be sent as a digital signal to a device such as a laser imager, where it is used to produce hard copy on a film. Lastly, the digital signal may be sent to a *picture archiving and communications system* (PACS). This system has many functions: it provides long-term storage facilities for the digital image, and communicates with the departmental and hospital computer networks.

E.3 STORAGE AND TRANSMISSION OF DIGITISED IMAGES

As mentioned, digitised images may be stored on suitable optical disks as part of a PACS. Once stored, the information can be recalled by radiology staff or by staff in other parts of the hospital and its outstations for examination, if the PACS system permits this. By inserting the appropriate codes into a computer network, digital images may also be sent from one part of the

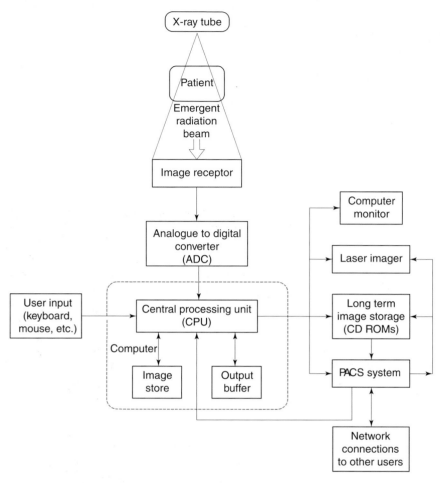

Figure E.4 Block diagram of the major components of a digital imaging system. Note the picture archiving and communication system (PACS) component of the system functions as an interface between the system and its long-term storage. It also permits communication between the internal departmental network and other hospital and external users.

country to another using a suitable linking system, thus allowing the possibility of *teleradiology*. PACS systems are becoming much more common and in the not too distant future may replace the film used by the conventional system as the principal method of production and storage of radiographic images.

Appendix F

Ultrasound Imaging

INTRODUCTION

Sound waves are mechanical pressure waves and are a series of compressions and rarefactions in a medium. For instance, sound travelling through air will cause the tympanic membrane in our ears to vibrate and because of this we can appreciate the existence of sound. The frequency (f) of a sound wave is defined as the number of high- and low-pressure regions crossing a point in unit time. Frequency is measured in cycles per second (or Hertz). The wavelength (λ) is the distance between one rarefaction and the next. The higher the frequency of the vibration, the higher the pitch of the sound. The velocity (C) or speed of the wave in a medium is defined by the formula:

$$C = \lambda f \qquad\qquad \textit{Equation F.1}$$

The normal human ear is able to detect sound within the range of 20 Hz to 20 kHz. Frequencies above this are inaudible to us, although they can be heard by animals, e.g. bats, dogs and dolphins. For this reason such sounds are termed ultrasound. Medical imaging makes use of ultrasound in the frequency range of 1–20 MHz. The relatively slow wave velocity of ultrasound in tissue permits distance measurements to be made. These are listed in Table F.1.

F.1 PRODUCTION OF ULTRASOUND

In medical imaging ultrasound is produced using the piezoelectric effect. This is illustrated in Figure F.1. If a potential difference is applied

Table F.1	Ultrasound in tissues
Medium	Velocity (cm.s^{-1})
Water	1480
Fat	1450
Blood	1570
Kidney	1560
Soft tissue (average)	1540
Liver	1450
Muscle	1580
Bone	4080

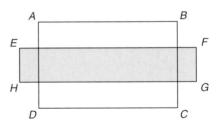

Figure F.1 When a potential is applied to the faces *AB* and *CD* it distorts to form the shape *EFGH*. Similarly, if mechanical stress applied to faces *AB* and *CD*, it then adopts the shape *EFGH*. This is known as the piezoelectric effect.

across the opposing faces of a suitable crystal (e.g. lead zicronate titonate, for instance) it will distort, as shown in Figure F.1. When potential is removed the crystal returns to its original shape as a series of oscillations. Conversely, if such a crystal is compressed by mechanical stress, a potential difference is produced between opposing faces. Thus the crystal can both produce and detect ultrasound.

F.2 PULSE-ECHO IMAGING

In pulse-echo imaging a device called a transducer is used to produce and detect ultrasound. This produces a pulse of ultrasound that lasts for approximately 1 microsecond; for the remaining 999 microseconds (999 μs) the transducer is capable of detecting the returning echoes. This process is repeated each millisecond (1 ms). The ultrasound wave travels through the patient and produces echoes at the interfaces of structures that have different acoustic impedance. The acoustic impedance of soft-tissue–air, bone–air and soft-tissue–bone interfaces is high and as a result almost total reflection of the wave occurs. Acoustic impedance (measured in Rayl's) of a substance is given by the equation:

$$Z = \rho c \qquad \text{Equation F.2}$$

where Z is the acoustic impedance, ρ is the density of the medium and c is the velocity of ultrasound travelling through that medium. By measuring the time from the transmission of the ultrasound pulse to the reception of the returning echo, the distance travelled by the ultrasound pulse and the returning echo from the interface to the transducer is recorded. The depth of the interface is calculated by the timing unit of the machine using the equation:

$$d = \tfrac{1}{2}ct \qquad \text{Equation F.3}$$

where d is the depth of the interface, c is the velocity of ultrasound in that tissue type and t is the time taken from the transmission of the ultrasound to the detection of the returning echo. The intensity of the echo is also recorded.

Figure F.2 is an example of a typical ultrasound machine. The function of the components shown is as follows:

- step-up transformer – increases the amplitude mains voltage
- the pulsing circuit, which 'clips' the supply into 1 millisecond pulses
- limiter – passes low-amplitude signals (echoes) but prevents the transmission pulse from passing into the receiver part of the unit
- log amplifier – increases the amplitude of input signals; weak signals are amplified more than the stronger ones
- time gain compensation – increases the output of the log amplifier to bring in synchronisation with lower amplitude of echoes from deeper structures and compensates for tissue attenuation of the echo
- rectifier – converts the negative half-cycles of the echo waveform into positive half-cycles before these signal passes to the demodulator
- demodulator – outputs the amplitude of the echo and the time delay from the transmission

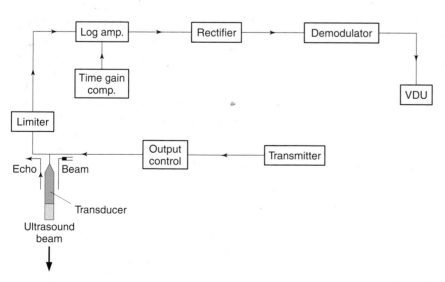

Figure F.2 Block diagram of the main components of an ultrasound machine, showing signal pathways for the transmitted pulse and the returning echo.

pulse. After further processing the signal is used to drive the visual display unit (VDU).

F2.1 Beam Attenuation

As the ultrasound beam passes through the tissues energy is lost through interactions (reflection and scattering) with objects in its path. The interactions that are of greatest importance in ultrasound imaging are those which result in the reflection of the beam as the transducer detects the returning echoes. Two types of reflection are involved. Specular reflection occurs from large interfaces between two different body tissues, e.g. the edge of the liver or kidney where the beam passes into the second tissue and is reflected back into the first tissue. The greater the difference in the impedance ($z_1 - z_2$) of the tissues, the greater the bias to reflection.

The direction of the reflected beam (or echo) follows the laws of reflection. The incident beam must be perpendicular to the interface to produce an echo that can be received by the transducer (i.e. when the angles of incidence and reflection are both zero).

Diffuse scattering occurs as the sound wave interacts with objects smaller than its wavelength; interface roughness and small variations in acoustic impedance within body organs are a common cause of this type of reflection. As the name implies, the echoes are produced in all directions and have very low amplitude. Such echoes do not form part of the useful image and only serve to increase the width of the beam, bringing about a further reduction in beam intensity.

F.3 DOPPLER ULTRASOUND

Echoes returning from a moving structure demonstrate a frequency shift bringing about a

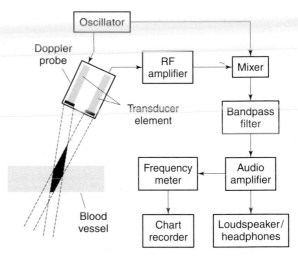

Figure F.3 Block diagram showing the main components of a typical Doppler scanning unit. RF, radiofrequency.

change in the pitch of the sound in a manner similar to the change in pitch of an ambulance siren as it approaches and passes a stationary observer. The Doppler effect depends on the velocity and direction of the movement: pitch increases as the structure moves toward the probe and decreases as it moves away. The probe differs from that used in pulse-echo imaging in that it is divided into two acoustically insulated transducers, one transmitting continuously and the other receiving (Figure F.3). Spectral analysis of the echoes is carried out by a fast Fourier transformation analyser and may be passed to a speaker producing an audible indication of the Doppler shift or the information may be displayed in 'false' colour on the unit's VDU. Imaging using the Doppler effect is utilised in imaging many vascular structures where movement of the blood cells relative to the transducer is measured.

Appendix G

Positron Emission Tomography (PET) Scanning

G.1 REVISION OF POSITRON PHYSICS

As was discussed in Chapter 27, if a nucleus has too few neutrons for stability, it is possible for the nucleus to achieve a more stable configuration by the emission of a positron. Positrons are the antiparticles of electrons and the positron and an electron will interact (within a very short distance in tissue), annihilating each other and producing two photons of annihilation radiation. These photons each have an energy of 0.51 MeV (511 keV) and detection of these photons forms the basis of positron emission tomography (PET). Each photon is produce at an angle close to $90°$ to the direction of travel of the positron (see Fig. 27.7).

G.2 DETECTION OF POSITRONS

If a positron-emitting radionuclide is introduced into the patient it can be labelled in such a way that it concentrates in specific structures. The number of positrons emitted by these structures can be related to the activity of the cells within the structure. If we surround the patient with a ring of positron detectors (Figure G.1), then each annihilation radiation from the positron–electron interaction can be registered and the intersections of these points can be back-projected to indicate the position of the positron-emitting tissue in the patient.

G.3 TYPES OF COINCIDENCE

For the annihilation radiation from the positron–electron interactions to give useful

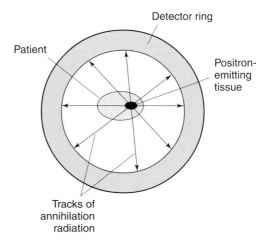

Figure G.1 Detection of annihilation radiation from a positron-emitting source within the patient.

information, the two photons must travel in straight lines from the source of the radiation to the detectors. The photons in Figure G.2A are of this type. Because the photons all travel with the velocity of electromagnetic radiation, they will each be detected by a detector at almost the same time – within < 10 nanoseconds (10×10^{-9} s) of each other. These photons are said to be co-incident. It is possible for one of the photons to be scattered (Figure G.2B). If the position of these two photons were back-projected it would be an incorrect position for the origin of the annihilation radiation. Because the scattered photon travels along a slightly longer route, the two photons will not be detected within 10×10^{-9}s of each other and so they are not said to be coincident and the imaging computer can be programmed to ignore them. Similarly, in Figure G2C, one of the photons has been absorbed.

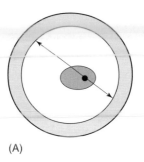
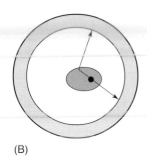
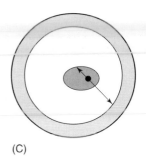

Figure G.2   Types of coincidence. (A) True coincidence. (B) One of the photons is scattered. (C) One of the photons is absorbed. This makes (B) and (C) false coincidences.

(A)   (B)   (C)

Because there is no matching coincident photon, the imaging computer will again ignore this event.

G.4 DETECTOR MATERIALS

In the gamma camera (see Appendix B) the radiation is detected using a sodium iodide crystal. The radiation from technetium-99m has an energy of 140 keV. The energy of the annihilation radiation from the positron–electron interaction is 511 keV. The greater energy of this radiation requires a material of higher density and/or higher atomic number. Bismuth germinate (BGO) is the material of choice for the detector crystals.

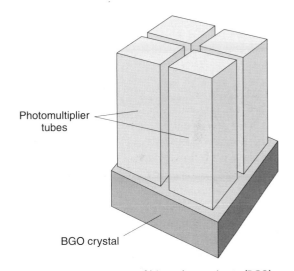

Photomultiplier tubes

BGO crystal

Figure G.3   Arrangement of bismuth germinate (BGO) crystal and photomultiplier tubes to make an imaging block.

G.5 DETECTOR MECHANISMS

The basic components of the detector mechanism are BGO crystals over which photomultiplier tubes are positioned, as shown in Figure G.3. These arrangements are known as blocks. Each photomultiplier tube detects the light emission as the result of the radiation photons interacting with the crystal. Groups of blocks (Figure G.4) arranged with shared electronics form detector cassettes and a number of these detector cassettes form a detector ring around the patient. Normally there is more than one ring so that we can detect information from a number of slices simultaneously. To avoid oblique rays from one slice interfering with the image on another ring, the rings are separated by septa made of lead or tungsten (Figure G.5).

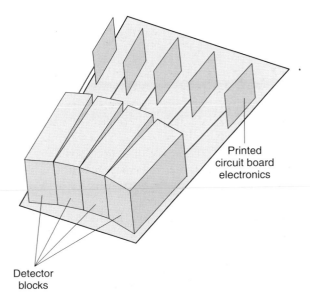

Printed circuit board electronics

Detector blocks

Figure G.4   Arrangement of imaging blocks to make an imaging cassette.

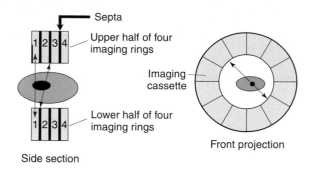

Figure G.5   Arrangement of detection rings separated by septa which avoid detection of oblique rays.

G.6 RADIONUCLIDES USED IN PET

Three common radionuclides used in PET imaging are identified below:

1. 18-fluorodeoxyglucose (FDG) is a useful nuclide for cerebral metabolism and can also be used to demonstrate tumour activity
2. $^{13}NH_3$ is useful for myocardial perfusion.
3. $H_2^{15}O$ is useful for imaging of cerebral blood flow patterns.

Appendix H

Modulation Transfer Function (MTF)

Modulation transfer function (MTF) is a mathematical method of assessing the resolving power of an imaging system, whether it be optical, radiographic or radioactive (e.g. gamma camera: see Appendix B.3). The use of the MTF for this purpose was pioneered in the field of optics when it was discovered that a lens that was excellent at imaging the structure of very fine objects was not necessarily as good as another lens of lower resolving power when imaging coarser (i.e. larger) objects.

DEFINITION

The MTF of an image is a numerical value determined by the division of the modulation (m_i) of the recorded image by the modulation of the stimulus (m_0):

$$\text{MTF } (v) = m_i/m_0 \qquad \textit{Equation H.1}$$

H.1 MODULATION AND SPATIAL FREQUENCIES

As can be seen from the definition, the process of modulation is inherent in any description of the MTF and will therefore be considered first. Modulation is linked to spatial frequency. Consider the sine wave shown in Figure H.1, which has a wavelength of X.

The spatial frequency of this waveform is the number of cycles per unit length (say v cycles per cm), and is therefore given by $1/x$. The *modulation* of the object, m_0, is defined as:

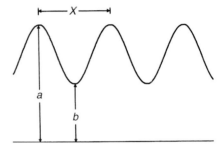

Figure H.1 The definition of modulation (see text).

$$m_0 = (a - b)/(a + b) \qquad \textit{Equation H.2}$$

where a and b are the height of the peaks and troughs of the waveform, respectively.

The units in which amplitude of the sine wave is recorded will differ with the application, e.g. X-ray intensity in radiography, light intensity for optical lenses, level of activity for gamma cameras or optical density for photographic film.

If it is supposed that an absorber is placed in the path of an X-ray beam such that it would produce a sinusoidal variation of intensity of the transmitted beam, then a perfect imaging system would produce a sine wave of the *same* modulation.

The *image modulation* would then be the same as the *object modulation*. However, in practice, the relative amplitude of the image modulation is reduced by the finite size of the focal spot. In addition, the recorded image is also affected by the characteristics of the film/screen combination (or other image receptor). This tends to spread the image on to a larger area than theoretically desirable. Thus, the peaks of the sinusoidal exposure tend to contribute to the troughs, so that an overall reduction in amplitude (and therefore modulation) is experienced.

This effect of a reduction in image modulation is small when the sinusoidal object has a long wavelength (low spatial frequency), but is of increasing importance as the wavelength is reduced to about 1 mm or less (spatial frequencies of 10 per cm or more). The image modulation therefore depends upon the spatial frequency of the object, and this forms the basis of the MTF, described below.

H.2 MTF AND SPATIAL FREQUENCY

As seen, the MTF (Equation H.1) is defined as:

$$\text{MTF}(v) = m_i/m_0$$

In a perfect imaging system, the image is an exact copy of the object and so has the same modulation at all spatial frequencies. The MTF is therefore always unity for such a system. However, as the spatial frequency increases, it is to be expected that the imaging of fine detail (high spatial frequencies) would be worse (because of geometric distortion; Figure H.2A) and the image modulation is reduced (Figure H.2B).

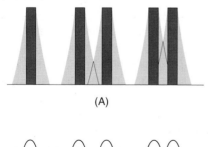

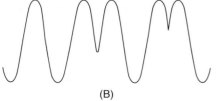

(A)

(B)

Figure H.2 The effect of increasing line-pairs per centimeter on spatial frequency. (A) Increasing geometric distortion as line-pair per millimetre increases; (B) the sine wave plot of the densities produced by (A).

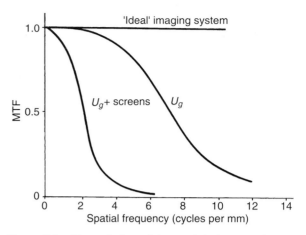

Figure H.3 The variation of the modulation transfer function (MTF) with spatial frequency for an ideal system, that due to geometric unsharpness (U_g), and that due to geometric unsharpness and screens (U_g + screens).

The graph shown in Figure H.3 shows three examples: (1) an 'ideal' imaging system, where the MTF is 1 and is independent of the spatial frequency; (2) a curve where the MTF is reduced at the higher frequencies due to geometric unsharpness (U_g) only; and (3) a curve obtained when using a film/screen recording medium ($U_g + U_s$).

The MTF is particularly useful in separating the individual causes of image degradation. MTFs due to each cause may be measured separately (MTF_1, etc.) and may be combined to produce the overall MTF of the system:

$$\text{MTF} = \text{MTF}_1 \times \text{MTF}_2... \qquad \textit{Equation H.3}$$

It thus becomes possible to predict the response of the overall system with various combinations of focal spot size, film/screen combinations, etc. if the MTF of each is known.

H.3 OBJECTS AS SPATIAL FREQUENCIES

A sinusoidal object does not bear much similarity to the objects that are normally radiographed. However, it may be shown that the shape of any object may be obtained from the summation of sine and cosine waves of different amplitudes and frequencies (Fourier's theorem). Thus, if the MTF of the X-ray unit is known at each frequency, the overall response to the object may be determined.

As an example of the summation of amplitudes of different frequencies forming a shape, consider the flat-topped object shown by the dashed lines in Figure H.4A. The height of the object may be considered to represent the degree of absorption of the X-rays by the object, and its width as the physical size of the object. It may be shown that such a shape may be obtained by adding an infinite series of cosine waves (which are just sine waves displaced by 90°) of increasing frequency (f), where the amplitudes are given by:

$$g = \sin{(\pi f d)}/(2\pi f) \qquad Equation\ H.4$$

The sum of the first 500 terms of such amplitudes is shown in Figure H.4A. The effect of including 2500 terms (i.e. containing higher frequencies) is shown in Figure H.4B, where a closer approximation to the square shape is obtained. The agreement is exact when an infinite number of terms is included. However, the higher spatial frequencies present in the object are poorly reproduced in the image, because the MTF is low at high frequencies. Since the high frequencies are responsible for the squareness of the corners for objects, such as shown in Figure H.3, sharp objects will be shown as being slightly blurred or out of focus. This is in accordance with the concept of *unsharpness*, as discussed earlier, and the two approaches are just two ways of looking at the same thing. The MTF is more mathematically rigorous as a complete description of the imaging properties of the X-ray unit, but even this does not consider other problems such as statistical 'noise' within the image, known as *quantum mottle*.

H.4 MEASUREMENT OF MTF

In practice it is difficult to manufacture sinusoidal objects in the numbers and wavelengths required and it would also be very time-consuming to measure the image modulation for every combination of frequency, position of absorber and image receptor for every object recorded. Fortunately, there is no need to do this: an intensity curve can be obtained by 'shining' an X-ray beam through a very narrow slit (Figure H.5).

Since the width of the slot is known, the blur or line spread function (LSF) of these images can be calculated, after taking into consideration all other factors affecting the blur produced. These calculations are carried out by complex computer programs, the explanation of which is beyond the scope of this book. Once the LSF is known it can in turn be used to calculate the MFT of the recorded image.

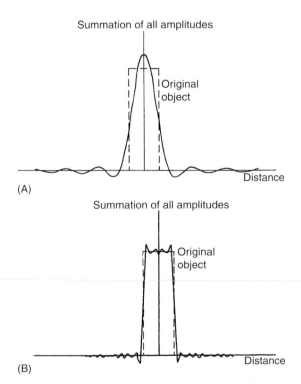

Figure H.4   The representation of a 'square' object (dashed lines) by the summation of frequencies of different amplitudes: (A) 500 terms; (B) 2500 terms. An infinite number of terms reproduces the object exactly.

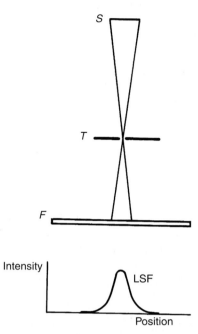

Figure H.5   The line spread function (LSF). *S*, source of X-rays; *T*, test object with narrow slit; *F*, image-recording medium.

Appendix I

SI Base Units

International System of Units (SI) base units were discussed in Chapter 6. Below are the precise definitions of these units.

MASS

The unit of mass is the *kilogram*. The mass of 1 kilogram is equal to the mass of the international platinum-iridium prototype of the kilogram.

LENGTH

The unit of length is the *metre*. The metre is the length equal to 1 650 763.73 wavelengths in a vacuum of the radiation corresponding to the transition between the levels $2p_{10}$ and $5d_5$ of the krypton-86 atom.

TIME

The unit of time is the *second*. The second is the duration of 9 192 631 770 periods of the radiation corresponding to the transition between the two hyperfine levels of the ground state of the caesium-133 atom.

ELECTRIC CURRENT

The unit of electric current is the *ampere*. The ampere is the constant current which, if maintained in two straight parallel conductors of infinite length, of negligible circular cross-section and placed 1 metre apart in a vacuum, would produce between these conductors a force equal to 2×10^{-7} newton per metre of length.

TEMPERATURE

The unit of temperature is the *kelvin*. The kelvin is the fraction 1/273.16 of the thermodynamic temperature of the triple point of water.

LUMINOUS INTENSITY

The unit of luminous intensity is the *candela.* The candela is the luminous intensity, in the perpendicular direction, of the surface of 1/600 000 square metres of a black body at the temperature of freezing platinum under a pressure of 101 325 newtons per square metre.

AMOUNT OF SUBSTANCE

The unit of amount of substance is the *mole*. The mole is the amount of substance of a system which contains as many elementary entities as there are atoms in 0.012 kilogram of carbon-12.

Tables

Table A Powers of 10

Prefix	Symbol	Factor
exa	E	10^{18}
peta	P	10^{15}
tera	T	10^{12}
giga	G	10^{9}
mega	M	10^{6}
kilo	k	10^{3}
milli	m	10^{-3}
micro	μ	10^{-6}
nano	n	10^{-9}
pico	p	10^{-12}
femto	f	10^{-15}
atto	a	10^{-18}

Table C Important conversion factors

1 atomic mass unit (amu)	$= 1.66 \times 10^{-27}$ kg
1 electron volt (eV)	$= 1.60 \times 10^{-19}$ J
1 joule (J)	$= 6.24 \times 10^{18}$ eV
Electron mass	$= 0.511$ MeV
Proton mass	$= 938$ MeV
Neutron mass	$= 940$ MeV
1 angstrom (Å)	$= 0.1$ nm

Table B Physical constants

Quantity	Value
Avogadro's number, N_A	6.02×10^{23} mol^{-1} [a]
Velocity of light in a vacuum, c	3.00×10^{8} m.s^{-1}
Permittivity of vacuum, ε_0	8.8×10^{-12} F.m^{-1}
Permeability of vacuum, μ_0	1.26×10^{-6} H.m^{-1}
Electron rest mass, m_e	9.11×10^{-31} kg
Proton rest mass, m_p	1.672×10^{-27} kg
Neutron rest mass, m_n	1.675×10^{-27} kg
Planck's constant, h	6.63×10^{-34} J.s
Electronic charge, e	-1.60×10^{-19} C

[a] Or 6.02×10^{26} (kg.mol)$^{-1}$.

Table D	Greek symbols and their common usage		

Name	Symbol Capital	Lower case	Usage
Alpha	A	α	α-particle (He nucleus); also lower-case alpha (α) is the 'flip' angle in MRI
Beta	B	β	β-particle (electron or positron)
Gamma	Γ	γ	γ-rays; also the gyromagnetic ratio in MRI
Delta	Δ	δ	Δx or δx used to indicate the change in x
Epsilon	E	ε	
Zeta	Z	ζ	
Eta	H	η	
Theta	Θ	θ	Used to represent an angle
Iota	I	ι	
Kappa	K	κ	
Lambda	V	λ	(λ) Wavelength; decay constant
Mu	M	μ	(μ) Total linear attenuation coefficient
Nu	N	ν	(ν) Frequency of electromagnetic radiation
Xi	Ξ	ξ	
Omicron	O	o	
Pi	Π	π	(π) Linear attenuation coefficient for pair production
Rho	P	ρ	(ρ) Density of matter
Sigma	Σ	σ	(σ) Standard deviation or linear attenuation coefficient for the Compton effect or (Σ) summation of terms
Tau	T	τ	(τ) Linear attenuation coefficient for photoelectric absorption
Upsilon	Y	υ	
Phi	Φ	φ	Used to represent an angle
Chi	X	χ	
Psi	Ψ	ψ	
Omega	Ω	ω	Symbol for resistance and impedance in ohm (Ω); ω is also the precessional frequency in MRI

MRI, magnetic resonance imaging.

Table E Periodic table of the elements

Period	1	2	3	4	5	6	7	8	9	10	11	12	13	14	15	16	17	18
1	1 H																	2 He
2	3 Li	4 Be											5 B	6 C	7 N	8 O	9 F	10 Ne
3	11 Na	12 Mg											13 Al	14 Si	15 P	16 S	17 Cl	18 Ar
4	19 K	20 Ca	21 Sc	22 Ti	23 V	24 Cr	25 Mn	26 Fe	27 Co	28 Ni	29 Cu	30 Zn	31 Ga	32 Ge	33 As	34 Se	35 Br	36 Kr
5	37 Rb	38 Sr	39 Y	40 Zr	41 Nb	42 Mo	43 Tc	44 Ru	45 Rh	46 Pd	47 Ag	48 Cd	49 In	50 Sn	51 Sb	52 Te	53 I	54 Xe
6	55 Cs	56 Ba	71 Lu *	72 Hf	73 Ta	74 W	75 Re	76 Os	77 Ir	78 Pt	79 Au	80 Hg	81 Tl	82 Pb	83 Bi	84 Po	85 At	86 Rn
7	87 Fr	88 Ra	103 Lr **	104 Rf	105 Db	106 Sg	107 Bh	108 Hs	109 Mt	110 Uun	111 Rg	112 Uub	113 Uut	114 Uuq	115 Uup	116 Uuh	117 Uus	118 Uuo

*Lanthanoids	57 La	58 Ce	59 Pr	60 Nd	61 Pn	62 Sm	63 Eu	64 Gd	65 Tb	66 Dy	67 Ho	68 Er	69 Tm	70 Yb
**Actinoids	89 Ac	90 Th	91 Pa	92 U	93 Np	94 Pu	95 Am	96 Cm	97 Bk	98 Cf	99 Es	100 Fm	101 Md	102 No

Note: Elements with atomic numbers 117 and 118 have been named and their position in the periodic table is shown but they have not been created at the time of writing of this text. Previous claims, made in 1999, to have created element 118 have now been withdrawn. Element 111 has now been renamed roentgenium (Rg).

Table F Electron configuration of elements

Element	Atomic no.	Symbol/Shell	K	L	M	N	O	P	Q
			Number of electrons in shells						
Hydrogen	1	H	1						
Helium	2	He	2						
Lithium	3	Li	2	1					
Beryllium	4	Be	2	2					
Boron	5	B	2	3					
Carbon	6	C	2	4					
Nitrogen	7	N	2	5					
Oxygen	8	O	2	6					
Fluorine	9	F	2	7					
Neon	10	Ne	2	8					
Sodium	11	Na	2	8	1				
Magnesium	12	Mg	2	8	2				
Aluminium	13	Al	2	8	3				
Silicon	14	Si	2	8	4				
Phosphorus	15	P	2	8	5				
Sulphur	16	S	2	8	6				
Chlorine	17	Cl	2	8	7				
Argon	18	Ar	2	8	8				
Potassium	19	K	2	8	8	1			
Calcium	20	Ca	2	8	8	2			
Scandium	21	Sc	2	8	9	2			
Titanium	22	Ti	2	8	10	2			
Vanadium	23	V	2	8	11	2			
Chromium	24	Cr	2	8	13	1			
Manganese	25	Mn	2	8	13	2			
Iron	26	Fe	2	8	14	2			
Cobalt	27	Co	2	8	15	2			
Nickel	28	Ni	2	8	16	2			
Copper	29	Cu	2	8	18	1			
Zinc	30	Zn	2	8	18	2			
Gallium	31	Ga	2	8	18	3			
Germanium	32	Ge	2	8	18	4			
Arsenic	33	As	2	8	18	5			
Selenium	34	Se	2	8	18	6			
Bromine	35	Br	2	8	18	7			
Krypton	36	Kr	2	8	18	8			
Rubidium	37	Rb	2	8	18	8	1		
Strontium	38	Sr	2	8	18	8	2		

Table F Electron configuration of elements—(Cont'd)

Element	Atomic no.	Symbol/Shell	K	L	M	N	O	P	Q
					Number of electrons in shells				
Yttrium	39	Y	2	8	18	9	2		
Zirconium	40	Zr	2	8	18	10	2		
Niobium	41	Nb	2	8	18	12	1		
Molybdenum	42	Mo	2	8	18	13	1		
Technetium	43	Tc	2	8	18	14	1		
Ruthenium	44	Ru	2	8	18	15	1		
Rhodium	45	Rh	2	8	18	16	1		
Palladium	46	Pd	2	8	18	18			
Silver	47	Ag	2	8	18	18	1		
Cadmium	48	Cd	2	8	18	18	2		
Indium	49	In	2	8	18	18	3		
Tin	50	Sn	2	8	18	18	4		
Antimony	51	Sb	2	8	18	18	5		
Tellurium	52	Te	2	8	18	18	6		
Iodine	53	I	2	8	18	18	7		
Xenon	54	Xe	2	8	18	18	8		
Caesium	55	Cs	2	8	18	18	8	1	
Barium	56	Ba	2	8	18	18	8	2	
Lanthanum	57	La	2	8	18	18	9	2	
Cerium	58	Ce	2	8	18	20	8	2	
Praseodymium	59	Pr	2	8	18	21	8	2	
Neodymium	60	Nd	2	8	18	22	8	2	
Promethium	61	Pm	2	8	18	23	8	2	
Samarium	62	Sm	2	8	18	24	8	2	
Europium	63	Eu	2	8	18	25	8	2	
Gadolinium	64	Gd	2	8	18	25	9	2	
Terbium	65	Tb	2	8	18	26	9	2	
Dysprosium	66	Dy	2	8	18	28	8	2	
Holmium	67	Ho	2	8	18	29	8	2	
Erbium	68	Er	2	8	18	30	8	2	
Thulium	69	Tm	2	8	18	31	8	2	
Ytterbium	70	Yb	2	8	18	32	8	2	
Lutetium	71	Lu	2	8	18	32	9	2	
Hafnium	72	Hf	2	8	18	32	10	2	
Tantalum	73	Ta	2	8	18	32	11	2	
Tungsten	74	Wo	2	8	18	32	12	2	
Rhenium	75	Re	2	8	18	32	13	2	
Osmium	76	Os	2	8	18	32	14	2	

Continued

Table F   Electron configuration of elements—(Cont'd)

Element	Atomic no.	Symbol/Shell	K	L	M	N	O	P	Q
			\multicolumn{7}{c}{Number of electrons in shells}						
Iridium	77	Ir	2	8	18	32	15	2	
Platinum	78	Pt	2	8	18	32	17	1	
Gold	79	Au	2	8	18	32	18	1	
Mercury	80	Hg	2	8	18	32	18	2	
Thallium	81	Tl	2	8	18	32	18	3	
Lead	82	Pb	2	8	18	32	18	4	
Bisuth	83	Bi	2	8	18	32	18	5	
Polonium	84	Po	2	8	18	32	18	6	
Astatine	85	At	2	8	18	32	18	7	
Radon	86	Ra	2	8	18	32	18	8	
Francium	87	Fr	2	8	18	32	18	8	1
Radium	88	Ra	2	8	18	32	18	8	2
Actinium	89	Ac	2	8	18	32	18	9	2
Thorium	90	Th	2	8	18	32	18	10	2
Protactinium	91	Pa	2	8	18	32	20	9	2
Uranium	92	U	2	8	18	32	21	9	2
Neptunium	93	Np	2	8	18	32	23	8	2
Plutonium	94	Pu	2	8	18	32	24	8	2
Americium	95	Am	2	8	18	32	25	8	2
Curium	96	Cm	2	8	18	32	25	9	2
Berkelium	97	Bk	2	8	18	32	27	8	2
Californium	98	Cf	2	8	18	32	28	8	2
Einsteinium	99	Es	2	8	18	32	29	8	2
Fermium	100	Fm	2	8	18	32	30	8	2
Mendelevium	101	Md	2	8	18	32	31	8	2
Nobelium	102	No	2	8	18	32	32	8	2
Lawrencium	103	Lw	2	8	18	32	32	9	2
Rutherfordium	104	Rf	2	8	18	32	32	10	2
Dudnium	105	Dd	2	8	18	32	32	11	2
Saeborgium	106	Sg	2	8	18	32	32	12	2
Bohrium	107	Bh	2	8	18	32	32	13	2
Hassium	108	Hs	2	8	18	32	32	14	2
Meitnerium	109	Mt	2	8	18	32	32	15	2
Ununillium	110	Uun	2	8	18	32	32	17	1
Roentgenium	111	Rg	2	8	18	32	32	18	1
Uunbium	112	Uub	2	8	18	32	32	18	2
Ununtrium	113	Uut	2	8	18	32	32	18	3
Ununquadium	114	Uuq	2	8	18	32	32	18	4
Ununpentium	115	Uup	2	8	18	32	32	18	5
Ununquadium	116	Uuh	2	8	18	32	32	18	6
Uunvseptium	117	Uus	2	8	18	32	32	18	7
Ununoctium	118	Uno	2	8	18	32	32	18	8

Note: Elements with atomic numbers 117 and 118 have been named in the table and their configuration is shown, although they have not been created at the time of writing. Claims to have created element 118, made in 1999, have been withdrawn. The element has been renamed roentgenium (Rg).

Answers to self-tests

CHAPTER 2

a. Fine 3.46 × 0.6 mm; broad 6.91 × 1.2 mm
If your answer differs substantially from the outline answer, refer to Section 2.3.

b. 2.5 × 3.0 cm
If your answer differs substantially from the outline answer, refer to Section 2.4.

c. 1.02 cm
If your answer differs substantially from the outline answer, refer to Section 2.5.

d. (i) 0.043 mm

   (ii) 0.021 mm
If your answer differs substantially from the outline answer, refer to Section 2.6.

e. (i) The images of points on the plane of the fulcrum move at the same velocity as the film and are thus sharp. The images of points above the plane of the fulcrum move with a higher velocity than the film, whereas those of points below the plane of the fulcrum move with a lower velocity than the film. Because their velocity differs from that of the film they will show movement unsharpness.

   (ii) The tomographic angle and the tomographic layer thickness are inversely related, i.e. as the tomographic angle is increased, so the layer thickness decreases.
If your answer differs substantially from the outline answer, refer to Section 2.8.

CHAPTER 3

a. The intensity of a beam of electromagnetic radiation at a point is the total energy per second flowing past that point when normalised to a unit area.
If your answer differs substantially from the outline answer, refer to Section 3.2.

b. The intensity of the radiation emitted from a small isotropic source is inversely proportional to the square of the distance from the source, provided there is negligible absorption or scattering of the radiation by the medium through which it passes.
If your answer differs substantially from the outline answer, refer to Section 3.3.

c. (i) 0.8 mGy.s^{-1}

   (ii) 300 cm
If your answer differs substantially from the outline answer, refer to Section 3.5.

d. 6 mAs
If your answer differs substantially from the outline answer, refer to Section 3.6.

CHAPTER 4

a. 17:00 on 17 February
If your answer differs substantially from the outline answer, refer to Section 4.5.

b. 121.58 days
If your answer differs substantially from the outline answer, refer to Section 4.5.

c. 67.2 MBq
If your answer differs substantially from the outline answer, refer to Section 4.5.

d. $1/t^1/_{2(eff)} = 1/t^1/_{2(phys)} + 1/t^1/_{2(biol)}$
If your answer differs substantially from the outline answer, refer to Section 4.6.

e. 19.8 mm
If your answer differs substantially from the outline answer, refer to Section 4.8.

f. (ii) 6 hours

(iii) 0.1155 h^{-1}

(iv) 0.24 MBq
If your answer differs substantially from the outline answer, refer to Section 4.10.

CHAPTER 5

a. Matter is neither created nor destroyed, but it may change its chemical form as the result of a chemical reaction.
If your answer differs substantially from the outline answer, refer to Section 5.2.

b. Energy can neither be created nor destroyed but can be changed from one form to another. The amount of energy in a system is thus constant.
If your answer differs substantially from the outline answer, refer to Section 5.3.

c. The total linear or rotational momentum in a given system is constant.
If your answer differs substantially from the outline answer, refer to Section 5.4.

d. *Law 1:* A body will remain at rest or will travel with a constant velocity unless acted upon by a net external force.

Law 2: The rate of change of momentum of a body is proportional to the applied force.

Law 3: The action of one body on a second body is always accompanied by an equal and opposite action of the second body on the first.
If your answer differs substantially from the outline answer, refer to Section 5.5.

e. 187.4×10^6 m.s^{-1}
If your answer differs substantially from the outline answer, refer to Section 5.5.

f. 0.262 kg
If your answer differs substantially from the outline answer, refer to Section 5.6.

CHAPTER 6

a. Velocity = *metre per second*; acceleration = *metre per second per second*; force = *newton*; pressure = *pascal*; weight = *newton*; energy = *joule*; power = *watt*.
If your answer differs substantially from the outline answer, refer to Table 6.2.

b. Exposure generates 7500 HU. As the maximum heat storage capacity of the anode disc is 10 000 HU, a second exposure would generate a total heat of 15 000 HU, which is beyond the capacity of the disc.
If your answer differs substantially from the outline answer, refer to Section 6.4.

CHAPTER 7

a. 0.1; 10%
If your answer differs substantially from the outline answer, refer to Section 7.3.3.

b. 6%
If your answer differs substantially from the outline answer, refer to Section 7.3.4.

c. (i) 100%

(ii) 50%

(iii) 10%

(iv) 2%

(v) 1%
If your answer differs substantially from the outline answer, refer to Section 7.3.3.

d. (i) = 10%

(ii) = approximately 21%
If your answer differs substantially from the outline answer, refer to Section 7.3.4.

e. (i) Mean = 36; median = 36

(ii) Mean = 9; median = 10

(iii) Mean = 47.7; median = 47
If your answer differs substantially from the outline answer, refer to Section 7.4.1.

f. Mean = 70.07; standard deviation = 1.111; standard error = 0.035; 2 standard deviation limits = 69.85–70.29
If your answer differs substantially from the outline answer, refer to Section 7.4.1.

CHAPTER 8

a. When thermal energy is applied, this causes increased vibrational energy in the atoms of the bar. Because of this they occupy more room, causing an expansion of the bar.
If your answer differs substantially from the outline answer, refer to Section 8.3.

b. 373 K
If your answer differs substantially from the outline answer, refer to Section 8.3.1.

c. 840 W
If your answer differs substantially from the outline answer, refer to Section 8.3.2.

d. The temperature rise in the molybdenum disc will be half of the temperature rise produced in the tungsten disc.
If your answer differs substantially from the outline answer, refer to Section 8.3.2.

e. Kinetic energy is given to the atoms at the point of heating. These atoms transfer some of their vibrational energy to neighbouring atoms. Heat is transmitted along the structure by these interatomic collisions.
If your answer differs substantially from the outline answer, refer to Section 8.4.1.

f. Heat is transferred to atoms at its point of application by conduction. These atoms have increased vibrational energy and so occupy more space. This causes a decrease in the density of the fluid and so it will rise because of hydrostatic pressure. The rising molecules will dissipate heat to the surrounding molecules. In this way convection currents are established and the whole of the fluid is heated.
If your answer differs substantially from the outline answer, refer to Section 8.4.2.

g. When atoms are heated they increase their vibrational energy. Atoms may get rid of this energy in the form of photons of electromagnetic radiation in the infrared part of the spectrum. These photons are absorbed by other bodies and so the energy is transferred.
If your answer differs substantially from the outline answer, refer to Section 8.4.3.

h. *Stationary anode:* heat is dissipated from the target by conduction to the copper anode and along the copper anode to the oil by conduction. *Rotating anode:* heat is dissipated from the anode disc by radiation to the oil. In both types heat is dissipated through the oil by convection, through the housing by conduction and to the air in the X-ray room by convection.
If your answer differs substantially from the outline answer, refer to Section 8.7.1 and 8.7.2.

CHAPTER 9

a. The general properties of electrical charges are as follows:

- Charges can be considered as being of two types: positive and negative

- The smallest unit of negative charge that can exist in isolation is that possessed by an electron and the smallest unit of positive charge that can exist in isolation is that possessed by the proton

- Electrical charges exert forces on each other even when they are separated by a vacuum. The forces are mutual, equal and opposite

- Like charges (i.e. charges of the same sign) *repel* each other while unlike charges (of opposite signs) *attract* each other

- The magnitude of the mutual forces between the charges is influenced by:

  o the magnitude of the individual charges

  o the medium in which they are embedded, being greatest when the medium is a vacuum

  o the inverse square of the distance between the charged bodies

- Electrical charges may flow *induced* in a body by the proximity of a charged body, leading to a force of attraction between the two bodies

- Electrical charges may flow easily in some materials (called *electrical conductors*) and with difficulty in other materials (called *electrical insulators*). Both types of material are capable of having charges induced in them

- When electrical charges move they produce a magnetic field.

If your answer differs substantially from the outline answer, refer to Section 9.3.

b. The force is proportional to the magnitude of each of the charges and inversely proportional to the square of the distance between them.
If your answer differs substantially from the outline answer, refer to Section 9.4.

c. (i) *Conductor*. Proximity of a positively charged body will attract electrons on to the surface of the conductor next to the charged body. This leaves positive charges on the opposite surface. A state of equilibrium is set up where the force of attraction on the electrons from the positively charged body is equal to the attraction from the positive charges on the opposite surface of the conductor. At this point there is no further flow of charge.

(ii) *Insulator*. This involves a description of the action of a positively charged body on the molecules of an insulator either to produce molecular distortion or to cause rotation of polar molecules so that they align with the electrical field.
If your answer differs substantially from the outline answer, refer to Sections 9.7.1 and 9.7.2.

d. Earth is assumed to be electrically neutral in that it contains equal numbers of positive and negative charges. Thus there is no force between neutral earth and a unit positive charge and so no work is needed to move the latter towards earth. As no work is done, the electrical potential of earth is zero.
If your answer differs substantially from the outline answer, refer to Section 9.8.1.

e. (i) On a conducting sphere the charges experience mutual repulsion so that we get a regular distribution of charge on the external surface of the sphere.

(ii) On an irregularly shaped body the charges repel each other so that the distribution of charge varies with the radius of curvature of the body surface. The highest concentration of charge is on the parts of the body with the smallest radius of curvature.
If your answer differs substantially from the outline answer, refer to Sections 9.8.5 and 9.9.

CHAPTER 10

a. An electrical conductor will readily allow the flow of electric charge whereas an insulator will have a very large resistance to the flow of charge. This is explained by the fact that conductors have an ample supply of electrons in the conduction band whereas, in insulators, the conduction band is empty of electrons.
If your answer differs substantially from the outline answer, refer to Section 10.3.

b. Length of the conductor ($R \propto l$); cross-sectional area ($R \propto 1/A$); resistivity ($R \propto \rho$) *and* temperature ($R \propto T$).
If your answer differs substantially from the outline answer, refer to Section 10.7.1.

c. 2 metres
If your answer differs substantially from the outline answer, refer to Section 10.7.1.

d. *Ohm's law* states that the current flowing through a metallic conductor is proportional to the potential difference that exists across it, provided that all physical conditions remain constant.

A body is said to have an electrical resistance of 1 *ohm* if a potential difference of 1 volt across it produces an electrical current through it of 1 ampere.
If your answer differs substantially from the outline answer, refer to Section 10.8.

e. $R = 24\ \Omega$; $I = 0.25$ A; $I_1 = 0.2$ A; $I_2 = 0.05$ A; $V_1 = 2$ V; $V_2 = 4$ V.
If your answer differs substantially from the outline answer, refer to Section 10.8.

f. Energy = 30 kJ; power = 250 W.
If your answer differs substantially from the outline answer, refer to Section 10.9.

g. Volt drop in the cables is 20 V and the potential difference across the set is 380 V.
If your answer differs substantially from the outline answer, refer to Section 10.10.

CHAPTER 11

a. $F = m_1 m_2 / 4\pi \mu_0 d^2$
If your answer differs substantially from the outline answer, refer to Section 11.2.1.

b. This requires a diagram similar to Figure 11.3. *If your answer differs substantially from the outline answer, refer to Section 11.3.*

c. The three terms refer to the magnetism induced in a material as a result of an external magnetic field.

In *diamagnetism*, the electrons orbiting a nucleus have their orbits changed as a result of the external magnetic field. They remain in this condition until the field is removed and then revert to their original orbitals. Thus all materials are diamagnetic. The magnetic induction produced within the sample opposes the applied magnetic field and so the relative permeability is less than unity.

In *paramagnetism* the atoms of the material can be considered as elementary bar magnets since the magnetic effect of the electrons complement each other. Such materials are rapidly demagnetised at room temperature when the external magnetic field is removed. Materials have a temperature above which the paramagnetic effect is lost and only the diamagnetic effect remains. Paramagnetic materials have a relative permeability of just over unity.

Ferromagnetic materials are easily magnetised. The atoms within the material rotate as domains when influenced by an external magnetic field. Such materials have relative permeabilities measured in hundreds or thousands.
If your answer differs substantially from the outline answer, refer to Section 11.6.

d. In ferromagnetic materials, the induced magnetism always lags behind the magnetising force because of the frictional forces between magnetic domains. This phenomenon is known as hysteresis.
If your answer differs substantially from the outline answer, refer to Section 11.7.

e. Spins are aligned parallel and antiparallel to the main magnetic field, which is called B_0. The net or overall magnetisation is parallel to the main magnetic field, at 0°, in the longitudinal plane. The spins are also precessing or rotating, all out of phase. On the application of a radio-frequency pulse, some of the spins gain sufficient energy for their magnetic vector to oppose B_0. This pushes the overall magnetisation into the transverse plane, facing towards the receiver coil. This magnetisation is still rotating. When the radiofrequency pulse is turned off, two processes take place simultaneously: (1) the overall magnetisation slowly relaxes back to the longitudinal plane, in the process of T_1 relaxation; and (2) the spins dephase, in the process of T_2 relaxation.
If your answer differs substantially from the outline answer, refer to Sections 11.8.2 and 11.8.3.

f. In proton density weighting the image intensity corresponds directly to the number of protons in the imaging voxel. Such images are usually of relatively low contrast, although fluid-containing tissues such as oedema will show up bright. In the brain, grey matter will show up brighter than white matter. T_1 and T_2 weighting are minimised.

In T_1 weighting fat normally appears bright and fluid appears dark. These images are good for demonstrating anatomy. Signal differences due to the longitudinal relaxation process are maximised and T_2 weighting is minimised.

In T_2 weighting fat appears grey and fluid appears bright. These images are good for demonstrating pathology. Many pathologies, such as oedema, abscess, inflammation, tumours and cysts, have an increased fluid content. Signal differences due to transverse relaxation are maximised and T_1 weighting is minimised.
If your answer differs substantially from the outline answer, refer to Section 11.8.3.

CHAPTER 12

a. In a bar magnet the atomic magnets predominantly face in one direction and so produce a magnetic field, as shown in Figure 11.3. When electrons flow through a wire, they produce a magnetic field, as shown in Figure 12.3A. By comparing the two diagrams the similarities between the two fields can be seen.
If your answer differs substantially from the outline answer, refer to Sections 11.3 and 12.6.

b. Iron has higher magnetic permeability than air and so there is an increase in the lines of magnetic force in the vicinity of the iron core. As the current through the solenoid is

increased, so the magnetising force is also increased. This is initially accompanied by an increase in the magnetic intensity as the molecular magnets align with the magnetic field. Eventually the point is reached where there is no further increase in the magnetic intensity as all the molecular magnets have now aligned with the field from the solenoid – magnetic saturation has been produced.
If your answer differs substantially from the outline answer, refer to Sections 12.6 and 11.6.3.

c. This requires a diagram similar to Figure 12.5. When switch S is open, no current flows through the solenoid and so the soft iron piece M is held in the position shown by the spring P. Contacts C_1 and C_3 are in contact, while C_1 and C_2 are 'open'. When S is closed, the current passing through the solenoid magnetises the soft iron core, which attracts M by induced magnetism. M pivots about O so that the arm L lifts C_1 away from C_3 and into contact with C_2. Thus, if the external circuit is joined, current will flow between C_1 and C_2 but no current will flow between C_1 and C_3. Opening S reduces the current in the solenoid to zero and hence restores the system to its original condition, since M loses its magnetism and is pulled quickly away under the action of the spring P (C_1 and C_3 are closed and C_1 and C_2 are open).
If your answer differs substantially from the outline answer, refer to Section 12.7.

CHAPTER 13

a. Electromagnetic induction is where electricity is produced by the interlinking of a conductor with a changing magnetic field. Electromagnetism is the production of a magnetic field by the passage of an electric current.
If your answer differs substantially from the outline answer, refer to Section 13.2.

b. Faraday's first law states: a change in the magnetic flux linked with a conductor induces an EMF in the conductor. This means that the conductor must be in close proximity to the magnetic field (to produce linkage) and that the magnitude or position of the magnetic field relative to the conductor must be changing in order to produce an EMF.

Faraday's second law states: the magnitude of the induced EMF is proportional to the rate of change of the magnetic flux linkage. This means that the EMF will alter if the strength of the magnet alters, if the rate of change of the magnetic field alters and if the linkage between the magnetic field and the conductor alters.

Lenz's law states: the direction of the induced current in a conductor caused by a changing magnetic flux is such that its own magnetic field opposes the changing magnetic flux. This means that when an EMF is induced in a conductor this will be in such a way as to cause a current to flow which will have an associated magnetic field in opposition to the changing magnetic flux which created it.

The magnitude of the induced EMF depends on:

- the magnitude of the magnetic flux

- the efficiency by which this flux is interlinked with the conductor (e.g. how many turns there are in the coil)

- the rate of change of the magnetic flux.
  If your answer differs substantially from the outline answer, refer to Sections 13.4 and 13.5.

c. If a conductor is moved through a magnetic field but no external circuit is connected to the ends of the conductor, an EMF will be generated in the conductor but no current will flow through it.
If your answer differs substantially from the outline answer, refer to Section 13.4.

d. If the conductor is moved in the direction indicated, the EMF will be such as to cause a flow of electrons into the page. The maximum EMF is produced when the conductor is moved at right angles to the magnetic field. Zero EMF is produced if the conductor is moved parallel to the magnetic field.
If your answer differs substantially from the outline answer, refer to Section 13.6.

e. (i) When the magnet moves downwards above the wire the current induced in the wire will be in a clockwise direction.

(ii) When the magnet moves downwards below the wire the current in the wire will be in an anticlockwise direction.

If your answer differs substantially from the outline answer, refer to Section 13.6.

f. If a changing current is passed through one conductor, then this will produce a changing magnetic field around this conductor. If a second conductor is placed within this changing magnetic field, then (by Faraday's laws) an EMF will be generated in the conductor and a current will flow in it if the conducting loop is complete. By Lenz's law this current will be in the opposite direction to the original current. The size of this secondary current will vary with the magnetic field – it will be a current of changing magnitude as there is a changing magnetic field. This changing secondary current will produce its own changing magnetic field which will induce an EMF and current in the first conductor. Thus *each conductor induces electricity in the other* and the effect is known as *mutual induction*.

If a solenoid is connected across a source of EMF, current flow starts to build up in the solenoid. As this current increases, *each turn* of the solenoid produces a changing magnetic flux which is linked to the *other turns* of the solenoid. Thus from Faraday's and Lenz's laws, an EMF in the opposite direction to the EMF from the source will be induced in the solenoid – this is known as a *back-EMF*. This effect is known as *self-induction*.

A mutual inductance of 1 *henry* exists between two conductors if 1 volt is induced in one conductor where there is a current change of 1 ampere per second in the other.

A conductor has a self-inductance of 1 *henry* if a back-EMF of 1 volt is induced when the current flowing through it changes at 1 ampere per second.
If your answer differs substantially from the outline answer, refer to Sections 13.7 and 13.8.

g. This requires a simple diagram similar to Figure 13.6 and an explanation as follows. Consider the situation where the coil shown is rotated in a clockwise direction. Thus, from the initial position, side X of the coil will move upwards through the magnetic field and side Y will move downwards. At this point in its movement the coil is cutting the maximum number of lines of flux as it is moving at right angles to the flux lines, and so the maximum EMF will be

generated. We can see that electrons will travel towards us on side X and away from us on side Y. Thus an excess of electrons will exist at brush A and a shortage of electrons will exist at brush B – brush A is negative and brush B is positive. This situation is shown as position 1 on the graph. Now consider the situation when the coil had turned in a clockwise direction from its initial position through 90° – this is the second position of the coil shown. In this position both side X and side Y of the coil are moving parallel with the lines of magnetic flux and so no current is generated – this is shown as 2 on the graph. In position 3 the coil has rotated through 180° from its original position. Side X of the coil is now moving downwards through the magnetic field and side Y is moving upwards. As in position 1, a maximum number of lines of flux are being cut as the conductor is moving at right angles to the flux, and so, again, the maximum EMF will be generated. The polarity of A and B is now the reverse of position 1. In position 4 the conductor is again moving parallel to the lines of flux so no EMF is generated. The conductor then returns to position 1 and so one cycle is complete. The process is then repeated. The type of current shown in the graph is known as an *alternating current*.

In cases where there is no external circuit connected, then no current is able to flow and only sufficient work to overcome the frictional resistance is necessary to keep the rotational movement at the same speed. As soon as an external circuit is connected, then a current is able to flow in the circuit and in the winding. This current will flow in such a direction as to oppose the motion of the coil. This means that mechanical work must be performed to overcome this resisting force, i.e. mechanical energy is converted into electrical energy.

The effect of suddenly increasing the electrical load demanded from the generator is suddenly to increase the opposition to its rotation. Hence the generator slows down momentarily and the induced EMF (which depends on the speed of rotation) is reduced. Thus we find that, in times of increased demand on the generators, there is a drop in the voltage they supply.
If your answer differs substantially from the outline answer, refer to Section 13.9.

CHAPTER 14

a. A sinusoidal alternating current is one where the current can be illustrated in graphical form to describe a sine wave. A graph similar to the one in Figure 14.2 should be included.
If your answer differs substantially from the outline answer, refer to Section 14.4.

b. The *peak* value of the current is the same as the amplitude and represents the maximum positive or negative value of the current. The *average* value of the current is the mean current which flows during a complete cycle. The *RMS* value of the current is that value of constant current which, flowing for the same time, would produce the same expenditure of electrical energy in a circuit.

For an alternating current: $I_{AV} = 0$; $I_{RMS} = 0.707I_p$

For a full-wave rectified current: $I_{AV} = 0.636I_p$; $I_{RMS} = 0.707I_p$
If your answer differs substantially from the outline answer, refer to Sections 14.4.1, 14.4.2 and 14.4.3.

c. (i) RMS current = 0.1 A

(ii) Peak current = 0.1414 A

(iii) Average current = 0

(iv) Average power = 1 W
If your answer differs substantially from the outline answer, refer to Sections 14.4.1, 14.4.2 and 14.4.3.

d. Impedance = 46 1 Ω; phase angle = 29.9°; peak current = 6.5 A.
If your answer differs substantially from the outline answer, refer to Section 14.7.4.

e. The resonance frequency for a circuit is that frequency of the supply to the circuit which results in the highest current flow through the circuit for a given potential across its ends. The resonance frequency for the circuit given is 39.8 Hz.
If your answer differs substantially from the outline answer, refer to Section 14.7.4.

f. Line voltages = 398 V; phase voltages = 230 V.
If your answer differs substantially from the outline answer, refer to Section 14.8.1.

CHAPTER 15

a. A current-carrying conductor will experience a force when placed in a magnetic field.
If your answer differs substantially from the outline answer, refer to Section 15.2.

b. The magnitude of the force is proportional to:

• the magnetic flux density (B)

• the magnitude of the electric current (I)

• the length of the wire (l)

• the sine of the angle between the magnetic field and the wire (sin θ).

The equation is $F = BIl \sin θ$
If your answer differs substantially from the outline answer, refer to Section 15.3.

c. A diagram similar to Figure 15.4 is required. A simplified DC electric motor is shown in the diagram where a battery is connected to a coil of wire *KLMN* via brushes *B* at a commutator *C*. The coil of wire is in the magnetic field of a permanent magnet, the direction of whose field is from left to right in the figure. When the current is switched on, the electron flow is in the direction indicated in the diagram, and the coil is affected by a clockwise force due to the motor principle (i.e. an *upward* force on *KL* and a *downward* force on *MN*). The commutator *C* turns with the coil *KLMN* so that the current always flows in the same direction relative to the permanent magnet. Hence the coil always experiences a clockwise force and keeps turning. Without the commutator, *KLMN* would eventually stop at right angles to the permanent magnetic field.
If your answer differs substantially from the outline answer, refer to Section 15.6.

d. Three uses might include:

• drive motors for mobile X-ray machines

• production of the rotation of the rotating anode X-ray tube

• electron beam scanning in the television monitor

or other reasonable examples.
If your answer differs substantially from the outline answer, refer to Section 15.9.

CHAPTER 16

a. Capacitance is the ratio of the charge on the body to its potential. The unit of capacitance is the *farad*. The capacitance of a body is 1 *farad* if a charge of 1 coulomb held by the body results in a potential of 1 volt.
If your answer differs substantially from the outline answer, refer to Section 16.3.

b. 80×10^{-3} C, 70 kV
If your answer differs substantially from the outline answer, refer to Section 16.3.

c. The capacitance depends on the area of the plates, A, the separation of the plates, d, and the dielectric constant, K, of the material between the plates. The equation is $C = \varepsilon_0 KA/d$.
If your answer differs substantially from the outline answer, refer to Section 16.4.

d. (i) Connect the three capacitors in parallel.

(ii) Connect the three capacitors in series.
If your answer differs substantially from the outline answer, refer to Section 16.5 and 16.6.

e. 20 μF
If your answer differs substantially from the outline answer, refer to Section 16.5 and 16.6.

f. 27.38 V; 273.8 μC
If your answer differs substantially from the outline answer, refer to Section 16.8.

CHAPTER 17

a. 55 kV$_{RMS}$; 77.8 kVp
If your answer differs substantially from the outline answer, refer to Section 17.3 or Section 14.4.3 to convert RMS value to peak value.

b. The efficiency of a transformer is the ratio of the output power to the input power.

The primary current is 0.2 A$_{RMS}$.
If your answer differs substantially from the outline answer, refer to Section 17.5.

c. When a current flows through the secondary of the high-tension transformer there is a volt drop because of the resistance of the secondary winding given by $V = IR$, where R is the resistance of the secondary winding and I is the current through it. The potential difference across the secondary is $V_0 - IR$ where V_0 is the off-load voltage. Thus an increase in current produces an increase in IR and thus a reduction in the output voltage.
If your answer differs substantially from the outline answer, refer to Section 17.6.3.

d. 98 kV
If your answer differs substantially from the outline answer, refer to Section 17.6.3.

e. (i) 600 turns

(ii) 120 V

(iii) 640 turns
If your answer differs substantially from the outline answer, refer to Section 17.7.

f. Transformer rating is the maximum combination of voltage and current which a transformer can withstand for a specific time without damage to the transformer. If the voltage is exceeded, then the insulation in the transformer may be insufficient for the electrical potential involved, thus leading to insulation breakdown. If too large a current flows for too long a time, then there may be overheating of either the transformer core or the transformer windings. Some transformers as part of their normal function generate significant amounts of heat. Such transformers are cooled by immersing the transformer in an oil bath.
If your answer differs substantially from the outline answer, refer to Section 17.9.

CHAPTER 18

a. An intrinsic semiconductor is a chemically pure semiconductor which is also assumed to have perfect regularity of atoms within its crystal lattice. In such materials there is a narrow gap between the valence band and the conduction band so that, at normal room temperatures, many electrons have sufficient energy to jump up to the conduction band and so take part in electrical conductivity.
If your answer differs substantially from the outline answer, refer to Section 18.3.

b. If small amounts of trivalent or pentavalent impurities are added to an intrinsic semiconductor, its conductivity is greatly increased. It is now classed as an extrinsic

semiconductor. If the impurity added is a trivalent impurity, then the substance is a P-type semiconductor, whereas a pentavalent impurity produces an N-type semiconductor.
If your answer differs substantially from the outline answer, refer to Sections 18.4 to 18.4.2.

c. In the P-type semiconductor the majority carriers are positive holes in the valence band and the minority carriers are thermally generated free electrons in the conduction band. In the N-type semiconductor the majority carriers are free electrons in the conduction band and the minority carriers are free holes in the valence band.
If your answer differs substantially from the outline answer, refer to Sections 18.4.1 and 18.4.2.

d. A *PN* junction is produced when a P-type semiconductor and an N-type semiconductor are heat-fused together. When P- and N-types are brought together and heat-fused in intimate contact, then free electrons from the N-type and free positive holes from the P-type are able to penetrate across the boundary between them. This diffusion of charge across the barrier results in recombination of the positive holes and the free electrons (the free electrons drop into the positive holes so that their charges are cancelled). Thus for a short distance on either side of the *PN* junction (about 0.5×10^{-6} m) no free carriers exist – this is therefore known as a *depletion layer*. However, a net charge exists on either side of the junction because the N-type has lost electrons and the P-type has lost positive holes. Thus there is a negatively charged area just within the P-type region and a positively charged area just within the N-type region. The two peaks of charge increase in size until no further net flow of majority carriers takes place. For example, a free electron from the N-type will only be able to pass over to the P-type if it has sufficient energy to overcome the repulsion of the negative peak at the *PN* junction. The charge distribution produces its own potential difference, known as the *potential barrier*, since it acts in opposition to the flow of majority carriers from either side of the barrier. When the *PN* junction is forward-biased, the potential barrier is lowered, so free charges readily cross the junction. If the *PN* junction is reverse-biased, the height of the potential

barrier is increased, thus preventing any charge flow across the barrier.
If your answer differs substantially from the outline answer, refer to Section 18.5.

e. The solid-state rectifier has the following advantages over the thermionic diode valve:

- It contains no filament and thus has a longer life, consumes less power and produces less heat.

- It is smaller in size than the thermionic diode, thus enabling the production of a more compact X-ray unit.

- It has a smaller forward voltage drop, thus enabling a higher kVp to be applied to the X-ray tube.

- The reverse current is less than a vacuum diode and so it is a more efficient rectifier.
If your answer differs substantially from the outline answer, refer to Section 18.5.4.

f. When electrons are injected into the base from the emitter across the *NP* junction, they become *minority carriers* within the base and so readily cross the collector-to-base *PN* junction. This process is so efficient that approximately 98% of the electrons injected into the base from the emitter are able to diffuse across the base and form the collector current. The remaining 2% form the base current. This ratio of approximately 50:1 for the collector current and the base current remains constant for a particular transistor. Thus the base current may be used to control the collector current, as an increase in the base current will allow a subsequent increase in the collector current.
If your answer differs substantially from the outline answer, refer to Section 18.6.1.

g. This requires a diagram similar to Figure 18.13 together with the following explanation.

Junctions J_1 and J_3 are forward-biased but junction J_2 is reverse-biased. Consequently, if the thyristor is connected into a circuit, only a small leakage current flows through it – it behaves as an open switch. If a positive pulse is applied to the P-type layer (the gate) at junction J_1, then positive holes are injected into the P-type material and flow across the junction J_1 so that the potential barrier at that junction is greatly reduced. The reduced potential difference across J_1 means that a higher reverse potential difference than before exists

across J_2 and, if high enough, will cause electrical breakdown to occur at this junction due to the avalanche effect. Once this breakdown occurs, a large current may flow through the thyristor – it behaves as a closed switch. It is not possible to switch the thyristor off by applying a negative pulse to the gate but it will switch off when the potential difference across it is zero – the avalanching effect can no longer be maintained under such conditions.
If your answer differs substantially from the outline answer, refer to Section 18.7.

CHAPTER 19

a. In the X-ray unit it is necessary to step up voltage before it is applied across the X-ray tube and it is also necessary to step down voltage before it is applied across the tube filament. The most convenient method of achieving this is to use a transformer which requires an AC supply. The X-ray tube will only produce useful X-rays when the anode is positive and the cathode is negative, and so it is desirable to have a unidirectional supply to the tube. This is achieved by the use of rectification.
If your answer differs substantially from the outline answer, refer to Section 19.2.

b. The self-rectified unit has the following advantages and disadvantages:

- The circuit is simple and thus little can go wrong.

- The unit is relatively inexpensive

- Because it is possible to incorporate the circuit in a single tank, the need for external high-tension cables is eliminated, decreasing production costs

- The output of self-rectified units as low as this is necessary to keep the anode temperature below 1500°C to prevent thermionic emission form the anode. If this occurred the X-ray tube would be irreparable.

If your answer differs substantially from the outline answer, refer to Section 19.3.

c. A diagram similar to Figure 19.2B is required with an explanation to indicate that during one half-cycle the electron movement is through one pair of diodes and through the other pair in the other half-cycle. For both half-cycles, electrons can flow through the X-ray tube from cathode to anode.
If your answer differs substantially from the outline answer, refer to Section 19.4.

d. Voltage ripple is the difference between the peak and the lowest value of the voltage waveform expressed as a percentage figure.

Because the energy of the electrons in the cathode beam is directly related to the maximum energy of the X-ray photon that could be produced when the electron interacts with the atoms of the anode target, the effective energy (or quality) of an X-ray beam is related to the voltage across the X-ray tube. The greater the ripple, the lower the effective energy of the X-ray beam and the higher the absorbed radiation dose to the patient.

High-tension capacitors are placed between the rectification circuit and the X-ray tube. Capacitors are devices that store electrical charge, with pulsating voltage.

Charge is stored as the voltage rises and as the voltage falls the capacitor discharges. Thus, the discharge from the capacitor slows the rate at which the voltage falls. A diagram similar to Figure 19.5 would help with the explanation.
If your answer differs substantially from the outline answer, refer to Section 19.6.

e. Medium-frequency rectification provides a near-DC supply to the X-ray tube. Because of this the effective voltage across the X-ray tube is almost the same as the peak voltage. This is reflected in the X-ray beam produced and the percentage of high-energy photons in the beam is increased. This in turn means that for a given exposure less dose is delivered to the patient. In addition the increase in frequency brought about by the inverter improves transformer efficiency and permits resonant transformers to be used: this reduces transformer losses. This in turn permits the high-tension transformer to be smaller and lighter, reducing the overall size of the X-ray unit required. Another important factor is that the system can be used with battery, single-phase or three-phase supplies and that regardless of the supply the output remains unchanged.
If your answer differs substantially from the outline answer, refer to Section 19.7.

CHAPTER 20

a. During the 'prep' stage of the exposure sequence two major things happen:

- The appropriate filament of the X-ray tube is raised to its working temperature so that it emits the required number of electrons by thermionic emission, thus allowing the tube current (mA) to flow during the exposure

- The anode is made to rotate at the required speed prior to the exposure being made.
If your answer differs substantially from the outline answer, refer to Section 20.2.

b. This requires a simple diagram similar to Figure 20.2, followed by a description similar to the one below.

This type of switching has no moving parts and utilises two thyristors as a flip-flop circuit to perform the switching sequence. Two thyristors are required to switch an alternating supply as each conducts the half-cycle when that thyristor is forward biased. At the end of each half-cycle each thyristor will cease to conduct as the potential difference across it drops to zero, and so a pulse must be applied to its gate if it is required to conduct during the next half-cycle when it is forward biased. Thus during the exposure the timer is simply required to permit the passage of a train of synchronised pulses to the gates of the thyristors slightly later than the mains zero to ensure their continued conduction. At the end of the exposure the timer stops this chain of pulses and the thyristors cease to conduct at the end of the next half-cycle. This means the system is inertia free and allows accuracy of one voltage pulse (i.e. an exposure time of 0.01 seconds in the case of a two-pulse unit).
If your answer differs substantially from the outline answer, refer to Section 20.3.1.

c. X-rays are produced when electrons flow from the cathode to the anode of the X-ray tube. These electrons are normally focused on the target of the anode by a focusing cup which is at a negative potential equal to that of the filament. If a separate bias is applied to the focusing cup, then it is possible to make it more negative than the filament. Tubes offering this facility are known as grid-controlled tubes. If the focusing cup is made about 3 kV more negative than the filament, it will produce a sufficiently large electrostatic field to prevent any electrons from crossing the X-ray tube and therefore no exposure is made. When the bias is reduced to make it equal to that of the filament, electrons will flow across the tube and X-rays will be produced. At the end of the exposure the high negative bias is re-established on the focusing cup, stopping electron flow. The grid-controlled tube therefore acts as an electronic switch as well as a producer of X-rays. This arrangement is used in capacitor discharge units, and pulsed fluoroscopy units.
If your answer differs substantially from the outline answer, refer to Section 20.3.2.

d. This requires a simple diagram similar to Figure 20.4, followed by a description similar to the one below.

The time taken to charge a capacitor so that there is a predetermined potential across its plates is determined by the resistance in the line. When this trigger voltage is achieved a signal is sent to the switching system, which terminates the X-ray exposure by stopping current flow through the X-ray tube. With thyristor switching this is done by interrupting the chain of pulses to the gates of the thyristors. Thus at the end of the half-cycle the thyristors will cease to conduct and the exposure will terminate.
If your answer differs substantially from the outline answer, refer to Section 20.4.1.

e. This requires a simple diagram similar to Figure 20.5, and an explanation similar to the one below.

The capacitor is charged from two sources, V_1 and V_2. V_1 is a stable source of voltage (e.g. a rectified supply from the autotransformer); the amount of charge the capacitor receives from V_1 is controlled by the variable resistor, R. V_2 is a rectified supply from the mid-point of the high-tension transformer so that the amount of charge received from this source is directly related to the amount of charge passing through the X-ray tube (the mAs). The radiographer's selection of the mAs will determine the position of the variable resistance R, which in turn determines the charge contributed from V_2 and hence the charge passing through the X-ray tube during the exposure.
If your answer differs substantially from the outline answer, refer to Section 20.4.2.

f. Three types of automatic timer are:

1. Phototimers

2. Ionisation timers

3. Anatomically programmable timers.

With manually controlled timers the duration of the exposure is determined by the radiographer's selection of time or the selection of the mAs value to be delivered.

Autotimers are designed to produce a predetermined average density in the resultant image; this is determined by the sensing chamber selected or, in the case of anatomically programmable timers, by the body region and projection selected.
If your answer differs substantially from the outline answer, refer to Section 20.4.3.4.

g. The radiographer selects the appropriate chamber or chambers in relation to the region of interest in the radiograph.

On exposure a potential difference is applied across the outer and inner walls of the selected chambers, the capacitor in the timer is 'shorted' to remove any potential on it and radiation is produced at the X-ray tube.

The radiation beam passes through the patient and is attenuated by this process. The emergent attenuated beam passes through any secondary radiation grid used and through the selected chamber(s) to the film or image receptor where it produces the latent image.

As the radiation passes through the ionisation chamber it ionises the air in the chamber; the ions produced are attracted towards the chamber wall of the opposite potential. This movement of ions permits a small electrical current to flow between these potentials.

The current is amplified by a pre-amplifier and is added to a pre-set supply controlled by a variable resistor. This pre-set supply permits compensation to be made for the sensitivity of different image recording systems, e.g. reduced for 'slow' systems and increased for 'fast' systems.

The combined current is used to charge a capacitor, increasing the potential on the capacitor. When this potential rises to that of the switching device the switching device operates terminating the exposure.

At this point the potential applied across the walls of the selected chamber(s) is also removed.
If your answer differs substantially from the outline answer, refer to Section 20.4.3.

h. With manually controlled timers the duration of the exposure is determined by the radiographer's selection of time or the selection of the mAs value to be delivered.

This in turn depends on the patient, region of examination, pathology and the experience of the radiographer. The longer the duration of the exposure, for a given selection of factors, the greater the radiation dose received by the patient.

It is possible the radiographer may make an error in selection or that unexpected pathologies may be present which may result in the incorrect exposure being delivered, making it necessary to repeat the examination, delivering another radiation dose to the patient and increasing the total dose received for the examination.

Automatic timers terminate the exposure when sufficient radiation has been delivered to produce a required average film density, regardless of the individual patient, region of examination or any pathology present. Provided the appropriate chamber(s) or body part and projection are selected, the 'ideal' exposure will always be produced and the patient will receive the minimum dose required for the projection. This also eliminates repeat examinations due to incorrect exposure – another factor that contributes to the reduction of patient dose.
If your answer differs substantially from the outline answer, refer to Section 20.4.3.

CHAPTER 21

a. The functions of the major components are as follows:

- *Filament* – production of a given number of electrons by thermionic emission

- *Focusing cup* – this prevents the spread of the electron beam by the electrostatic repulsion of the electrons and focuses the electron beam on to the target at the anode

- *Target* – this is responsible for converting some of the kinetic energy of the electrons which cross the tube into X-rays

- *Anode* – the anode mass is responsible for removing heat from the target by conduction and dissipating this heat to the oil

- *Oil* – the oil has the functions of a coolant and an insulator

- *Expansion bellows* – these allow for the expansion of the oil when heated

- *Microswitch* – this prevents further X-ray exposures being made if the oil is overheated

- *Tube port* – this allows the useful X-ray beam to leave the tube

- *Lead lining* – this reduces the radiation leakage from the tube to the required limits

- *Tube shield* – this protects the components and holds them in place. It also restricts access to the 'live' components.

If your answer differs substantially from the outline answer, refer to Section 21.6.

b. A diagram similar to Figure 21.1 is required. The functions of the major components are as follows:

- *Filament* – production of a given number of electrons by thermionic emission

- *Focusing cup* – this prevents the spread of the electron beam by the electrostatic repulsion of the electrons and focuses the electron beam on to the target at the anode

- *Focal track* – this is responsible for converting some of the kinetic energy of the electrons which cross the tube into X-rays

- *Anode disc* – the anode disc is responsible for removing heat from the focal track by conduction and dissipating this heat to the oil by radiation

- *Anode stem* – this connects the anode disc to the rotor. It is designed to allow minimal heat dissipation through it by conduction

- *Rotor assembly* – this is responsive to the induced currents from the stator coils to produce a torque which rotates the disc

- *Ball bearings* – these allow rotation of the rotor which is free from vibration and only has limited frictional forces

- *Glass envelope* – holds components in place and preserves the vacuum

- *Stator coils* – these produce the rotating field which induces currents in the rotor to produce rotation of the anode of the tube.

- *Oil* – the oil has the functions of a coolant and an insulator

- *Expansion bellows* – these allow for the expansion of the oil when heated

- *Tube port* – this allows the useful X-ray beam to leave the tube

- *Lead lining* – this reduces the radiation leakage from the tube to the required limits

- *Tube shield* – this protects the components and holds them in place. It also restricts access to the 'live' components.

If your answer differs substantially from the outline answer, refer to Sections 21.5.1–21.5.2.

c. Tungsten is used in the construction of the filament because:

- Tungsten has a low thermionic work function and so will readily emit electrons by thermionic emission

- Tungsten has a low vapour pressure and so does not easily evaporate. This helps prolong the life of the filament as evaporation would cause the wire to become thin. It also prolongs the life of the tube as it prevents the formation of a tungsten film on the inner wall of the glass envelope

- Tungsten is a rugged metal which can be drawn into a thin wire which will not easily distort. This helps to maintain the shape of the filament helix over a period of time.

Tungsten is used in the construction of the target because:

- Tungsten has a high atomic number ($Z = 74$) and so is an efficient producer of X-rays

- Tungsten has a high melting point ($3387^\circ C$) so it can withstand the heat generated during the X-ray exposure without melting

- Tungsten has a low vapour pressure so it does not readily vaporise at its normal working temperature

- Tungsten can be readily machined to give the smooth surface required for X-ray production.

If your answer differs substantially from the outline answer, refer to Sections 21.5.2 and 21.5.4.

CHAPTER 22

a. The rating of an X-ray unit is the combination of exposure settings which the unit can withstand without incurring unacceptable damage.
If your answer differs substantially from the outline answer, refer to Section 22.2.

b. (i) If the focal spot size is increased, the electrons will dissipate their energy over a larger area. This will produce a smaller temperature rise and so will increase the rating.
If your answer differs substantially from the outline answer, refer to Section 22.3.

(ii) The heat produced at the target of the X-ray tube is related to the number of electrons striking the target per unit time (mA) and the energy of the electrons (related to the kVp). Thus, for a given exposure time, the mA and the kVp are reciprocal factors in that, if the mA is halved, the kVp can be doubled.
If your answer differs substantially from the outline answer, refer to Section 22.3, Insight.

(iii) For a given value of kVp and mA the amount of heat produced in the target is related to the exposure time. If the exposure time is very short, then insignificant cooling takes place at the target and the rating is principally affected by the target area. If the exposure time is long, then significant dissipation of heat from the target takes place and the rating is more affected by the thermal characteristics of the anode disc.
If your answer differs substantially from the outline answer, refer to Section 23.3.

(iv) The self-rectified circuit has the poorest rating while the constant-potential circuit has the best rating. The differences in rating are most marked at short exposure times. This is because the heating effect of individual pulses is most apparent in this situation. The more constant the heat production, the less likelihood of thermal damage to the target – hence the best rating

for constant potential. For longer exposure times, the thermal capacity of the anode disc is the dominating factor. This is independent of the type of rectification and so the curves all tend to come closer together as the exposure time increases.
If your answer differs substantially from the outline answer, refer to Section 22.3.

(v) If we increase the anode diameter, we also increase its circumference and often its mass. Increasing the circumference means that heat energy is now deposited over a larger area, reducing the heat load per unit area, leading to more efficient cooling. Any increase in the mass of the anode will increase its thermal capacity, permitting an increase in the amount of heat we can produce before damage occurs. Doubling the diameter of the disc will therefore increase its rating by as much as 50%, but extra mechanical stress on the rotor bearings imposes practical limitations on this concept.
If your answer differs substantially from the outline answer, refer to Section 22.3.2.

(vi) Doubling the speed of rotation will again increase the rating by about 40–50%. It should also be noticed that the difference in rating diminishes with longer exposure times since it is the overall thermal capacity of the anode that is the dominant factor.
If your answer differs substantially from the outline answer, refer to Section 22.3.2.

c. For short exposure times the rating is determined by the temperature rise at the target surface. This is affected by rectification, focal spot size, etc. and so all of the above will cause a separation of the curves at short exposure times. For longer exposure times, the rating is more affected by the thermal properties of the anode disc. As these are constant for any one tube, irrespective of the choice of focus, the curves therefore become closer together.
If your answer differs substantially from the outline answer, refer to Section 22.3.

d. With modern interlock protection circuits these circumstances are unlikely, as before each exposure is made the computer calculates the heat load generated, adding this to the heat load stored by the X-ray tube. However if the generator has been switched off this stored data is lost and the computer assumes that the X-ray tube is 'cold' and will permit the exposure. Under these circumstances, if the X-ray tube has a high stored heat load, the thermal loading of the X-ray tube can be exceeded. This event can be avoided by ensuring that the generator is not switched off during the working day.

If your answer differs substantially from the outline answer, refer to Section 22.5.

CHAPTER 23

a. Your answer should include the following points: the construction of the anode and the filtration of the primary beam in the diagnostic and orthovoltage tube inserts.
   If your answer differs substantially from the outline answer, refer to Sections 23.3.1–23.3.3, 21.5.2 and 21.6.2.

b. A simple list of the following components: gantry, stand, treatment head, magnetron, AFC, RF circulator, vacuum pump wave guides, accelerator section, bending magnet.
   If your answer differs substantially from the outline answer, refer to Figure 23.2.

c. An oscillating current flowing along a solid conductor will induce a back EMF, at high frequencies, this EMF will significantly reduce the current the conductor can carry.
   If your answer differs substantially from the outline answer, refer to Section 23.4.4.

d. With electron therapy the electron beam is spread to produce a 'flat' beam through the use of electron-scattering foil while, for X-ray therapy, this foil is removed and a bell-shaped flattening filter is placed after the transmission target.
   If your answer differs substantially from the outline answer, refer to Section 23.4.6.

CHAPTER 24

a. The mass of a body, m, and its energy, E (excluding potential energy), are related by the formula $E = mc^2$, where c is the velocity of electromagnetic radiation. Thus the energy of a body is proportional to its mass (and vice versa), since c is a constant. If we consider a stationary body with a rest mass m_0, then the rest energy of this body is given by $E_0 = m_0c^2$. If we now

consider this body travelling with a velocity V, then its energy is now E_v and Einstein's equation is $E_v = m_vc^2$. Since the energy of the body when moving, E_v, is greater than the energy of the body when at rest, E_0, and since c is a constant then m_v must be greater than m_0 – a body increases in mass as its velocity increases. For this reason it is usual to define the mass of the body when it has zero velocity as its *rest mass* and the mass of the body when it is travelling with a known velocity, V, as its *relativistic mass*.
   If your answer differs substantially from the outline answer, refer to Section 24.4.1.

b. Sometimes electromagnetic radiation behaves as 'packets' of energy which have an associated momentum. Such a packet of energy is called a photon or a quantum and the quantum theory predicts that the quantum will have an energy, E, given by $E = hv$ where h is a constant known as Planck's constant and v is the frequency of vibration of the associated wave. Thus, the electromagnetic wave may also behave like a particle, possessing energy and momentum. An electromagnetic wave may behave like a particle in the case of photoelectric absorption and an electron (a particle) behaves like a wave in part of the electron microscope.
   If your answer differs substantially from the outline answer, refer to Section 24.6.

c. The central point of the principle is that measuring one quantity affects another quantity so that it is never possible to measure both quantities simultaneously with complete accuracy.
   If your answer differs substantially from the outline answer, refer to Section 24.7.

CHAPTER 25

a. The general properties of all electromagnetic radiations are:

- The waves of the radiations are composed of transverse vibrations of electric and magnetic fields

- The vibrations have a wide range of wavelengths and frequencies

- All electromagnetic radiations travel through a vacuum with the same velocity – 3×10^8 m.s^{-1}

- All electromagnetic radiations travel in straight lines

- The radiations are unaffected by electric or magnetic fields

- The radiations may be polarised so that they vibrate in one plane only

- The radiations are able to produce constructive or destructive interference

- All the radiations obey the duality principle and so can either be considered as waves or as quanta with energy and momentum.

If your answer differs substantially from the outline answer, refer to Section 25.3.

b. (i) *Cycle* – one complete waveform (this can start from any point on the wave and end at the corresponding point on another wave)

(ii) *Wavelength* – the distance travelled in completing one cycle

(iii) *Frequency* – the number of cycles per second

(iv) *Amplitude* – the magnitude of the peak of the wave above the x-axis.

If your answer differs substantially from the outline answer, refer to Section 25.3.1.

c. $E = hc/\lambda$ or $E = 0.124/\lambda$

Using the equation: $E = 0.124/\lambda$

$$\lambda = 1.24/E$$

$$= 1.24/50 \text{ nm}$$

$$= 0.0248 \text{ nm}$$

Using the equation: $E = 0.124/\lambda$

$$\lambda = 1.24/0.0124 \text{ keV}$$

$$= 100 \text{ keV}$$

If your answer differs substantially from the outline answer, refer to Section 25.3.2.

d. Radiowaves, microwaves, infrared radiation, visible, ultraviolet radiation, X-rays and gamma-rays.

If your answer differs substantially from the outline answer, refer to Section 25.4.

e. When the anode of the X-ray tube is bombarded by electrons it emits both heat and light as well as X-rays. The X-ray spectrum is composed of a continuous or Bremsstrahlung spectrum upon which is superimposed a characteristic or line spectrum from the tungsten target. The absorption processes within the aluminium filter and the lead collimators also produce characteristic radiation from these elements, although these are of fairly low intensity. When the radiation beam passes through the patient, some of the photons are absorbed and some are scattered. The above processes produce a minute amount of heat and other characteristic radiations from the elements which make up the body tissues. When the transmitted X-ray beam strikes the intensifying screens in the cassette, these produce fluorescent radiation in the ultraviolet and visible parts of the spectrum. This is principally responsible for the production of the radiographic image on the film.

If your answer differs substantially from the outline answer, refer to Section 25.6.

f. A wide range of answers are possible. Some of these might include:

- The emission of light from image intensifiers when bombarded with X-rays

- The emission of light from cathode ray tubes and television monitors when the phosphors are bombarded by electrons

- The emission of light from fluorescent tubes to allow us to view radiographs

- The emission of X-rays and gamma-rays from certain radioisotopes which allow imaging or treatment of organs

- The emission of light from sodium iodide crystals (in gamma cameras and CT scanners) when bombarded with gamma-rays or X-rays

- The emission of light from photostimulable plates when scanned using a laser beam

- The use of a laser beam to 'write' information on to the film in a laser imager.

If your answer differs substantially from the outline answer, refer to Section 25.6.

CHAPTER 26

a. This requires a simple planetary model diagram of the nitrogen atom to demonstrate that the nucleus contains seven protons and seven neutrons. The K-shell contains two electrons and the L-shell contains five electrons.

If your answer differs substantially from the outline answer, refer to Section 26.2.

b. (i) A *nuclide* is a nucleus with a particular value of atomic mass number and atomic number.

(ii) A *radionuclide* is a nuclide where the atomic nucleus is unstable and therefore likely to undergo radioactive decay.

(iii) An *isotope* is a nucleus which has the same atomic number but a different mass number compared to another nucleus, e.g. $^{14}_{6}C$ and $^{12}_{6}C$ are both isotopes of carbon.

(iv) An *isobar* is a nucleus which has the same atomic mass number as another nucleus, e.g. ^{14}C and ^{14}N are isobars.

(v) The *atomic number* of an element is the number of protons in the atomic nucleus.

(vi) The *atomic mass number* is the total number of nucleons (protons and neutrons) in the nucleus.

If your answer differs substantially from the outline answer, refer to Section 26.3 and Table 26.2.

c. (i) The *discrete electron orbital* is the pathway followed by a particular electron around the atomic nucleus.

(ii) These orbitals are grouped together to give *electron shells*, e.g. the two electrons in the K-shell each have discrete electron orbitals.

(iii) Electrons in a particular shell have an *electron-binding energy* which is the amount of work which must be done to remove the electron from that shell and create a free electron. The electron-binding energy varies with electron shell (K being highest) and also increases, for a shell, with the atomic number of the element.

If your answer differs substantially from the outline answer, refer to Section 26.4 and 26.7.

d. There are two Bury–Bohr rules:

- An electron shell, n, cannot contain more than $2n^2$ electrons

- The outer shell cannot contain more than eight electrons.

Using these rules we can say that potassium will have the following electron configuration:

K-shell   2

L-shell   8

M-shell   8

N-shell   1

If your answer differs substantially from the outline answer, refer to Section 26.5.

e. (i) *Ionic bonds*. This type of bond is caused when one or more electrons are transferred from one atom to another, forming charged atoms (*ions*) which are attracted to one another by electrostatic attraction, thus forming the bond. After the electron exchange, the shells of each ion appear to be closed.

(ii) *Covalent bonds*. These bonds are formed by the apparent sharing of electrons such that each atom appears to increase its number of electrons, thus forming an apparently closed shell.

If your answer differs substantially from the outline answer, refer to Section 26.5.

f. If the electron within an orbital is given sufficient energy to cause it to move to a higher energy level but not overcome its binding energy, then the process is called *excitation*. The excited electron will return to its original orbital with the emission of a photon of electromagnetic radiation. In *ionisation* the electron is given sufficient energy to overcome its binding energy and leave the atom. The atom has now lost one of its electrons and so becomes a positive ion.

If your answer differs substantially from the outline answer, refer to Section 26.6.

CHAPTER 27

a. For the spontaneous emission of an alpha (α) particle from a nucleus, the nuclide must have an atomic mass number greater than 150. The nucleus must also have too few neutrons for the number of protons – a higher neutron-to-proton ratio would be required to produce nuclear stability. The alpha-particle consists of two protons and two neutrons tightly bound together (a helium nucleus). It may be considered as a free particle having high kinetic energy, which is trapped in the nucleus. Thus the daughter nucleus has two protons and two neutrons fewer than the parent nucleus.

The mechanism of production of the α-particle is quite complex. The nucleus depends on a balance of disruptive electrostatic (Coulomb) forces and attractive forces between the nucleons caused by the short-range nuclear forces. In very large nuclei there is a large amount of electrostatic repulsion between the protons which extends across the whole nucleus. This is balanced by the short-range nuclear force which exists between adjacent nucleons. Thus, if the nucleus becomes elongated, the electrostatic forces dominate and the nucleus becomes even more elongated. This process continues until the nucleus divides into two fragments, the daughter nuclide and the α-particle.

An example of α-decay is the decay of bismuth-212 to thallium-208 with the emission of an α-particle, as shown in the equation below:

$$^{212}_{83}Bi \rightarrow ^{208}_{81}Tl + ^{4}_{2}\alpha$$

If your answer differs substantially from the outline answer, refer to Section 27.4.

b. *Negatron (β^-) emission.* β^--particles are emitted from nuclei which have too many neutrons for nuclear stability. Nucleons are being constantly changed from proton to neutron and back within the atomic nucleus. A neutron may be thought of as consisting of a proton and a negatron:

$$n \rightarrow p^+ + \beta^-$$

It appears that in nuclei which have too many neutrons, there is a finite possibility that a neutron becomes isolated within the nucleus and then decays to form a proton and a negatron. The proton rejoins the nucleus and the negatron is ejected. This transformation results in the atomic mass number remaining unchanged (the combined number of protons and neutrons is still the same) but the atomic number will increase by one as one extra proton has been added to the nucleus (this results in the formation of a different element with the consequent rearrangement of electron orbitals to suit the new element).

An example of β^--particle decay is where carbon-14 decays to form nitrogen with the emission of a β^--particle.

$$^{14}_{6}C \rightarrow ^{14}_{7}N + \beta^-$$

Positron (β^+) emission. Protons are continuously changing into neutrons and back. In these reactions we can consider a proton as consisting of a neutron and a positron.

$$p^+ \rightarrow n + \beta^+$$

Positron emission takes place from nuclei that have too many protons to achieve stability. In such cases, protons appear to become isolated within the nucleus and then decay to form a neutron which rejoins the nucleus and a positron which is ejected from the nucleus. In this reaction the atomic mass number will remain the same but the atomic number will decrease by one (the total number of protons and neutrons is unchanged but one proton has been converted into a neutron).

An example of such a reaction is the decay of carbon-11 to boron, as shown below:

$$^{11}_{6}C \rightarrow ^{11}_{5}B + \beta^+$$

If your answer differs substantially from the outline answer, refer to Sections 27.5.1 and 27.5.2.

c. When cobalt-60 decays with the emission of a β^--particle the daughter nucleus is left in an excited state. The $^{60}_{28}Ni$ nucleus is left at an energy 2.5 MeV above its ground state. It immediately decays to its ground state in two jumps:

• it decays to 1.33 MeV above its ground state by the emission of a 1.17 MeV gamma-ray

• it then drops to its ground state by the emission of a second gamma-ray of energy 1.33 MeV.

In the case of $^{60}_{27}Co$ decaying to $^{60}_{28}Ni$, the nucleus remains in an excited state before the emission of the gamma-rays for a time so short that it is incapable of accurate measurement. However, this is not always the case, and those excited states which last sufficiently long for their durations to be measured are known as *metastable states*. The transition from a metastable state to a more stable state is known as an *isomeric transition*.
If your answer differs substantially from the outline answer, refer to Sections 27.6 and 27.6.1.

d. If a nucleus of low mass number has too few neutrons for stability but has insufficient excess energy (<1.02 MeV) to eject a positron, then an alternative way by which the nucleus may undergo an isobaric transformation and lose energy is by electron capture. In this process the nucleus captures one of the orbiting electrons, the most likely being a capture of a K-shell electron.

The capture of an electron by the nucleus results in one of the protons in the nucleus changing into a neutron. During the process of electron capture a neutrino is emitted by the nucleus. The processes involved in electron capture may be shown thus:

$$p^+ + e^- \rightarrow n + \nu$$

If your answer differs substantially from the outline answer, refer to Section 27.7.

e. The short-range forces holding the nucleus together exist between adjacent nucleons, whereas the Coulomb forces act across the whole of the nucleus. This fact becomes increasingly important as the size of the nucleus increases. A very large nucleus may be pictured rather like a liquid drop in which the nucleons are moving about with very high energy and continuously deforming the shape of the nucleus.

During this process, it is possible for the nucleus to become very elongated and then to break into two fragments – usually of fairly similar sizes. Such a phenomenon is known as *spontaneous fission* and can occur for very large nuclei, e.g. thorium-232 is capable of spontaneous fission. As well as the *fission fragments* from such a reaction, one or more neutrons are usually liberated and the whole fission process is accompanied by the release of large amounts of energy.

Neutron-activated fission is a more controllable process than spontaneous fission. This occurs as a result of a heavy nucleus capturing an incoming neutron and then breaking into large fragments in a similar way to spontaneous fission. An example of such a reaction is the disintegration of $^{238}_{92}U$ into two fission fragments of $^{145}_{56}Ba$ and $^{94}_{36}Kr$ if the uranium-238 nucleus is made to absorb a neutron. The fission of the nucleus is normally accompanied by the release of gamma-rays and neutrons. Both of the fissile fragments are extremely rich in neutrons and so each will usually release a neutron. The neutrons from both of the above processes can now react with two $^{238}_{92}U$ nuclei, resulting in the release of four fissile fragments and four

neutrons and so a *chain reaction* can be set up. Such a process is accompanied by the release of large amounts of energy.
If your answer differs substantially from the outline answer, refer to Section 27.9.

f. This requires a diagram similar to Figure 27.15 accompanied by the following description. If molybdenum-98 is placed in a neutron stream, the nuclei of the molybdenum atoms can be made to absorb the neutrons to produce molybdenum-99. The capture of a neutron raises the energy of the resulting molybdenum-99 nuclei and each loses this energy by the prompt emission of a gamma-ray. The reaction may be shown using the equation below:

$$^{98}_{42}Mo + n \rightarrow {}^{99}_{42}Mo + \gamma$$

A molybdenum-99/alumina column is in the centre of the generator. The molybdenum-99 has a half-life of 67 hours and decays to form technetium-99m by β⁻-particle emission, as shown below:

$$^{99}_{42}Mo \rightarrow {}^{99}_{43}Tc^m + \beta^- + \bar{\nu}$$

The $^{99}_{43}Tc^m$ is eluted from the generator at regular intervals as sodium pertechnetate. This isotope, which is in liquid form, may then be used for a number of radionuclide imaging situations. The $^{99}_{43}Tc^m$ decays to $^{99}_{43}Tc$ by the emission of a gamma-ray of energy 140 keV. The metastable isotope has a half-life of 6 hours.
If your answer differs substantially from the outline answer, refer to Section 27.11.1.

g. The ideal radionuclide for imaging should:

- have a short half-life – approximately twice the length of time from injection into the patient to completion of the scan – the half-life of $^{99}_{43}Tc^m$ is 6 hours

- emit gamma-rays of relatively low energy, so that these are easily detected and do not pose a major hazard to others because of their penetrating power – the gamma-rays emitted from $^{99}_{43}Tc^m$ have an energy of 140 keV

- emit no particles as part of its decay pattern as these add significantly to the patient dose – 90% of the radiation from $^{99}_{43}Tc^m$ is in the form of gamma radiation; the remaining

10% consists of energy emitted as a result of internal conversion, X-rays and Auger electrons

- be readily labelled to allow its uptake by specific organs – $^{99}_{43}Tc^m$ is readily labelled

- be readily excreted by the patient – $^{99}_{43}Tc^m$ is readily excreted by the patient, normally through the urinary system, although other routes are possible, depending on the labelling

- be easily generated in the radiopharmacy – $^{99}_{43}Tc^m$ is readily generated in the radiopharmacy using a technetium generator.

If your answer differs substantially from the outline answer, refer to Section 27.12.

CHAPTER 28

a. This requires a diagram similar to Figure 28.1 accompanied by the following text. There are a number of ways in which high-energy electrons from the filament of the X-ray tube may lose their energy when they collide with the atoms of the target. These are:

the loss of energy by the electrons from the filament because of interactions between them and the outer electrons surrounding the atoms of the target material

the loss of energy by electrons from the filament because of interactions between them and the nuclei of the atoms of the target material

the loss of energy by electrons from the filament because of interactions between them and individual electrons of the target atoms.
If your answer differs substantially from the outline answer, refer to Section 28.2.

b. To produce Bremsstrahlung radiation, electrons which are accelerated from the filament of the X-ray tube must interact with the positive nucleus of the atoms of the tube target. When such a quantum is emitted, the kinetic energy of the electron is suddenly reduced by an amount equal to the energy of the quantum, and so the electron is suddenly slowed down or *braked*. This is an example of an inelastic interaction since the total kinetic energy of the

electron and of the nucleus are not conserved because some energy is removed by the emission of the quantum of radiation. The energy of the quantum may be in the X-ray part of the electromagnetic spectrum and the radiation is known as *braking* or *Bremsstrahlung radiation*. The exact energy of this quantum will vary and may be very small if the electron does not lose much energy in its interaction with the nucleus, or it may be up to the total kinetic energy of the electron if it is involved in a direct collision with the nucleus. This means that the Bremsstrahlung radiation will form a continuous spectrum.
If your answer differs substantially from the outline answer, refer to Section 28.4.2.

c. If the energy of the electrons accelerated across the tube from the filament is greater than the binding energy of a particular orbital electron, it is possible for a filament electron to be involved in an inelastic collision with one of the orbital electrons of the target atoms. The orbital electron will be given sufficient energy to overcome its binding energy and thus be liberated from the atom. This causes a vacancy in the electron shell involved, e.g. the *K*-shell. This vacancy is quickly filled by one of the outer electrons undergoing a quantum jump downwards to fill the vacancy and emitting a quantum of electromagnetic radiation in the process. The energy of the quantum emitted is given by:

$E = E_1 - E_2$

where E_1 is the energy of the electron before the jump and E_2 is the energy of the electron after the jump. As this energy varies for the same transition in different materials it is known as *characteristic radiation* as it is characteristic of the material emitting the radiation.
If your answer differs substantially from the outline answer, refer to Section 28.5.

d. This requires a diagram similar to Figure 28.6 accompanied by the following description. The energy of the Bremsstrahlung radiation is expressed in keV and lies somewhere between zero and a maximum value. This maximum photon energy is achieved if an electron which has the maximum kinetic energy gives up all its energy to form a single photon. The value of this photon in the case of the beam will be 100 keV as the maximum potential across the X-ray tube will be 100 kVp. The Bremsstrahlung radiation is a continuous spectrum. The intensity of the low-energy photons within this spectrum is decreased because of absorption of these photons by the target material. The average energy of the X-ray beam is about one-third to one-half of its maximum energy. The total intensity of the beam – the quantity of the radiation – is given by the area under the curve. The energies of the K, L, M, etc. lines are always in the same position, although the energy of lines from M onwards is so small that it is likely to be totally absorbed in the X-ray tube. These discrete energies form a line spectrum – the exact energy of the line is determined by the difference between the initial energy of the electron and its final energy. The line spectra will not be produced in this case for all lines from K outwards as the energy of the electrons from the filament is sufficiently large to displace any electron from its orbital within the tungsten target atom.

The relationship between the kVp across the tube and the minimum wavelength is given by the equation:

$$\lambda_{min} = 1.24/kVp$$

If your answer differs substantially from the outline answer, refer to Section 28.6.

CHAPTER 29

a. The quality of the radiation is a measure of the penetrating power of the X-ray beam. The more penetrating the X-ray beam, the higher the beam quality. The quantity of the radiation is a measure of the number of X-ray photons present in a beam of radiation. The larger the number of photons present, the greater the quantity of radiation.
If your answer differs substantially from the outline answer, refer to Section 29.2.

b. This should have a graph similar to Figure 29.1. The tube current is a measure of the number of electrons crossing the X-ray tube in unit time. An increase in the number of electrons per unit time (with all other factors remaining unchanged) produces an increase in the chance of producing X-ray photons and thus will produce an increase in the intensity or quantity of the radiation. A

reduction in the tube current has the opposite effect. As the energy of the electrons is unaffected by the tube current, then the quality of the X-ray beam is not affected by the mA.
If your answer differs substantially from the outline answer, refer to Section 29.3.

c. This should be accompanied by a graph similar to Figure 29.2. An increase in the potential difference across the X-ray tube will produce an increase in the kinetic energy of the electrons at the point of contact with the target. This has two effects on the Bremsstrahlung spectrum:

- As the electrons have more energy, they are more likely to have some of this energy converted into X-ray photons – thus there will be an increase in the quantity of radiation from the tube

- As the electrons have an increase in their energy, there will be an increase in the average energy of the photons in the X-ray beam – thus there will be an increase in the quality of the X-ray beam.

The use of a lower kVp has the opposite effect. The use of a lower kVp may also mean that the kinetic energy of the filament electrons may be less than the binding energy of the K-shell electrons of the target atoms and so no characteristic radiation will be produced as a result of quantum leaps by electrons to fill the vacancy in the K-shell (see graph for lower kVp in Figure 29.2).
If your answer differs substantially from the outline answer, refer to Section 29.4.

d. This should be accompanied by a graph similar to Figure 29.3. The higher the atomic number of the target material, the more positive the nucleus of each target atom. This means that the material is more efficient at producing radiation by the Bremsstrahlung process. Thus, the quantity of the Bremsstrahlung radiation is affected, but not the quality. A material with a higher atomic number will also produce characteristic radiation at a higher photon energy than is produced by a target of a lower atomic number. This has a marginal effect on the quality of the overall spectrum from the X-ray tube.
If your answer differs substantially from the outline answer, refer to Section 29.5.

e. This should be accompanied by a graph similar to Figure 29.4B. The closer the waveform across the X-ray tube is to a constant potential, the higher the average kinetic energy of the electrons at the point of contact with the target. This will produce an increase in the quality and in the quantity of the radiation from the tube.
If your answer differs substantially from the outline answer, refer to Section 29.6.

f. This should be accompanied by a diagram similar to Figure 29.5. Filtration absorbs X-ray photons by the photoelectric effect. Thus, there is a selective absorption of low-energy photons compared with high-energy photons. As a result, the average photon energy of a beam is increased – filtration increases the quality of the radiation beam. However, as some of the photons have been absorbed by the filter, there are fewer photons in the beam after filtration than there were before filtration – filtration produces a reduction in the quantity of a beam of radiation.
If your answer differs substantially from the outline answer, refer to Section 29.7.

CHAPTER 30

a. (i) If we measure the intensity of the radiation before it enters an attenuator and measure the intensity again when it leaves the attenuator, we find that there is less intensity at the point of exit than there was at the point of entrance. This reduction in intensity is known as attenuation.

   (ii) When the beam of radiation passes through matter, some of the energy of the photons may be transferred to the atoms of the material. This process is known as absorption.

   (iii) When a beam of radiation passes through matter, some of the photons may interact with atoms of the material and, as a consequence of this interaction, the photons may be deflected from their original paths. This may or may not be accompanied by a loss of energy. This process is known as scattering.
If your answer differs substantially from the outline answer, refer to Section 30.2.

b. The total linear attenuation coefficient, μ, is the fraction of the radiation removed from a beam per unit thickness of an attenuating medium. This would be used as a measure of attenuation when it is important to establish the amount of radiation attenuated along a straight line.

The total mass attenuation coefficient, μ/ρ, is the fraction of the radiation removed from a beam of unit cross-sectional area as it passes through unit mass of a medium. This measure of attenuation would be used if we wish to see how the photon energy influences the amount of attenuation, as it is independent of the state of the medium.
If your answer differs substantially from the outline answer, refer to Sections 30.2.2 and 30.2.3.

c. In photoelectric absorption the photon interacts with a bound electron. The maximum chance of the process occurring is when the energy of the photon is equal to or just greater than the binding energy of the particular electron shell. The photon displaces the electron from its orbital, some of the photon energy being used to overcome the binding energy of the electron and the rest being given to the electron as kinetic energy. The vacancy is filled by electrons further from the nucleus undergoing quantum jumps and giving off characteristic radiation. The mass attenuation coefficient due to the photoelectric effect (τ/ρ) is influenced by the atomic number of the absorber and by the energy of the incident photon, as shown in the following equation:

$$\tau/\rho \propto Z^3/E^3$$

If your answer differs substantially from the outline answer, refer to Section 30.5.

d. In Compton scattering the photon interacts with a free electron. As a result of this interaction, the photon is deflected from its path and loses some of its energy which the electron gets as kinetic energy. As the photon is deflected from its path, it is said to be scattered. The likelihood of the process occurring depends on the electron density of the attenuator and the energy of the incident photon, as shown in the equation below:

$$\sigma/\rho \propto \text{electron density}/E$$

As the electron density of all materials (with the exception of hydrogen) is approximately the same, the amount of Compton scattering is largely unaffected by the material.

If your answer differs substantially from the outline answer, refer to Section 30.6.

e. Pair production involves an interaction between a high-energy photon ($\geq$1.02 MeV) and the field around an atomic nucleus. This interaction results in the energy of the photon being converted to matter in the form of an electron and positron pair. Any excess energy is given to the pair as kinetic energy. The positron will eventually interact with an electron and both will be annihilated, producing two photons, each of energy 0.51 MeV. These photons are known as annihilation radiation. The likelihood of the process occurring is linked to the photon energy and the atomic number of the attenuator by the equation shown below:

$$\pi/\rho \propto (E - 1.02)Z$$

If your answer differs substantially from the outline answer, refer to Section 30.7.

CHAPTER 31

a. If a substance is bombarded with high-energy radiation and the atoms of the substance absorb the radiation, this will cause an increase in the energy of some of the electrons within the atoms of the absorber. If this energy is re-emitted in the form of light, then the whole process is called luminescence. If the light emission stops within 10^{-8} s of the end of the radiation bombardment, then the process can be termed fluorescence; if it continues beyond this point then it is known as phosphorescence or afterglow.
If your answer differs substantially from the outline answer, refer to Section 31.3.

b. When an X-ray photon is involved in a photoelectric interaction with an atom of a phosphor crystal then this liberates an electron and gives it kinetic energy. This electron will now move within the conduction band, leaving a hole in the valence band. As the electron passes close to other atoms it liberates further electrons and so a large number of electrons will enter the conduction band. Some of the electrons in this band will collide with one another and so will lose small amounts of energy and will thus adjust their energy to the upper energy level of the luminescent centre. At the same time, some holes in the valence band will raise their energy to the lower level of the luminescent centre. Some of the electrons at the upper level of the centre will perform quantum jumps to neutralise the holes at the lower level of the centre and in so doing will give up energy in the visible part of the spectrum. As a result of one photoelectric interaction, a large number of electrons can perform this transition; thus the number of light photons liberated is much greater than the number of X-ray photons absorbed.
If your answer differs substantially from the outline answer, refer to Section 31.3.1.

c. When an X-ray photon is involved in a photoelectric interaction with an atom of a phosphor crystal, this liberates an electron and gives it kinetic energy. This electron will now move within the conduction band, leaving a hole in the valence band. As the electron passes close to other atoms it liberates further electrons and so a large number of electrons will enter the conduction band. Some of the electrons in this band will collide with one another and so will lose small amounts of energy and will thus drop into the deep traps in the forbidden energy gap. Thus, the number of electrons in the traps is proportional to the amount of radiation. If the substance is heated, these electrons can have their energy raised to allow them to re-enter the conduction band and some will adjust to the energy level of the luminescent centre. At the same time, some holes in the valence band will raise their energy to the lower level of the luminescent centre. Some of the electrons at the upper level of the centre will perform quantum jumps to neutralise the holes at the lower level of the centre and in so doing will give up energy in the visible part of the spectrum. The number of light photons liberated is proportional to the number of X-ray photons absorbed.
If your answer differs substantially from the outline answer, refer to Section 31.4.

d. A diagram similar to Figure 31.4 would help the description. The intensifying screen consists of a base material – normally a flexible plastic – which provides support for the rest of the system. On one side of this is coated a substratum layer which may be reflective or absorptive depending on the function of the screen. The phosphor layer is coated on top of the substratum layer and consists of phosphor crystals in a binder material.

The binder may be clear or tinted and may also contain carbon microgranules. On the outer surface of the screen is a clear supercoat which protects the phosphor from abrasion and from chemical contamination.
If your answer differs substantially from the outline answer, refer to Section 31.5.1.

e. When an X-ray photon is involved in a photoelectric interaction with an atom of a barium fluorohalide crystal, this liberates an electron and gives it kinetic energy. This electron will now move to the conduction band, leaving a hole in the valence band. As the electron passes close to other atoms it liberates further electrons and so a large number of electrons will enter the conduction band. Some of the electrons in this band will collide with one another and so will lose small amounts of energy and will thus drop into the deep traps in the forbidden energy gap. Thus, the number of electrons in the traps is proportional to the amount of radiation. If the substance is scanned with a laser beam, then these electrons can have their energy raised to allow them to re-enter the conduction band and some will adjust to the energy level of the luminescent centre. At the same time, some holes in the valence band will raise their energy to the lower level of the luminescent centre. Some of the electrons at the upper level of the centre will perform quantum jumps to neutralise the holes at the lower level of the centre and in so doing will give up energy in the visible part of the spectrum. The number of light photons liberated is proportional to the number of X-ray photons absorbed. This light may be measured and used to produce a digitised image.
If your answer differs substantially from the outline answer, refer to Section 31.7.

CHAPTER 32

a. The density of bone is approximately twice that of soft tissue and so (if all the other factors are equal) bone will attenuate twice as much radiation as soft tissue. Bone and soft tissue also differ in atomic number. This is important for photoelectric absorption, as shown by the equation $\tau \propto \rho \times Z^3/E^3$. Since the atomic number of bone is approximately twice that of soft tissue, the combination of this with its higher density results in it attenuating about 16 times as much radiation as the same thickness of soft tissue. Because of this the intensity of the X-ray beam transmitted through bone will be less than that transmitted through soft tissue.
If your answer differs substantially from the outline answer, refer to Section 32.3.1.

b. The kVp selected affects the quality and the quantity of the radiation from the X-ray tube. Increasing the kVp will increase the average photon energy and so will cause an appreciable reduction in the amount of photoelectric absorption. This will cause a reduction in the contrast on the radiograph. An increase in the kVp also increases the amount of scattered radiation reaching the radiograph, again reducing the contrast. However, if the kVp selected is too low, then more dense structures such as bone will be underpenetrated. The kVp also affects the quantity of radiation which in turn affects the average density on the radiograph.
If your answer differs substantially from the outline answer, refer to Sections 32.3.5 and 32.6.

c. Scatter to the radiograph can be limited by:

- the use of collimation, thus limiting the amount of scatter formed

- the use of low-kVp techniques so that the scatter is largely absorbed by the patient – this does produce an increase in patient dose

- the use of a secondary radiation grid to absorb the scatter formed.
If your answer differs substantially from the outline answer, refer to Sections 32.3.3 and 32.3.4.

d. Characteristic curves may be used to compare the speed, contrast and film latitude of the two emulsions.
If your answer differs substantially from the outline answer, refer to Sections 32.5.2, 32.5.3 and 32.5.4.

CHAPTER 33

a. The exposure at a particular point in a beam of χ or γ radiation is a measure of the amount of ionisation which will occur as the beam passes through unit mass of air. The absorbed dose is a measure of the energy imparted to a unit mass of the medium as a result of the radiation beam

being directed at the medium. The dose-equivalent is the absorbed dose multiplied by the quality factor for the radiation. For the same exposure, different media will absorb different absorbed doses of radiation. The amount of biological damage to tissue is dependent on the dose equivalent and so it is necessary to convert the absorbed dose in gray to the dose-equivalent in sievert.
If your answer differs substantially from the outline answer, refer to Sections 33.3, 33.3.3 and 33.4.

b. The methods which can be used include calorimetry, the free air ionisation chamber or chemical methods of radiation dose measurement. One of these methods should then be described in detail.
If your answer differs substantially from the outline answer, refer to Sections 33.5.1, 33.5.2 and 33.5.3.

c. This requires a diagram similar to Figure 33.6. The chamber wall is made of graphite, bakelite or plastic and as it has an atomic number similar to air it is said to be air-equivalent, i.e. it absorbs the same amount of radiation as the same mass of air. When the wall absorbs radiation it emits electrons which will enter the air of the chamber and cause a loss of charge from the positive central electrode. The amount of charge lost is proportional to the radiation exposure to the chamber. This can then be corrected for the calibration factor against the standard chamber. When we know the exposure we can calculate the absorbed dose in air as we know the energy required to produce an ion pair in air.
If your answer differs substantially from the outline answer, refer to Section 33.6.1.

d. Methods used include the thimble ionisation chamber, the Geiger–Müller counter, scintillation detectors, thermoluminescent dosemeters, photographic film and semiconductor detectors. One of these methods should then be described in detail.
If your answer differs substantially from the outline answer, refer to Sections 33.6.1–33.6.6.

CHAPTER 34

a. When a photon of ionising radiation interacts with an atom of a tissue cell, the photon can have sufficient energy to cause ionisation of the atom. The secondary electrons emitted by this process may also have sufficient energy to ionise other atoms. The free radicals produced by such ionisations can produce new chemicals within the cell. If the original chemical was important to the cell function, this new chemical can cause a change in the cell's function – a biological effect of radiation.
If your answer differs substantially from the outline answer, refer to Section 34.4.

b. Both stochastic and deterministic effects are possible biological effects of ionising radiation. The effects are contrasted in the table overleaf:

Stochastic effects	Deterministic effects
No safe lower limit below which the effect will not occur	Threshold limit exists below which the effect will not occur
The greater the dose received, the greater the risk of the effect occurring	The effect always occurs once the threshold has been exceeded
The severity of the effect when it occurs is not related to the dose received	The greater the dose received above the threshold, the more severe the effect

If your answer differs substantially from the outline answer, refer to Sections 34.4.1 and 34.4.2.

c. As the sum of the weighting factors of all the organs is unity, the effective whole-body dose is 2×1 mSv = 2 mSv.
If your answer differs substantially from the outline answer, refer to Section 34.8.

d. The factors to be considered include:

- the effective half-life of the material
- the level of the radioactivity in the body organs
- whether the level is uniform or if there is increased uptake by certain organs
- the decay system of the radionuclide
- the quality factor(s) of the radiation(s) emitted during the decay
- the size of the organs involved
- the weighting factor of the organs involved.

If your answer differs substantially from the outline answer, refer to Section 34.9.

e. (i)   20 mSv

 (ii)   6 mSv

 (iii) 1 mSv

 (iv) 13 mSv in 3 months

 (v)   10 mSv during the declared period of a pregnancy.
 If your answer differs substantially from the outline answer, refer to Table 34.4 A and B.

f. A classified radiation worker is someone who is likely to receive a dose of radiation which exceeds more than three-tenths of any relevant dose limit. The person concerned must be over 18 years of age, must be medically fit to be a classified person and must be informed of his/her classification.
 If your answer differs substantially from the outline answer, refer to Section 34.10.

g. The three general principles are:

 • Every practice resulting in an exposure to ionising radiation should be justified by the advantages it produces

 • All exposures should be kept as low as reasonably achievable (ALARA)

 • The sum of the doses and committed doses should not exceed specified limits.
 If your answer differs substantially from the outline answer, refer to Section 34.11.

h. The radiation protection advisor is usually responsible for ensuring that the employer complies with the current radiation protection legislation. Duties would include giving advice on:

 • dosimetry and monitoring

 • the designation and control of restricted areas

 • drawing up systems of work and local rules

 • investigation of radiation incidents

 • ensuring adequate training and update of radiation workers

 • commenting on the design of new, or modification of old, premises from a radiation protection aspect

 • preparation of contingency plans

 • selection and training of radiation protection supervisors (RPSs).

RPSs are persons directly involved in working with ionising radiation on a day-to-day basis. It is normal to have an RPS in each department to ensure safe working practice within that department. All RPSs must have sufficient knowledge and experience to allow them to carry out their duties in their department.
If your answer differs substantially from the outline answer, refer to Section 34.11.1.

i. The three common methods of personnel monitoring are:

 • the film-badge method

 • thermoluminescent dosimetry

 • the use of pocket dosemeters.

The advantages and disadvantages depend on the method selected. The main advantage of the film-badge method is that there is a permanent record of the dose received, as the film is kept after processing. The disadvantages include the fact that the reading is obtained some time after the exposure to radiation, the film is expensive and it will deteriorate if not stored in proper conditions prior to processing. A similar list of advantages and disadvantages for TLD or pocket dosemeters is acceptable.
If your answer differs substantially from the outline answer, refer to Section 34.11.3.

j. A controlled area is one where the instantaneous dose rate exceeds $7.5 \propto Sv \cdot h^{-1}$ or where an adult employee is likely to receive more than three-tenths of any relevant dose limit. The following have access to such an area:

 • classified radiation workers

 • other workers for whom there is a written scheme of work

 • patients undergoing diagnostic or therapeutic procedures.
If your answer differs substantially from the outline answer, refer to Section 34.11.4.

k. The radiation field size may be limited by the use of collimation. The fastest film/intensifying screen combination consistent with good image quality should be used. The number of repeat examinations should be eliminated/reduced by the use of good radiographic technique (positioning, exposure, patient preparation, etc.). There should be consistent optimum film processing. The highest practicable kV_p for the particular examination should be used. Autotimers should (if possible) be used to control exposure time. Gonad shields shoould be used where appropriate. An appropriate secondary radiation grid should be selected. It may be possible to use compression or tissue displacement for obese patients. Digital techniques should be used where appropriate.

If your answer differs substantially from the outline answer, refer to Section 34.11.5.

Index

A

Absolute electrical potential, 76
Absolute standards, 325, 328
Absorbed dose, 320
  absolute measurement, 325–328
    calorimetry, 325
    chemical methods, 327–328
    free-air ionisation chamber,
      325–327
  in air see Air kerma
  biological effects and, 323, 343
  definition, 321
  dose equivalent and, 323–325
  effects of different media, 322–323
  and exposure, 320–322
  and kerma, 322
  relative measurement, 328
    Gieger-Müller counter, 329–330
    photographic film, 331
    scintillation detectors, 330
    semiconductor detectors, 331
    thermoluminescent dosimetry
      (TLD), 330–331
    thimble ionisation chamber,
      328–329
Absorption, 4, 281
  attenutation and, 287
  coefficient see Mass absorption
    coefficient
  edges, 290, 296
  inverse square law and, 20, 21
  photoelectric see Photoelectric
    absorption
  X-ray photons, 284, 285, 287
Acceleration, 45, 46
Acceptor impurity, 167
Accuracy, 52–53
  of diagnostic test/evaluation, 59,
    60
Acoustic impedance, 392
Afterglow see Phosphorescence
Afterloading, 6

Air
  absorbed dose in, 320, 322–323
  equivalence, 328, 330
  magnetic properties, 96
  mass attenuation coefficients,
    295–296
  in radiation dosimetry, 320
Air kerma, 277, 278, 320
ALARA (ALARP) principle, 337–338,
  344, 345, 351
Algebraic symbols, 357
Alpha-particles, 238, 239
  biological effects, 323, 324
  committed dose, 342
  emission, 248–249, 260
Alternating current (AC), 118,
  120–133
  capacitors and, 146
  circuits, 124–126
    capacitors, 127, 146
    impedance, 125–126
    inductors, 127–128
    phase angle, 125, 128
    phase difference, 125
    power, 126
    reactance, 125–126
    resistors, 126
    resonance (RLC in series),
      128–129
    three-phase, 130–132
  generators, 114, 117–118
  induction motors, 138–139, 148
  irregular, 121
  sinusoidal, 121–125
  square-wave, 121
  switching, 173–174
  transformers see Transformers
  types, 120–121
  X-ray tube, 124, 177
Aluminium, 197, 281
  doping, 167
  equivalent, millimetres of, 281
  filtration, 198, 215, 234, 281, 282
Amount of substance, 42, 45, 401

Ampere, 45, 49, 84
  definition, 137, 401
  see also mA
Amplitude
  electromagnetic radiation, 230,
    231
  sinusoidal AC waveform, 122
Analogue image, 387
Analogue-to-digital converter
  (ADC), 388, 389
Annihilation radiation, 225, 251, 252
  detection, 394
  positron emission tomography
    (PET), 394
Anode, 10, 199–200
  angle, 10, 200
  compound, 202
  cooling, 210, 211, 212
  diameter, 210
  disc, 199
  heat storage capacity, 211
  heating, 210, 211
  magnetron, 217
  speed of rotation, 210
  stationary anode tube, 202
  stem, 200
Anode heel effect, 21, 200–201
Antimony doping, 166
Antineutrino, 252
Antiparticles, 251, 252
Argon, 242
Arsenic doping, 166
Atom, 94
  Bohr model, 224, 271
  cross-section (to radiation), 285
  energy levels, 100
  excitation, 243, 272, 273
  ground state, 243
  ionisation, 244, 272, 273
  magnetisation, 98, 106, 108
  nucleus see Nucleus, atomic
  planetary model, 237
  quantum physics model, 237
  structure, 80, 81, 237–245

Atomic mass number, 239
  beta decay, 250
  nuclear stability, 247
Atomic number, 239, 240, 242
  air compared with muscle, 320
  alpha decay, 248
  beta decay, 250
  bone versus soft tissue, 307, 308
  in electron capture, 255
  nuclear stability, 247, 248
  photoelectric absorption and,
    290
  target material, 272, 279
Attenuation, 281
  absorption and, 287
  coefficients see Linear attenuation
    coefficient; Mass attenuation
    coefficient
  exponential law, 31–32
  half-value thickness (HVT),
    32–33
  tenth-value thickness (TVT), 33
  X-ray beam, 284, 285, 287
    by body, 306, 307–309
    importance in radiography,
      294–296
    photon energy and, 275
  processes, 287
  see also Absorption; Scatter(ing)
Auger electrons, 251, 254–255
Autotransformer, 151, 158–160
  functions, 159–160
  losses, 159
  regulation, 159
Avalanching, electron, 171, 173
Average current, 122
Average voltage, 122
Avogadro's equation, 257
Avogadro's hypothesis, 42
Avogadro's number, 42, 403

B

Back-EMF, 116, 138
Barium sulphate plaster, 351
Barriers, X-ray room design, 351
Base measurement units, 44
Base plus fog, 312
Becquerel, 28, 247
Bending magnet, linear accelerator,
  218–219
Beta-particles, 6, 7
  biological effects, 324
  committed dose, 342
  emission, 249–252, 260
    neutrinos, 252
    pure, 250

liquid scintillation counting,
    374–376
  see also Negatrons; Positrons
Biangular tube, 201
Bias, 56
Binding energy (BE)
  electron shells, 244–245
  in internal conversion, 254
  nuclear (NBE), 240
  per nucleon, 240
Biological effects, 4, 5, 334
  deterministic (non-stochastic),
    337, 340–341
  genetic, 336–337
  stochastic, 335–337, 340–341
  type of radiation and, 323
Biot and Savart's law, 108
Biparietal diameter, 59
Bismuth, 248
  magnetic properties, 96, 97
Bismuth germinate (BGO), 395
Bismuth-212 decay, 249, 256
Bismuth-214 decay, 256
Black body radiation, 66–67
Blur (line spread function; LSF), 399
Bone
  attenuation of X-ray beam, 307,
    308
  photoelectric absorption, 291
Brachytherapy, 5–6
Brackets (maths), 360
Braking radiation see
    Bremsstrahlung radiation
Breakdown voltage, 171
Bremsstrahlung radiation, 67, 205,
    234
  production, 271–272, 273, 274,
    275, 278, 279
Bucky (Potter–Bucky) diaphragm,
    310
Bury–Bohr rules, 242

C

Cables
  high-tension, 197, 202
  mains, resistance, 90
  power loss, 90–91
Caesium iodide, 304
Caesium-131 decay, 255
Caesium-137 decay, 264
Calcium tungstate ($CaWO_4$), 300,
    303, 304
Calculations in examinations,
    367–368
Calculators, 367–368
Calorimetry, 325

Cancer
  radiation-induced, 335–336
  treatment, 5, 6
Candela, 45, 401
Capacitance, 127, 141–143
  capacitors in parallel, 144
  capacitors in series, 144–145
  definitions, 142
  parallel-plate capacitor, 143–144
  total or equivalent, 144, 145
  units, 142
Capacitance reactance, 127
Capacitor discharge mobile units,
    146, 147
Capacitor resistor circuit
  charging, 145
  discharging, 146
  time-constant, 145–146
Capacitors, 141–149
  in AC circuits, 127, 146
  charging, 145, 146
  discharging, 146
  in parallel, 144
  parallel-plate, 143–144
  in radiography, 146–148
  in series, 144–145
  voltage smoothing, 146, 147–148,
    180–181, 182, 183
Carbon
  atomic structure, 238, 239
  isotopes, 239–240
  see also Graphite
Carbon-11 decay, 250, 252
Carbon-13
  magnetic resonance imaging, 100
  magnetic sensitivity, 100
Carbon-14, 240
  clinical use, 264
  decay, 248, 250, 252
Cathode, 10, 201–202
  magnetron, 217
  rotating anode tube, 201–202
  stationary anode tube, 202
Cathode ray tube, 235
Celsius scale, 63
Characteristic curve
  emulsion/film, 311–313
    important features, 312
    uses, 312–313
  PN junction, 171
Characteristic radiation, 244, 256
  production, 272–273, 274
  target materials, 279
Chemical bonds, 81
Chernobyl nuclear accident, 259
Chromium-51, 264
Chromosomal damage, 336
Cobalt, magnetic properties, 96
Cobalt-57, 264

Cobalt-58, 255, 264
Cobalt-60, 250, 253, 264
Coefficient of variation, 57
Coercive force, 155, 156
Coherent (elastic) scattering,
    287–289, 296
Collector, 171, 172
Collimation, 309
    orthovoltage beam, 216
Committed dose, 342–343
    equivalent, 342
Committed effective dose, 342
Commutator, 137, 138
Compensating circuits, 159
Compton peak, 373
Compton scattering, 214, 251, 288,
    291–293, 296, 297
    attenuation/absorption/scatter
        coefficients, 292–293
    conservation of momentum, 225
    importance in radiography,
        294–296, 308, 309
    process, 291–293
Compton wavelength shift, 291
Computed tomography (CT)
        scanning, 235, 377–382
    gantry, 377
    image reconstruction, 382
    multislice, 382
    quantum noise reduction, 58–59
    radiation dose, 377–379
    scanning process, 379–380
    spiral, 380–381
Computers, digital imaging, 388–389
Conduction
    electrical, electron theory, 80,
        81–83, 106–107
    thermal, 65
        rotatory anode tube, 70
        stationary anode tube, 68, 69
Conduction band, 81
    N-type semiconductors, 166, 167
    photoelectric interactions, 300,
        301, 304
    semiconductors, 83, 164, 165
    silicon, 165
Conductors, electrical, 73, 85
    charge distribution
        irregularly shaped, 77–78
        spherical shape, 77
    electromagnetic induction,
        113–114
    electron arrangements, 82, 164
    good, 81
    induction, 74, 75
    magnetic fields, 107–108
    motor principle, 135
Conservation of energy, law of, 40,
    114, 224–225

Conservation of matter (mass), law
    of, 39–40
Conservation of momentum, law of,
    40, 225
Constant potential generator,
    180–181
Constant potential (voltage) circuits,
    178, 180–182
Constant-voltage transformer, 151,
    160
Constants, physical, 403
Contamination monitors, 330
Contrast
    comparison between images,
        312–313
    exposure selection to omptimise,
        313–314
    radiographic image, 309, 310, 311
Controlled areas, 344, 349
Convection (of heat), 65–66
    currents, 66
    stationary anode tube, 69
Converison factors, 403
Convoluted back-projection, 382
Copper
    disc, AC induction motor, 138, 139
    filtration, 215, 281–282
    losses, transformer, 153–154
    stationary anode tube, 202
    thermal properties, 65, 69
Copper-63 fission, 258
Coronal discharge, 78
Cosine, 366
Coulomb, 73
    per kilogram of air, 320
Coulomb force, 77, 247, 248, 256,
    257
Coulomb potential, 77
Coulomb's law, 73
Covalent bonds, 165, 243
Cross-multiplication, 361–362
CT scanning see Computed
        tomography (CT) scanning
Curie, 247
Curie temperature, 98
Current, 83–84, 401
    alternating see Alternating
        current
    average, 122
    convention for representation,
        107
    'conventional', 106, 107
    DC electric motor, 138
    direct see Direct current
    effective/root mean square (RMS),
        123
    electron flow, 106–107
    filament heating, 204
    mains, 124

minimising power loss, 90–91
Ohm's law, 86, 87, 88
peak, 122
RLC circuits, 128
secondary of a transformer,
    152–153
units, 45, 49–50, 84
wattless, 126
X-ray tube see X-ray tube, current
Cycle
    electromagnetic radiation, 230
    sinusoidal AC waveform, 121
Cyclotron, medical, 259, 262–263

D

DC see Direct current
De Broglie wavelength, 224, 226
    electron orbitals, 241–242
Dead time, 330
Decay constant, 28–30
Decay curves, 28
Decay, radioactive, 27, 240, 246
    alpha, 248–249
    beta, 249–252
    branching scheme, 247, 256
    decay scheme, 247, 248
    electron capture, 255–256
    exponential nature, 27
    gamma, 253–255
    half-life and, 28–30
    internal conversion, 254
    law of, 27, 240
    nuclide chart, 247–248
    summary of effects, 259, 260
Deceleration, 46
Delay circuit, 185–186
Delta connections, 130, 180
Delta-rays, 273, 320
Densitometer, 311
Detectors, radiation, 328–331
Deterministic effects of radiation,
    337, 340–341
Detriment, 337–338
Diagnostic radiography, 3
    radiation protection, 344, 351
    statistical methods, 58–59
Diagnostic X-ray tubes
    construction, 195–206
    filtration, 281
    X-ray production, 272
Diamagnetic materials, 97
Diamagnetism, 97
Diaphragm, 4
    light-beam, 196, 197, 198
    penumbra, 15
    Potter–Bucky, 310

Dielectric constant, 74, 144
Dielectrics, 75–76, 143–144
Diethylenetriaminepentaacetic acid (DTPA), 263
Digital imaging, 387–390
  coding, 388
  definition, 387
  process, 388–389
  quantization, 388
  scanning, 388
  storage and transmission of images, 389–390
Digital-to-analogue converter (DAC), 389
Diode
  PN junction, 168, 170–171
  solid-state, 174
Direct current (DC), 80–92, 120
  capacitors and, 145
  constant, 120
  electric motor, 137–138
  pulsatile, 121
  types, 120–121
Division, 359–360
Donor impurities, 166
Doping, 165, 166
  junction transistor, 171
  pentavalent elements, 166
Doppler effect, 393
Doppler ultrasound imaging, 393
Dose, 7
  -dependent radiation effects, 337
  absorbed see Absorbed dose
  ALARA (ALARP) principle, 337–338
  average population, 7, 319–320, 333, 334
  calculation, 59
  committed, 342–343, 345
  CT scanning, 377–379
  effective, 341–342
  genetically significant, 336–337
  limits, 343
  maximum permissible, 339
  measurement see Absorbed dose
  minimisation methods, 350
  monitoring, 345
  potential, 344
  radiotherapy (dose fractionation), 5
  records, 344
  review of procedures, 59–60
  units, 320–323
Dose equivalent, 323–325
  committed, 342
  effective, 341
  units, 343
Dose rate, 324

Dose-equivalent limits, 334, 335, 339–341
  specific organs, 343
Dose-rate meters, 322
Dosemeters, 322
  absolute standards, 325
  chemical, 327–328
  Fricke, 327
  personal, 344
  pocket, 347, 348–349
  secondary standards, 325
  substandards, 325
  types, 328–331
Dosimetry, 7, 319–332
  service, 344
Drain, field effect transistors, 172
Dual-focus tube, 201
Duality, wave–particle see Wave–particle duality

E

Echo planar imaging, 383
Eddy currents, transformer core, 152, 154–155
Effective current, 123
Effective dose, 341–342
  committed, 342
  limits, 342
Effective dose equivalent, 341
Effective voltage, 123
Einstein, Albert, 224, 233
Elastic collisions, 40
  in X-ray production, 270, 271
Elastic scattering, 287–289, 296, 297
  interactions, 288
Electric capacity see Capacitance
Electric current see Current
Electric 'lines of force', 74, 95
Electric motors
  AC induction, 138–139, 148
  DC, 137–138
  in radiography, 139
  see also Motor principle
Electrical charge(s)
  attraction, 73
  distribution
    on conducting sphere, 77
    on irregularly shaped conductor, 77–78
  force between two, 73–74
  induction, 73, 74–76
  magnetic poles comparison, 93–94
  negative, 73
  positive, 73

properties, 72–73
  repulsion, 73
  see also Electrostatics
Electrical circuit, 83
Electrical dipole, 75
Electrical energy, 89–90
Electrical field strength, 74
Electrical mains see Mains
Electrical potential, 76–77
  absolute, 76
  conducting sphere, 77
  point charge, 77
  units, 77
  zero, 76
Electrical power see Power, electrical
Electrical safety
  filament transformer, 202
  X-ray tube shield, 196, 197–198
Electricity, 4
  direct current (DC), 80–92, 120–121
Electromagnet, 108
Electromagnetic fields
  interaction between two, 136–137
  MRI signal production, 101, 102
Electromagnetic induction, 112–119
  AC generator, 117–118
  AC induction motor, 138–139
  DC electric motor, 138
  definition, 112
  Faraday's laws see Faraday's laws
  Lenz's law see Lenz's law
  mutual, 115–116
  necessary conditions, 113
  self-, 116–117
  sign convention, 114–115
Electromagnetic radiation, 4, 228–236
  attenuation by matter, 31–32
  interactions with matter, 229
  interference, 231
  linear progapation, 230–231
  polarisation, 231
  properties, 229–232
    particle-like, 231–232
    wave-like, 229–231
  in radiography, 234–235
Electromagnetic relay, 109–110
Electromagnetic spectrum, 232, 233
Electromagnetism, 106–119
  Biot and Savart's law, 108
  circular coil of wire, 107–108, 109
  definition, 112
  in medical imaging, 99
  motor, 135
  solenoid, 108, 109
  straigh wire, 107, 109

Electromotive force (EMF), 84, 113
  AC generator, 117, 118
  back (back-EMF), 116, 138
  DC electric motor, 138
  Faraday's law, 113, 114
  in mutual induction, 115
Electron microscope, 226
Electron-volt (eV), 50
Electronic charge, 239, 403
Electronic equilibrium, 321
Electronic switch, 173, 174
Electron(s), 73, 100, 238, 239
  acceptors, 242
  Auger, 251, 254–255
  avalanching, 171, 173
  braking, 271
  capture, 255–256, 260
  conduction band, 81
  in conductors, 81, 82
  configurations of elements, 242,
    243, 406–408
  converted, 254
  density, 292, 296
  donors, 242
  energy bands, 81
  energy levels, 81
  energy loss in X-ray tube,
    269–270
  focusing, 204
  free, 291
  in insulators, 81, 83
  interactions with matter, 269–270
  linear accelerator production,
    216, 218–219
  loosely and tightly bound, 81
  magnetic deflection, 139–140
  orbitals (shells), 94, 238, 241–242,
    243
    binding energy, 244–245
    changes, 243–244
    configurations, 242
    in electrical conduction, 81
    fluorescent radiation emission
      and, 254
    internal conversion and, 254
    maximum number of electrons,
      242
    see also K-shell; L-shell; M-shell
  rest mass, 403
  in semiconductors, 81, 83, 164
  spin-up/spin-down, 100
  theory of electrical conduction,
    80, 81–83, 106–107
  thermionic emission, 202–203
  traps, 300, 301, 304, 305
  valence, 165
  valence band, 81
  see also Negatrons

Electrostatics, 72–79
  electrical field strength, 74
  electrical potential, 76–77
  induction of charge, 73, 74–76
  permittivity/relative permittivity,
    74
  see also Electrical charge(s)
Elements, 239
  characteristic radiation, 244
  chemical reactivity, 242
  electron configuration, 242,
    243–244, 406–408
  periodic table, 242–243, 405
EMF see Electromotive force
Emitter, 171, 172
Employees see Radiation workers
Employer, duties of, 349–350
Emulsion
  characteristic curve, 311–313
  contrast, comparing, 312–313
  radiographic image pattern, 311
  see also Film
Endoscopy, 3–4
Energy, 4
  AC circuit, 123
  alpha dacay, 249
  beta decay, 250, 251, 252
  binding see Binding energy
  Bremsstrahlung radiation, 274,
    275
  characteristic radiation, 272–273
  electrical, 89–90
  gamma decay, 253, 254
  heat, 63–64
  kinetic see Kinetic energy
  law of conservation, 40, 114,
    224–225
  nucelar fission, 257
  photon, 231, 274
  potential, 47, 76
  units, 45, 47, 89
  X-ray beam see X-ray beam,
    energy/photon energy
Environmental monitoring, 345
Epidemiology, 59
Equations, solving, 360–362
Errors, 52–56
  combining, 54–55
  fractional/percentage, 54
  measurement, 52–53
  observational, 53
  potential sources, 56
  practical examples, 55–56
  in a product, 54–55
  in a quotient, 55
  random, 53–54
  in a sum, 55
  systematic, 53–54

Euratom Directives, 334
Evaporation, 68
Exchange forces, 240
Excitation, atom, 243, 272, 273
Excitation pulse, 383
Experimental errors see Errors
Exponential decay, 26, 27
Exponential growth, 25, 26
Exponential law, 25–25, 145
  attenuation of electromagnetic
    radiation by matter, 31–32
  definition, 27
  description, 25–27
  logarithmic form, 33–34
  radioactive decay, 27
Exposure
  absorbed dose and, 320–322
  air kerma and, 320
  circuits, 185–192
  definition, 320
  measurement methods, 325–328
  range/film latitude, 312–313
  relative photographic, 311–312
  selection, 313–314
  switching, 185–192
  timing, 188–191
  transformer rating, 160–161
  units, 320–323
  X-ray beam quantity and, 277
  X-ray tube preparation, 185–186
Exposure rate, 320
Extrapolation, 366
Eye, laser hazards, 234

F

Farad, 127, 142, 143
  definition, 142
Faraday's laws, 113–114, 138
  first, 113, 114
  mutual induction, 115, 116
  second, 113, 114
  transformers, 151, 152–153
Ferromagnetic materials, 97, 98
  hysteresis, 98, 99
  magnetic domains, 98
Ferromagnetism, 98–99
Fetus
  assessing maturity, 59
  protection, 338, 343
  radiosensitivity, 336, 338
Field effect transistor (FET), 171,
  172–173
Field size, 9, 11–12
Filament transformer, 150, 177,
  202

Filaments, 199–200, 201
    broad focus, 201
    configuration, 201, 202
    electron emission, 202–203
    heating current, 204
    rotating anode tube, 201
    stationary anode tube, 202
Film
    latitude, 312–313
    radiation detection, 331
    speed, 313
    X-ray image production, 311
    see also Emulsion
Film badges, 331, 347, 348
Filtration, 4
    added, 198, 215, 281
    inherent, 198, 215, 281
    orthovoltage X-ray tube beam,
        215
    therapeutic X-ray tube beam, 281
    total, 198, 281
    X-ray beam effects, 279, 280–282
Fission see Nuclear fission
Fleming's hand rules, 114, 135
Flip angle, 383
Flip-flop circuit, 174
Fluorescence, 233, 235, 298–299
    activators, 299
    mechanism, 299–300
    in radiography, 301–304
Fluorescent radiation, 254, 255, 256
Fluorescent screens, 5, 301–304
Fluorescent tubes, 235, 304
Fluorescent yield, 255
Fluorine, 242
Fluorine-19
    magnetic resonance imaging, 100
    magnetic sensitivity, 100
18-Fluorodeoxyglucose (FDG), 396
Fluoroscopy
    good radiographic practice, 350
    image intensifiers, 304
    transformer ratings, 160–161
Focus, 10–11
    broad, 201
    effective (apparent), 10–11, 199,
        200
    fine, 202
    real, 10–11, 199, 200
    X-ray tube rating and, 208, 209
Focus to diaphragm distance (FDD), 9
    field size and, 11
Focus to film distance (FFD), 9
    field size and, 11–12
    geometric unsharpness, 14–15
    image magnification, 12, 13
    mAs settings and, 22
Focus to object distance (FOD), 9
    geometric unsharpness, 14
Focus to skin distance (FSD), 9

Focusing cup, 187, 201, 202
'Fog' level, 312
Forbidden energy gap (E), 81, 301,
    304
Force, 45, 46
Forward bias, 169
Fractions, 357–358
    addition, 358
    indices, 362–363
    multiplying and dividing, 359–360
Frame store, 389
Free induction decay, 103
Free-air ionisation chamber, 325–327
Frequency, 391
    electromagnetic radiation, 230
    resonance, 129
    sinusoidal AC waveform, 122
Frequency-encoding gradient, 385
Fricke dosemeter, 327
Fringe field, 385

G

Gadolinium oxybromide, terbium-
    activated, 302, 303
Gadolinium oxysulphide, 300
    terbium-activated, 303
Gadolinium-based contrast agents,
    98
Gallium-68, 264
Gamma camera, 235, 374
Gamma-rays, 232, 233, 235, 250
    clinical applications, 263, 264
    emission, 253–255, 260
        internal conversion, 254
        metastable states/isometric
            transitions, 253
    line spectra, 253
    scintillation counting, 373
'Gassy tube' effect, 68, 199
Gauss (G), 96
Geiger–Müller counter, 329–330
Generators
    AC, 117–118
    constant potential, 180–181
    medium-frequency, 182–183
    orthovoltage, 214–216
    six-pulse, 180
    three-phase see Three-phase
        generators
    twelve-pulse, 180
X-ray see X-ray generators
Genetic effects, 336–337
Geometric unsharpness (Ug), 13–15
    calculation, 14
    see also Penumbra
Geometry, 9–17
    definitions, 9

penumbra, 13–15
    triangles, 366–367
Germanium, 166
Glass
    envelope, 198–199
    thermal conductivity, 65
Gonads
    dose, 337, 341
    weighting factors, 341
Good radiographic practice, 350
Gradient echo imaging, 104
Gradient-echo pulse sequence, 383
Graphite
    in rotating anode disc, 199, 200
    thermal properties, 69, 70
    see also Carbon
Graphs, 364–366
Gratz bridge circuit, 178, 183
Gray, 321
Greek symbols, 404
Grid bias, 187
Grid factor, 310
Grid lattice, 310
Grid ratio, 310
Grid, secondary radiation, 5,
    309–310, 313
Grid-controlled X-ray tube, 187
    dose limitation, 187
Ground state, atomic, 243
Gyromagentic ratio, 101

H

Half-life, 28–30
    biological, 30–31, 342
    effective, 30–31, 342
    physical, 30–31, 342
Half-value thickness (HVT), 32–33,
    278
Health and Safety Executive (HSE),
    334–335, 345
Heat, 62–71
    capacity, specific, 63–64
    emission by anode, 234
    energy, 63–64
        units, 63–64
    evaporation and vaporisation, 68
    generation
        autotransformers, 159
        high-tension transformers, 160,
            161
        X-ray tube target, 270–271, 273
    loss from X-ray tube, 68–70, 200
    storage capacity, anode, 211
    transfer mechanisms, 64–67
Heat units (HU), 49, 50–51
Heisenberg's uncertainty principle,
    226

Henry, 94, 116
High-tension cables, 197, 202
High-tension transformers (HTT),
        150, 177, 182, 183
    compensating circuits, 159
    heat generation, 160, 161
    input voltage, 159, 160
    rating, 126, 160–161
Housing see Shield
HU (heat units), 49, 50–51
Hydrogen
    atomic structure, 241
    effects of magnetic field (proton
        precession), 99
    electron density, 292
    magnetic resonance imaging, 99,
        100, 101
    magnetic sensitivity, 100
    see also Tritium
Hysteresis, 98, 99
    loops, 155
        area, 155
        soft iron and steel, 155–156
        subsidiary, 156
    transformer losses and, 154,
        155–157

I

Image
    analogue, 387
    CT scanning, 382
    digital, 387
    magnetic resonance imaging
        (MRI), 384–385
    magnification, 12–13
    matrix, 387, 388
    modulation, 397
    modulation transfer function
        (MTF), 397–400
    radiographic see Radiographic
        imaging
Image intensifiers, 235, 304
Impedance, 125–126
    acoustic, 392
    in RLC circuits, 128
Incidents, notification of, 345
Indices see Powers
Indium-113m, 264
Induction motors, AC, 138–139, 148
Inductors, in AC circuits, 127–128
Inelastic collisions, 40, 270
    Bremsstrahlung radiation,
        271–272
    characteristic radiation, 272–273
    in Compton scattering, 291
    photoelectric absorption, 289

Inertia, 47
Infinity, 76
Infrared radiation, 66, 232, 233
Inherent filtration, 198, 281
Insert, 196, 197, 198–199
    envelope, 198–199
    orthovoltage units, 215
    rotating anode tube, 198–199
    stationary anode tube, 202
Insulators, electrical, 73, 85
    electron arrangements, 83
    energy bands, 83, 164
    induction, 75–76
        molecular distortion, 75
        polar molecules, 75–76
        perfect, 81
Integrated circuits (ICs), 165, 171,
        174
Intensification factor, 304
Intensifying screens, 301–302
    comparison, 303–304
    construction, 302
    fast, 302
    high-resolution (detail), 302
    phosphor materials, 303
    substratum layer, 302
    supercoat, 302
    X-ray image production, 311
Intensity of magnetism, 97
Intensity of radiation, 19–20
    inverse square law, 20, 21
    relationship to distance, 21
Intensity, X-ray beam, 180, 274, 277
    definition, 278
    factors affecting, 277–283
    fraction transmitted, 308
    incident (I_0), 307
    photon energy and, 274
    transmitted (I_T), 307
Interference, 231
    constructive, 231
    destructive, 231
Internal conversion, 254, 260
    coefficient, 254
International Commission for
        Radiation Protection (ICRP),
        334, 338, 339, 341
International System of Units see SI
    units
Interpolation, 366
Inverse proportion, 364, 365
Inverse square law, 19–24
    conditions of application, 20
    electrical charge and, 73, 74
    mAs and, 21–23
    mathematical proof, 20–21
    statement, 20
    X-ray beam and, 21
Iodine-125, 264

Iodine-131, 264
    scintillation counting, 373
    therapy, 6–7, 264
Iodine-132, 264
Ionic bonds, 243
Ionisation, 244, 273, 335
    biological effects and, 324,
        335–337
    secondary, 320, 335
Ionisation chamber
    free-air, 325–327
    solid-state, 331
    thimble, 328–329
Ionising radiation
    artificial sources, 7, 334
    biological effects see Biological
        effects
    natural, 333, 334
    primary/secondary, 7
    protection see Radiation
        protection
    sources of exposure, 7, 319, 333,
        334
    see also Gamma-rays; X-rays
Ionising Radiation (Medical
        Exposure) Regulations 2000
        (IR(ME)R 2000), 58, 334, 335,
        345, 346
    duties of designated individuals,
        349–350
Ionising Radiation Regulations 1999
        (IRR 1999), 334, 335, 345, 346
    dose limits, 342, 343
    employees, 235, 343, 344
    local rules, 346–347
    work area designation, 349
Ions, 80, 243
    positive, 254
Iridium-192, 264
Iron
    loss, transformer, 154
    magnetic properties, 96, 98
    soft, 155, 156
Iron-59, 264
Irox oxide contrast agent, 98
Isobar, 239
Isodose lines, 5
Isometric transitions, 253
Isotopes, 239
    nuclear medicine, 6–7
    nuclide chart, 247–248
    within human body, 100
Isotropic source, 20

J

Joule, 47, 89

K

K capture, 255
K space, 385
K-characteristic radiations, 273, 274
K-shell, 238, 242
  binding energy, 244
Kelvin, 45, 63, 401
Kerma, 321
  air *see* Air kerma
KeV (kiloelectron-volt), 49, 50, 296
Kilogram, 45, 401
Kilovolt (kV), 50
  peak (maximum) *see* kVp
Kinetic energy (KE), 47
  annihilation radiation, 251
  calculation, 41
  in internal conversion, 254
  in X-ray production, 270, 271
Krypton, 242
Krypton-81m, 264
kV, 50
  orthovoltage units, 215
kV selector, 159–160
kVA, 126
kVp (maximum kilovoltage), 49, 50, 122, 124, 204–205
  effect on X-ray beam, 278–279, 282
  effect on X-ray image, 310–311
  maximum photon energy and, 274
  scatter radiation and, 309
  selection, 313–314
  X-ray tube rating and, 208, 209

L

L-capture, 255
L-characteristic radiations, 273, 274
L-shell, 238, 242
  binding energy, 244
Laboratory technicians, 344
Lamination, transformer core, 154–155
Lanthanum oxybromide, terbium-activated, 299, 303
Lanthanum oxysulphide, terbium-activated, 303
Larmor equation, 101
Larmor frequency, 99, 101–102
Lasers, 20, 232–234
  basic physics, 232–233
  hazards, 234

optical pumping, 233
  in radiography, 235
Last menstrual period (LMP), 339
Latent period, radiation-induced cancer, 336
Lattice density, 310
Laws of physics *see* Physical laws
Lead, 234
  equivalents, 351
  mass attenuation coefficients, 295–296
  photoelectric absorption, 289, 290
  for radiation protection, 351
  secondary radiation grid, 309, 310
Lead lining
  orthovoltage tube insert, 215
  tube housing, 197
Length, 45, 401
Lenz's law, 97, 114, 118, 138, 139
  mutual induction, 115
  transformers, 151, 152–153
Leukaemia, radiation-induced, 336
Light, 230, 231, 232, 233
  emission by anode, 234
  polarisation, 231
  velocity, 403
Light amplification by stimulated emission of radiation *see* Lasers
Light-beam diaphragm, 12
Line focus principle, 10, 199–200
Line spread function (LSF), 399
Linear accelerator, 216–219
  accelerating waveguide, 217–218
  bending magnet, 218–219
  magnetron, 216–217
  radiofrequency circulator, 217
  treatment head, 218–219
  waveguides, 217
Linear attenuation coefficient, 287
  bone versus soft tissue, 307, 308
  pair production, 294
  photoelectric effect, 290–291
  total μ, 32, 286, 287
Linear expansivity, 67
Liquid scintillation counting, 374–376
Lithium fluoride, 301, 330
Local rules, 344, 346–347
Logarithms, 368
Logic circuits, 174
Longitudinal relaxation, 103
Luminescence, 298–305
  definition, 298
Luminous intensity, 45, 401

M

M-shell, 242
mA (milliamperes), 49, 50, 84, 124
  effect on X-ray beam, 278, 282
  filament heating current and, 204
  half-wave/full-wave rectification, 179
  meter, 124
  orthovoltage units, 215
  selection, 314
  X-ray tube rating, 208, 209
Magnetic domains, 98
Magnetic fields, 94
  circular coil of wire, 107–108
  electron beam deflection, 139–140
  interaction of two, 136–137
  lines of force, 94, 95, 107–108
  motor principle, 134
  solenoid, 108
  straight wire, 107
Magnetic flux, 94, 95, 113
  losses of transformer, 154
  transformers, 13, 151, 152
Magnetic flux density, 95, 96
  Biot and Savart's law, 108–109
  coil of wire, 107–108, 109
  motor principle, 135
  solenoid, 108, 109
  straight wire, 109
  transformer, 151
Magnetic flux linkage, 113–114
  AC induction motor, 139
  Faraday's law, 114
Magnetic moment, 96
Magnetic poles, 93–94
  force between, 94
Magnetic resonance imaging (MRI), 97, 99–104, 383–386
  coil design, 385–386
  contrast agents, 98
  free induction decay, 103
  image production, 384–385
  image weighting (T_1/T_2 processes), 102–103
  longitudinal (spin-lattice) relaxation, 103
  magnetic field strength, 96, 97
  magnets, 82, 97, 385–386
  nuclear spins, 100–101
  principle, 99–100
  pulse sequences, 383
  radiofrequency (RF) pulse, 101, 102, 103, 104, 383, 384–385
  receiver, 102, 129
  safety, 97, 386

signal production, 101–102
transmit coil, 102
transverse (spin-spin) relaxation, 103
Magnetic resonance spectroscopy (MRS), 99, 101, 385
Magnetic saturation, 98
Magnetising force (H), 95, 99
Magnetism, 93–94
induction, 95–97
diamagnetic materials, 97
ferromagnetic materials, 98–99
hysteresis, 99
intensity, 96–97
in medical imaging, 99
types of materials, 97–99
Magnetron, 216–217
Magnets
magnetic resonance imaging (MRI), 82, 97, 385–386
permanent, 385–386
resistive, 385
superconductor, 385
Magnification, image, 12–13
Mains
-independent X-ray units, 91
cable resistance, 90–91
resistance compensator
adjustable, 91
static, 91
voltage compensator, 118, 159
voltage and current, 124
Majority carriers, 169
N-type semiconductors, 167
P-type semiconductors, 167
transistors, 172, 173
mAs (milliampere-seconds), 49, 50, 84
-based timer, 188–190
inverse square law and, 21–23
Mass, 45, 47, 401
law of conservation, 39–40
relativistic, 224
rest, 224, 403
Mass absorption coefficient
absorbed dose and, 323
air and bone, 323
air and muscle, 320
Compton scattering, 292
pair production, 294
photoelectric effect, 290
total (μρ), 286, 287, 295–296
Mass attenuation coefficient
Compton scattering, 292
pair production, 294
Mass scattering coefficient
Compton scattering, 293
pair production, 294

Mass-energy equivalence, 224–225, 251
Mathematics, 357–371
Matrix, image, 387, 388
Matter
electromagnetic radiation interactions, 229
electron interactions, 269–270
law of conservation, 39–40
X-ray interactions, 284–297
Mean, 57
Measurement
error, 52–53
units see Units of measurement
Median, 57
Medical surveillance, radiation workers, 344
Menstrual period, last (LMP), 339
Metal envelope, 199
Metastable states, 253
Metre, 45, 401
Microfarad, 143
Microprocessors, 163, 174
monitoring rating, 212
Microwaves, 233
Milliampere-seconds see mAs
Millicoulombs, 49, 84
see also mAs
Minority carriers, 169
N-type semiconductors, 167
P-type semiconductors, 167
PN junction, 169, 170, 171
transistors, 172
Mobile X-ray machines, 140
Mobile X-ray units
adjustable mains resistance compensator, 91
capacitor discharge, 146, 147
mains-independent, 91
power source, 182–183
X-ray generator, 182–183
Mode, 57
Modulation, 397–398
Modulation transfer function (MTF), 397–400
definition, 397
measurement, 399
objects as spatial frequencies, 398–399
spatial frequency and, 398
Mole, 42, 45, 401
Molybdenum
in rotating anode disc, 199, 200
thermal properties, 65, 69, 70
X-ray beam quality/quantity, 279
Molybdenum-98, technetium-99m generation, 259, 261
Molybdenum-99 decay, 262

Momentum, 45, 48
law of conservation, 40, 225
Newton's second law, 40, 41
Monitoring, 7
Motion
Newton's laws see Newton's laws of motion
rotational, 47
translational, 47
Motor principle, 134–140
definition, 135
direction of force on conductor, 135
convention, 135–136
interaction of two electromagnetic fields, 136–137
magnetic deflection of electron beam, 139–140
magnitude of force on conductor, 135
in radiography, 140
Motors see Electric motors
Movement unsharpness (Um), 14
MRI see Magnetic resonance imaging
Multiplication, 359–360
Mumetal, magnetic properties, 96
Mutual inductance (M), 116
transformer, 151

N

N-shell, 242
National Radiological Protection Board (NRPB), 339
Natural radiation sources, 7, 319, 333, 334
Negative numbers, multiplying and dividing, 359
Negatrons (β⁻), 249
emission, 249–250, 252, 260
Neon, 242
Neutrino, 239, 252
Neutron number, 239
Neutron-activated fission, 257
Neutrons, 238, 239, 240, 241
beta decay process, 249–250
biological effects, 324
delayed, 258
prompt, 258
rest mass, 403
spin, 100
Newton, 41, 46
Newton's laws of motion, 40–42, 47
first, 40
second, 40, 41, 46
third, 40–41, 42, 73

Nickel
    focusing cup, 201
    magnetic properties, 96
Nickel-60 decay, 253
Noise pulses, 373
Normal distribution, 57
NPN junction transistor, 171–172
NPNP thyristor, 173–174
Nuclear binding energy (NBE), 240
Nuclear fission, 256–259, 260
    fragments, 257
    neutron-activated, 257
    in nuclear reactor, 258–259
    spontaneous, 257
Nuclear magnetic resonance (NMR),
        99, 100, 383
Nuclear medicine, 5, 6–7, 31, 263
    radiation protection, 344
Nuclear reactor, 258–259
Nuclear shells, 240
Nuclear transformation, 247
    radioactive *see* Decay, radioactive
Nucleon, 239
    binding energy per, 240
Nucleus, atomic, 238–241
    short-range forces, 240
    spin properties, 100
    stability, 240–241, 246–248
    terminology, 239
Nuclide, 239
Nuclide chart, 247–248

O

Object to film distance (OFD), 9
    geometric unsharpness, 14–15
    image magnification, 12
Occupancy factor, 351
Occupational exposure, 344, 345
Ohms, 85, 87
Ohm's law, 86–89
    AC circuits, 123–124
    calculations using, 88–89
    resistors in parallel, 87–88
    resistors in series, 87
Operator, duties of, 350
Optical density, 311
    optimising, 314
Optical pumping, 233
Organs, weighting factors, 341
Orthovoltage generators, 214–216
Orthovoltage unit, 215–216
    beam
        collimation, 216
        filtration, 215–216
    X-ray tube, 215
Ovaries, 341

Ovum, radiosensitivity, 338
Oxygen-17
    magnetic resonance imaging,
        100
    magnetic sensitivity, 100

P

Pair production, 225, 288, 293–294,
        296, 297
    attenuation/absorption/scatter
        coefficients, 294
    importance in radiography,
        294–296
Paramagnetic materials, 97
    magnetic resonance imaging
        contrast, 98
Paramagnetism, 97–98
Particles
    subatomic, 238, 239, 240
    as waves, 224, 226
Pascal, 46
Patients
    dose limits, 342
    dose minimisation, 350
Pauli exclusion principle, 242
Peak current (voltage), 122
Pentavalent impurity, 166
Penumbra, 13–15
    from diaphragms, 15
    see also Geometric unsharpness
Percentages, 358
Period (*T*), sinusoidal AC waveform,
        122
Periodic table of elements,
        242–243, 405
Permalloy, 156
Permeability (μ), 96, 97
    relative (μ_r), 96, 97, 98
    vacuum (μ_0), 96, 403
Permittivity, 74
    relative, 74
    vacuum, 73, 403
Personnel *see* Radiation workers
Personnel monitoring, 345, 347–349
Pertechnetate, 263
Phase angle, 125, 128
Phase difference, 125
Phase voltages, 130, 131
Phase-array coils, 386
Phase-encoding gradient, 385
Phosphorescence, 298–299
    mechanisms, 300–301
    in radiography, 301
Phosphors, 299
    activators, 299
    in fluorescent tubes, 304

fluoroscopic image intensifiers,
        304
    in intensifying screens, 302, 303
    measures of efficiency, 300
    television monitors, 304
Phosphorus
    doping, 166
    nuclear magnetic resonance, 100
Phosphorus-31
    magnetic resonance spectroscopy,
        202
    magnetic sensitivity, 100
Phosphorus-32, 264
Photoelectric absorption, 244, 251,
        281, 282, 288, 289–291, 296,
        297
    attenuation/absorption
        coefficients, 290–291
    importance in radiography,
        294–296, 308, 309
Photoelectric effect, 255
Photoelectron, 289
Photofission, 258
Photographic exposure, relative,
        311–312
Photographic film *see* Film
Photographic unsharpness (*Up*), 14
Photomultiplier tubes, 304, 372–373
    scintillation detectors, 330
Photons, 225, 231, 239
    coincident, 394–395
    energy, 231, 275, 278
    inducing fission, 258
    wavelength, 231, 274–275
    see also Quantum
Photostimulable plates, 235, 305
Photostimulation, 298, 304–305
Phototimers, 190
Physical constants, 403
Physical laws
    classical, 39–43, 223–224
    modern, 223–227
Pi meson, 239, 240–241
Picofarad, 143
Picture archiving and
        communications system
        (PACS), 389, 390
Piezoelectric effect, 391
Pinch-off potential, 173
Pixels, 387, 388
Planck's constant, 225, 231, 403
Planck's quantum hypothesis,
        223–224
Platinum, magnetic properties, 96, 98
PN junction, 168–171
    characteristic, 171
    depletion layer, 169, 170
    diode, 168, 170–171
        characteristic curve, 171

forward bias, 169
  minority carriers, 169, 170, 171
  potential barrier, 169, 171
  reverse bias, 170, 171
  see also Thyristor; Transistor
PNP junction transistor, 171
Polarisation, 231
Population, 56
Positive ions, 254
Positron emission tomography (PET)
  scanning, 259, 263, 394–396
  annihilation radiation detection,
    394, 395
  detector materials, 395
  detector mechanisms, 395
  radionuclides, 396
  types of coincidence, 394–395
Positrons β⁺, 239, 250, 394
  clinical applications, 263, 264
  detection, 394
  emission, 250–251, 260, 394
  fate, 251
Potassium-43, 264
Potential barrier, PN junction, 169,
    171
Potential difference (PD), 76, 83,
    84–85
  capacitance and, 142, 143
  definition, 77, 84
  peak see kVp
  units, 77
  see also Voltage
Potential energy, 47, 48, 76
Potter-Bucky diaphragm, 310
Power, electrical, 89–90
  in AC circuits, 126
  losses
    in autotransmformers, 159
    in cables, 90–91
    in transformers, 153–158
  in a resistor, 89
  units, 45, 48, 89
Power factor, 126
Powers (indices), 362–364
  of 10, 363–364, 403
  combining, 362
  fractional, 362–363
  negative, 362
  to different bases, 363
Practitioner, duties of, 350
Precession, 99
Precision, 53
Pregnant women, 336, 338, 339
Pressure, 45, 46
Principal quantum number, 242
Proportion
  direct, 364, 365
  inverse, 364, 365
Proportionality, 364

Proton density, 102
Protons, 73, 81, 238, 239, 240, 241
  beta decay process, 249–250
  biological effects, 324
  inducing fission, 258
  precession within magnetic field,
    99
  rest mass, 403
  spin, 100
Public see Patients
Pulse height analyser (PHA), 373
Pulse-echo imaging, 392–393
Pythagoras' theorem, 128

Q

Quality control, 58
Quality factor, 324
Quantum, 225, 239
  jump, 254, 273, 300
  Plank's hypothesis, 223–224
  see also Photons
Quantum conversion efficiency
  (QCE), 300
Quantum detection efficiency (QDE),
  300
Quantum mottle, 399
Quantum noise, 58
Quantum number, principal, 242
Quantum theory, 224
Quarks, 238
Quasielectronic equilibrium, 321

R

Radiation of heat, 65
  rotating anode tube, 69, 70
  stationary anode tube, 69
Radiation protection, 7, 333–353
  ALARA (ALARP) principle,
    337–338
  committed dose, 342–343, 345
  detriment, 337–338
  dose-equivalent limits, 339–341
  effective dose, 341–342
  Ionizing Radiation Regulations,
    334–335
  practical aspects, 345–351
  purpose and scope, 333–334
  radiation worker designation,
    343–345
  risk–benefit, 337–338
  women of reproductive capacity,
    338–339
  X-ray tube shield, 196, 197, 198

Radiation protection advisers (RPA),
    344, 345, 347, 349
Radiation protection supervisors
    (RPS), 346, 347
Radiation treatment see Therapeutic
    radiography
Radiation workers, 343–345
  classified designation, 345
  dose limits, 342, 343
  dose minimisation methods, 351
  dose monitoring, 345, 347–349
  medical surveillance, 344
  overexposure, 345
  records, 344, 345
  regulations affecting, 345–347
Radio waves, 67, 232, 233
Radioactive decay see Decay,
    radioactive
Radioactive disintegration, 247
Radioactive equilibrium, 262
Radioactive sources, brachytherapy,
    5
Radioactivity, 246–265
  measures, 28, 247
Radiobiology see Biological effects
Radiofrequency circulator, 217
Radiofrequency coils, 386
Radiofrequency (RF) pulse, 101,
    102, 103, 104, 383, 384–385
Radiographic imaging, 4–5, 306–314
  attenuation of X-ray beam by
    body, 306, 307–309
  characteristic curve for an
    emulsion, 311–313
  digital image manipulation, 313,
    314
  exposure selection, 313–314
  geometric aspects, 9–17
  kVp effect, 310–311
  magnification, 12–13
  radiographic image pattern, 311
  scatter, 309
    limiting formation, 309
    removal, 309–310
  X-ray image pattern, 307–311
Radioimmunoassay, 264
Radioisotope, 235, 239, 240
Radionuclides, 239, 240
  artificial production, 259,
    261–263
    cyclotron, 262–263
    growth of activity, 261–262
    technetium generator, 259,
      261
  clinically useful, 263, 264
  decay see Decay, radioactive
  decay curve, 28
  dose minimisation, 253
  half-life, 28–30

Radionuclides (cont'd)
  for imaging, 263
    positron emission tomography
      (PET), 396
  labelled, 263
  metastable, 253
  specific activity, 247
  for therapy, 264
Radiopharmaceuticals, 263
Radiotherapy see Therapeutic
  radiography
Random errors, 53–54
Random sampling, 56, 57
Raster, 140
Rating
  charts, 365–366
  definition, 207–208
  rotating anode tubes, 210
  stationary anode tubes, 210
  transformer, 126, 160–161
  X-ray unit see X-ray unit rating
Rayleigh scattering, 287, 296
Reactance, 125–126
  capacitance, 127, 128
  inductive, 128
  in RLC circuits, 128
Real focal spot, 10
Receiver coil, 102
Recombination, electrons, 164
Records, radiation workers, 344,
  345
Rectification, 122, 177–183
  constant potential circuits,
    180–182
  full-wave, 122
    current waveforms, 179
    four-diode, 178–179
  half-wave, 122, 178
    current waveforms, 179
  in modern X-ray generator, 182
  three-phase, 180
  voltage smoothing, 148, 180–181,
    182, 183
  X-ray beam effect, 282
  X-ray tube rating and, 209
Rectifiers, 165
  silicon-controlled (SCR), 173, 186
  solid-state, 170
Reentrant seals, 198
Referrer, duties of, 350
Refraction, 232
Refractive index, 230
Regulation, 85
  autotransformer, 159
  transformer, 154, 157–158
Relative biological effectiveness
  (RBE), 324–325
Relative photographic exposure,
  311–312

Remanence, 155, 156
Resistance, 85–86
  AC circuits, 125, 126
  factors affecting, 85–86
  mains cable, 90–91
  minimising power loss, 90
  Ohm's law, 86–89
  shape/cross sectional area
    relationship, 85–86
  specific (ρ), 86
  temperature coefficient (α), 86
  temperature relationship, 82, 83,
    85, 86
  type of substance and, 85, 86
Resistivity (ρ), 86
Resistors
  in AC circuits, 126
  charging a capacitor through,
    146
  discharging a capacitor through,
    146
  in parallel, 87–88
  in series, 87
Resonance, 129
  circuits, 128–129
  frequency, 101, 129
    magnetron, 217
Rest mass, 224, 403
Reverse bias, 170, 171
Review of procedures, 59–60
Rhenium
  in rotating anode disc, 199
  thermal properties, 69, 70
Risk
  accepatable, 340
  levels, 334, 339, 340
Risk factors, 336
Risk–benefit principle, 337–338
RLC (resonance) circuits, 128–129
RMS see Root mean square
Room design, 350–351
Root mean square (RMS) values
  current, 123
  voltage, 123, 124
Rotating anode X-ray tube, 195
  AC induction motor, 139, 140
  anode assembly, 199–200
  cathode assembly, 201–202
  heat loss mechanism, 69–70,
    200
  insert, 198–199
  rating, 210
  shield, 197
Rotor
  AC induction motor, 139
  rotating anode tube, 200
Rubber, thermal conductivity,
  65
Rutherford, 237, 238

S

Safety
  electrical, 196, 197–198, 199, 202
  lasers, 234
  magnetic resonance imaging, 97,
    386
  see also Radiation protection
Sampling, random, 56
Scalar quantities, 46
Scaling factor, 324
Scatter(ing), 4, 281, 284, 285
  coefficient see Mass scattering
    coefficient
  Compton see Compton scattering
  elastic (coherent, Rayleigh,
    classical), 287–289, 296
  inverse square law and, 20, 21
  limiting formation, 309
  protection from, 198
  radiographic image degradation,
    309
  radiotherapy units, 214–215
  removal, 309–310
  X-ray photons, 287
Scintillation counters, 304, 372–376
  components, 372–373
  liquid, 374–376
  use in medicine, 373–374
  see also Gamma camera
Scintillation detectors, 330
Scintillation efficiency (ScE), 300
Seals, reentrant, 198
Second, 45, 401
Secondary ionisations, 320
Secondary radiation grid, 5,
  309–310, 313
Secondary standard unit, 329
Secondary standards, 325, 329
Selenium-75, 264
Self inductance (L), 116
Self-induction, 116–117
  autotransformer, 158
Semiconductors, 163–176
  devices in radiography, 174
  electron arrangements, 81, 83,
    164
  extrinsic, 166–168
  intrinsic, 164–166, 168
  N-type, 166, 168
    diagramatic representation,
      168
  P-type, 166, 167–168
    diagramatic representation,
      168
  PN junction see PN junction
  positive holes, 164, 166, 167
  properties, 168

radiation detectors, 331
silicon, 165–166
temperature–conductivity
    relationships, 83, 164,
    167–168, 169, 171
thyristors, 173–174
transistors, 171–173
Sensitivity, 59, 60
    magnetic resonance imaging, 103
Sensitometry, 312
Shield (housing), 196
    construction, 196–198
    electrical safety, 196, 197–198, 199
    radiation safety, 196, 197, 198
SI units, 45–51
    base, 45–48, 401
    derived, 45–46
    fundamental, 45
Sieverts (Sv), 324, 343
Silicon, 165–166, 171
    chips, 163, 171, 174
    doping, 165, 166, 167
Silicon-controlled rectifier (SCR),
    173, 186
Similar triangles proof of inverse
    square law, 20–21
Simulator, 5
Sine, 366
Sine wave, 367
Sinusoidal alternating current (AC),
    121–124
    average, 122, 123
    cycle, 121
    definitions, 121
    effective (root mean square;
        RMS), 123
    peak, 122
    rectification, 122
Skewness
    negative, 57
    positive, 57
Sodium, 242
Sodium iodide, 235, 304, 330
    in scintillation counters (NaI(Tl)),
        372–373, 374
    thyroid uptake, 373–374
Soft tissue
    attenuation of X-ray beam, 307,
        308
    photoelectric absorption, 291
Solenoid, 108
    electromagnetic induction, 113,
        114
    electromagnetic relay, 109–110
    magnetic flux density, 109
    in motor principle, 134
    self-induction, 116
Solid-state diode, 174
Solid-state multiplication, 171

Solid-state rectifiers, 170
Solid-state switches, 110
Somatic effects, 337
Source, field effect transistors, 172
Space charge effect, 203
Spatial frequency, 397
Specific activity, radioactive sample,
    247
Specific heat capacity, 63–64
Specificity, 59, 60
    magnetic resonance imaging, 103
Speed, 45, 46
    imaging system, 313
Speed class, 304
Spin down, 100, 101
Spin up, 100, 101
Spin-echo imaging, 104
Spin-echo pulse sequence, 383
Spiral CT scanning, 380–381
Stalloy, 156
    magnetic properties, 96, 98
Standard deviation, 57
Standard error of the mean (SEM),
    58
Standard measurement units, 44
Star connections, 130, 131, 180
Static electrical charges see
    Electrostatics
Stationary anode X-ray tube, 195
    anode, 202
    cathode and filament(s), 202
    heat loss mechanisms, 68–69
    insert, 202
    orthovoltage units, 215
    ratings, 210
Statistics, 56–60
    descriptive, 56
    inferential, 56
    measures of location/deviation,
        57–60
    radiographic applications, 58–59
Stator coils, AC induction motor,
    139
Steel, 155, 156
    stainless, focusing cap, 201
Stefan's law, 67, 69
Stochastic effects, 335–337, 340–341
Storage, digitised images, 389–390
Substandard unit, 329
Substandards, 325
Substratum layer, intensifying
    screens, 302
Suffixes, 357
Sulphur-35, 264
Supercoat, intensifying screens, 302
Superconductor, 82
    magnets, 385
    temperature–conductivity
        relationships, 82

Superparamagnetic materials, 98
Supervised areas, 349
Switching
    electrical, 83
    electromagnetic relay, 109–110
    exposure, 185
        prepare sequence, 186
        primary, 186
        secondary, 186–187
        solid-state/electronic, 186
        thyristors, 173, 174
Systematic errors, 53–54

T

T_1/T_2 sequences, magnetic resonance
    imaging, 102–103, 383
Tangent, 366
Tantalum-182, 264
Target, 202
    interactions with electrons,
        269–270
        nuclei of target atoms, 271–272
        outer electrons of target atoms,
            270–271
    material effects, 279, 282
    mechanisms of X-ray production,
        270–272
    thickness effects, 275
    see also Tungsten
Target angle, 10, 200
Technetium-99m, 253, 254, 255,
    262
    clinical applications, 263, 264
    generator, 259, 261
Teleradiology, 390
Teletherapy, 5
Television monitors, 140, 235, 304
Temperature, 63–64
    absolute zero, 63
    demagnetising effect, 97, 98
    electrical resistance and, 82, 83,
        85, 86
    monitoring, 212
    scales, 63
    semiconductor conductivity and,
        83, 164, 167–168, 169, 171
    thermionic emission and, 178,
        202, 203
    units, 45, 63–64, 401
Temperature coefficient of
    resistance (α), 86
Ten-day rule, 339
Tenth-value thickness (TVT), 33
Tesla (T), 95, 96, 135
Testes, 341
Thallium (Tl) impurities, 372

Therapeutic radiography, 3–7
  applicator size, 12
  dose calculation, 59
  jaws (of unit) position, 12
  linear accelerators, 216
  orthovoltage treatment, 214–215
  radiation protection, 344, 351
  statistical methods, 58–59
  treatment field alterations, 12
  X-ray beam filtering/hardening,
    281
Thermal capacity, 63–64
  X-ray tube rating and, 209
Thermal conductivity, 65
Thermal equilibrium, 63
Thermal expansion, 67–68
Thermionic emission, 202–203
  space charge effect, 203
  temperature and, 178, 202, 203
Thermoluminescence, 301
Thermoluminescent dosemeter
    badge, 348
Thermoluminescent dosimetry (TLD),
    330–331, 347, 348
Thimble isolation chamber, 328–329
Thorium-232, 257
Three-phase AC circuits, 130–132
  in radiography, 131
  star and delta connections, 130,
    131, 180
  windings, 130, 131
Three-phase four-wire supply, 131
Three-phase generators, 130–131,
    132, 180
  in radiography, 131
  six-pulse, 180
Three-phase rectification, 180, 182
Thyristors, 165, 168, 173–174
  gate, 173
  for switching, 186, 188
  use in radiography, 174
Thyroid gland
  iodine uptake, 373–374
  therapy of overactive, 6–7
Time, 45, 401
Time to echo (TE), 383
Time to repetition (TR), 383
Timers, 146
  anatomically programmed, 191
  automatic, 189, 190–191
  guard, 191
  ionisation, 190
  mAs, 188–190
  phototimers, 190
  time-based, 188, 189
Timing exposure, 188–191
Tin, filtration, 215
Tissues
  radiosensitivity, 336

ultrasound velocities, 391
  weighting factors, 341
  see also Bone; Soft tissue
Tomography, linear, 15–17
  angle adjustment, 15, 17
  fulcrum height adjustment, 15,
    16–17
  layer thickness, 17
  principles, 15–16
  see also Computed tomography
    (CT) scanning
Transducer, ultrasound, 392
Transformers, 98, 124, 150–162
  alternating current (AC), 114
  constant-voltage, 160
  core, 151
    eddy currents, 152, 154–155
    iron losses, 154
    lamination, 154–155
  efficiency, 153
  Faraday's and Lenz's laws and,
    151, 152–153
  filament, 150, 177, 202
  high-tension see High-tension
    transformers
  ideal, 151–152
  losses, 153–158
  in practice, 153
  primary (input) side, 151
  in radiography, 150
  rating, 126, 160–161
  regulation, 15, 157–158
  secondary (output) side, 151
  step-down, 124, 150, 152
  step-up, 124, 150, 152
  turns ratio, 152
  voltage gain, 152
  see also Autotransformer
Transistor, 171–173
  field effect (FET), 171, 172–173
  NPN junction, 171–172
  PNP junction, 171
  use in radiography, 174
Transistors, 165, 168
Transmission, 4
Transmit bandwidth, 384–385
Transmit coil, 102
Transverse relaxation, 103
Triac, 174
  use in radiography, 174
Triangles
  geometry, 366–367
  right-angled, 366
  similarity, 367
Trigonometry, 9, 366–367
Triode smoothing, 181
Tritium (^{3}H), 264
Trivalent elements, doping,
    167

Tungsten, 178
  compound anode, 202
  current, 204
  filaments, 201
  rotating anode disc, 199
  target see Target
  thermal properties, 65, 69, 70
  thermionic emission, 203, 204
  vaporisation, 68, 199
  X-ray beam quality/quantity,
    279
  X-ray production, 270, 272, 273
Turns ratio, 152

U

Ultrasound, 391–393
  beam attenuation, 393
  Doppler imaging, 393
  production, 391–392
  pulse-echo imaging, 392–393
Ultraviolet radiation, 232, 233
Units of measurement, 44–51
  SI units, 45–51
  used in radiography, 48–51
Unsharpness, 399
  geometric see Geometric
    unsharpness
  movement (Um), 14
  photographic (Up), 14
  total (Ut), 15
Uranium decay, 247, 248, 257
Uranium-238 fission, 257, 258
Use factor, 351

V

Vacuum
  electrical changes in, 73
  heat transfer through, 66
  magnetic properties, 96
  permittivity, 73
Valence band, 81
  N-type semiconductors, 166,
    167
  P-type semiconductors, 167
  photoelectric interactions, 300,
    301, 304
  positive holes, 164
  semiconductors, 83, 164, 165
  silicon, 165
Valence electrons, 165
Valency, 243
Valency bond, 243
Vaporisation, 68

Variable
  dependent, 365
  independent, 365
Vector diagram, 125, 126, 127, 128
Vector quantitites, 46, 368–369
Velocity, 391
  electromagentic radiation, 229,
    230, 231
  light, 403
  Newton's first law, 40, 41
  SI units, 45, 46
Very large-scale integration (VLSI),
    163, 174
Volt, 76–77
Voltage
  average, 122
  constant, 178, 180
  effective/root mean square (RMS),
    123, 124
  gain, 152
  line, 131
  mains, 124
  peak, 122
  phase, 130, 131
  pulsating unidirectional, 179, 180
  ripple, 147, 180, 181, 183
  smoothing, 146, 147–148
  wattless, 126
  X-ray tube, 124, 177–178,
    204–205
  zener (breakdown), 171
  see also kVp
Volume coils, 386
Voxel, 102, 384

W

Water, magnetic properties, 96
Watt, 48, 89
Wattless current, 126
Wattless voltage, 126
Wave–particle duality, 224, 225–226
  electromagnetic radiation, 229–231
  electron orbitals, 241
  particles as waves, 226
  waves as particles, 225–226
Waveguides, 217
  accelerating, 217–218
Wavelength, 230, 231, 232, 391
  shifter, 375
Waves, electromagnetic, 229
Weber (Wb), 94, 95
Weight, 45, 47
Weighting factors, 341
Windowing technique, 380

Women of reproductive capacity,
    336, 338–339
  dose limits, 343
Work, 45, 47
Work areas designation, 349
Work function, 203
Workers see Radiation workers

X

X-ray beam
  attenuation see Attenuation,
    X-ray beam
  energy/photon energy, 274, 275,
    278
    average, 274, 310
    effective, 180
    maximum, 274
  filtration, 198, 279, 280–282
  intensity see Intensity, X-ray beam
  inverse square law and, 21
  kVp changes and, 278–279, 282
  mA changes and, 278, 282
  quality, 274, 277
    definition, 278
    factors affecting, 277–283
  quantity, 274, 277
    definition, 277
    factors affecting, 277–283
  rectification effects, 279–280, 282
  target material effects, 279, 282
X-ray diffraction of crystals, 289
X-ray generators, 4, 182–183
  computed tomography (CT), 377
  switching section, 186–187
  timing section, 188–191
X-ray room design, 350–351
X-ray spectrum, 234, 273–275
  filtration effects, 281
  kVp changes and, 278–279
  mA changes and, 278
  rectification effects, 279–280
  target material effects, 279, 282
X-ray tube, 4
  AC flow, 124, 177
  components, 196
  constant potential circuits, 180–182
  construction, 196
  current, 124
    filament heating current and,
      204
    half-wave/full-wave rectification
      comparison, 179
    see also mA
  design trends, 205

  electron focusing, 204
  'gassy', 68, 199
  grid-controlled, 187
  heat loss, 68–70
  insert, 196, 198–199, 202
  monitoring and protection,
    207–213
  orthovoltage units, 215
  preparation for exposure,
    185–186
  principles of operation, 202–205
  rating see X-ray unit rating
  shield (housing), 196–198
  space charge effect, 203
  target see Target
  thermionic emission, 202–203
  voltage, 124, 177–178, 204–205
    see also kVp; Rectification
  X-ray production, 205, 269–276
  see also Rotating anode X-ray
    tube; Stationary anode X-ray
    tube
X-ray unit rating, 207–208
  automatic monitoring, 212–213
  charts, 365–366
  definition, 207–208
  factors affecting, 208
  multiple exposures, 210–212
  single exposures, 208–210
X-rays, 4, 232, 233
  biological effects, 323, 324
  emission, 254–255, 271–272
  interactions with matter, 284–297
    importance to radiography,
      294–296
    probability and cross-sections,
      285
    see also Absorption;
      Attenuation; Scatter(ing)
  production, 205, 269–276
Xenon-133, 264

Y

Yttrium-90, 264

Z

Zener voltage, 171
Zero index, 363
Zero potential, 76